Human Anatomy 1

General Anatomy, Special Anatomy:
Limbs, Trunk Wall, Head and Neck

H. Frick · H. Leonhardt · D. Starck

Translated by David B. Meyer

417 colored illustrations

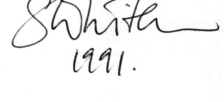

1991
Georg Thieme Verlag
Stuttgart · New York

Thieme Medical Publishers, Inc.,
New York

Library of Congress Cataloging-in-Publication Data
Frick, Hans, Prof. Dr. med.
[Allgemeine Anatomie, spezielle Anatomie, English]
Human anatomy/H. Frick, H. Leonhardt, D. Starck: translated by David B.
Meyer, p. cm.
Translation of: Allgemeine Anatomie: Spezielle Anatomie. 3., überarbeitete Aufl.
1987.
Includes bibliographical references.
Includes indexes.
Contents: v. 1. Limbs, Trunk Wall, Head and Neck—v. 2. Viscera and nervous
system.
1. Human anatomy. I. Leonhardt, Helmut. II. Starck, Dietrich, 1908-.
III. Title.
[DNLM: 1. Anatomy. 2. Anatomy, Regional. QS 4 F897a]
QM23.2.F7513 1990, 811—dc20, DNLM/DLC
90-10972

Prof. Dr. med. HANS FRICK
Anatomische Anstalt der Universität München
Pettenkoferstr. 11
8000 München 2, West Germany

Prof. Dr. med. HELMUT LEONHARDT
Anatomisches Institut der Universität zu Kiel
Olshausenstr. 40
2300 Kiel, West Germany

Prof. Dr. med. Dr. phil. h. c. DIETRICH STARCK
Zentrum für Morphologie der Universität
Frankfurt, Theodor-Stern-Kai 7
6000 Frankfurt am Main, West Germany

1st German ed. 1977
2nd German ed. 1980
3rd German ed. 1987
1st Greek ed. 1985
1st Spanish ed. 1981

DAVID B. MEYER, Ph.D.
Dept. of Anatomy
and Cell Biology
Wayne State University
540 East Canfield Avenue
Detroit, MI 48201, USA

This book is an authorized and revised translation from the third revised German edition, published and copyrighted 1987 by Georg Thieme Verlag, Stuttgart, Germany. Title of the German edition: Allgemeine Anatomie. Spezielle Anatomie I. Extremitäten, Rumpfwand, Kopf, Hals.

© 1991 Georg Thieme Verlag, Rüdigerstraße 14, D-7000 Stuttgart 30, Germany
Thieme Medical Publishers, Inc., 381 Park Avenue South, New York, N.Y. 10016
Typesetting: Macmillan India Ltd., Bangalore 25, on Monotype Lasercomp
Printed in Germany by Appl, Wemding

ISBN 3-13-732401-7 (Georg Thieme Verlag, Stuttgart)
ISBN 0-86577-3076 (Thieme Medical Publishers, Inc., New York)   1 2 3 4 5 6

Preface

The present two-volume treatise on human anatomy is introduced to the English-speaking reader with the conviction that it provides a compact packaging of easily accessible, up-to-date and clinically correlated anatomical information for the medical student, practitioner and researcher. Utilizing the internationally accepted terminology from Nomina Anatomica as well as superbly illustrated and clearly labeled drawings (in color when appropriate), these two textbooks present a valuable and precise account of human anatomy (systematic, regional and topographical) in a readily transportable flexibook format that is not otherwise available in the English language at present. Flexibooks of this type are enjoying much popularity in Europe and will no doubt become a welcome addition to the libraries of English-speaking students and faculty.

Furthermore, Professors Frick, Leonhardt and Starck are to be commended for their fine integration of gross and microscopic anatomy, which provides the reader with a comprehensible insight into the normal (as well as disturbed) physiology of the human body. Clinically correlated anatomical data abound throughout the two volumes and strongly emphasize even further the relevance of understanding and visualizing the detailed structure of the human body and its component parts.

Detroit, Michigan   *David B. Meyer*
Fall 1990

Contents

Volume 1 of *Human Anatomy* was written in the course of close collaboration
between the authors. The writing and selection of the illustrations for the various
chapters were carried out as follows:
1, 2, and 8–10 by H. FRICK;
3–7 by H. LEONHARDT;
11A by D. STARCK and H. FRICK;
11B, C and 12 by H. LEONHARDT and H. FRICK.

The illustrations were drawn by:
Mr. R. BRAMMER (Denzlingen), Figures
212–216, 224b, c, 233, 234, 237–239, 241, 243–245, 251, 252, 263, 264, 266, 271,
280–284, 286;
Ms. ERHARD (Munich), Figures
269, 273;
Ms. KLEBE (Munich), Figures
277, 278;
Mr. S. NÜSSEL (Munich), Figures
6, 8, 10, 13, 15, 17, 69b, 76, 77, 79–96, 98–109, 118, 123–127, 130–132, 139, 140,

144–149, 153–161, 186–188, 193, 194, 197, 200–203, 205–207, 211, 217, 218, 228, 230, 248–250, 253, 254, 257, 260, 265, 267, 268, 274;
Ms. ROSER (Frankfurt), Figure
240;
Mr. H. RUSS (Munich), Figures
1–5, 7, 9, 11, 12, 14, 16, 18–67, 69a, 72–74, 78, 97, 110–117, 119–122, 128, 129, 133–138, 141–143, 150–152, 162–185, 189–192, 195, 196, 198, 199, 204, 208–210, 255, 256, 258, 259, 261, 270, 272, 275, 276, 279;
Mr. SCHNEEBERGER (Frankfurt), Figures
224a, 231, 232;
Mr. SCHNELLBÄCHER (Frankfurt), Figures
219–222, 225–227, 229, 235, 236, 242, 246, 247;
Ms. SUTT (Munich), Figures
262, 265.

General Human Anatomy

1. Structural Plan

1. Form and Structure

Form is the *external shape* of an organism or its parts; **structure** denotes the *inner construction* (ranging from macroscopic to submicroscopic).

The *human body* is characterized by the *vertebrate structural plan* and *mammalian features*. Its specific human character is due to the *structural adaptations* which have resulted from the adoption of erect posture – with its associated bipedal movement and standing – as well as from the strong development of the cerebral hemispheres.

Typical vertebrate features in the human are: bilateral symmetry; regional organization of the body; embryonic anlagen of serially arranged branchial pouches; the early embryonic development of a *notochord* as an axial skeleton and its replacement by a bony vertebral column; the topographical relationship between the central nervous system and the axial skeleton, the formation of large sense organs; the bony skeleton; the metameric organization of the body wall musculature and, in relation to it, the nerves, blood vessels and skeleton of the body wall.

Typical mammalian features are: the development of a secondary jaw (temporomandibular) articulation; the formation of an undivided cranial vault consisting of membrane (covering) and cartilage (replacement) bones; the development of muscularized lips and cheeks, as well as specialized integumentary glands (mammary glands); the organization of a circulatory system (warmbloodedness with the formation of a hairy coat, rudimentary, of course, in the human); the prenatal development within the uterus (with the formation of a *placenta*); and, most important, the specific formation of a telencephalon with the dominance of a new type of cerebral cortex, the *neopallium*.

A *typical human feature* is erect posture; it causes the lordotic curvature of the lumbar vertebral column, the oval shape of the thorax when viewed transversely, the broad expansive hip bones which, with the sacrum, form a ring-shaped, closed pelvis inserted tightly into the body wall, and the typical arching of the human foot. With the simultaneous enlargement of the telencephalic hemispheres into the cerebrum, the capacity of the cranium increases. The large occipital foramen (*foramen magnum*), through which the cranial cavity opens into the vertebral canal, has been displaced basally. The arm has become a grasping apparatus, whereas the legs alone serve for locomotion and bear the weight of the body. By the enlargement of the hip bone and the angling off of the ilium and ischium, the prerequisites have been created to enable the middle and least gluteal muscles to balance the pelvis (and with it the trunk), even when supported by one leg. The line of gravity in the upright standing position lies near the hip joint, not far in front of the vertebral column (Fig. **166 c**), so that balance can be maintained with minimal muscle activity.

A typical human characteristic is the formation of a buttock and its demarcation by a gluteal fold. The round construction of the pelvis in human phylogeny must not only satisfy the altered statics and locomotion, but – in the case of the female pelvis – must also provide a sufficiently large birth canal for the relatively large head of the human newborn.

a) Organization of the Human Body

Regional organization into body segments. In the human the following are distinguished:
– the **main body** consisting of **head**, **neck** and **trunk**, as well as
– the paired **upper** and **lower limbs** (extremities).

The **trunk** can be divided into **thorax** and **abdomen**. The lower division of the trunk is generally marked off as the *pelvis*, to whose wall structure parts of the body wall and the lower limbs contribute. The portion of the neck and trunk directed backwards is termed the *dorsum*.

The skeleton of the **head**, the *skull* (*cranium*), encloses the *cranial cavity* which harbors the brain. The *thoracic cavity* is enclosed by the thoracic wall, the *abdominal cavity* by the abdominal and pelvic walls.

The **thoracic cavity** (Fig. 33) is separated from the abdominal cavity by the diaphragm and harbors the right and left *pleural cavities*, as well as the *mediastinal space* (mediastinum). Each pleural cavity is lined by a serous membrane (*parietal pleura*) and contains the lungs (right or left) which are covered by the visceral layer of the pleura (*visceral pleura*). In the mediastinum lies the *pericardial cavity*, which encloses the heart.

In the **abdominal cavity** (Figs. 33 and 34) the *peritoneum* marks off the *peritoneal cavity* with its parietal layer (*parietal peritoneum*). It harbors the liver, the spleen, and parts of the intestine, which are (nearly) surrounded by the visceral layer of the peritoneum (*visceral peritoneum*). In some places the thin connective tissue layer between the abdominal wall and the parietal peritoneum widens greatly to contain organs. That part of the abdominal cavity situated outside of the peritoneal cavity is termed the *extraperitoneal space*. It can be further divided into a *retroperitoneal space* (behind the peritoneal space and containing, among others, the kidneys and suprarenals) and a *retropubic space* (behind the pubic symphysis, in front of the urinary bladder).

The **pelvic cavity** is a downward continuation of the abdominal cavity extending as far as the pelvic floor. In topographical and applied anatomy, the segment of the abdominal cavity (peritoneal cavity + extraperitoneal space) situated below the linea terminalis is designated separately as the space of the lesser pelvis, usually abbreviated as *lesser pelvis*. The organs "anchored" at the pelvic wall and on the pelvic floor form the *pelvic viscera*.

Functional organization into organ systems. The preceding *regional organization* into body segments is paralleled by a *functional* organization into organ systems.

Organs are (higher) functional units composed of several tissues which possess a definite shape and structure and carry out specific tasks. Organs which work together in the discharge of complex functions can be grouped together into *apparatuses* and *systems*.

Since one and the same organ regularly contributes to a series of different processes (for example, skeletal muscle in the retention and movement of skeletal parts, in metabolism and in heat production), such classifications will always be somewhat arbitrary and simplifying; yet they facilitate an understanding of the construction of the human body.

The following apparatuses and systems can be distinguished:

Locomotor apparatus
passive parts: skeleton and skeletal connections
active parts: skeletal musculature

Viscera
Metabolic apparatus
   Circulatory system
   Endocrine system
   Digestive system
   Respiratory system
   Urinary system
Genital apparatus   ⎫
   Reproductive system ⎬ Urogenital apparatus
               ⎭

Communication apparatus
   Nervous system
   Sense organs
   Skin

The metabolic and genital apparatuses are designated as the *viscera*. Anatomically, they are the organs (or parts of organ systems) situated in the thoracic and abdominal cavities with their connections to the outside world and to the periphery of the body. Physiologically, the viscera could be denoted as the organ systems which, on the one hand, serve the construction and support of the individual, on the other hand, the species.

Organization of this book into "General Anatomy" and "Special Anatomy". In the description of human anatomy, either the regional organization (*topographical anatomy*) or the functional arrangement (*functional* *anatomy*) can be emphasized. Since the physician must frequently be concerned with the anatomy of all parts of the body, topographical anatomy is considered as the true *medical* anatomy.

The ideal, classic approach to teaching anatomy formerly proceeded through set steps. After the theory of the three "systems" (*locomotor apparatus, viscera, nervous system*) had been presented, *topography* was taught as the synoptical "final touch". The time allotted to the teaching of anatomy, however, no longer permits this approach in most cases, a situation reflected in the organization of these two volumes.

In *Special Anatomy* (Part 2 of Volume 1, and Volume 2), *topographically-oriented anatomy* is the focal point. It assumes a knowledge of systemic anatomy. When an organ can be assigned exclusively or largely to a certain body region (e.g. the liver to the abdominal region), its specific systemic structure can be discussed within a topographical framework. In those cases, however, in which a broader knowledge of functional (systemic) anatomy is necessary, it will be furnished in the *General Anatomy* section.

Since the locomotor apparatus, blood and lymphatic vessels, nerves and skin occur in all regions of the body, their structure is discussed in *General Anatomy*. Mucous and serous membranes, as well as glands, are likewise constituents of several systems of the viscera (endocrine, digestive, respiratory, urinary and reproductive). Indeed, in form and function all are specific to a system (organ-specific), yet to avoid repetition general information regarding overlapping systems is discussed in *General Anatomy*.

General Anatomy thus provides basic information on systemic anatomical aspects essential for understanding *Special Anatomy* which cannot be included there. Since systemic anatomy only overlaps in certain regions, *General Anatomy* discusses the systems in *selected chapters* which do not reflect the complete systemic anatomy. For a total picture of the systemic *and* topographical anatomy of the human body, both parts must be consulted.

b) Axes and Planes

Relative Positions and Directions

Many axes can be arbitrarily positioned through the human body, cutting it at different angles and into many planes. For reasons of standardization, however, three main axes placed perpendicular to one another – and the planes they define – are used as "spatial coordinates" (Fig. 1).

The three main axes are:
- a *longitudinal axis,* which runs in a longitudinal direction in humans standing upright and is perpendicular to the standing surface;
- a *transverse axis,* which passes transversely through the body and connects the corresponding points of both sides to one another;

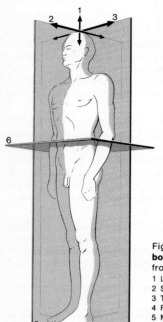

Fig. 1. **Main axes and planes of the human body** – bilateral symmetry, view from left side and in front

1 Longitudinal axis
2 Sagittal axis
3 Transverse axis
4 Frontal plane
5 Median plane
6 Transverse plane

– a *sagittal axis* – perpendicular to both of the preceding axes – which runs through the anterior and posterior body wall in the direction of an arrow aimed perpendicular to the body.

Sagittal planes represent all vertical planes of the human body which are placed sagittally.

The *median plane* is that sagittal plane which divides the body into two equal halves.

Transverse planes are all cross-sectional planes of the body. (Each plane is defined by a transverse and a sagittal axis.)

Frontal planes lie parallel to the face and are, therefore, perpendicular to both of the preceding planes.

Specific terms are used for the *designation of the position or the direction* of structural parts of the body:

at the trunk:

cranial or superior	toward the head
caudal or inferior	toward the rump
ventral or anterior	toward the front (abdominal side)
dorsal or posterior	toward the back
medial	toward the median plane
median	in the median plane
lateral	away from the median plane
central	toward the body interior
peripheral	toward the body surface
deep	away from the surface of the body
superficial	near the surface of the body

at the limbs:

proximal	toward the trunk
distal	toward the end of the limb
radial	toward the radius (thumb side)
ulnar	toward the ulna (little finger side)
tibial	toward the tibia (big toe side)
fibular	toward the fibula (little toe side)
palmar	toward the palm of the hand
plantar	toward the sole of the foot
dorsal	toward the back of the hand (foot)

When a position is designated, reference points are always used: "The esophagus lies dorsal to the trachea, but ventral to the vertebral column."

c) Body Weight, Body Size (Stature), Proportions

(Based in part on data from G. H. Lowrey, Growth and Development of Children, 8th ed., 1986, Yearbook, Chicago.)

The **body weight** of a mature newborn child (neonate) varies usually between 2810 g (6.2 lbs) and 4130 g (9.1 lbs). The mean birth weight for males is 3400 g (7.5 lbs), for females 3360 g (7.4 lbs).

In rare cases, the body weight amounts to only around 2500 g in full-term births; in about 10%, it is more than 4000 g. The average **height** (Fig. **2**) of newborn boys is about 19.9″ (50.6 cm) and of newborn girls 19.8″ (50.2 cm).

At the end of growth, the average body weight in 18-year-old boys in the United States amounts to 139 lbs (63.05 kg), whereas 18-year-old girls average 119.9 lbs (54.39 kg).

Body weight depends on stature (body size) (Fig. **3**), the state of nutrition and the function of the endocrine glands. The influence of age on body weight is slight. *Body size* is influenced by genetic factors to a greater degree than body weight.

Extreme values are usually caused by hypo- or hyperfunction of the endocrine glands (pituitary, thyroid, gonads). As a rule of thumb, body

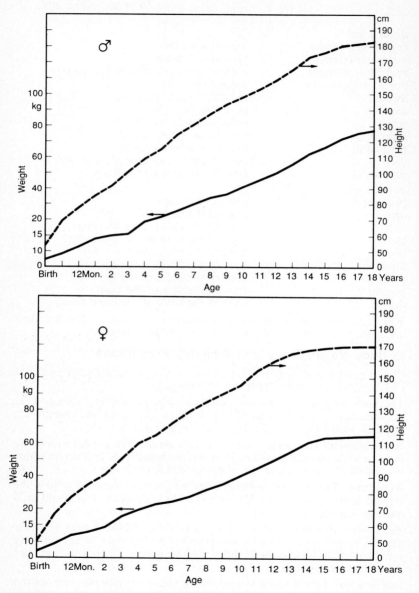

Fig. 2a, b. **Average stature of boys (♂) and girls (♀).** Height: - - - ; weight: ———. Data after G. H. Lowrey, Growth and Development of children, 8th ed. 1986, Yearbook, Chicago

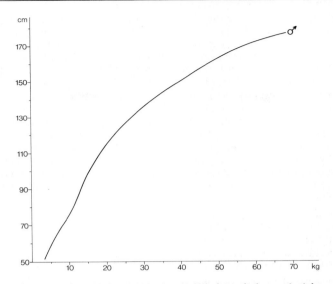

Fig. 3. **Relations between stature and body weight in boys during postnatal development** (data after Kunze)

weight (expressed in kg) in the adult male should amount to no more than the body size in cm minus 100. For females (more graceful body structure), this is somewhat less.

In the case of *under-average growth* (*microsomia*), body size lies between a mean value of -1σ and -3σ. At maturity this corresponds to a height ranging between 170.5 and 157.5 cm in males and between 161.5 and 150.5 cm in females. In the case of *dwarfism* (*nanism*) mature height is less than the mean value -3σ, i.e. less than 157.5 cm. (♂) or 150.5 (♀). *Above-average growth* (*macrosomia*) represents a body length with mean values between $+1\sigma$ and $+3\sigma$. A body size exceeding this is considered *gigantism*. Macrosomia exists, therefore, when males measure between 183.5 and 196.5 cm, females between 172.5 and 183.5 cm. Gigantism represents a body size of more than 196.5 cm (♂) or 183.5 cm. (♀).

Secular trends. Since the time of the Revolutionary War, stature and other measurements of Americans have, until recently, been increasing, whereas maturation (as indicated, for instance, by the onset of menstruation in girls) has been at an earlier age.

Growth, which is terminated in girls at 17–18 years, in boys at 18–19 years, takes place in spurts which are fixed genetically and can be modified (to a limited extent) by environmental factors.

The rate of growth is high in the first year of life (especially in the first six months). From the 3rd to the 10th (♀) or 12th (♂) year of life, *absolute* growth remains rather constant (around 5–6 cm in length and about 2.5 kg in weight per year), while *relative* growth decreases. Around the 6th year of life, a distinct inhibition of growth can occur. A new growth spurt ("prepuberal growth") takes place in girls aged 10–12, in boys aged 12–14.

In the United States, *puberty,* as indicated by the first menstrual period (*menarche*), commences in girls at 12.6 years of age on the average; 100 years ago it was 15.5 years of age. Boys reach puberty about two years later than girls. In most individuals, the onset of puberty is preceded for a few months by a spurt in growth called the adolescent growth spurt, and puberty is followed by a deceleration in growth rates. Individuals vary in the rates and times of these events, and the variations are related to nutritional factors. Therefore, growth and maturation are correlated with other indices of social and economic status.

The *birth weight* of 3400 g for a male neonate
– is doubled within 5 months,
– is tripled in about 12 months,
– is 7-fold in about 7 years,
– is 11-fold in about 12 years.

The *birth size* of 50.6 cm for a male neonate is increased
– 1.5 times in about a year,
– 2-fold in about 4 years,
– 2.5 times in about 8 years,
– 3-fold in about 13 years.

The *body size* of a boy amounts to
– 87.5 cm (34.4″) at 2 years of age = 50% of his definitive size,
– 96.2 cm (37.9″) at 3 years of age = 55% of his definitive size,
– 124.1 cm (48.9″) at 7 years of age = 71% of his definitive size,
– 149.6 cm (58.0″) at 12 years of age = 86% of his definitive size.

Proportions and proportional changes. A large man is not the scale model of a small man, much less still that of a child. Organs, organ systems and body parts are developed during pre- and postnatal ontogenesis (individual development before and after birth) at different times (heterochronous growth). Proportional changes and proportional differences arising thereby are designated as *allometry.* The growth of the head – correlated with the development of the brain – advances ahead of the other body parts. The growth of the limbs is delayed in its onset and thus continues longer.

The vertical height of the head in the newborn child amounts to about $\frac{1}{4}$ of the total body length. In a 6-year-old child it amounts to $\frac{1}{6}$, and in the adult it becomes about $\frac{1}{8}$ (Fig. **4**) of the total body length. The middle of the body lies at the level of the navel in the neonate and at half the distance between the navel and pubic symphysis in a 6-year-old child. In

Height of the head ¼   ⅙   ⅛   body length

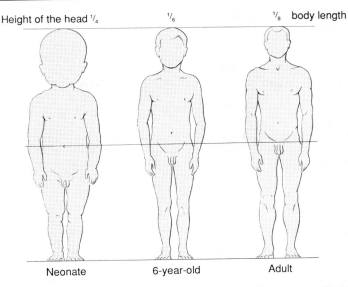

Neonate   6-year-old   Adult

Fig. 4. **Proportions and proportional changes in postnatal ontogenesis** (modified after Stratz)

the adult female it is at the upper margin of the pubic symphysis and in the adult male at the lower margin.

Lengths of the trunk and lower limbs (especially the femur) are not strictly correlated, however, with the result that there can be "standing giants" or "sitting giants".

In the newborn, the legs are shorter than the arms, whereas in the adult the legs are distinctly longer. The circumferences of the head and chest are roughly proportional in the newborn (35 cm); in the adult they differ considerably (56–60 cm to more than 75 cm, respectively).

2. The Norm, Variability, Malformation

The Norm. In this textbook *normal* anatomy, i.e. the structure of the *healthy* human body, is described. The *typical* shape, the typical structure, i.e. the most *frequently* observed structural characteristics (statistical norm), are considered as the *norm*. The particular feature designated as the norm can be formed in all healthy men in the manner described. It can occur in a majority or only in a minority, as long as it is the most frequently encountered form of the part of a organ, organ, etc., under discussion.

Variations or *variants* are deviations in anatomical structures from that described as the norm, which do not reduce the adaptability of an organism to its natural environment (or at least not to an extent worth mentioning). There is a gradual transition from a variation to a *pathological* change with functional disturbance.

The human organism – like all biological objects – exhibits considerable variability. The variation can affect only a limited region (e.g. altered series of branches of an artery) or can involve a larger body region (e.g. mirror-image position of inner organs, situs inversus).

Malformations represent permanent variations from the normal structure or fine structure of the human body which result from a disturbance in morphological development. The course of development can be retarded, excessive or defective. Malformations can be caused by a change of genotype or by external (exogenous) influences which affect the developing organism.

3. Bilateral Symmetry

At first glance the human body appears to be formed as a mirrored image (Fig. 1). A more careful inspection reveals, however, that *bilateral symmetry*, a typical vertebrate characteristic, is not strictly realized. Even the paired limbs are only apparently symmetrical.

In a right-handed person, the right arm is more muscular and heavier, the left leg often a slight degree longer. The face does not comprise completely mirrored halves. If one constructs a full-face photograph by photomontage utilizing only one facial half and its copied mirror image, a different, "strange"-looking face results. Numerous unpaired organs, like the heart, stomach, liver, spleen, large and small intestines, lie more or less eccentric. Even paired organs (e.g. lungs, kidneys, suprarenals) exhibit asymmetry of form or position. Bilateral symmetry in the human body is restricted to the minimum required for the maintenance of balance in bipedal standing and walking.

4. Metamerism of the Body Wall and Branchiomerism

Metamerism of the body wall refers to the construction of the trunk wall from essentially similar segments (*metameres*), which follow one another in a craniocaudal direction and which consist of a muscle segment, together with its vascular and nerve supply, a segment of the axial skeleton, and a skin segment.

In the neck region this metameric arrangement is attained postnatally in the short cervical muscles and the cervical vertebrae. Body cavities, together with their contents, are never arranged metamerically. The detailed structure of the central nervous system also exhibits no primary segmentation.

The sinuous movements of primitive vertebrates necessitate a segmentally-arranged musculature of the trunk wall and a corresponding segmentation of the axial skeleton. Also in humans, the anlagen (blastemae) for the fixed, autochthonous musculature of the trunk wall and the elements of the axial skeleton are organized segmentally. This primary metamerism of the trunk wall musculature leads to the formation of *segmental vessels* (intercostal and lumbar arteries and veins) and *segmental nerves* (spinal nerves) (Figs. **25** and **49**). A secondary effect is the segmentation of the axial skeleton.

The metameric construction of the body wall is not visible in some regions since segmental muscles unite into larger individual muscles (long back muscles, abdominal muscles, ventral cervical muscules) during embryonic development and muscles of the upper limb encroach upon the trunk wall. In the adult the metamerism of the body wall can still be recognized in the unisegmental short dorsal muscles and the intercostal muscles, in the segmental vessels and nerves, as well as in the segmental organization of the vertebral column and ribs.

Branchiomerism represents the serial, craniocaudally-directed origin of certain structural elements of the branchial region of the intestine (pharynx) in the formation of the vertebrate head and neck, e.g. the embryonic development of the pharyngeal (branchial) arches, pouches and clefts. Branchiomerism and metamerism of the trunk wall occur independent of each other, although somites (dorsal) and pharyngeal pouches (ventral) slide over one another in the boundary region and therefore lie in the same transverse section. Branchiomerism also leads – temporarily or permanently – to the formation of segmental structural parts (pharyngeal arches = branchial arches, branchial muscles, branchial arch arteries, branchial nerves). The serial origin of the pharyngeal arches, however, has nothing to do with the segmental organization of the spinal nerves. The head and trunk are organized differently. The formation of the head (*cephalogenesis*) and trunk (*notogenesis*) are two processes which are independent of each other.

5. Primary and Secondary Sexual Characteristics

The **primary sexual characteristics** are the *primary* (testes, ovaries) and *secondary sexual **organs*** (excretory genital tracts + external genitalia) which are formed during prenatal development.

Secondary sexual characteristics are formed during puberty. They are also designated as *accessory sexual organs* and imply sexually distinguished features and structural characteristics (in different body regions) which have no direct sexual function. The formation of the secondary sexual characteristics is initiated directly by an increased secretion of hormones from the pituitary gland (gonadotropins) which stimulate the hormone-producing sites in the gonads to an increased production of androgens and estrogens.

The most striking secondary sexual characteristics of the female are the mammary glands, between which the median furrow of the thoracic wall is deepened to form the bosom. In addition to the typical difference in size, there are also differences in proportion between males and females. The skeleton and skeletal musculature are more strongly developed in males; the increased deposition of subcutaneous fat lends a rounder and softer appearance to the female body. Striking masculine features are the heavier development of facial hair, the different formation and localization of body hair and the more visible "Adam's apple".

The female pelvis is lower and broader than that of the male; the pubic angle is rounded and greater than 90° (Fig. **118**). The male trunk is broad in the shoulder region and distinctly narrower at the hips, whereas in females the widths of the shoulder and hips are more similar to each other.

6. Body Form and Composition

Bodily form varies among individuals. Besides differences based on age and sex, there are marked differences based on the extent and disposition of body fat and the degree of development of muscles and other tissues.

The older idea that the variations could largely be subsumed under three body types has largely given way to an attempt to measure the body components responsible for the obvious variations. Thus, the use of a skinfold caliper to measure subcutaneous fat at various body sites may supplement the information about fatness adduced from body weight or BMI (Body Mass Index = weight/stature) and indicate something of the fat pattern (whether the fat is relatively more prominent on the limbs or trunk, upper or lower parts of the body, etc.). Likewise, where the facilities are available, bioelectric impedance, electrical conductivity, body specific gravity (by densitometric methods), whole body K and body water determinations give objective information on the extent of these variations and are increasingly used in sports medicine and some other clinical specialities.

The attempt to evaluate body types subjectively gave way to estimates of somatotype on highly standardized nude photographs and then by measurements on photographs, and the idea of constitutional types has survived in clinical use because the differences in body composition and the patterns of distribution, especially of subcutaneous fat, seen in this way, do vary in different chronic diseases. But these features are now known to vary greatly throughout the life span, to depend on nutrition, and generally to result from, rather than to predispose to, specific diseases.

2. Locomotor Apparatus

Bony and cartilaginous skeletal elements joined by connective tissue structures form the supporting framework of the body, the **skeleton**, whose parts are moved or held in a fixed position by the **skeletal musculature**. The skeletal and muscular systems are subsumed under the general category, **locomotor apparatus**.

The *passive locomotor apparatus* consists of the skeleton and the skeletal connections. The *active locomotor apparatus* consists of the skeletal musculature.

There are over **200 bones** in the human body. The number cannot be determined precisely: supernumerary bones (→ vertebra, p. 451), for example, can appear; sutural (wormian) bones can develop in the cranial sutures, or accessory bones (e.g. os trigonum) can be formed; the customary union of the two frontal bones may not take place; the number of sesamoid bones varies; and, finally, the diaphysial and epiphysial bones which have not yet united osseously in the tubular bones of juveniles are counted as separate bones.

Under pathological conditions, *heterotopic bones* can also be formed in atypical places (e.g. rider's bone in the adductor of the thigh).

A. Elements and Structural Principles of the Skeleton

1. Structural Materials of the Skeleton

In the adult the skeletal elements consist almost exclusively of *osseous tissue. Cartilaginous tissue* covers only the articulating ends of the bones, forms the costal cartilages in the sternal portion of the ribs, provides the nasal cartilage as part of the nasal skeleton, and forms the cartilaginous end of the xiphoid process of the sternum.

A connective tissue covering surrounds the skeletal elements like a stocking, except for the articular cartilage. At bones it is designated as *periosteum* and at cartilage as *perichondrium*. The periosteum and perichondrium serve to nourish the skeletal tissue, confine the skeletal elements and place them in touch with their environment.

In cross-section, each bone exhibits a cortical layer (*substantia corticalis*), and a meshwork of bony trabeculae (*substantia spongiosa*) enclosed by it (Figs. **6 a** and **9**). The thickness of the corticalis and the density of the spongiosa vary according to bone type.

The inner surface of the bony tissue is lined by a thin layer of flattened connective tissue cells (*endosteum*), which lines both the spongy trabeculae and the Haversian and Volkmann's canals (→ p. 17).

Bone marrow lies in the meshlike spaces of the spongy bone. Macroscopically visible openings in the corticalis (*nutrient foramina*) carry blood vessels (*nutrient vessels*) and nerves to the bone marrow and spongiosa.

Osseous tissue consists of *bone cells* (*osteocytes*) (700–800/mm^2 in cross-sections of lamellar bone) and an organic, calcified *osseous ground substance*.

Osteocytes are connected by numerous branched processes which form a network. Osteocytes reside in bony cavities, their processes in bony canaliculi.

Mineral salts (especially hydroxyapatite = complex calcium phosphate compound) are deposited in the ground substance (= collagenous fibrils and organic cement substance [glycosaminoglycans, proteoglycans]).

The dry substance of adult bone contains about one-third organic material (mostly collagen) and two-thirds inorganic constituents.

The mineral salts can be dissolved out of bone by immersion in weak acid. The residue of the organic ground substance consists of collagen fibrils and shrunken osteocytes. *Decalcified bone* retains its external form, but loses its compressive strength. It is pliable and can be cut. When the organic matrix is removed by heating (calcining), the external form is also generally preserved. *Calcinated bone*, however, is glassy, brittle and shatters upon slight pressure.

In embryonic bone the collagenous fibrils form a network: *network bone* (fibrous bone). By the end of the first decade of life, this network bone has been largely rebuilt and replaced by the (presumably) stronger *lamellar bone*. Network bone is preserved only in the region of the cranial sutures, the osseous labyrinth, and the zones of tendinous radiation.

In *lamellar bone* (Fig. **5**) the collagenous fibrils are grouped into lamellae about 5–10 μm thick within a cement substance, in which they course approximately parallel. The angle of ascent and the direction in which the fibrils are wound change from lamella to lamella. The structural unit of lamellar bone – the most typical example can be seen in the compacta of long bones – is the *osteon* (Haversian system), the totality of all *Haversian lamellae*, which are arranged (more or less) concentrically around a bony canal, the *Haversian canal* (*central canal*). Haversian canals (∅ about 20–200 μm) contain 1–2 blood vessels (capillaries or postcapillary veins, more rarely arterioles) and, like these vessels, form an acute-angled, branched tubular network.

Osteons are, therefore, not a structural unit limited on all sides, but segments (0.5 cm to ca. 2 cm long) of a continuous system. The space between them is bounded by fractional pieces of former Haversian systems, *interstitial lamellae* (brecciated structure of bone; breccia = stones from rock debris united by a cement mass). Toward the surface

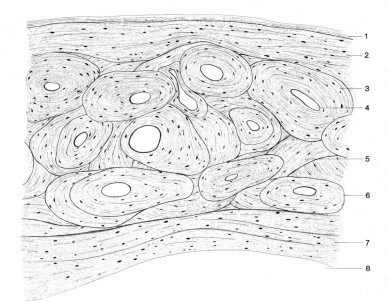

Fig. 5. **Transverse section through compacta of a long bone**

1 Periosteum	5 Interstitial lamellae
2 External general lamellae	6 Cement line
3 Osteon (Haversian system)	7 Internal general lamellae
4 Haversian canal	8 Marrow cavity

and toward the marrow cavity, the framework of osteons and interstitial lamellae is enclosed by external and internal *general lamellae* (basic lamellae).

The external general lamellae course parallel to the surface, but do not enclose the entire circumference of the bone. The internal general lamellae continue into the trabecular network of the spongiosa. Cement lines (fibril-poor organic matrix) demarcate the various lamellar systems. The spongiosa can differ markedly from this structural pattern of lamellar bone and in many bones are formed exclusively of lamellar systems resembling interstitial lamellae.

Vascular supply of bone. Blood vessels to supply the bone pass through the external general lamellae from the periosteum. They course in *Volkmann's canals* (perforating canals) which are not surrounded by lamellae, continue into the Haversian canals, and also communicate with the vessels of the bone marrow.

Strength of bone. Bones are firm, hard and (when stressed within certain physiological limits) elastic organs. The compressive strength of lamellar bone exceeds the tensile strength (in the compacta of long, tubular bones about 15 or $10\,kg/mm^2$). The ability to withstand torsion is less. In comparison to hyaline cartilage, osseous tissue can be stressed nearly tenfold more by pressure or tension.

The lamellar structure of osseous tissue increases the strength of bone. Compression and tensile stress cause compressed areas to appear between the lamellae with their different wrapping of fibrils; these have a stiffening effect. Collagenous fibrils are stretched in bone (in contrast to connective tissue, in which they are wavy); they are "harnessed". The tensed bundles of collagenous fibrils maintain a certain compressive strength through their intimate union with the stored (embedded), inorganic crystals.

Bone remodeling. Immediately after the beginning of embryonic bone formation, the destruction of osseous tissue by bone-eating cells, *osteoclasts* (large, short-lived, multinucleated cells), sets in. Irregular indentations (Howship's lacunae) appear on the bony trabeculae. Bone is reconstructed continuously throughout life. In the growth phase, new bone formation predominates. In old age, bone becomes generally thinner and more brittle owing to the relatively stronger destruction. The trabeculae of the spongiosa become rarefied, and the basic construction of the trabecular network becomes more clearly delineated. (The water content of bone is reduced in the elderly, and the inorganic components decrease.)

In the case of reduced stress (longer bed rest or immobilization, a longer period in weightless space), but also in the case of hormonal changes (decreased secretion of estrogen after menopause), osseous tissue is more rapidly decomposed (osteoporosis), and bones can break more readily.

In addition to continuous bone remodeling, changes in bone shape and in the architecture of the spongiosa occur when mechanical conditions are altered (fracture, operative procedures on the locomotor apparatus).

An important role in normal and disturbed bone formation is played by hormones (especially parathormone) and vitamins (vitamin A in bone remodeling, vitamin C in the formation of ground substance, vitamin D in the mineralization of osseous tissue).

Cartilaginous tissue. In the skeletal system, *hyaline cartilage* appears almost exclusively as cartilaginous tissue. It is elastic under pressure, sectionable and transparent in thin slices. The water-rich hyaline cartilage $(60-70\% \; H_2O)$ consists of *cartilage cells, chondrocytes* (usually arranged in small groups), and an amorphous *cartilage ground substance* (sulfated glycosaminoglycans), in which "masked" (not directly visible in the light microscope) *collagenous fibers* are deposited.

Chondrocytes are spherical or ovoid and become flattened at surfaces which contact neighboring cells. In mature cartilage, they are surrounded by a strongly basophilic cartilaginous capsule (wall of the cartilage cavity, in which the iso-genous cartilage cells, i.e. chondrocytes derived from a mother cell, reside) and by the likewise distinctly basophilic cartilaginous corona. Together with the cartilage capsule and cartilage cells, the corona forms a *territory*, or *chondrone*. Between the territories lies the *interterritorial matrix*, which is less basophilic. The territorial organization results from the irregular distribution of chondroitin sulfuric acids, which are especially concentrated in the cartilaginous capsule, but also in the territories.

Studies with the polarizing microscope show that the collagenous fibers are densely wound around the territories like a shell. In the interterritorial region the collagenous fibers intersect, and externally they continue into the bundles of collagenous fibrils of the perichondrium. The chondrones, as pressure-compressible bodies, represent the functional building blocks of hyaline cartilage, which are linked by interterritorial fibril tracts into structural units of increasing order (two packs, four packs, etc. up to the perichondrium).

Cartilage is (almost) free of blood vessels and possesses neither lymphatic vessels nor nerves. Nourishment is obtained by diffusion from the perichondrium, in the case of articular cartilage from the synovial fluid (synovia).

With increasing age, degenerative changes appear. In the central parts of large pieces of cartilage, a demasking of the fibers can occur (asbestos fibrillation) and mineral salts can be deposited.

The **perichondrium,** which graduates into the cartilage without sharp boundaries, consists of tense connective tissue containing elastic networks, blood vessels and nerves.

Hyaline cartilage grows interstitially (by division of chondroblasts) and appositionally (from the perichondrium).

Fibrocartilage covers the articular surfaces of the temporomandibular and clavicular joints and occurs in the intervertebral discs and pubic symphysis. Between compact (unmasked) collagenous fibers there are small islands of sparse cartilaginous matrix which enclose a chondrocyte (or rows of chondrocytes). In the intervertebral discs, chondromucoid is deposited sparsely around the "cartilage cells".

The **periosteum** (Figs. **5** and **6a**), a faintly shiny, slightly yellowish *membrane*, surrounds the osseous tissue like a stocking and provides a surface for attaching tendons and ligaments. It consists of two layers which can only be clearly distinguished in growing bones: an external fibrous layer, *stratum fibrosum* (a reticulum of collagenous fibers with an elastic network), and an internal cell-rich, osteogenic (cambium) layer, *stratum osteogenicum*, bordering directly on the osseous tissue and containing blood vessels and nerves.

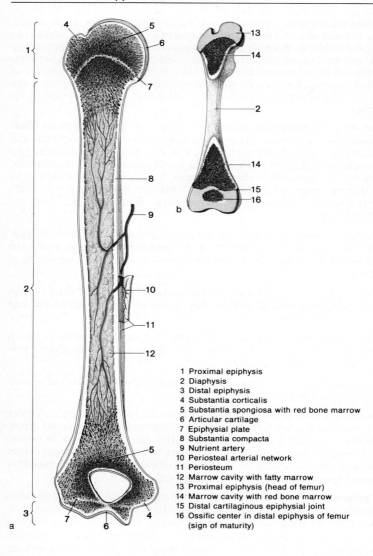

1 Proximal epiphysis
2 Diaphysis
3 Distal epiphysis
4 Substantia corticalis
5 Substantia spongiosa with red bone marrow
6 Articular cartilage
7 Epiphysial plate
8 Substantia compacta
9 Nutrient artery
10 Periosteal arterial network
11 Periosteum
12 Marrow cavity with fatty marrow
13 Proximal epiphysis (head of femur)
14 Marrow cavity with red bone marrow
15 Distal cartilaginous epiphysial joint
16 Ossific center in distal epiphysis of femur
   (sign of maturity)

Fig. 6. **Longitudinal sections through long bones**
a Tubular bone (humerus) of adult
b Proximal and distal ends of long bone (femur) of newborn child

During bone formation, the osteoblasts in the osteogenic layer of the periosteum become differentiated and lay down bone ground substance (growth in thickness of bone). The fibrous layer is fixed by bundles of collagenous fibers, *Sharpey's fibers* (*perforating fibers*), radiating into the general lamellae. At the articular end, it continues into the stratum fibrosum of the joint capsule.

Blood vessels pass from the periosteal vascular network into Volkmann's canals. Myelinated and non-myelinated nerve fibers pass into the osseous tissue from the nerve plexuses of the periosteum, which is richly innervated and very sensitive to pain.

Osseous tissue which is no longer covered by periosteum as a result of a fracture or a surgical procedure is resorbed by increased osteoclastic activity.

In **fracture healing**, the periosteum, the connective tissue cells in the Haversian canals, and the reticular tissue of the bone marrow are of particular importance. From these connective tissue structures a cell-rich and highly vascular supporting tissue, the connective tissue *callus*, first develops on and between the broken ends of the bones. Then connective tissue cells differentiate into osteoblasts, and mineral salts are deposited in the ground substance. Later, the bony callus (network bone) formed in this manner becomes transformed into lamellar bone. (The duration of fracture healing is weeks to months.)

If the ends of bones are not sufficiently fixed, osseous tissue cannot become differentiated, and a *pseudo-arthrosis* arises in the fibrous tissue connecting the ends of the fracture.

When the fracture ends are closely matched and well fixed through special operative procedures (osteosynthesis) so that no noteworthy osseous space results, no callus is formed. A (callus-free) fracture healing parallels bone remodeling.

Bone marrow. The marrow spaces of bone contain bone marrow (Fig. **6**), the total mass of which amounts to almost 5% of body weight. In the adult, red (blood-forming) bone marrow, which fills all the marrow spaces of a child's bones, is present only in the short and flat bones and in the epiphyses of tubular bones (Fig. **30c**). In the marrow cavities of the diaphyses it has been converted into fatty marrow. In healthy adults the quantity of red and fatty marrow is roughly equal.

The bone marrow is supplied with blood by the nutrient vessels (Fig. **6a**). The capillaries flow into wide-lumened sinuses, whose endothelial cells (lining cells) are able to phagocytize and store.

2. Types of Bone

On the basis of external shape, bones are classified as *short, long* and *flat*. These succinct divisions correspond to typical structural differences.

Short bones (vertebral bodies, carpals and tarsals) usually have a thin cortical layer which surrounds a framework of spongy trabeculae. A centralized marrow cavity is absent; the bone marrow is organized in various ways by means of trabeculae of spongiosa.

Long bones (tubular bones: humerus, radius, ulna, femur, tibia, fibula, metacarpals, metatarsals) possess a tubular-shaped middle part (*diaphysis*), the cortical layer of which is formed as a massive layer of compact bone (*substantia compacta*, Fig. **6a**). Sparse and extraordinarily fine trabeculae of spongiosa are present in the bone marrow. The end pieces (*epiphyses*) consist of spongiosa which is covered by a more or less thin corticalis.

The diaphysial region bordering on the epiphysis is termed the *metaphysis*.

Flat bones exhibit certain structural differences owing to different types of mechanical stress. The bones of the cranial vault and ribs possess robust layers of compacta at their outer and inner surfaces, between which a hard bony network of trabeculae spreads out. In the bones of the cranial vault this central layer is termed *diploë* (Fig. **8**).

In the scapula and hip bone the structural frame consists of a strong compacta which encloses a slight amount of spongy bone. In contrast, the central portions of the wing of the ilium and scapula and the thin bony plates in the skull (e.g. in the ethmoid) consist only of a uniform layer of bone.

3. Cartilage and Membrane Bones

During embryonic development, most skeletal elements appear first as cartilage. It is superseded by *cartilage (replacement) bone* during pre- and postnatal ontogenesis by means of *endochondral ossification*. Degeneration and replacement of the skeletal elements preformed in cartilage begin at about the 7th embryonic week and are completely finished only at the beginning of the third decade of life. The clavicle, the bones of the skull, and almost all of the bones of the facial skeleton develop directly from the mesenchyme by means of *intramembranous ossification*. They are designated as *membrane (covering) bones*.

The mode of histogenesis (intramembranous or endochondral ossification) however, is not as important as it might seem on the basis of the above characteristics for classifying bone as cartilage or membrane-bone. On the contrary, membrane bones are derivatives of the bony outer skeleton (exoskeleton) of primitive vertebrates, whereas cartilage bones are descendants of the inner skeleton (endoskeleton) of lower vertebrates which perhaps consisted of a primitive mucous cartilage.

Bone which is formed directly in connective tissue, but in close connection with cartilaginous preformed bones, is known as *incremental bone* (e.g. shaping of the fine pattern of the petrous bone, lateral wall of facial canal; completion of the incisura ovalis into the foramen ovale of the greater wing of the sphenoid, etc.). This *incremental bone*, which is not preformed in cartilage, is morphologically, however, cartilage bone. In mammals, some cartilage bones are combined with membrane bones into mixed bones. The squamous part of the occipital bone contains, for example, the interparietal, which is a membrane bone, and in the temporal bone the squamous and tympanic parts are membrane bones, the petrous part and styloid process cartilage bones.

4. Bone Growth

The **longitudinal growth of tubular bones** is accomplished by the interstitial *growth of cartilage* which takes place in the proliferative or growth zones at the border region between the diaphysis and epiphysis. Here, cartilaginous tissue is newly formed by active cell division and concurrently destroyed from the diaphysial side, later also from the epiphysial side, to be replaced by bone. In this way a *cartilaginous epiphysial joint* (epiphysial disc or plate, Figs. **6b** and **9**) is formed. As soon as cartilage destruction proceeds faster than cartilage growth, the cartilaginous joint becomes thinner. Longitudinal growth ceases when the cartilaginous epiphysial disc completely decomposes and is replaced by a *bony epiphysial line* (Fig. **6a**). For the epiphyses of different tubular bones this point in time is between the 13th and 25th years of life.

As long as the epiphysis is still cartilaginous, it also grows interstitially. The contribution to growth in length afforded by the cartilage between the epiphysial ossific centers and the articular surfaces is slight. In the case of short bones (without cartilaginous epiphysial joints) growth takes place in a proliferative zone of the cartilage adjacent to the ossific center.

The **growth in thickness of tubular bones** occurs without the participation of cartilage and takes place as the appositional growth of bone from the osteogenic layer of the periosteum. At the same time osteoclasts destroy bone from within so that the compacta does not become disproportionately thick. Concomitantly, the marrow cavity is enlarged.

The **areal growth of the flat bones** of the cranial vault takes place at the margins in the cranial sutures. At the same time, finely balanced bony deposition and destruction occur at the external and internal surfaces of these bones and produce the remodeling essential for the growing skull. The bones of the cranial vault, still single-layered in the newborn, become triple-layered.

Bone growth is influenced by hormones.

Castration prior to puberty leads to eunuchoid gigantism, vitamin D deficiency to disturbed ossification. Traumatic separation of the epiphyses (e.g. detachment of the head of the humerus due to faulty obstetrics) or disease of the epiphysial joint causes a disturbance in the growth of the injured or diseased skeletal elements.

Centers of ossification. The ossification of the skeleton proceeds from so-called centers of ossification. These ossific centers are also termed *osseous nuclei* or *loci* (Fig. **6b**) and are demonstrable radiographically because of the deposition of calcium salts. They typically appear in definite prenatal or postnatal developmental stages, partly within narrowly-defined, partly within very broad intervals. The osseous nuclei in the distal epiphysis of the femur and in the proximal epiphysis of the tibia are formed in the last fetal month and are valuable as indicators of terminal maturity.

Ossific centers appear in the short bones of the limbs (exclusive of the talus, calcaneus, cuboid) and in most epiphyses of the long tubular bones only after birth. Ossific loci in the *apophyses* (bony processes for the attachment of muscles and ligaments, Fig. **9**) usually appear only in the second decade of life. On the basis of the number, form and size of the radiologically-discernible ossific centers in a specific age group, the physician can estimate the degree of *skeletal maturity*.

5. Functional Structure of Bone

The bony skeleton is designed as a *light structure*, i.e. constructed with relatively *minimal material*. A bone contains only as much structural material as is necessary for the highest stress expected under normal conditions, plus a certain safety margin (the back-up system of the engineer). Any excess in bony tissue would not be economical, for bone mass must not only be put in motion but also nourished – even when at rest. This consumes energy, as does the continuous physiological rebuilding of the fine structure. As bone is a relatively minimal construction, it follows of necessity that the relation between the strength of bone and the highest stress appearing under physiological conditions must be equal in all places. Bone is – in the engineer's definition – a body of equal strength.

Since the skeleton fulfills its function with a minimal expenditure of material (maximum-minimum principle), it is designated as *functionally adapted*. According to Roux, the founder of the theory of **functional adaptation,** there is an "adaptation to the function by practice of it" which leads both to a *functional structure* and to a *functional shape* of the skeletal elements.

The structural analysis of a knee joint ankylosis (ossified union of the femur and tibia) provided proof for the correctness of this assertion. The spongy architecture deviating from the norm in this preparation illustrates the tension trajectories, which can be demonstrated in a model of the ankylosed knee joint made from homogeneous material when suitable pressure is applied using the optical tension experiment. The transformation of the spongy architecture which takes place after ankylosis can be traced to two factors: *hypertrophic activity* of bone, in which bone substance is deposited at those points in the spongy trabeculae where mechanical stress is increased (within a physiological region), and *inactivity atrophy*, in which osseous tissue is destroyed where stress is decreased. This results in a rearrangement of the trabeculae, a process which can only then be stopped when the axis of the trabeculae runs in the direction of the stressing force. These construction principles are probably valid for the entire spongiosa architecture of the human skeleton.

In all those bones whose *architecture of the spongiosa* has already been thoroughly investigated (especially the coxal end of the femur, vertebral body) the spongiosa forms a *trajectoral framework*. The spongy trabeculae (frequently also tubules, plates, shells, etc.) are always so arranged or become so reconstructed that they undergo an axial compressive or tensile stress, but no bending stress.

As *trajectories* (Fig. **7b**), lines are noted in the statics which indicate, at each position of a body, the directions of the greatest compression or the greatest traction which agree mostly with the course of greatest compressive or greatest tensile stress.

Tensile and compressive stress trajectories intersect at right angles and can be demonstrated in transparent, homogeneous bodies with the help of optical tension methods.

In experiments with models of the coxal end of the femur or a vertebral body, for example, it could be shown that the course of tension in homogeneous bodies corresponds to the arrangement of the spongy trabeculae in these bones (Figs. **7a,b**). Also the *compacta* of tubular bones is functional, although not formed trajectorally (Figs. **7c,d**). Maximum tensions here always run in a longitudinal direction. They can be optimally absorbed by the longitudinally-directed tracts of osteons.

The orientation of osteons demonstrable with the help of split line methods can be interpreted as a growth structure. The longitudinal course of osteon tracts corresponds to the direction of the tensile stresses which appear in the periosteal tube as a result of the longitudinal expansion caused by epiphysial growth. A causal explanation, however, for the longitudinal orientation of osteons in the lamellar bone that replaces the original woven bone formed by the periosteum cannot be given at this time.

For the *long tubular bones*, evidence could be produced that they have a *functional shape*, in addition to the *functional structure* mentioned above. Their thick form is predisposed for reducing the amount of bending stress on the one hand and for maximally absorbing the bending tensions with a minimum of material on the other. The tubular form of the diaphysis represents an optimal form of material distribution for the bending requirements of long tubular bones. Protection against fracture can be increased by the development of bony ridges ($\rightarrow$ linea aspera of the femur).

Likewise, in the long tubular bones the axial curvature of the shaft is adapted in the best possible way for bending stresses, both in the sagittal and in the frontal planes.

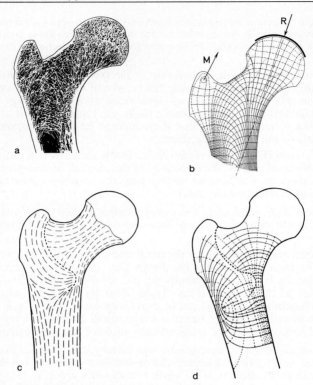

Fig. 7. **Proximal end of right femur**
a Sawed section of neck of femur in the frontal plane
b Course of stress trajectories in model (synthetic plastic plate) weighted analogous to
   the proximal end of femur of the supporting leg. Compressive stress trajectories =
   solid lines; tensile stress trajectories = dotted lines; R = result from body weight and
   muscle strength; M = direction of muscle pull of adductors of hip joint
c Course of cleavage lines at posterior surface
d Course of stress trajectories at posterior surface (lacquer line picture). Cleavage lines
   and stress trajectories do not correspond in their course at the surface of the bone
(b–d after *Pauwels*)

Thus, for example, the sagittal axial curvature of the human femur resembles the
axial form of levers with low curvature which are subjected to a static stress similar
to that of the femur. In the case of growing bones, a change of axial form is
possible in the region of ossification of the cartilaginous epiphysial joint. If this is
stressed on bending, it seeks to regulate itself by an unequal growth of bone
perpendicular to the direction of all the forces influencing it. The axial direction of

the newly formed bone is thereby altered: functional adjustment by growth in length. An example of this is the transformation of the physiological bowleg of an infant to the physiological knock-knee of a six-year-old child.

A decisive reduction of bending stresses in the shaft of long, tubular bones is attained by the **tension belt**. The task of skeletal muscles is to move the skeletal parts or hold them in a certain position. In a contracted state they act simultaneously as bracings (*tension belts*) against the bending stresses to which tubular bones are exposed when burdened eccentrically by body weight and added weights (e.g. reduction of stress on the femur in a standing position through the iliotibial tract, Figs. **128** and **129**). The contraction of muscles acting as a tension belt leads, therefore, to relief of pressure and not to increased stress.

Without the tension belt formed by muscles and ligaments the pre-requisites for the functional structure of bone would not exist, for it organizes a relatively uniform stress on the skeletal elements independent of the position of the limb. The quality of stress thereby remains the same for a specific bone in the various joint positions and in the different phases of movement. Thus, only the quantity of static or dynamic stress can be changed.

An increase in the amount of stress in the physiological range is at least controlled by the multiple safeguards with which the skeletal system is designed. Moreover, the impact forces accompanying dynamic stress are absorbed partly by the muscles, which stretch like coiled springs and thereby slow the impact.

B. Connections of Skeletal Parts

The *continuous* union of skeletal pieces by a filling tissue is termed a suture (*synarthrosis*), whereas the *discontinuous* union, i.e. a union enclosing a space, is called a (true) *joint* (*synovial articulation, diarthrosis*). Sutures are primarily sites of growth (e.g. cranial sutures), their flexibility being generally slight. (Contrary examples are, among others, the quite movable connections of the vertebral bodies.) True joints are sites of movement of the skeleton. Rigid joints (*amphiarthroses*), of course, permit no noteworthy movement.

1. Sutures

According to the type of filling tissue, the following sutures are distinguished:
- *syndesmoses, fibrous articulations* (union by collagenous or elastic connective tissue), and
- *synchondroses, cartilaginous joints* (union by cartilaginous tissue).

A **syndesmosis** (fibrous joint) can be developed as a *ligamentous* union (e.g. stylohyoid ligament, ligamentum flavum, interosseous membranes) or as a *bony suture* (e.g. sutures of the cranial bones, Fig. **8**).

In *plane sutures* the bones border on each other with smooth marginal surfaces. In the abundant *serrated sutures*, the toothed bony margins interdigitate into one another, whereas in *squamous sutures* they are tapered and overlap like scales.

The connective tissue anchoring of the roots of the teeth into the bony alveolus is known as a *gomphosis*.

A **synchondrosis** (cartilaginous joint) is, for example, the union of the osseous first rib with the sternum by hyaline cartilage (costal cartilage) or the union of two vertebral bodies by the fibrocartilaginous intervertebral disc. The connection of the bony diaphysis and the epiphysis of a tubular bone by the cartilaginous epiphysial disc also represents a synchondrosis, as does the cartilaginous union of the hip bones (pubic symphysis). After birth, however, a longitudinal fissure filled with synovial fluid rather regularly appears in these cartilaginous joints, which are then known as *hemiarthroses* (Fig. **118**).

If the original filling tissue in a skeletal union is replaced by bone, a *synostosis* then exists (e.g. ossification of the cranial sutures).

2. Joints

The characteristic feature of a (true) joint is the separation of the articulating skeletal pieces by a cavity.

In all human joints except the temporomandibular and vertebral arch joints, the *articular cavity* is formed by dehiscence within a uniform mesenchymal blastema, from which arise the primordia of the skeletal elements and the joint capsule (with the joint ligaments): *joint segmentation*. In the case of the (secondary) temporomandibular articulation in man (and mammals in general), the joint cavity is formed from a mucosal bursa between two extensively differentiated skeletal parts (mandible and squamous part of the temporal): *joint accumulation*.

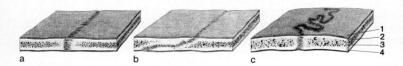

Fig. 8. **Bony sutures**
a Plane suture (example: median palatine suture)
b Squamous suture (example: parietotemporal suture)
c Serrated suture (example: sagittal suture)

1 Periosteum
2 External lamina (outer "layer" of bone of cranial vault)
3 Diploë
4 Internal lamina (inner "layer" of bone of cranial vault)

a) Structure and Histology of Joints

In joints (Fig. **9**), the skeletal pieces are connected by the *joint capsule* (*articular capsule*), a continuation of the periosteal tube. The *joint surfaces* (*articular surfaces*) are separated by a capillary-sized fissure, the *joint cavity* or joint space (*articular cavity*). A true cavity originates, however, only when the fissure is enlarged, e.g. by an accumulation of fluid or by the opening of the joint.

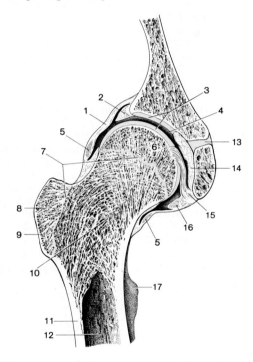

Fig. 9. **Structure of a synovial joint**, shown in a section through the hip joint of a 15-year-old (the terms in parentheses refer to the hip joint)

 1 Articular capsule
 2 Articular (acetabular) lip
 3 Articular cartilage (lunate surface, head of femur)
 4 Articular cavity (joint space shown widened)
 5 Articular ligament (zona orbicularis)
 6 Epiphysis (head of femur)
 7 Cartilaginous epiphysial or apophysial plates
 8 Process (greater trochanter)
 9 Substantia corticalis
10 Substantia spongiosa (in neck of femur)
11 Substantia compacta (body of femur)
12 Medullary cavity
13 Synchondrosis between ilium and pubis
14 Fat pad in acetabular fossa
15 Ligament of head of femur
16 Transverse acetabular ligament
17 Lesser trochanter

The **joint cavity** contains a small amount of a viscous, mucin-containing fluid, *synovial fluid* (*synovia*), which is secreted by the connective tissue cells of the synovial membrane lining the joint cavity. The synovia, rich in hyaluronic acid and therefore viscous, reduces the friction at the articular surfaces. It also plays an important role in the nourishment of the articular cartilages.

The **articular surfaces** possess a cartilaginous covering of avascular, (usually) hyaline cartilage, which varies in thickness (usually between 0.2 and 0.5 mm, up to 6 mm at the patella) and is often also unequally thick in the various areas of an articular surface. It forms a smooth surface so that friction is largely reduced. The articular cartilage distributes the joint pressure to the underlying spongiosa, whereby the surfaces of the cartilage are reversibly deformed and adapted to one another. No elasticity worth mentioning occurs, since the deformability of cartilage is too slight and the thickness of the cartilage layer is insufficient to absorb impacts.

Toward the osseous tissue, the **articular cartilage** exhibits a stratified alteration of its structure. Toward the margin, the superficial, tangential layer of fibers is continuously united with the periosteum. In it lie the "tangential fibers", the apex of the bow of collagenous fibers, whose two ends are anchored to the calcification zone bordering the osseous tissue (Fig. 10). The fiber arcades in the broad radial zone aim directly upwards toward the articular surface, bend over in the transition zone and run a short distance parallel to the surface in the tangential zone before returning downwards. With respect to the glenoid cavity, it has been shown that the tangential fibers are so directed that they counteract a surface expansion of the cartilage.

Intermittent distortions in the shape of cartilage cells, which result from the physiological stress of a joint, are the *stimulus for mainte-*

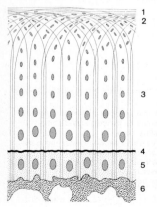

Fig. 10. **Arrangement of collagenous fibers in articular cartilage** (only individual fibril tracts are shown)

1 Tangential fiber layer (uncalcified hyaline cartilage)
2 Transition zone (uncalcified hyaline cartilage)
3 Radial zone (uncalcified hyaline cartilage)
4 Limiting layer (calcified hyaline cartilage)
5 Calcification zone (calcified hyaline cartilage)
6 Bone

nance of joint cartilage. In joints placed at rest, degenerative changes of the articular surfaces can be observed after only a few days; they are no longer adequately moistened with synovia and thus are no longer sufficiently nourished. When there is an unphysiological distribution of pressure (e.g. in the knee joint of the bowlegged or knock-kneed), the overstressed cartilage areas undergo considerable wear and pathological changes. Since the articular cartilage is nourished only by diffusion (mainly from the synovia), degenerative changes (arthroses) are common in the elderly. The regenerative capacity of articular cartilage is slight (absent perichondrium).

The **articular capsule** (Fig. 9) provides an airtight seal for the joint cavity. It consists of an outer *fibrous layer* and an *inner joint membrane* (*synovial membrane*) lining the joint cavity. Since the articular capsule has a rich sensory innervation which extends into the deeper layers of the inner membrane of the joint, injuries are extremely painful. Small lamellar corpuscles (Golgi-Mazzoni bodies) reside in the capsule and its vicinity as sense organs which provide information regarding the orientation of the joint.

The *fibrous membrane* consists of bundles of collagenous fibrils which alternate direction in the individual fiber layers.

When a joint is rested for a longer period, the connective tissue fibers shorten, the joint capsule shrinks (joint contracture) and the mobility of the joint is reduced.

Strong, superficially-situated tracts of the external fibrous layer whose fibrils run in the same direction can be defined as *articular ligaments*. They strengthen the capsular wall.

The *synovial membrane* is richer in cells and poorer in fibers than the outer layer. It contains fat cells in variable amounts and lines the articular cavity with connective tissue cells which form here and there an epithelioid, often stratified, union of cells. The inner surface of the synovial membrane is enlarged by richly vascularized *synovial folds* and by (only microscopically visible) *synovial villi*, which often are branched and able to contain capillaries. The synovial membrane not only secretes synovia but, at the same time, possesses considerable capacity for absorption.

When there is an excessive production of synovia (e.g. as a result of a chronic irritation of the synovial membrane), joint effusion occurs. At weak points in the fibrous membrane, the inner membrane can bulge outward so that a *synovial cyst* is formed.

Intra-articular discs are developed in several joints. As *articular discs*, they divide the joint space completely into two cavities; as *articular menisci* they do so only partially. The superficial portion of the intra-articular discs resembles fibrocartilage in its histology; the central part consists of tendinous tissue. Discs and menisci form floating joint surfaces (temporomandibular and knee joints), enlarge the contact area of the articulating surfaces and allow a better distribution of joint pressure. In the shoulder and hip joints, the cartilage-covered joint cavity is surrounded and enlarged by an annular connective tissue projection, the *articular lip* (Fig. 9). Like the intra-articular discs, the articular lips are aneural and (almost) avascular.

Coherence of joint surfaces. All human joints are "pressure closed". The articular contact is caused by the joint surfaces always pressing on each other as a result of muscular pull and the weight of bearing or moving body or limb segments. The coherence of joints is thus ensured by *muscle power*.

Atmospheric pressure, which is frequently assigned a considerable role in the coherence of joints, can only be effective when there is negative pressure in the interior of the joint. Negative pressure, however, occurs only when external forces seek to separate the epiphyses from one another without the tension of the musculature preventing it. Under physiological conditions, this state does not occur in the living. (Moreover, a longer-lasting negative pressure would produce an effusion in the joint cavity which would undo the action of atmospheric pressure on the joint contacts.) Other mechanisms (e.g. adhesion, check ligaments or tension of skin or fascia) have no significance at all for the coherence of joint surfaces.

b) Joint Types

Joints can be classified according to different criteria. Depending upon the number of skeletal elements articulating at a joint cavity, there are *simple* and *compound* joints. According to the shape of the joint surfaces, they can be further classified into *ball-and-socket* (*spheroidal*), *ellipsoid*, *saddle* and *hinge* joints.

In **ball-and-socket joints** (Fig. 11a), a more or less spherical joint *head* (convex-shaped articular surface) articulates with a correspondingly concave joint *socket* (e.g. shoulder joint). The midpoint of the ball is the pivot of the joint, through which many arbitrary axes can be drawn. Nonetheless, all movements of a skeletal piece in a ball-and-socket joint can be imagined to be composed of movements around *three axes* placed perpendicular to each other, one of which must correspond to the longitudinal axis of the skeletal element. The three axes of this three-dimensional axial crossing each represent a cardinal axis around which the joint can move, i.e. it is an articulation allowing movements around three *cardinal axes*. The ball-and-socket joint, therefore, has three degrees of freedom, whereby a *degree of freedom* implies the possibility of movement around a cardinal axis.

A ball-and-socket joint in which the socket embraces the joint head beyond the equator of the ball (e.g. hip joint) is termed an *enarthrosis*.

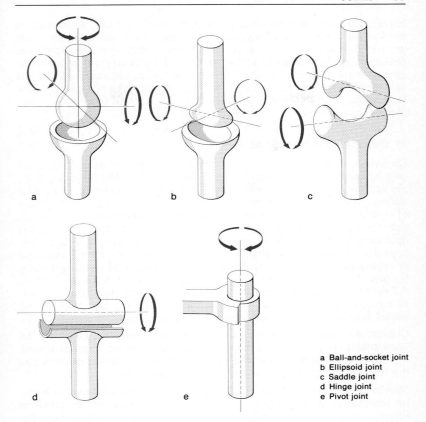

a Ball-and-socket joint
b Ellipsoid joint
c Saddle joint
d Hinge joint
e Pivot joint

Fig. 11. **Forms of joints**
Arrows indicate direction in which skeletal element can be moved around respective axis

Ellipsoid (Fig. **11 b**) and **saddle** (Fig. **11 c**) **joints** are *biaxial* joints in the sense mentioned above. In the ellipsoid joint, the joint head is curved convexly in two planes perpendicular to one another, and the joint socket is shaped concavely in the corresponding planes (e.g. proximal wrist joint). In the saddle joint, the articular surfaces of the head and socket are formed convexly in one plane and concavely in a plane perpendicular to it (e.g. carpometacarpal joint of the thumb).

In **hinge joints** (*ginglymus*, Fig. **11 d**), only movements in *one plane* are possible. Displacements in the direction of the axis of rotation are hindered by collateral ligaments. The humero-ulnar joint, which can be cited as an example of a hinge joint, possesses a spiral-shaped guidance groove. The angle of ascent of the spiral, however, is so slight that deviations of the median axis resulting from it are of no great importance, and thus the distinction of a "spiral joint" is unnecessary. When the movements in a uniaxial joint, i.e. in a hinge joint, take place around the longitudinal axis of the skeletal piece, it is also referred to as a *pivot joint* (Fig. 11e, e.g. median atlanto-axial joint).

c) General Mechanics of Joints

Directions of movement. The direction of joint movements is defined not only by the shape of the articulating surfaces, but also to a large degree by the arrangement of the muscles and ligamentous structures. In applied science, joints are "areally determined" and possess fixed axes or points of rotation. In contrast to these, joints in the living human are "pressure determined", i.e. the directions and types of movement are primarily determined by the total forces acting on the respective bones. The articular surfaces are usually more or less incongruent, their form often deviating considerably from the surface shape of ideal rotating bodies. Strictly speaking, therefore, the axes of movement are not exactly fixed. All details concerning the course of the axes or the position of the points of rotation in the joints of living humans, therefore, can describe the actual situation only in a simplified schematic fashion.

Clinical measurement of the range of movement takes place from the "anatomical position". The patient stands erect, looks straight ahead, the arms hanging down with the palms of the hands facing forward and the feet standing parallel and close to one another.

Movement around the longitudinal axis of a bone is described as external or internal *rotation*, external or internal *circumduction*, external or internal *torsion*. *Abduction* leads the skeletal piece away from the body (or from the reference element), perpendicular to the axis of flexion; *adduction* brings the skeletal piece toward the body (or toward the reference element). In the case of *flexion* (*bending*), (the longitudinal axes of) both articulating skeletal pieces are angled down toward one another perpendicular to the plane of abduction. *Extension* (*straightening*) is the opposite movement. Flexion at the shoulder and hip joints is usually termed *anteversion*, extension is usually termed *retroversion*.

Abduction and adduction take place around a cardinal axis lying in a sagittal plane, whereas flexion and extension occur around a cardinal axis lying in a frontal plane, provided the articulating limb segments are neither externally nor internally rotated. *Circumduction* is a circular movement which results from the combination of movements around the cardinal axes (e.g. rotation of the arms and legs). Thereby, the moved segment describes a cone, while the distal point of the limb describes a circle or an oval. Movements around each cardinal axis are always designated as *cardinal movements*; circumduction, on the other hand, is not a cardinal movement.

Joint inhibition. The inhibition of joint movement, i.e. the limiting of the extent of a movement, can have different causes. In the case of *bone inhibition*, two bones in a definite joint arrangement push against one other so that a continuation of movement is impossible. This is rare, but can occur, for example, in extreme extension of the elbow joint by the olecranon striking the olecranon fossa. In the case of *ligamentous inhibition*, a ligamentous tract is so stretched by a movement that the movement comes to a standstill automatically (e.g. stretching of the iliofemoral ligament during extension of the hip joint). The (passive) movement of the tibia in the knee joint is inhibited as soon as the calf and the posterior surface of the thigh are touched: *soft tissue inhibition* (mass inhibition).

If the limit of distensibility of a muscle is reached by a specific joint position, a continuation of movement is impossible: *muscle inhibition* (Fig. **17 b**).

The joint position which must be reached in order to inhibit a certain movement varies from individual to individual and can change in the course of an individual's life. The small child is more flexible than the adult. Soft tissue inhibition in the forward bending of the trunk commences earlier in the obese than in the lean person. In "body building", the extent of movement in certain joints (e.g. elbow joint) is restricted by mass inhibition. In trained athletes, muscle inhibition is less than in the untrained. For certain acrobats (contortionists) who practice extreme movements from earliest childhood, ligamentous inhibition appears to be largely neutralized. Joint diseases, but also cutaneous scars, can lead to a pathological limitation of movement.

C. General Myology

1. Elements and Principal Structures of Skeletal Muscle

Skeletal muscles (Fig. **12a**) consist of variously shaped *muscle bellies*, whose contractile structural parts can be shortened or elongated, and usually distinctly narrower *tendons*, which are attached to the skeleton or to connective tissue structures of the locomotor apparatus (fascia, interosseous membranes) and which transfer the muscular pull directly or indirectly to the skeletal parts. In general, the proximal (at the extremities) or cephalic (at the trunk) site of attachment is referred to as the *origin* of the muscle, the opposite attachment as the *insertion*.

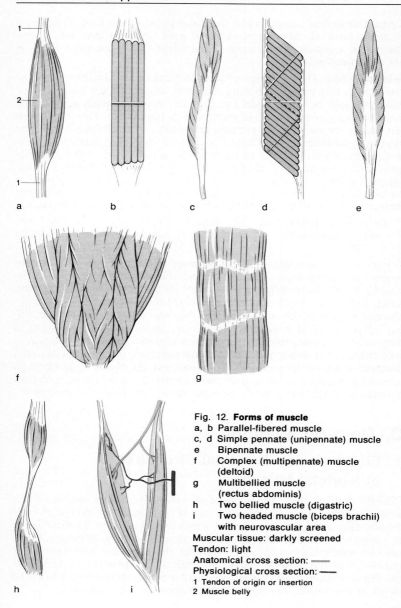

Fig. 12. **Forms of muscle**
a, b Parallel-fibered muscle
c, d Simple pennate (unipennate) muscle
e   Bipennate muscle
f   Complex (multipennate) muscle
      (deltoid)
g   Multibellied muscle
      (rectus abdominis)
h   Two bellied muscle (digastric)
i   Two headed muscle (biceps brachii)
      with neurovascular area
Muscular tissue: darkly screened
Tendon: light
Anatomical cross section: ━━━
Physiological cross section: ━━━
1 Tendon of origin or insertion
2 Muscle belly

Origin and insertion are defined purely conventionally. They must not be regarded as "fixed points" or "mobile points", since the origin can be moved in relation to the insertion, the insertion can be moved in relation to the origin, or both attachment sites of the muscle can be moved reciprocally.

In muscles with divided origins, the individual origin portion is termed the *head*; two-*headed* or several-*headed* muscles are distinguished (e.g. biceps brachii [Fig. **12i**], quadriceps femoris). If the origin is undivided but the muscle belly has an intermediate tendon, we refer to two-*bellied* or several-*bellied* muscles (e.g. digastric [Fig. **12h**], rectus abdominis [Fig. **12g**]).

The **muscle belly** consists of cross-striated muscle fibers which are grouped into bundles of increasing organization by connective tissue structures (*endomysium, perimysium*). Thus, they form a unit, the parts of which are mutually mobile.

Striated muscle fibers ($\varnothing$ 10–100 µm, length up to over 10 cm) form the *structural units* of skeletal muscle. As contractile elements, they contain in their cytoplasm (*sarcoplasm*) myofibrils ($\varnothing$ 0.5–1 µm), which create the cross-striation phenomenon. The myofibrils consist of smaller units, the *myofilaments* (actin and myosin filaments). The nuclei of the muscle fibers (20–40/mm long) lie close to the margins. The sarcoplasm is covered by a *sarcolemma*.

The *endomysium* encloses each individual muscle fiber. The delicate connective tissue covering, consisting predominantly of reticular fibers, carries numerous, mostly longitudinally-directed, blood capillaries and nerve fibers. The **endomysium** groups several individual fibers into a *primary bundle* which is enclosed by the *internal perimysium* (Fig. **13**). The primary bundle is the *functional unit* of skeletal muscle. The internal perimysium forms the sliding interface between primary bundles. Several primary bundles are combined into macroscopically-visible *secondary bundles* (fleshy fibers) by a somewhat stronger connective tissue covering, the *external perimysium* (carrying blood vessels and nerves). The border of the muscle and its fascial connections are taken over by the *epimysium*.

The connective tissue framework which borders the contractile elements carries nerves and blood vessels to the muscle fibers via circumscribed entry sites (*neurovascular areas*, Fig. **12 i**). It also harbors the nervous apparatus of muscle sense, the muscle spindle.

Fascia. The surface of a muscle is enclosed by a firm connective tissue covering, the *muscle fascia* (Fig. **13**), which isolates the muscle from its neighbors and, at the same time, provides a movable interface with them, frequently also serving as surface of origin. Several muscles can be enclosed by a common *group fascia* which is in communication with the individual muscle fascia and, moreover, is attached to bones. Thus, osteofibrous *muscle compartments* are formed in which individual muscles or their parts can be displaced one against the other and be controlled at the same time. Some muscles are also attached to regions of the group fascia that are tendinous in structure.

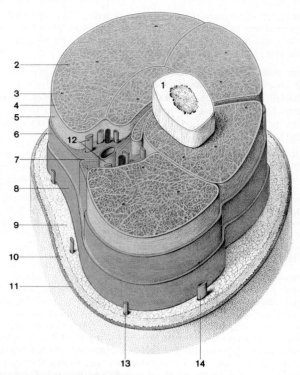

Fig. 13. **Connective tissue investments of skeletal muscle,**
shown in cross section through middle third of (left) arm (⟶ Fig. 88)
(Muscle fibers and connective tissue structures within the muscle not according to scale)

1 Humerus
2 Muscle fibers covered by endomysium, grouped
  into primary bundles by internal perimysium
3 External perimysium carrying blood vessels and
  nerves
4 Epimysium
5 Muscle fascia
6 Group fascia united with bone by intermuscular
  septum (7) to form an osteofibrous muscle compartment

8 Brachial fascia
9 Subcutaneous connective tissue
10, 11 *Skin*
10 Dermis
11 Epidermis
12 Deep vessels and nerves
13 Cutaneous nerve
14 Cutaneous vein

Increased muscular activity leads to compensatory *hypertrophy* of the skeletal musculature, the muscle fibers becoming thicker (the number of fibers remaining constant). Decreased use (immobilization, muscle paralysis) produces disuse *atrophy*.

The ability of skeletal muscle to regenerate is slight in humans. A connective tissue scar replaces destroyed muscle tissue.

A **tendon** consists of tense bundles of collagenous fibers which are parallel in short tendons and arranged in spiral windings in long cords. It is only sparsely vascularized.

The fibers of tendons are attached to tubular-shaped indentations of the plasmalemma. Tendinous fibers (= bundles of collagenous fibers) are fixed to the basal lamina at the base of the invaginations of the sarcolemma, whereas the actin filaments are attached to the plasmalemma from within. Collagenous fibrils pass from the sarcolemmal tubules into the tendinous fibers.

The **muscle-tendon connection** does not occur at one place, but is staggered. The tendon lies on the surface of the muscle belly as a more or less broad tendinous sheath or is inserted between muscle bundles. The tendon fibers never follow the direction of the muscle fibers – not even in muscle with "parallel fibers". On the contrary, the muscle fiber bundles form acute angles of different sizes (*feather angles*) with the tendon. When the muscle fibers contract, the feather angle becomes greater. In this way, space is obtained for the increased thickness of the contracting muscle fibers without the tendon fibers being pressed apart. Broad-surfaced tendinous plates are referred to as **aponeuroses.**

The bundles of tendinous fibers of resting muscle are somewhat compressed in the longitudinal direction and slightly "wavy" owing to elastic fibers. This undulation is first assimilated at the beginning of the contraction of the muscle fibers before the muscle pulls on the bone, which allows the movement to be effected more gently, more flowingly. The tendon fibers – like the muscle fibers – are grouped by connective tissue coverings (*peritendinea*) into bundles of increasing degrees of organization. The peritendineum forms a connective tissue casing system which unites the sliding tendon bundles with each other. It contains tendon spindles as stretch receptors – arranged chiefly at the muscle-tendon border.

The attachment of a muscle is always tendinous, yet the "tendon" can be so short that it cannot be recognized macroscopically. This is then described as a "fleshy" origin or insertion of a muscle. The union of tendons with bones is formed differently depending upon the cross-sectional size of tendons and the types of attachments. Origins and insertions involving large surfaces radiate into the periosteum and become united with the bones (Sharpey's fibers) through this bony covering. Tendons with small cross-sections which are attached at rough areas of bone or its prominences are anchored directly to the bone. The periosteum exhibits gaps corresponding to the sites of tendinous attachments. The tendon fibers penetrating into the bone are enclosed by cartilaginous tissue, the deep layer of which is calcified and meshed with the bone on its lower surface. The cartilage cushion prevents the enclosed segment of the tendon fibers from being bent acutely at the surface of the bone toward the free portion of the tendon, thereby injuring the tendon. The fan-shaped bending and spreading of the tendon fibers shortly before they penetrate into the bone serve the same purpose.

In many tendons, fiber tracts situated toward the margins are deflected in the direction of the bony axis, whereas the central bundles meet with the bone at an angle of maximally 90 degrees. It is assumed that in each phase of movement only those fibers of the tendon fan are tensed which course in the tract direction of the free tendon segments. In this interpretation, tension is not lost in the fibers which extend at a "dangerous angle" (i.e. bent more or less acutely) into the embedded portion of the tendon, whose direction is fixed. On the contrary, in the network of the tendinous fan built up from primary bundles, it is transferred to fiber tracts with a more favorable course direction. The structural changes of the tendon in the tendinous fan thus make possible the complete utilization of muscle power acting in the direction of the pull of the tendon, although only a part of the tendinous fiber bundle is tensed at any given time.

The anchoring of the enclosed part of the tendon in the bone is very firm. If the tendon is torn at this site, a small piece of bone is always torn out with it (strain fracture).

2. General Muscle Mechanics

Parallel-fibered and pennate muscles are distinguished according to the size of the feather angle. In **parallel-fibered** muscle (Fig. **12a,b**) the feather angle is small. In **pennate** muscle (Fig. **12c–f**), it is not difficult to recognize macroscopically the oblique attachments of the muscle fibers to the tendon. The greater the feather angle of a muscle, the more muscle fibers can be attached to an equal length of tendon. Pennate muscles can be simple (unipennate), double-sided (bipennate, e.g. rectus femoris) or complex (multipennate, e.g. deltoid), depending on whether the muscle fibers approach the tendon from one or two sides, or whether several tendinous layers are inserted between the bundles of muscle fibers.

In parallel-fibered muscle with its minimum feather angle, *tendon strength* (a term not quite happily chosen, but current in physiological work, which characterizes the portion of muscle power acting in the direction of the pull of the tendon) and *muscle power* are approximately equal. In pennate muscle, the greater the feather angle, the less is the tendon strength in comparison to muscle power. The (absolute) muscle power of a muscle depends upon the total cross-section of all muscle fibers. The *work* of a muscle is the product of the tendon strength and the lift, i.e. it is determined by the number of fibers, the feather angle, and the shortening capacity of the muscle fibers.

The total cross-sectional surface of all muscle fibers is called the **physiological cross-section** of the muscle (Fig. **12b,d**). It runs perpendicular to the longitudinal axis of each muscle fiber. The *anatomical cross-section*, on the other hand, lies in the middle of the muscle at a right angle to its longitudinal axis. It coincides with the physiological cross-section only in parallel-fibered muscles. The *lift* of a muscle is determined by the length of the muscle fibers and by their feather angle. Stretched muscle fibers can contract to maximally 30–50% of their initial length. In parallel-fibered muscle, the lift corresponds approximately to the contractive ability of the stretched muscle.

The "windup" in pitching, adequately – perhaps maximally – stretches the muscle fibers which carry out the motion of the throw. With their contraction, the total shortening capacity of the affected muscles, i.e. their maximal lift, can then be effective.

The **direction of muscle pull** (Fig. **14**) is determined by the *effective terminal extension* of the tendon. If the muscle belly and the origin and insertion tendons lie in a straight line, the direction of the pull of the muscle corresponds to a straight line connecting the middle of the muscle origin with the middle of the muscle insertion (*principal line*). If, however, the tendon is carried around an abutment (fulcrum, *hypomochlion*), only the direction of the section lying between the fulcrum and the insertion is decisive for the direction of muscle pull.

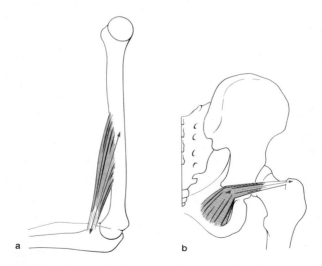

Fig. 14. **Direction of muscle pull** (◀——▶), virtual lever arm (——)
a Direction of muscle pull corresponds to principal line (example: brachialis)
b Direction of muscle pull corresponds to effective terminal extension of tendon situated between hypomochlion and muscle attachment (example: obturator internus)

The *torque* of a muscle is the product of tendon strength and virtual lever arm. The virtual lever arm is equal to the perpendicular distance between the principal line (or the straight line drawn through the effective terminal section of the tendon) and the axis of rotation or the point of rotation of the joint (Fig. **14 a**). It varies with a change in position of the joint and is greatest in the position in which the tendon of insertion (the tendon of origin when the muscle origin is near a joint) meets the bone at a right angle. The tendon strength becomes less with increasing shortness.

3. Auxiliary Support of Muscles

Muscles and tendons are extraordinarily sensitive to friction and to localized pressure. They are protected from such mechanical injuries by mucous bursae, by tendons and tendon sheaths, and by sesamoid bones.

Mucous bursae (*synovial bursae*) are cleft-like spaces of different sizes enclosed by connective tissue. Those located near joints can communicate with the articular cavities (Fig. **83**). Their connective tissue capsule is comparable to the joint capsule; their lumen contains a slight amount of *synovia*, which is secreted by the inner layer of the wall, the synovial membrane. Mucous bursae lie between bony processes and skin, muscles, tendons or fascia. They decrease friction in the case of displacements and protect the above structures from localized pressure. Like water cushions, they act as pressure distributors. At the attachments of many tendons, mucous bursae are inserted between the bone and the segment of tendon near the bone. On the one hand, they fill up the space created by the enlargement of the attachment angle of the tendon; on the other hand, they prevent an acute-angled bending of the tendon at the transition between the segment enclosed in bone and the free tendon.

Tendon sheaths (*vaginae tendinum*, Fig. **15**), are double-walled connective tissue tubes, which enclose the tendons for shorter or longer distances and prevent friction with bony or ligamentous structures. The *inner* (*synovial*) *layer*, which lies directly on the tendons, and the *outer* (*fibrous*) *layer*, which is usually strengthened by rigid connective tissue, are separated by a sliding fissure containing synovia. Both layers of the tendon sheath are united at their proximal and distal ends and are able to communicate with one another by a *mesotendon* which – like a type of mesentery – conveys blood vessels and nerves. In the region of the carpals and tarsals, on the palmar side of the fingers and plantar side of the toes, the tendon sheaths are fixed to the bones. Their outer wall is strengthened by strong fibrous sheaths (*vaginae fibrosae*) so that the tendons glide in osteofibrous canals which determine their direction and do not permit them to separate from the bone.

Tendon sheaths and mucous bursae can become inflamed (e.g. through chronic irritation). In stenotypists, tendovaginitis occurs rela-

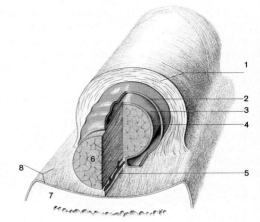

Fig. 15 **Tendon sheaths**
1 Fibrous layer
2 Synovial layer, external sheath
3 Synovial cavity
4 Synovial layer, internal sheath
5 Mesotendineum (vascularized)
6 Tendon
7 Bone
8 Periosteum

tively often at the extensor tendons in the region of the proximal wrist joint. People who work on their knees (tile layers) are frequently afflicted with bursitis in the mucous bursae in front of the patella (prepatellar bursa) or in front of the tibial tuberosity (tibial tuberosity bursa).

Sesamoid bones. In tendons which glide directly on bone and possess no tendon sheaths, cartilage cells infiltrate the surface facing the bone. *Sesamoid bones* (Figs. **98a** and **120c**) can also appear in tendons or joint capsules as small (hand, foot) or large bones (patella). Some sesamoid bones are formed constantly, others are quite variable.

4. Muscles at Rest and in Motion

At rest, all muscles also possess a certain tension, a *tonus*. It varies from person to person, from time to time, and from muscle to muscle. The tonus of the muscles which are regulated by the nervous system determines the carriage of the body (erect or relaxed). Many muscles have the primary task of maintaining a certain position in the body parts concerned (*holding muscles*: e.g. soleus; short foot muscles). Their activity is more concerned with adapting tonicity to the situation than with contraction.

In the execution of a movement, several muscles regularly work together (*synergists*). Frequently, coordinated movements are produced by *muscle chains*, which pass over several joints and which contract individually either in succession or simultaneously. *Antagonists*, i.e. muscles which counter the intended movement, are as important as the synergists in shaping movement. By a gradual diminution of their tension, they enable the synergists to complete the movement.

When two opposed muscles are attached at almost the same site on a skeletal element, the skeletal piece can be guided by them like a sling: *muscle sling* (Fig. **16**). The skeletal piece between the two muscles is called a bony inscription.

Synergists and antagonists are *functional groups*, into which the individual muscles are divided with respect to their action on a certain joint. They do not necessarily correspond to genetic muscle groups. At hinge joints there are *benders* (*flexors*) and *stretchers* (*extensors*) which frequently, but not always, coincide with genetic groups of flexors and extensors. At ball and socket joints, the potential movements are more versatile thus increasing possibilities for the cooperation of individual muscles. They can be grouped into *flexors* and *extensors*, *abductors* and *adductors*, *external* and *internal rotators*.

Only through the greatest exertion do all fibers of a muscle contract simultaneously. In general, only a part of a muscle fiber bundle is actively involved in each phase of movement. The organization of a muscle in fiber bundles and the further recognizable division of many muscles into portions whose origins, fiber directions and attachments deviate slightly already equip the individual muscle with many combinations of the muscle fiber groups active in a phase of movement.

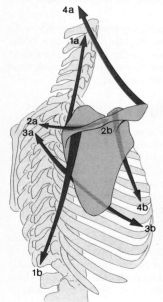

Fig. 16. **Guidance of scapula by muscle slings**
1 Vertical muscle sling: levator scapulae (a) – ascending part of trapezius (b)
2 Horizontal muscle sling: transverse part of trapezius (a) – middle part of serratus anterior (b)
3 Oblique muscle sling: rhomboideus (a) – pulling of inferior part of serratus anterior (b)
4 Oblique muscle sling: descending part of trapezius (a) – pectoralis minor (b)

In the execution of a movement, however, partial components of several muscles work together, whose number and combination can vary during the course of movement, so that the possibilities for gradation and modification of a movement are extraordinarily great. The usual data concerning origin, insertion and "function" of a muscle provide, therefore, only a modest illustration of the actual process.

Active and passive muscle insufficiency. In general, multijointed muscles cannot be shortened to such an extent that they bring into final position all the joints over which they move. In maximal contraction, they become *actively insufficient* (Fig. **17c, d**). Conversely, multijointed muscles usually cannot be stretched in such a way that all the joints which are passed over can be brought into final position by the antagonists. This insufficient extensibility of multijointed muscles is known as *passive insufficiency* (Fig. **17a, b**). It causes a muscular suppression of movement (→ p. 35). Among others, the long flexors and extensors of the fingers and the ischiocrural muscles are examples of actively and passively insufficient muscles.

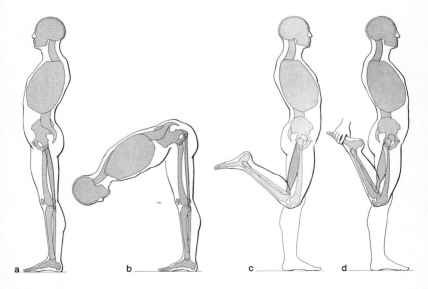

Fig. 17. **Passive and active muscle insufficiency**
When the knee joint is extended, the ischiocrural musculature (a) cannot be stretched to such an extent that maximum flexion of the hip joint is possible (b): passive insufficiency. When the hip joint is extended, it cannot be shortened sufficiently to permit maximum flexion of the knee joint (c): active insufficiency. An additional flexion of about 20–30° is possible (d) when supplemented by an external force.

A powerful closure of the fist is only possible when the wrist joint is extended (dorsally flexed) at the same time. Otherwise, the long flexors of the fingers are actively insufficient (grasping a horizontal bar, carrying a suitcase). When bending the trunk forward with knees extended, those who are untrained cannot touch the floor with the tips of their fingers because the flexors of the knee joint pulling from the ischium to the tibia (ischiocrural muscles) are passively insufficient and cannot be sufficiently extended.

3. Circulatory System

A. Elements and Structural Principles of the Circulatory System

The biological functions of cells and tissues of all organs are maintained by a *transport system*. *Routes of transport* are the blood and lymphatic vessels; *vehicles of transport* are the blood and lymph. Blood *transports*, among other things, respiratory gases, nutrients, hormones, protective substances, metabolic wastes and heat. Lymph transports, for example, portions of extracellular tissue fluids and metabolic products back into the blood vascular system.

Blood vessels form a *closed channel* for the *circulation* of blood; the transport system is therefore known as the *circulatory system*. The bloodstream is organized into a *large (systemic)* and a *small (pulmonary) circuit* (Fig. **18**).

The **heart** is located at the points of transition in the bloodstream between the *systemic circulation* and the *pulmonary circulation*. It lies – figuratively speaking – at the crossing of both circles of a figure 8.

On the basis of its construction, the heart is the pump for the simultaneous movement of blood in both circuits. The heart is divided into a *right* and a *left* half, also shortened to "right heart" and "left heart". Each half of the heart is further divided into an *atrium* and *ventricle*. The *atria* receive the blood *entering* the heart – the *right atrium* from the *systemic*, the *left atrium* from the *pulmonary circulation*. The *ventricles* expel the blood *back*, the *right ventricle* into the *pulmonary circuit* (pump for the small circuit), the *left ventricle* into the *systemic* (pump for the large circuit). The expulsion of blood is caused by the simultaneous and rhythmic contractions (*systole*) of the middle, muscular layer of the heart wall (myocardium) of both ventricles.

Arteries, **capillaries** and **veins**. All vessels that carry blood *away from the heart* are called *arteries*, those that carry it *to the heart*, *veins*. Arteries and veins are defined according to their role as *transport segments* in the circulatory system and not according to the oxygen content of their blood flow. In the *pulmonary circuit*, oxygen-poor, deoxygenated blood flows in the arteries, oxygen-rich, oxygenated blood in the veins. In the *systemic circuit*, on the other hand, the arteries transport oxygen-rich, the veins oxygen-poor blood. Hair-fine *capillaries* are the *oxygen exchange sections* of the circulation between the ends of arteries and the beginning of veins. *Arterioles* form the transition between arteries and capillaries, and *venules* that between capillaries and veins. Whereas blood in the various *veins of*

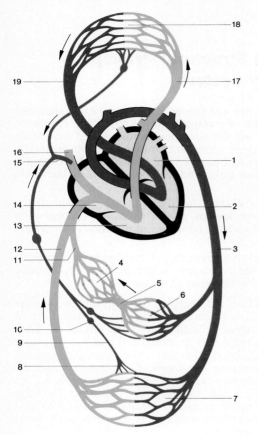

Fig 18. **Systemic and pulmonary circulations**
Vessels with oxygen-rich blood ▬▬ , with oxygen-poor blood ▬▬

1–16 *Systemic circulation*
1 Left atrium
2 Left ventricle
3 Aorta
4 Capillary beds in liver supplied by portal vein (5) which receives blood from capillary beds of unpaired abdominal organs (6)
7 Capillary beds of trunk wall
8 Lymphatic capillaries
9 Lymphatic vessels
10 Lymph nodes
11 Hepatic vein
12 Inferior vena cava
13 Right ventricle
14 Right atrium
15 Opening of central lymphatic trunk
16 Superior vena cava
17–19 *Pulmonary circulation*
17 Pulmonary arteries
18 Capillary beds of lungs
19 Pulmonary veins

the pulmonary circulation does not differ, blood found in the different parts of the *venous portion of the systemic circuit* varies in composition. For example, the blood in the renal vein is poorer in metabolic wastes than that in other veins, the venous blood of endocrine glands is richer in hormones, that of the liver is warmer than the venous blood of other organs. The systemic circulation consists of numerous parallel *circulatory parts* with heterogeneous functional tasks. All arise directly or indirectly from the aorta and empty into the venae cavae. In the capillary region the arterial blood assumes the character of venous blood.

Bloodstream. All the blood vessels of a circuit comprise a closed, multi-branched tubular system, the *bloodstream*, consisting of segments of different caliber and wall structure – arteries, capillaries, veins. Under normal conditions, i.e. when the vessel walls are intact, blood does not leave the bloodstream at any point except the spleen. (Menstrual bleeding results from damage to the vascular wall occurring in the physiological course of the cycle).

An active *exchange* of blood plasma and other blood constituents with the surrounding tissue takes place, of course, predominantly in the *capillary section* of the circuit. In the blood-forming organs (red bone marrow, lymph nodes, spleen, etc.) young cells enter the blood. In the capillary segments containing so-called phagocytic cells (phagocytes) – primarily in the liver – the debris of destroyed cells is eliminated. Certain defense cells of the blood (lymphocytes) regularly wander back to the organs of their formation and from these again into the blood (lymphocyte recirculation). Blood components, which are relatively stable in their proportions, are subjected to a constant replacement in connection with the functions of the blood. In addition, there are daily and seasonal variations in the composition of the blood. This uninterrupted exchange of blood constituents takes place through the *intact vessel wall*, principally in the capillary segment of the circuit. Bleeding, on the other hand, in which blood leaves the bloodstream, requires an injury to the vascular wall.

Public vessels, private vessels. The work of numerous organs is closely connected with the circulation of blood (e.g. the heart acts as a circulatory pump, in the kidneys decomposed substances are filtered from the blood, in the liver nutrients from the intestine are exposed to metabolism); these organs are interpolated in the bloodstream. Those blood vessels of organs which directly *serve the total organism* are termed *public vessels*. In order to be able to fulfill their functions, however, the organs themselves must be supplied by blood vessels, by *organ-specific private vessels*. (The public vessels of the heart, for example, are the superior and inferior venae cavae, the aorta and the pulmonary artery; the private vessels are the coronary vessels).

Blood vessel walls. *General structure* (Fig. **19a**). Basically, the wall of blood vessels is comprised of *three layers*.

The *inner layer* (*tunica intima*) serves mainly for the regulation of *exchange of material*. It consists of endothelial cells, flat cells which border the vascular lumen, and of a thin membrane of fine connective tissue fibers; in arteries, elastic networks are added.

The *middle layer* (*tunica media*) is primarily concerned with the motor activity of the vessel. It contains smooth muscle cells and elastic networks in varying composition.

The *outer layer* (*tunica externa* or *adventitia*) facilitates the incorporation of the vessels into the surrounding tissues and is composed chiefly of connective tissue elements (cells and fibers).

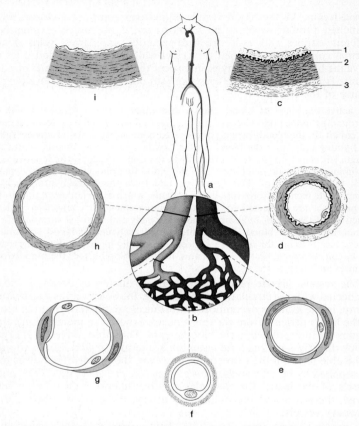

Fig. 19. Structure of blood vessels in different segments of the systemic circulation
Dashed lines indicate site of vascular cross sections (c–i)
Vessels walls are increasingly magnified toward capillaries
a Arterial (——) and venous (——) divisions of systemic circulation
b Arterial branches and venous roots in communication with capillary bed
c Artery close to heart (aorta)
d Artery distant from heart
e Arteriole
f Capillary
g Venule
h Vein distant from heart
i Vein close to heart from lower half of body (inferior vena cava)
1 Tunica intima
2 Tunica media
3 Tunica externa (adventitia)

The three layers of the wall are formed differently in arteries and veins in accommodation of their different tasks in the circulation; the wall of capillaries is reduced to just the tunica intima.

1. Elements of the Circulatory System

a) Arteries

The **arteries** are transport segments and possess, therefore, a strongly developed tunica media (Fig. **19c, d**).

Elastic membranes predominate in *arteries located near the heart*; they are stretched during systole of the heart by the ejected volume of blood (increase in pressure) and, contracting during relaxation, push the blood column further = *arteries of the elastic type* (hydraulic reservoir function). The discontinuous output of the heart is thus transformed into a continuous stream.

The *pulse wave* brought about by systole leads to caliber fluctuations which are deadened in the surrounding loose connective tissue. In directly adjoining bones, e.g. on the inner surface of the cranial vault, furrows and canals are formed owing to the pulse wave.

A diseased, enlarged arterial segment, an aneurysm, can erode adjacent bone up to complete disintegration.

In *arteries located far from the heart*, the tunica media is composed primarily of *smooth muscle tissue* which can constrict and dilate these arteries and thus regulate the circulation of blood to regions supplied by them = *arteries of the muscular type*.

Arteries are under an elastic *longitudinal tension*. Arteries that pass over the flexor side of joints are adapted to the shortening of the course segment occurring during flexion by a decrease in their longitudinal tension; they are withdrawn in this way from the flexion angle.

If a small artery is severed in the living, it can spring back into the connective tissue by virtue of its elastic longitudinal tension. The internal elastic membrane can turn the severed end of the artery inward into the vascular lumen and, thus, temporarily prevent bleeding until a blood clot is formed. In the elderly, when the elasticity of the arterial wall decreases, the artery becomes lengthened and tortuous.

At many sites in the body the arteries are primarily *tortuous*, e.g. the facial artery in the cheek, the vertebral artery before its entrance into the posterior cranial fossa. Such *reserve lengths* permit deformities or movements of the affected body parts (e.g. deformation of the cheek and rotary movements of the head).

Arterial collateral routes. Medium-sized and small peripheral arteries frequently have connections with one another (*anastomoses*) which can lead to the formation of an arterial network (*rete arteriosum*). If the anastomoses form a parallel route to the main vascular stream, they are called *collaterals*. In the case of a deficiency in this main vascular system (occlusion, ligation), they can feed the capillary region dependent on it by forming a *collateral circulation*.

The surgeon must estimate the possibility of a collateral circulation before ligating an artery, and, if necessary, select the place of ligature which assures the blood supply via collaterals. The gradual closure of a vessel, in contrast to a sudden closure, promotes the development of a collateral circulation.

Terminal arteries are those arteries which, when occluded, cannot be supplanted by (anatomically present) collaterals in their supply region (e.g. the terminal branches of intestinal arteries still coursing in the mesentery). *Functional terminal arteries* are those in regions, in which collaterals are indeed present anatomically but, according to general experience, cannot provide an adequate blood supply (e.g. branches of the coronary arteries).

When a terminal artery is occluded (e.g. by a blood clot, *embolus*), bloodlessness (*ischemia*) arises in the dependent supply region which leads to a local destruction of tissues (*infarct*). Organs vulnerable to infarcts are lungs, liver, spleen, kidneys, brain, heart and retina of the eye. Yet experience teaches that arterial collateral routes can be formed also in these organs when arterial occlusion is gradual.

Special constrictive arteries can be inserted ahead of the capillary region and temporarily exclude the capillaries from the circulation; they are microscopically small. As an occluding arrangement, some arteries possess longitudinally-directed, muscle-like cells in their intima which project into the lumen like a cushion (*cushion artery*). Such arteries occur in endocrine organs and in genital cavernous bodies.

Spiral arteries. In some organs, arteries take a corkscrew-like, spiral or strongly tortuous course. On the one hand, this comprises a *reserve length* for the artery which facilitates a brief volume change to the organ, for example, in the helicine arteries of the penis. On the other hand, spiral arteries also occur in organs which undergo no volume change, e.g. in the hilum of the ovary, or they retain their tortuous course in the case of slow volume change, e.g. in the uterus; the significance of this type of spiral artery is not known.

Arterioles (Fig. **19e**), as the smallest arteries ($\varnothing$ about 30 µm), are connected to the capillary bed. Their tunica media consists chiefly of muscular tissue. The terminal end of the arteriole, which branches off into capillaries, is therefore also called the "precapillary sphincter".

Arteriovenous anastomoses are shunt connections which transport the blood from the smallest arteries to the smallest veins by by-passing the capillaries. They function to regulate the circulation.

b) Capillaries

Capillaries (Fig 19f) possess a diameter of 4 to about 15 μm. The deformable blood corpuscles, the diameters of which are insignificantly larger than that of the narrowest capillaries (erythrocyte diameter 7.6 μm), are compressed by the capillaries; they slide along the capillary endothelium. The capillaries form an extensively branched network, collectively called *capillary bed* (Fig. **19b**). The capillary wall consists only of an endothelial tube which is surrounded by a basal lamina of glycoprotein. Individual cells (*pericytes*) lie here and there on the endothelial tube.

Rete mirabile is an *additional capillary bed* which is *inserted* in the arterial or venous segment of a partial circuit. The total of all capillary loops of the renal corpuscles is the arterial rete mirabile; the liver possesses a venous rete mirabile.

While the *diameter* of the individual vessels regularly decreases from arteries to capillaries, the *total cross-section* of the vessels increases by continual branching from about 4.5 cm^2 (main aorta) to about 4500 cm^2 (capillaries, which, of course, are not all carrying blood at the same time). The greatest increase in total cross-section takes place at the transition from arterioles to capillaries. At the same time, the *blood pressure* in this region undergoes the strongest decrease, from about 85 mmHg to about 15 mmHg. The *circulation of blood* is strongly retarded.

c) Veins

Veins (Fig. **19h, i**), as a rule, have a thinner wall than corresponding arteries, and this is adequate for the lower blood pressure in the venous segment. In the wall of veins, smooth muscle tissue produces a venous tone; elastic networks, on the other hand, play a lesser role. The layers of the vessel wall are not clearly delimited. The tunica media is often weakly developed, whereas the tunica adventitia exhibits strong tracts of longitudinal muscle. Moreover, the structure of the wall of veins is largely determined by the different hemodynamic relations in the individual parts of the body, veins in the lower segments of the body possessing more muscular tissue (higher internal pressure) than those of the upper body parts; veins which do not undergo caliber fluctuations owing to the nature of their incorporation (e.g. veins in the liver) have a weakly developed wall.

Venous valves, muscle pumps and (perhaps also to a small degree) *arteriovenous coupling* play a role in the *transport of venous blood back to the heart* – in addition to other, locally determined factors.

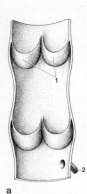 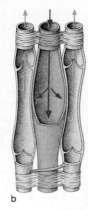

Fig. 20. **Venous valves and arteriovenous coupling**
a Vein, longitudinally sectioned and opened
b Two companion veins flank an artery, the pulse wave of which compresses the venous lumina. The lower venous valve is closed, the upper remains open so that venous blood is moved toward the heart
1 Pouch-shaped venous valves
2 Opening of smaller vein

a   b

Venous flaps are pocket-shaped folds of the intima which act like a valve (Fig. **20**). The openings of the pockets are directed toward the heart. They release the blood stream toward the heart, but, by unfolding, hinder the back flow. Venous flaps occur in all small and medium-sized veins except the veins of the head, vertebral canal and most of the viscera.

The valvular function of the venous flaps requires an adequate *tonicity* of the venous wall. If this is absent, the cross section of the vein increases, and the venous flap becomes insufficient. A venous reflux develops, which additionally strains and expands the venous wall and leads to the formation of varicose veins (*varices*).

Muscle pumps are defined as the action of pressure which muscles of the locomotor apparatus exert on veins by contraction. The muscle pump produces a displacement of the blood, which is directed toward the heart by the venous flaps. The incorporation of vessels into fissures and gaps of the muscle apparatus promotes this process; bodily movement increases the return of venous blood to the heart. Deep-lying veins of the locomotor apparatus are more exposed to muscle pumps than cutaneous veins, where a backward damming-up of venous blood, therefore, occurs sooner. (The backward damming-up facilitates the localization of cutaneous veins for injections).

Arteriovenous coupling. The small and medium-sized veins, which travel with the arteries – usually doubled – as accompanying veins (Fig. **20b**), are attached to the arteries by adventitial connective tissue (perivascular sheaths). It is assumed that the pulse wave from the artery can compress the lumina of the veins through this arteriovenous coupling and thus move the blood column. The efficiency of this mechanism, however, is not undisputed.

Venules (Fig. **19g**) are the smallest veins which receive blood from the capillary bed. The diameter of venules is only slightly larger than that of capillaries, yet the endothelial tube of venules is surrounded by smooth muscle cells – at first isolated – which can exert a sphincter action.

Throttle veins occur shortly after a capillary region and are microscopically small. Their walls contain thick ring-shaped or longitudinally-directed tracts of smooth muscle, whose contraction causes blood to dam up in the connected capillary bed. Throttle veins are found in endocrine glands, in the nasal mucosa and in the sex organs.

Venous collateral routes are more numerous and essentially more variable than arterial collaterals. Peripheral veins frequently form *venous networks* and *venous plexuses*.

Venous collateral pathways exist in the trunk wall, at the neck and in the limbs in the form of deep veins accompanying the arteries and superficial cutaneous veins that do not usually follow the course of the arteries; both routes are united with one another by anastomoses. As a rule, the interruption of a vein does not affect the venous drainage of a region.

Venous sinuses, in general colloquial usage, are microscopically small, widened vascular spaces in the *venous* segment of the circulation (e.g. in the suprarenal medulla). **Sinusoids** are enlarged *capillary spaces* (e.g. in the liver lobules). In the region of the *skull* there are macroscopically visible, rigid blood conduits which are enclosed by the firm dura mater; they are known as *venous sinuses of the dura mater*.

d) Lymphatic Vessels and Lymph Nodes

Lymphatic vessels arise from peripheral, capillary, *lymphatic networks* which are fed by *lymphatic capillaries*. These begin "blind" in the connective tissue of organs, i.e. without permanent communication with the intercellular spaces. *Lymph* and *intercellular tissue fluids* are constituted differently. The wall of lymphatic capillaries and networks consists of a low endothelium.

Lymphatic vessels are as fine as hair. Some accompany the deep arteries and veins of the locomotor apparatus and organs; others course superficially in the subcutaneous connective tissue, whereby they follow approximately the course of the cutaneous veins. Numerous connections are present between the superficial and deep lymphatic vessels.

The lymphatic vessels carry lymph *toward the heart* into the venous blood. The larger *lymphatic tracts* which run parallel and are scarcely branched ultimately empty into the *venous angle* (confluence of subclavian and internal jugular veins) on each side by means of collecting trunks (*thoracic duct* and the *lymphatic trunk*). Accordingly, lymphatic vessels are *parallel pathways to the venous segment* of the circulation.

In an inflammation of the lymphatic tracts in the subcutaneous connective tissue, these become visible through the skin as red stripes (lymphangitis, in the vernacular, "blood poisoning"). The pertinent (regional) lymph nodes are usually also painfully enlarged.

The **wall of lymphatic vessels** consists of an endothelial tube surrounded by a thin layer of smooth muscle cell bundles. The wall structures of larger lymphatic trunks are somewhat like the thinner veins. On account of their thin wall, lymphatic vessels are difficult to dissect. They are composed of valvular segments, portions of a vessel only a few millimeters to centimeters long. A pocket flap lies at the thick origin of a valve segment, thus causing the lymph vessels to resemble a string of beads (Fig. 21).

Lymph vessels possess their own pump. By contraction of the valvular segments, the lymph is pushed toward the heart from segment to segment.

Lymph nodes. Several lymph node stations are frequently inserted in series in the course of lymphatic vessels (Fig. 21), and act as biological filters, through which the lymph, on its route from the periphery, must pass. These stations consist of one or several lymph nodes which are variable in size, usually some millimeters.

The *lymph nodes* (Fig. 22) are generally bean-shaped and possess a *hilum* at which blood vessels enter and leave. The lymph node is enclosed by a *connective tissue capsule* and in its interior contains sponge-like, reticular connective tissue. In these meshes, massive numbers of *lymphocytes* are deposited, which are congregated in *nodules,* circular-shaped under the capsule and cord-like in the center and toward the hilum. Beneath the capsule a *marginal sinus* remains largely free of lymphocytes. The capsule is penetrated by numerous *afferent lymphatic vessels*, which bring lymph into the marginal sinus. The lymph then travels through *intermediate* and *medullary sinuses* before entering a few *efferent lymphatic vessels* which leave the lymph node at the hilum. The lymph nodes are thus places where lymph tracts converge and are united into larger lymph tracts.

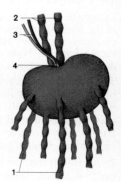

Fig. 21. **Lymph nodes**
1 Afferent lymphatic vessels
2 Efferent lymphatic vessels
3 Blood vessels
4 Hilum of lymph node

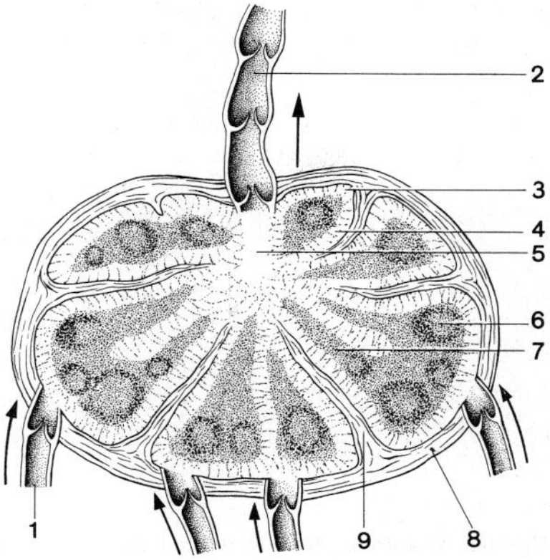

Fig. 22. Section through lymph node
Arrows indicate direction of lymph flow
1 Afferent lymphatic vessel
2 Efferent lymphatic vessel with pouched valves
3 Subcapsular (marginal) sinus
4 Perinodular, cortical (intermediate) sinus
5 Medullary sinus
6 Lymphatic nodule
7 Medullary cord
8 Connective tissue capsule
9 Connective tissue trabecula (septum)

In the lymph nodes, the lymph delivers foreign particles (e.g. bacteria) to phagocytes and, at the same time, picks up lymphocytes which ultimately reach the venous blood. Lymph nodes are *organs of the specific defense system* for the organism (→ Specific Defense System, p. 77).

Regional lymph nodes (Fig. 23) are the *first* to receive lymph from a body region or an organ. An organ or a region can give off lymph to several regional lymph nodes lying at different places, and a lymph node can receive lymph from several organs. Thus, "regional lymph nodes" can serve several organs or regions. The relationship of regional lymph nodes to organs or regions is very constant; it scarcely varies.

In the spread of an infection by lymph tracts, or colonization of a malignant tumor, the regional lymph nodes are the first to be attacked. Knowledge of their position and areas of drainage is therefore extremely important for the evaluation of such diseases.

Collecting lymph nodes (Fig. 23) are the lymph nodes inserted *after* the regional lymph nodes; they receive lymph from several regional nodes. As a result, plexuses of lymphatic vessel arise in the region of the collecting lymph nodes shortly before they drain into the central lymphatic trunks.

2. Structural Principles of the Circulatory System

Peripheral pathways of conduction are the *blood vessels* and *nerves* on their way between their central organ (heart and central nervous system) and the "peripheral" organs, referred to as the target organs of the vessels and nerves. The peripheral conduction paths are branched in a typical, but variable way. The branches arising from the progressive ramifications are given special *names* which, as a rule, indicate the target organs.

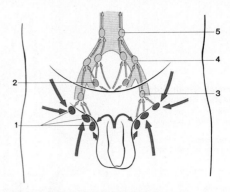

Fig. 23. Regional lymph nodes and collecting lymph nodes
Arrows indicate direction of flow of lymph

1,2 Regional lymph nodes
1 Superficial inguinal lymph nodes in groin (Drainage area: skin caudal to navel, external genitalia, anus)
2 Internal iliac lymph nodes at internal iliac artery (Drainage area: pelvic organs)
3–5 Collecting lymph nodes

3 Deep inguinal lymph nodes at femoral artery and external iliac lymph nodes at external iliac artery
4 Common iliac lymph nodes at common iliac artery
5 Lumbar lymph nodes at aorta and inferior vena cava

Examples: the *common carotid artery* divides into the *external* carotid (which branches chiefly *outside* of the cranial cavity) and *internal* carotid (which branches *inside* of the cranial cavity) arteries. The external carotid artery branches into the *maxillary* (in the region of the *maxilla*) and *temporal* (in the *temporal* region) arteries. The temporal artery gives off a *frontal* branch (to the *front* of the temporal region) and a *parietal* branch (to the *back* of the temporal region), etc.

In the course of *dissection*, the (larger) peripheral conduction paths are revealed by dissecting away the surrounding connective tissue.

Within the target organ, the conduction paths support the functioning of the organ; they become part of the organ structure. Thus, for example, the vascular structures of the liver, kidney, and spleen are so organ-specific that these organs can already be identified merely by their vascular organization, both macroscopically (in injection preparations, in which the vessels are filled with a coagulated mass, or in a radiological vascular demonstration) and microscopically. Organ-specific vessels and nerves are no longer regarded as peripheral conduction paths in the true sense; they are discussed with the structure of the individual organs.

Neurovascular pathways. Vessels and nerves can be damaged by compression, overstretching, torsion, shearing movements – especially in the vicinity of joints – and, therefore, need to be protected. In the peripheral conduction pathways, they usually course together in connective tissue spaces (*neurovascular pathways*) which, owing to their incorporation (e.g. in muscle and fascial recesses, bony canals) provide protection to the vessels and nerves against mechanical damage.

Neurovascular pathways are especially pronounced in the limbs and in the neck. In the limbs they frequently can be followed up to their entrance into the *neurovascular areas* of the muscles.

The *connective tissue* of the neurovascular pathways surrounds the peripheral conduction paths in some places with a dense connective tissue sheath – especially conspicuous in the neck. In these cases the conduction path bundle as a whole is displaceable into the surrounding looser connective tissue.

The neurovascular pathways can spread inflammation (cellulitis) over great distances.

The *neurovascular pathways* usually cross over joints on the flexion side. They always cross in such a way, however, that they are not exposed to any stretching during movement at the joints, which would cause the vessels to occlude and the nerves to overstretch. In joints that can be flexed at acute angles (e.g. knee joint), the conduction pathways are incorporated into a deformable body of fat which, in the case of flexion, is drawn out of the danger zone together with the conduction pathways by the elastic shortening of the arteries.

In *searching* for neurovascular pathways, attention should be directed to the fascial and muscular compartments, muscle gaps and skeletal elements. If neurovascular pathways are attached to muscle for a long distance, the muscle is termed a *conducting muscle*.

Particular consideration should be given to segments in proximity to bone. The conduction paths are endangered by fractures at these sites. During operations, organs are displaced toward the side of the conduction paths in order to protect them.

Subfascial conduction tracts course principally in the neurovascular pathways. Epifascial vessels and nerves, on the other hand, do not usually follow distinctly marked neurovascular pathways, although cutaneous nerves and veins commonly course together in the subcutaneous connective tissue. The small cutaneous arteries, however, usually have no connection with these.

In body segments which are *slightly flexible* or rigid (e.g. thoracic, abdominal and pelvic cavities or head), the connective-tissue conduction tracts are extensive and broad. Yet, cord-shaped neurovascular pathways can also be formed here in adaptation to an anatomical reality, e.g. at the openings of the cranial base or the pelvic wall.

In the case of *movable* (displaceable) inner organs of the abdominal and pelvic cavities, the conduction tracts are arranged in a cord-like manner, and enter or leave at circumscribed places (in the hilum of the organ). The conduction path cord in these cases lies (generally) in the axis, around which a rotary movement of the organ can take place.

Since the attention of the physician is frequently directed to the entire neurovascular bundle of a body part, the sections on the individual body regions will refer, as far as possible, to the neurovascular routes and neurovascular layers common to the conduction tracts.

The *large vascular trunks of the body*, except the superior vena cava, rest upon the *vertebral column*. Since the *chief lymphatic trunk* and the *large nerve trunks of the spinal cord*, the spinal nerves coming from the vertebral canal, also course in the connective tissue space in front of and beside the vertebral column, the latter becomes the large *central neurovascular route of the body*.

B. Structural Plan of the Circulatory System

1. Prenatal Circulation

In the *circulation before birth* (**prenatal circulation**), gaseous exchange, as well as the exchange of nutrients, metabolic wastes, etc., takes place in the *placenta*. The vessels of the embryonic and fetal placenta are inserted into the *systemic circulation* as a partial circulation, whereas the pulmonary circulation is largely functionless since the lungs do not respire.

Fetal circulation (Fig. 24). The oxygenated blood in the *placenta* flows into the (originally left) *umbilical vein* below the liver. The smaller part of the blood is conducted through the liver; the larger portion, however, is carried over a short (*first*) *shunt*, the *ductus venosus*, along the under-surface of the liver into the strongly de-oxygenated blood of the inferior vena cava. The (mixed) blood arrives at the right atrium. From here it is transported – by a ridge-like flap at the opening of the inferior vena cava – over a (*second*) *valve-like short shunt* in the atrial septum (*foramen ovale*) into the left atrium and the left ventricle. Part of the blood flows back into the fetal body via the aorta, part into the *placenta* via two *umbilical arteries*. The de-oxygenated blood flowing into the right ventricle from the head, neck and arms via the superior vena cava crosses in front of the blood stream coming into the right ventricle from the inferior vena cava, then flows via the pulmonary trunk and a (*third*) *shunt* (*ductus arteriosus*) into the aorta; the lungs are only slightly supplied with blood.

The liver receives the most oxygen-rich blood. The blood is richer in oxygen before the opening of the ductus arteriosus into the aorta than after it. The head and upper limbs are better supplied with oxygen than the lower half of the body.

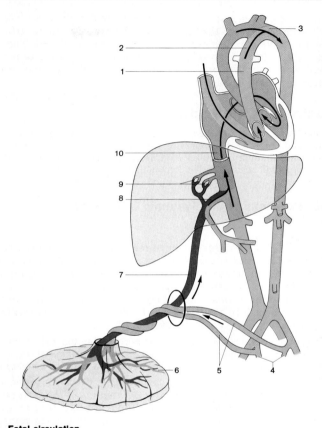

Fig. 24. Fetal circulation

1 Pulmonary trunk	6 Placenta
2 Ductus arteriosus	7 Umbilical vein
3 Aorta	8 Ductus venosus
4 Internal iliac artery	9 Hepatic vessels
5 Umbilical arteries	10 Inferior vena cava

The conversion from prenatal to postnatal circulation takes place immediately after birth. Through the closure of the umbilical vessels (contraction of their wall, ligation of the umbilical cord), the blood pressure rises in the aorta concomitant with an increase in the CO_2 partial pressure in the blood. This stimulates the respiratory center in the brain and initiates pulmonary respiration. In the process, the lungs expand, and the resistance in the pulmonary circulation diminishes. Owing to the pressure gradient, the blood entering the pulmonary circulation is increased. The blood flowing back from the lungs raises the pressure in the left atrium, whereby the valve-like foramen ovale is mechanically closed. The ductus venosus and ductus arteriosus are closed mainly by contraction of their muscular walls. In this way the flow relationships of the postnatal circulation are established.

2. Postnatal Circulation

In the following a *synopsis* of the large arterial and venous trunks of the systemic circulation and their direct branches or tributaries, as well as the large vascular trunks of the pulmonary circulation is presented. Their spatial relations and further divisions will be discussed in conjunction with the individual regions of the body.

a) Arterial Trunks of the Systemic Circulation

Aorta

The **aorta** (Fig. 25), the *large artery of the body*, carries blood directly or indirectly to all arteries of the systemic circulation. It originates from the *left ventricle*, passing first upwards to the right as the *ascending aorta* until it reaches the level of the sternal angle where it forms an arch (*arch of the aorta*) over the bifurcation of the pulmonary trunk and the root of the left lung. It then proceeds in a roughly sagittal direction backwards along the left side of the vertebral column (level of 4th thoracic vertebra).

In the distal segment of the arch of the aorta, after the exit of the direct branches, the aorta can be constricted slightly (*isthmus of the aorta*); a severe constriction or a closure (*isthmic stenosis*) can appear here as a malformation.

Thereafter, the aorta courses as the *descending aorta* down to the level of the 4th lumbar vertebra where it divides (*bifurcation of the aorta*) into the two common iliac arteries. Its stunted, caudal continuation proceeds to the coccyx as the *median sacral artery*. The descending aorta comprises a thoracic part (*thoracic aorta*) and an abdominal part (*abdominal aorta*); their boundary lies at the site of the aorta's penetration through the diaphragm.

The *direct branches* of the aorta can be arranged into *three groups* on the basis of their origin: one group arises partly from the *arteries of the pharyngeal arches*, another from the embryonic *segmental arteries* and a third from the embryonic *visceral arteries*.

Branches of the Ascending Aorta

The *direct branches of the ascending aorta* (visceral branches) are the **right** and **left coronary arteries**. They arise from the base of the aorta and supply the heart (as private arteries).

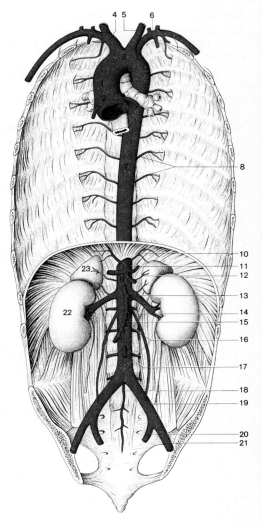

Fig. 25. **Direct branches of aorta**

1 Ascending aorta
2 *Branches of ascending aorta*
   Coronary arteries
3 Arch of aorta
4–6 *Branches of arch of aorta*
4 Brachiocephalic trunk (divides into right common carotid and right subclavian arteries)
5 Left common carotid artery
6 Left subclavian artery
7 Thoracic aorta
8 *Branches of thoracic aorta*
   Posterior intercostal arteries
9 Abdominal aorta
10–19 *Branches of abdominal aorta*
10 Inferior phrenic artery with superior suprarenal artery
11 Celiac trunk with left gastric, common hepatic and splenic (lienal) arteries
12 Middle suprarenal artery
13 Renal artery with inferior suprarenal artery
14 Testicular (ovarian) artery
15 Superior mesenteric artery
16 Lumbar arteries
17 Inferior mesenteric artery
18 Median sacral artery
19 Common iliac artery
20 Internal iliac artery
21 External iliac artery
22 Kidney
23 Suprarenal

Branches of the Arch of the Aorta

The *direct branches of the arch of the aorta*, which originates from the artery of the 4th left pharyngeal arch, are derivatives of pharyngeal arch arteries.

The **brachiocephalic trunk** divides behind the right medial clavicular joint into the *right common carotid artery* (for the right half of the head and neck) and into the *right subclavian artery* (for the right side of the neck, right shoulder and right arm)

The **thyroidea ima artery**, an unpaired artery with branches to the thyroid gland, thymus and trachea, occurs in about 10% of cases. It arises from the arch of the aorta or the brachiocephalic trunk.

The **left common carotid artery** supplies the left half of the neck and head.

The **left subclavian artery** branches to the left side of the neck, left shoulder and left arm.

Branches of the Descending Aorta

The *direct branches of the descending aorta* arise from the embryonic segmental and visceral arteries. The branches can be divided into the following three groups (Fig. **26**):

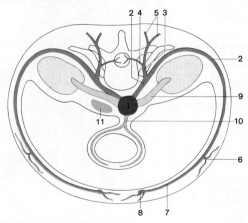

Fig. 26. **Direct branches of descending aorta**
1 Aorta
2 *Branch to trunk wall* (posterior intercostal artery)
3–6 Branches of posterior intercostal artery
3 Dorsal branch
4 Spinal branch
5 Medial cutaneous and ⎫
   lateral cutaneous branches ⎬ of dorsal ramus
6 Lateral cutaneous branch ⎭

7 Anterior intercostal branch, anastomoses with posterior intercostal artery
8 Internal thoracic artery
9 *Paired visceral branch* (renal artery)
10 *Unpaired visceral branch* (superior mesenteric artery)
11 Inferior vena cava

– *Trunk wall branches* (parietal branches) which arise from the aorta dorsally in a paired segmental arrangement,
– *Visceral branches* for viscera which develop in pairs. They arise laterally from the aorta in pairs, but without relation to the segments of the body wall,
– *Visceral branches* for viscera which develop unpaired from the anlage of the gastro-intestinal tract. They arise ventrally from the aorta unpaired and non-segmental.

Trunk Wall Branches of the Thoracic Aorta

The **posterior intercostal arteries** III – XI and the **subcostal artery** course in the corresponding segments of the trunk wall.

The **superior phrenic artery** passes from the thoracic cavity into the lumbar part of the diaphragm.

Visceral Branches of the Thoracic Aorta

Bronchial branches supply the wall of the bronchi, **esophageal branches**, the esophagus.

Pericardial branches for the pericardium and **mediastinal branches** for the posterior mediastinum are variably developed.

Trunk Wall Branches of the Abdominal Aorta

The **inferior phrenic artery** passes from below the diaphragm and gives off a branch to the suprarenal.

The **lumbar arteries**, four segmental arteries in the lumbar region corresponding to the intercostal arteries, supply, like the latter, the trunk wall. The fifth segmental artery arises from the median sacral artery as the *lumbar ima artery*.

The **common iliac artery** originates at the level of the 4th lumbar vertebra from the bifurcation of the aorta. It divides in front of the sacro-iliac joint into the *internal iliac artery*, which supplies the pelvic viscera and wall, and the *external iliac artery*, which gives off further branches to the anterior trunk wall before it passes beneath the inguinal ligament as the *femoral artery*.

The **median sacral artery** continues the course of the aorta as a thin artery on the middle of the anterior side of the sacrum.

Paired Visceral Branches of the Abdominal Aorta

The **middle suprarenal artery** passes to the suprarenal gland.

The **renal artery**, the largest lateral paired branch, arises almost at a right angle from the aorta at about the level of the 1st lumbar vertebra. It supplies the kidney and gives a branch to the suprarenal.

The **testicular (ovarian) artery** leaves the aorta below the exit of the renal artery and courses to the testis (ovary).

Unpaired Visceral Branches of the Abdominal Aorta

The **celiac trunk**, the first unpaired, ventral visceral artery of the abdominal aorta, arises in the area where the aorta penetrates the diaphragm. Its main branches (*left gastric, common hepatic* and *splenic arteries*) supply blood to the stomach, liver and spleen.

The **superior mesenteric artery**, the second unpaired, ventral visceral artery of the abdominal aorta, leaves the latter immediately below the celiac trunk and supplies the small and large intestines nearly to the left colic flexure.

The **inferior mesenteric artery**, the third unpaired, ventral visceral artery of the abdominal aorta, originates in the lower lumbar region and passes to the rest of the large intestine.

b) Venous Trunks of the Systemic Circulation

The blood from the systemic circulation flows via the *superior* and *inferior venae cavae* into the *right atrium* of the heart – only the blood from the heart wall is conveyed directly into the right atrium (coronary sinus). The venae cavae receive tributaries from the head, neck, limbs and viscera. Blood from the trunk wall (from the area of distribution of the paired segmental arteries of the trunk) is added to the venae cavae via two large longitudinal anastomoses (*azygos* and *hemiazygos veins*).

Superior Vena Cava

The **superior vena cava** (Figs. **27** and **28**) is 5–6 cm long and lies in the thoracic cavity behind the sternum, to the right beside the ascending aorta. At about the level of the 1st intercostal space, it arises from its two venous roots and receives the *azygos vein* as a *direct tributary*.

Left and **right brachiocephalic veins** form the two large venous roots of the superior vena cava. Since these lie to the right of the median plane, the left brachiocephalic vein is longer than the right. Each brachiocephalic vein arises through the confluence of the *internal jugular* and *subclavian veins*, which thereby form the venous angle. The internal jugular vein carries blood from the head and neck, the subclavian vein from the shoulder and arm. At each venous angle a large *lymphatic trunk* opens into the venous system, the long *thoracic duct* on the left, the very short *right lymphatic duct* on the right.

The **azygos vein** crosses the root of the right lung from dorsal to ventral and opens into the superior vena cava.

Inferior Vena Cava

The **inferior vena cava** (Figs. **27** and **28**) arises from its two venous roots at the level of the 5th lumbar vertebra. It passes cranialwards to the right in front of the vertebral column – and thus to the right of the aorta, indents the posterior surface of the liver and passes through the central tendon of the diaphragm into the right atrium of the heart. *Direct tributaries* of the inferior vena cava come from the trunk wall, as well as from the abdominal and pelvic viscera.

Right and **left common iliac veins** form the two large roots of the inferior vena cava. The confluence takes place to the right of the aortic bifurcation, whereby the left common iliac vein crosses the right common iliac artery dorsally.

Trunk Wall Tributaries of the Inferior Vena Cava

The **median sacral vein**, located in front of the sacrum, opens into the left common iliac vein or (less often) into the confluence of both common iliac veins.

Lumbar veins III and **IV** usually enter the inferior vena cava directly, whereas lumbar veins I and II empty into the *ascending lumbar vein*, and V into the *common iliac vein*.

The **inferior phrenic veins** collect blood from the abdominal surface of the diaphragm.

Paired Visceral Tributaries of the Inferior Vena Cava

The **renal veins**, coming from the kidney, open on both sides at about the level of the 1st lumbar vertebra. The left vein is longer than the right and usually crosses to the right, ventral to the aorta, into the inferior vena cava.

The **right testicular (ovarian) vein** from the right gonad empties into the inferior vena cava somewhat below the right renal vein, whereas the *left* vein opens into the renal vein.

The **right suprarenal vein**, the only vein of the right suprarenal gland, opens directly into the inferior vena cava. The *left suprarenal vein*, on the other hand, empties into the left renal vein.

Unpaired Visceral Tributaries of the Inferior Vena Cava

Three (or more) *liver veins* (**hepatic veins**) conduct the blood supplied to the liver – mainly by the portal vein – into the inferior vena cava. After a short course in the liver parenchyma, they open directly below the diaphragm.

The **portal vein** brings blood to the liver from the unpaired abdominal organs via three large venous roots: the *splenic vein* from the spleen, the *inferior mesenteric*

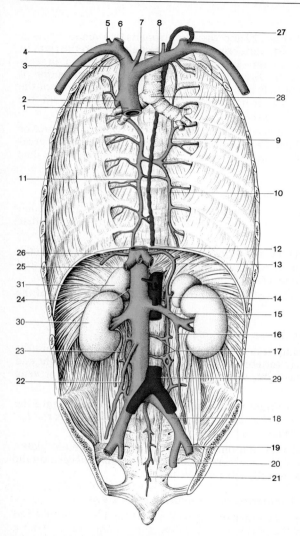

Fig. 27. **Venous trunks and their tributaries**

◀ 1 *Superior vena cava*   ▶
  2–11 Direct and indirect tributaries of superior
       vena cava
  2 Opening part of azygos vein
  3 Right brachiocephalic vein
  4 Right subclavian vein
  5 Right external jugular vein
  6 Right internal jugular vein
  7 Inferior thyroid vein
  8 Left brachiocephalic vein
  9 Accessory hemiazygos vein with posterior
    intercostal veins
  10 Hemiazygos vein with posterior intercostal
     veins
  11 Azygos vein with posterior intercostal veins
  11, 23 *Collateral venous pathways between
         superior and inferior venae cavae*
  12 *Inferior vena cava*
  13–26 Direct and indirect tributaries of inferior
        vena cava
  13 Left inferior phrenic vein
  14 Left suprarenal vein
  15 Left renal vein
  16 Left testicular (ovarian) vein
  17 Left lumbar veins
  18 Left common iliac vein
  19 Left external iliac vein
  20 Left internal iliac vein
  21 Median sacral vein
  22 Right testicular (ovarian) vein
  23 Right ascending lumbar vein
  24 Right suprarenal vein
  25 Hepatic veins
  26 Right inferior phrenic vein
  27 Arch of thoracic duct opening into
     venous angle
  28 Tracheal bifurcation
  29 Aortic bifurcation
  30 Kidney
  31 Suprarenal

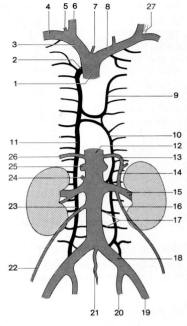

Fig. 28. **Venous trunks and their tributaries**

vein, which generally opens into the splenic vein, from the large intestine downward from the left colonic flexure, and the *superior mesenteric vein* from the small and the large intestines up to the left colonic flexure. Further tributaries of the portal vein come from the stomach and the gallbladder.

Azygos and Hemiazygos Veins

The **azygos** and **hemiazygos veins** (Figs. **27** and **28**), two veins about the size of a pencil running along the anterolateral surface of the vertebral column, begin on both sides of the lumbar region as **ascending lumbar veins**. These communicate with the *common iliac vein*, the venous root of the inferior vena cava. After penetrating the lumbar origin of the diaphragm, the *right* ascending lumbar vein becomes the *azygos vein*, the left, the *hemiazygos vein*. The hemiazygos vein crosses to the right behind the aorta, usually at the level of thoracic vertebrae 7–9, and opens into the *azygos vein*. The latter, after passing ventralward over the hilum of the right lung, finally opens into the superior vena cava. The original direction of the hemiazygos vein is continued cranialward by the **accessory hemiazygos vein**, which often establishes contact with the left brachiocephalic vein. The azygos and hemiazygos veins thus form a collateral pathway between the superior and inferior venae cavae.

Direct tributaries are received by the azygos and hemiazygos veins from the trunk wall and from the thoracic viscera.

Trunk Wall Tributaries of the Azygos and Hemiazygos Veins

Lumber veins I and **II** open into the ascending lumbar vein below the diaphragm.

The **posterior intercostal veins** come from the intercostal spaces.

Visceral Tributaries of the Azygos and Hemiazygos Veins

Esophageal branches carry blood from the esophagus, **bronchial branches** from the main bronchi and from the region of the hilum of the lung.

c) Arterial Trunks of Pulmonary Circulation

Pulmonary Trunk

The **pulmonary trunk** arises from the right ventricle and ascends in front of the ascending aorta to the left below the arch of the aorta; here it divides into the two pulmonary arteries (Fig. **18**).

The **right pulmonary artery** passes behind the ascending aorta at approximately a right angle to the right lung.

The **left pulmonary artery**, at first following the course of the pulmonary trunk, arrives at the left lung in front of the descending aorta. The *ligamentum arteriosum*, the connective tissue remains of the fetal *ductus arteriosus*, passes from the place of division of the pulmonary trunk (or the beginning of the left pulmonary artery) to the lower surface of the arch of the aorta.

d) Venous Trunks of Pulmonary Circulation

Pulmonary Veins

The **pulmonary veins**, usually two on each side, go from the hilum of the lungs to the left atrium of the heart (Fig. **18**).

e) Lymphatic Trunks of Systemic Circulation

Thoracic Duct

The **thoracic duct** (Fig. **29**) is the largest lymphatic trunk and about as thick as a pencil. It frequently begins with a dilatation (*cisterna chyli*) which lies in front of the vertebral column and behind the aorta at about the level of the 1st lumbar vertebra. The thoracic duct opens into the left venous angle with its arch (*arch of the thoracic duct*). A valve prevents here the reflux of blood into the thoracic duct.

The thoracic duct is frequently doubled here and there, more rarely multi-developed. When doubled in its entire length, the right trunk opens into the right venous angle. The cisterna chyli is variable, frequently incompletely shaped.

Direct tributaries enter the thoracic duct from the lower half of the body and from the left side of the upper half of the body (head, neck, body wall, as well as thoracic viscera).

The **right** and **left lumbar trunks**, which follow the course of the common iliac artery and vein and the aorta, carry lymph from the leg and pelvis to the cisterna chyli or to the thoracic duct.

The **intestinal trunk** brings lymph from the supply region of the superior

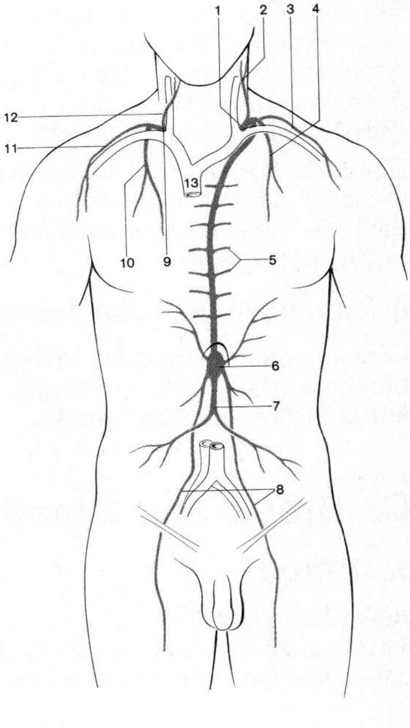

Fig. 29. Lymphatic trunks and their tributaries
1 *Thoracic duct* (opening of arch of thoracic duct into left venous angle)
2 Left jugular trunk
3 Left subclavian trunk
4 Left bronchomediastinal trunk
5 Intercostal lymphatic vessels
6 Cisterna chyli
7 Intestinal trunk
8 Lumbar trunks
9 *Right lymphatic duct* (opening into right venous angle)
10 Right bronchomediastinal trunk
11 Right subclavian trunk
12 Right jugular trunk
13 Superior vena cava

and inferior mesenteric arteries; it is (generally) an unpaired visceral tributary of the cisterna chyli.

Intercostal lymphatic vessels travel from the intercostal spaces to the thoracic duct.

Shortly before opening into the left venous angle, the *thoracic duct* receives the following lymphatic trunks from the upper half of the body, which can frequently also empty directly into the venous angle:

The **left jugular trunk** carries lymph from the left side of the head and neck; it courses with the internal jugular vein.

The **left bronchomediastinal trunk**, situated in the thoracic cavity near the vertebral column, transports lymph from the left (and right) lung, from the left half of the mediastinum and from the left thoracic wall.

The **left subclavian trunk** carries lymph from the left arm; it courses with the subclavian vein.

Right Lymphatic duct

The **right lymphatic duct** (Fig. 29), a short trunk hardly 1 cm long, carries lymph from an upper segment of the liver and from the right side of the upper half of the body – from the thoracic viscera, thoracic wall and mediastinum, arm, neck and head – to the right venous angle.

The *direct tributaries* of the right lymphatic duct – a recessively-formed *right lymphatic duct* due to the asymmetrical development of the human lymphatic vascular system – corresponds to those of the thoracic duct from the upper body half; they can also open directly into the right venous angle or into the right subclavian vein.

The *right jugular trunk* comes from the right side of the head and neck, the *right subclavian trunk* from the right arm,
the *right bronchomediastinal trunk* from the right lung and the right half of the mediastinum.

f) Lymphatic Vascular Trunks of the Pulmonary Circulation

Direct lymphatic vascular trunks of the pulmonary circulation pass from the lungs through the hilum and the pulmonary ligament to the **right** and **left bronchomediastinal trunks**.

C. Blood and Blood Cell Formation

1. Blood

Blood has multiple functions. It transports *oxygen, nutrients, metabolic wastes, carbon dioxide, heat, hormones, antibodies* and *defense cells*. It is concerned with the maintenance of the *internal milieu* of tissues.

Formed and unformed constituents of blood. The total circulating blood has a volume of about 5.61 (about 8% of the body weight). About *56% of the blood volume* constitutes the fluid, *unformed part* (*plasma*), which consists of over 90% water and 7–8% plasma proteins. In the plasma, among others, salts, nutrients, hormones, defense substances, and to a lesser degree also respiratory gases are transported. Blood plasma is coagulable. The remaining *44% of the blood volume* is occupied by *formed elements* – red and white blood corpuscles, as well as platelets.

a) Red Blood Corpuscles

The *red blood corpuscles* (**erythrocytes**) are equipped to transport *respiratory gas* because of their red blood pigment (*hemoglobin*); they fulfill their function *within* the blood vessels in the circulating blood. Over 90% of the dry substance consists of hemoglobin. Erythrocytes have a life span of about 3 months.

Reticulocytes are incompletely matured erythrocytes that still exhibit a slight content of basically-stained ribosomes. In normal blood, about 5–15% of the red blood corpuscles are reticulocytes. A substantial increase in the reticulocyte count indicates the expulsion of immature cells in an emergency situation, e.g. after blood loss.

b) White Blood Cells

The *white blood cells* (**leukocytes**) are representatives of the defense system. They perform their function mainly in the connective tissue *outside* of the blood vessels. The leukocytes in circulating blood are, for the most part, on the way from their place of formation to their place of action; they circulate "on call". Leukocytes are classified as *granulocytes*, *monocytes* and *lymphocytes*.

The **granulocytes** are subdivided on the basis of the different staining characteristics of their granules into *neutrophilic*, *eosinophilic* and *basophilic* granulocytes. They have different functions, but all undergo ameboid movement.

The **neutrophilic granulocytes**, *phagocytes*, are representatives of the nonspecific defense system; they *phagocytize* small particles, e.g. bacteria (→ nonspecific defense system, p. 77), which have invaded the body.

The **eosinophilic granulocytes,** likewise *phagocytes*, are specialized in the phagocytosis and destruction of products from the *specific defense system*; they are said to be able to inactivate histamine and thus are antagonists of the mast cells of connective tissue.

The **basophilic granulocytes** form *heparin*, which counteracts blood clotting and, on suitable stimulus, releases histamine. They are not considered to be phagocytic.

The **monocytes** (*blood macrophages*) – ameboid, motile cells – are involved in an activated form in the *nonspecific* and in the *specific defense systems* (→ p. 77).

The cells appearing in connective tissue as *histiocytes* (*tissue macrophages*) are activated monocytes. Also counted as macrophages are *Kupffer's stellate cells* of the liver capillaries and the *alveolar macrophages* of the lung, among others. The macrophages form the *mononuclear phagocyte system*, MPS (formerly also called *RES* or *RHS*).

The **lymphocytes** of the circulating blood are not a uniform cell population. They are cells of the *specific defense system* with distinct characters and with different potencies.

c) Blood Platelets

The **thrombocytes** are concerned with blood coagulation. When they decay, they release thrombokinase, an enzyme involved in coagulation.

d) Numerical Proportions

A mm^3 of blood contains *4.5–5 million erythrocytes* and *4000–8000 leukocytes*, as well as about *250,000 thrombocytes*. The *leukocytes* have a relatively constant numerical relationship to each other which is expressed in the differential blood count:

Granulocytes:	Neutrophils	55–68%
	Eosinophils	2.5– 3%
	Basophils	0.5– 1%
	Band cells (juvenile forms)	2– 3%
Monocytes		4– 5%
Lymphocytes		20–36%

Since the erythrocyte count depends on the oxygen requirements of the body and the oxygen supply, it can normally be raised by heavy bodily work or by staying at high altitudes for at least a week. A *pathological* increase in the erythrocyte count is called *polycythemia* and a decrease, *anemia*.

An increase (*leukocytosis*) or decrease (*leukopenia, agranulocytosis*) of the total leukocyte count and/or a change of percentile composition signals an alteration in the defense situation.

2. Formation of Blood Cells

Embryonic and *fetal blood cell formation* occurs in places other than the *postnatal* sites, where it is initiated only toward the end of fetal development. For simplicity, the term blood formation (hemopoiesis) is commonly used (instead of blood cell formation), and several *hemopoietic periods* are distinguished (Fig. **30**).

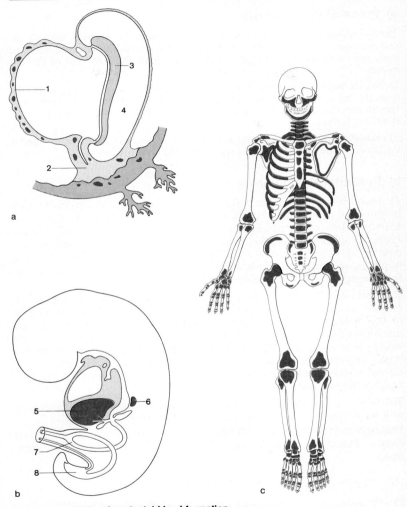

Fig. 30. **Prenatal and postnatal blood formation**
a Extra-embryonic blood formation (embryo, end of 3rd week, after *Starck*)
b Hepatosplenic blood formation (embryo, 6 weeks)
c Postnatal blood formation in adult (after *Rohr*)

1 Yolk sac	5 Liver
2 Connecting stalk	6 Spleen
3 Embryonic disc	7 Primary intestinal loop
4 Amniotic cavity	8 Cloaca

a) Prenatal Hemopoiesis

The *megaloblastic period* begins in the *embryonic connective tissue* of the yolk sac and allantois, then moves to the connective tissue of the embryo and leads to large, nucleated "erythrocytes" (*megaloblasts*). It lasts until about the end of the 2nd month.

During the **hepatosplenic period**, hemopoiesis occurs in the *liver* and *spleen* and lasts from the end of the 2nd to about the 8th fetal month (peaking at the beginning of the 4th month). Granulocytes and anucleated erythrocytes, finally also lymphocytes, are formed.

The **medullary period** occurs in the *bone marrow*. It begins in the 5th month and is continued as *postnatal myelopoiesis* (myeloid blood formation).

b) Postnatal Hemopoiesis

Postnatal hemopoiesis takes place in *red bone marrow* (*myelopoiesis*) which is contained at first in all bones. Toward the end of growth, however, red marrow is limited increasingly to the *short* and *flat* bones, as well as to the *epiphyses of long bones*, the remaining space being filled by yellow, fat-containing bone marrow (→ p. 21). Only the stem cells of *lymphocytes*, however, are formed in the bone marrow, the further lymphocyte derivatives being produced in the *lymphatic organs*.

Red and *white* blood cells, as well as *megakaryocytes*, from which *thrombocytes* are formed as (anuclear) fragments of the cell body, are developed in the bone marrow from homogeneous, pluripotential *stem cells*. By mitosis (differential cell division), precursor cells develop from them which are irreversibly unipotent and in each case initiate a developmental series (*erythropoiesis, granulopoiesis, monocytopoiesis, lymphopoiesis, thrombocytopoiesis*). The blood cells grow to maturity by way of "blasts" and additional intermediate forms.

The *lymphocytes* undergo additional transformations, however, in connection with the processes of *specific defense* after their formation.

Through mitotic poisons (cytostatic agents) and x-rays employed in cancer treatment, mitotically-active hemopoietic areas are also damaged.

D. Defense Systems of the Organism

White blood cells are the *vehicles for defensive action* of the organism directed toward pathogens and foreign substances entering from the outside, as well as toward genetic disturbances of cells from within. They carry out their function primarily in the *reticular* and in the *loose interstitial, connective tissue*.

1. Nonspecific Defense System

The cells of the *nonspecific defense system* render the infiltrated pathogens harmless by phagocytosis and intracellular, enzymatic destruction. Two cell types function in the nonspecific defense system: *neutrophilic granulocytes ("microphages")* and *macrophages*.

The *neutrophilic granulocytes*, "**microphages**" attracted by pathogens or cell debris, phagocytize particles that have infiltrated into the body or have been formed in it. During phagocytosis, granulocytes decay, giving rise to *pus corpuscles*. The enzymes released cause a softening of the inflammatory infiltrate (abscess).

The **macrophages** (connective tissue macrophages, exudate macrophages at the focus of inflammation, alveolar macrophages of the lung, Kupffer's stellate cells of the liver, histiocytic reticular cells in lymphatic organs), which derive from *monocytes*, phagocytize as mobile or sessile phagocytes. Some macrophages are then transported in the bloodstream to the lung alveoli, for example, where they are eliminated. Other macrophages – after phagocytizing antigenic particles which affect the specific defense system – can cooperate with T-lymphocytes in the *specific defense system*.

2. Specific Defense System

The *specific defense system* (*immune system*) is the *system of immunologically competent cells*. The immune system acts in a differentiated way, and its action requires an extended period. It enables the organism to distinguish between long-term substances of its own and certain foreign substances, the *antigens* (pathogens, foreign proteins and protein compounds), and to form defense substances (*antibodies*) against these. *Each antigen produces a specific (antigen-homologous) antibody*, which can be formed in the body for a long time, sometimes for decades, and which confers *immunity against the antigen*. The specific defense entails an *antigen-antibody reaction*, in which the antigen is chemically bound and made harmless. Proteins belonging to the body itself can also act as antigens if made "foreign" by external chemical action or by genetic defect; in this way the immune system exerts a *genetic control function*.

Cellular and humoral immunity. The specific defense system is developed in the 3rd–5th fetal month. It is localized *predominantly in the lymphatic organs*. The antibodies are always produced by cells – in *lymphocytes* or *lymphocyte derivatives* imprinted in a specific way. Yet, the antibodies can in one case be *discharged into the blood* (*humoral* immunity) and in another case be *retained at the cell surface*, thus remaining cell-bound (*cellular* immunity).

In *active prophylactic inoculation*, weakened antigens are transmitted which provoke a completely effective immunity (=active immunization). In *passive prophylactic inoculation*, on the other hand, (humoral) antibodies are supplied which were produced previously in another organism (=passive immunization). Since the antibodies in passive immunization rapidly decompose and are not replaced, its protection is short-lived.

a) Cells of the Specific Defense System

The cells of the *specific defense system* are the *immunologically competent T-lymphocytes* and *B-lymphocytes*. They function in cooperation with the *accessory cells of the specific defense system* (macrophages, specialized reticular cells of lymphatic organs, Langerhans' cells of the epidermis → p. 164). The T- and B-lymphocytes embody the *double action* of the immune system in the form of *cellular* and *humoral immunological response*. Both types of lymphocytes arise from primordial cells of the bone marrow and gradually develop their defensive properties (immunological competence) by way of precursor cells.

The **T-lymphocytes** (*t*hymus-dependent lymphocytes) are prepared for their task in the cortex of the thymus. There they "learn" to tolerate the body's (autologous) tissues (*T-lymphocyte tolerance* toward the host organism) and to develop defensive functions only against foreign substances (*antigens*). They leave the thymus either as *regulator cells* (*T-helper cells* or *T-suppressor cells*) or as *cytotoxic T-cells* and move through the bloodstream to the T-regions of lymphatic organs. From the latter the immunologically competent T-lymphocytes can re-enter the bloodstream via the lymphatic circulation and *recirculate*. T-lymphocytes are always on standby throughout the whole body (T-lymphocyte reservoir).

The *T-helper cells* stimulate B-lymphocytes to proliferate (cell division) and to secrete antibodies, either directly by cell-fixed factors or indirectly by soluble helper-factors. The B-cell response to most antigens depends on this T-cell help. Therefore, T-helper cells must be able to "recognize" the antigen. It is "presented" to them by accessory cells which adhere to it.

T-suppressor cells can, under certain circumstances, suppress the immunological response both of B-cells and of T-helper cells and cytotoxic T-cells.

The *cytotoxic T-cells* are able to decompose antigenic cells by direct contact ("cellular immunological response") without being damaged themselves. They are stimulated by T-helper cells.

The specificity of each of these functions is acquired with the first contact with an antigen (*primary contact*) through which T-cells are first activated into proliferating *T-immunoblasts*. "Memory cells", which can identify the triggering agent for a long period of time, also develop with the proliferation of T-immunoblasts.

The mature **B-lymphocytes** (*b*one marrow lymphocytes) possess membrane-bound antigen receptors (immunoglobulins).

The *primary contact* (in the case of activation by T-helper cells) can lead either directly or indirectly to plasma cell formation. *Plasma cells* produce humoral antibodies ("humoral immunological response") and secrete them.

In the case of *direct* formation of plasma cells, the B-cells give rise to proliferating *B-immunoblasts*, from which identical daughter cells arise (clone formation); the latter differentiate into plasma cells.

The *indirect* development of plasma cells occurs in the *lymphatic nodules* during the formation of a *germinal center* (secondary nodule). Here the B-lymphocytes are converted (via intermediate forms) into "memory cells" by forming receptors for the antigen in question. In the case of renewed contact with the same antigen (*secondary contact*), they react rapidly (even after years) by differentiation into plasma cells.

The **accessory cells** of the immune system are essential for the discharge of immunological information, as well as the immunological response. Phagocytizing and nonphagocytizing accessory cells are distinguished. The *phagocytizing accessory cells*, macrophages ($\rightarrow$ p. 77), can "present" the antigen to the immunologically-competent cells, among others. *Nonphagocytizing accessory cells* (specific reticular cells) facilitate the colonization of T-lymphocytes (in the T-region) and B-lymphocytes (in the B-region) of lymphatic organs.

For organ transplants and dental prostheses, metals and artificial substances must be used which are not antigenic in nature and which do not cause the body's own protein to become "foreign" to it.

An excessive specific defense reaction is termed an *allergy* or *anaphylaxis*. In the case of *auto-aggressive disorders*, the specific defense system is directed against organs or tissues of its host. In the case of *immunological suppression* (by means of chemical cytostatic drugs, x-rays, withdrawal of lymphocytes, administration of the adrenocortical hormone, cortisol), the cellular immunological response can be restrained.

b) Lymphatic Organs

The lymphatic organs (Fig. 31) are the *thymus* (located behind the sternum, above the heart), *tonsils* (at the entrance to the pharynx), *lymph nodes*, *spleen* (in the upper left part of the abdomen) and the *lymphatic constituents of the mucous membranes*. As producers of lymphocytes, the massive amount of these cells which they contain sets them apart from all other organs microscopically.

The **thymus** occupies a special position among the lymphatic organs inasmuch as without its participation (cellular) immunity cannot be

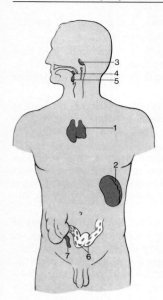

Fig. 31. **Lymphatic organs** (excluding lymph nodes)
1 *Control organ*: thymus
2 *Central organ in blood circulation*: spleen
3–5 *Organs in upper region of "foregut"*
3 Pharyngeal tonsil
4 Palatine tonsils
5 Lingual tonsil
6, 7 *Organs in lower region of gut*
6 Aggregated lymphatic nodules in mucosa of ileum
7 Vermiform appendix

established. This special status is also emphasized by the fact that the lymph nodule, the structural feature characteristic for the rest of the lymphatic organs, is absent in the thymus.

All **other lymphatic organs** have the following in common; the connective tissue of the lymphatic organs is *reticular connective tissue*, a spongy, cellular network reinforced by reticular fibers. The *lymphocytes* are aggregated in the interstices of the reticular connective tissue, preferably in *cords* and *lymphatic nodules*.

Lymphatic nodules are macroscopic, barely visible, spherical structures. They occur as isolated *solitary lymphatic nodules* in all mucous membranes. Accumulated as *aggregated lymphatic nodules*, they are especially evident in the mucosa of the lower small intestine and appendix, where they can form centimeter-long plates. In the lymph nodes, tonsils and spleen the lymphatic nodules also possess the character of aggregated lymphatic nodules. The appearance of the lymphatic nodules reflects their *participation in the specific defense processes*; from *primary nodules* arise *secondary nodules*.

Lymphatic vessels carry lymph and lymphocytes *from* the reticular connective tissue of the lymphatic organs. In addition, *lymph nodes* also possess *afferent* lymphatic vessels. Blood vessels serve for the nourishment of the lymphatic organs, as well as for the recirculation of lymphocytes.

Recirculation of lymphocytes: lymphocytes, which enter the blood from the lymph tract, stay there less than a day. They then return to the lymphatic organs through the wall of the postcapillary veins and, at a later point in time, are briefly washed out into the blood again with the lymph. About 98% of all lymphocytes are found in the *lymphatic organs.*

As representatives of the specific defense system, the *lymphatic organs*, except the regulatory thymus, are *localized at the danger sites*, the *invasion entrances of disease pathogens*. From these areas, the specific defense system can be "alerted" early in case of danger.

The **tonsils** represent the specific defense system as guardians of the air and food inlets into the body.

The **lymphatic tissue of the intestine,** especially the *aggregated lymphatic nodules* of the lower small intestine, is a defense against disease pathogens in those regions of the intestine in which the bactericidal hydrochloric acid of the stomach is no longer active.

The **lymph nodes** are inserted as biological filters in the lymph tracts coming from the external and internal surfaces of the body; they "inspect" the lymph coming from the periphery.

The **spleen** (*lien*) is distinguished from lymph nodes, tonsils and the lymphatic tissue of the intestine by its especially close relationship to blood vessels. The place of the spleen in the bloodstream corresponds to that of the lymph nodes in the lymph stream: it "inspects" the blood as the last "bastion." In addition the spleen continues to have an influence on the *composition of the blood.* It takes part in the formation and destruction of blood. It can store "off the track" *products of metabolism* (thesaurosis) and – in the case of insufficiency of bone marrow – can resume the *formation of blood* which it carried out in fetal life. The spleen therefore, is of abundant interest to the pathologist.

4. Mucous and Serous Membranes of the Viscera

The **viscera,** considered *functionally,* are the *organ systems of the metabolic and genital apparatuses* which are built up from the "inner organs".

Of the *circulatory system*, only the large organs, e.g. heart and spleen, are traditionally classified with the viscera; the peripheral blood vessels, on the other hand, are grouped with the peripheral nerves as *peripheral conduction paths* and excluded from the viscera.

With regard to the *incorporation* of the viscera in the body cavities, a distinction is made between *cranial, cervical, thoracic, abdominal* and *pelvic viscera.*

Tissue constituents. *Epithelial, connective, muscular* and *nervous tissues* are involved in the construction of the viscera.

Epithelial tissue covers the *inner* and, when the viscera are not embedded in connective tissue, the *outer surfaces* of the inner organs. In numerous viscera (e.g. in the liver, in all glands) the *specific* functional part is composed of epithelial tissue.

The *parenchyma* represents the *specific organ tissue*, in contrast to the nonspecific connective tissue stroma. In most organs the parenchyma consists of epithelial cells. In some organs (e.g. spleen) defense cells or precursor cells of blood elements form the parenchyma.

The **connective tissue** furnishes a *stromal network* in all organs which serves for stabilization. It carries blood vessels, lymphatic vessels and nerves, as well as "free cells of the connective tissue" which reside in its interstices.

The *stroma* represents the *loose* or the *reticular connective tissue* in the interior of the organ. It supports cells or cell groups of the parenchyma

Connective tissue surrounds the inner organs as a *fiber-rich organ capsule* (*tunica fibrosa*). In a few cases, an especially fiber-rich organ covering which therefore has a whitish sheen, is called the *tunica albuginea.* The external connective tissue layer of an organ embedded in connective tissue is termed the *tunica adventitia.*

Cartilage appears only in the *respiratory system*, where it can sporadically calcify or also ossify.

Smooth muscle produces the automotility found in all viscera – except in some cranial and cervical viscera, as well as the heart, in which striated muscle is found.

Smooth muscle occupies a portion of the wall structure of hollow organs as a special muscle layer (*tunica muscularis*).

Nervous tissue. *Efferent autonomic nerve cells* and fibers innervate the smooth muscle, as well as the glandular epithelial cells of the viscera.

The walls of many organs, especially those of the gastro-intestinal tract, contain autonomic nerve cells which, together with the autonomic nerve fibers, are called the "*intramural nervous system.*" The *afferent* nerve fibers of the viscera terminate in most cases as "free nerve endings." Structured *receptors* occur only exceptionally, for example, the smell and taste receptors of the cranial viscera and occasionally mechanoreceptors in the inner organs (e.g. lamellar corpuscles in the pancreas).

1. Elements and Structural Principles of the Mucous Membranes

The *inner surfaces* of viscera that develop as hollow organs, organs of the digestive and respiratory systems, as well as the urogenital apparatus, are lined by *mucous membranes* (Fig. 32); the organs of the circulatory system, on the orther hand, are lined by *endothelium*.

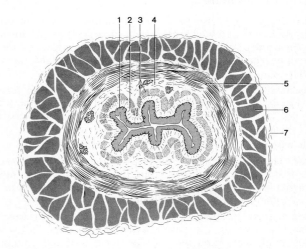

Fig. 32. **Mucous membrane as part of wall of a hollow organ** (esophagus)

1–3 *Mucous membrane layers*	5, 6 *Muscularis externa*
1 Epithelium	5 Circular layer
2 Lamina propria	6 Longitudinal layer
3 Muscularis mucosae	7 Adventitia
4 Submucosa	

The term "mucous membrane" reveals that this form of lining is closely related to the production of a *glandular secretion* – frequently mucus.

Each **mucous membrane** (short form: *mucosa*) is characteristic of its organ; mucous membranes therefore exhibit great differences. The organ specificity of a mucosa is so pronounced as a rule that an organ diagnosis can be made microscopically from the structure of this layer alone. Its constituents are:

– the *epithelial layer* (*mucosal epithelium*) which forms the inner lining of the mucosa;

– the *mucosal connective tissue* (*lamina propria*) which lies directly beneath the epithelium;

– the *mucosal muscle layer* (*muscularis mucosae*) which is developed distinctly only in the *digestive system* from the esophagus to the end of the intestine and which separates the lamina propria from the deeper-lying connective tissue (submucosa).

A *submucosa* can be clearly distinguished only when a muscularis mucosae is developed. It is not grouped with the mucosa, but is closely connected with it functionally.

a) Mucosal Epithelium

The *mucosal epithelial layer* (*mucosal epithelium*) consists of cells which are perfectly joined and which produce a superficial tissue closure in this way. As the border layer between the tissues of the organ and the surface, the epithelium has various *functions*, manifested in the degree of its *differentiation*.

The **classification** of epithelia generally conforms to the *form, stratification* and *differentiation of the free surface* of the epithelial cells, which may be *flat* (squamous), *cuboidal* or *columnar* and arranged in *single* (simple), *pseudostratified* and *stratified* layers.

Function. Mucosal epithelia protect, absorb and secrete.

Protection. The epithelium protects deeper-lying tissues from mechanical, thermal, and chemical influences. In the case of strong mechanical requirements (e.g. in the oral cavity, esophagus), the epithelium is multi-layered: *stratified, noncornified epithelium.*

Protection against the deposit of very small particles on the inner surface of organs (e.g. dust in the nasal cavity and trachea) is provided by numerous small cilia (*kinocilia*) on the surface of tall columnar cells arranged only in a simple or *pseudostratified layer*: *ciliated epithelium*, which is otherwise not very robust. The cilia beat in a coordinated fashion in the direction of an "exit" (e.g. toward the pharynx in the trachea and nasal cavity) and thus generate a fluid stream on the surface of the mucosa, which carries away the infiltrated particles.

In some organs the epithelium forms special *protective substances* against *chemical action* (e.g. against urine in the urinary bladder) which can also be secreted (e.g. against hydrochloric acid in the stomach). In this case protection is produced by secretion.

Resorption. Resorption occurs in numerous organs from the lumen into the interior of the organ. Mucosae which are particularly active in absorption (e.g. the small intestine) possess only a *simple columnar epithelium*, the luminal surface of which displays numerous, tiny *microvilli* distinctly visible only under the electron microscope. Appearing in the light microscope as a border, these microvilli greatly increase the resorptive surface area. A single-layered epithelium favors resorption. Stratified epithelium can likewise absorb substances, but to a lesser extent.

Secretion is the release of substances synthesized expressly for that purpose. Secretory epithelia are *tall columnar* or *cuboidal cells* arranged in a single layer. A *non-organ-specific* secretory capacity of epithelial cells of the mucosa is the production of *mucus* by *goblet cells*. In some organs (e.g. stomach), on the other hand, the mucosal epithelium secretes organ-specific substances.

The chief *biological significance of mucus* is to keep the mucosa moist and in many organs (e.g. the digestive system) to improve the gliding ability of the organ's contents. Mucus can also act chemically as a buffer.

In *glands*, secretory epithelial cells are grouped together like organs.

b) Connective Tissue of the Mucosa

The *mucosal connective tissue* consists of *loose* connective tissue, which in some organs (e.g. in the lower small intestine) may contain *reticular* connective tissue. It is separated from the epithelium by a *basal membrane* or at least by a *basal lamina*. The mucosal connective tissue is the transit site for the passage of substances between the blood vessels and the epithelial layer.

Some structures of the mucosal connective tissue are connected with the *functions of the mucosal epithelium. Arterioles* enter the mucosal connective tissue from small arteries of the submucosal connective tissue and carry nutrients to the *capillary network*. In many cases it is strongly developed and also organ-specific and releases, among other things, chemical substances (amino acids, sugar) from which secretory epithelial cells synthesize their secretions. *Venules* and *lymphatic capillaries* transport resorbed material into the veins and lymphatic vessels of the submucosal connective tissue. *Connective tissue fibers* stabilize the structure of the organ.

Other structures of the mucosal connective tissue, more or less strongly pronounced in the various organs, have a function as part of the specific defense system which is largely independent of the action of the epithelial layer. Lymphocytes, as well as other *cells of the defense system*, are embedded in the interstices of the reticular connective tissue at these sites, frequently in the form of solitary *lymphatic nodules*, in the lower small intestine as *aggregated lymphatic nodules*.

c) Muscularis mucosae

The *muscularis mucosae*, a distinctly pronounced arrangement occurring *only in the digestive system*, is composed of bundles of smooth muscle cells encircling the mucosa and crossing over one another in a spiral fashion. By means of the loose submucosal connective tissue, contraction of the muscularis mucosae can form *mucosal folds* independently of the external muscular wall of the intestinal tube (Fig. **32**). The muscularis mucosae makes automotility of the mucosa possible.

d) Submucosal Connective Tissue

The deeper-lying *submucosa, loose connective tissue* distinctly separated from the mucosal connective tissue by the muscularis mucosae only in the digestive system, is a *displaceable layer containing the conduction pathways* (Fig. **32**): blood vessels, networks of lymphatic vessels and autonomic nerve fibers. Together with their nerve cells, these form an extensive plexus in the digestive system which innervates the muscularis mucosae and the blood vessels of the mucosa.

2. Structural Principles of Serous Membranes and Serous Cavities

A *serous cavity* (Fig. **33**) is a capillary-sized, completely enclosed, polymorphic space which is lined by a *serous membrane* and contains a slight amount of *serous fluid*. The serous cavities in the thoracic, abdominal and pelvic spaces separates a part of the viscera of these spaces from the muscular and bony trunk wall and permit *displacements* of the viscera from the trunk wall and each other, as well as *alterations of the spatial conditions* of these viscera.

In most cases, the trunk wall is involved in alterations of the spatial state of the viscera (e.g. lung enlargement and continuous positional changes of the thorax in breathing; stomach enlargement and expansion of the abdominal wall in food ingestion).

Another part of the thoracic, abdominal and pelvic organs remains in a **connective tissue layer** of the thoracic, abdominal and pelvic spaces situated *outside* of the serous cavities (→ *mediastinum, extraperitoneal space*, Vol. 2). The mobility of these, as well as the cervical organs, results from their incorporation in loose connective tissue.

The *serous cavities* are the *pleural, pericardial* and *peritoneal cavities*.

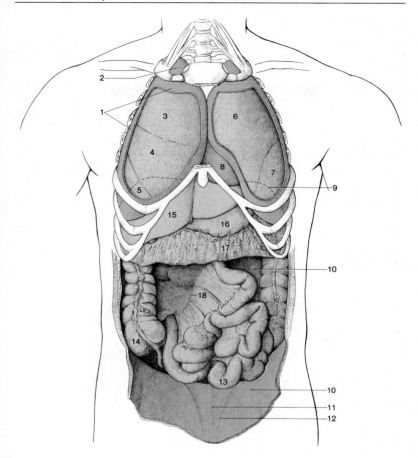

Fig. 33. **Serous cavities**
Pericardial cavity closed; pleural and peritoneal cavities opened

1 Costal pleura (windowed)
2 Pleural cupola (beneath scalenus anterior)
3–7 *Lungs*, covered by pleura
3 Right superior lobe
4 Middle lobe
5 Right inferior lobe
6 Left superior lobe
7 Left inferior lobe
8 Pericardium
9 Projection of dome of diaphragm
10 Parietal peritoneum

11 Median umbilical fold
12 Medial umbilical fold
13–18 *Abdominal viscera* covered by visceral
    peritoneum
13 Small intestine
14 Cecum with attached vermiform appendix
15 Liver
16 Stomach
17 Greater omentum
18 Root of mesentery

a) Serous Membranes

The *serous membrane* (short form: *serosa*) is thin, reddish in color and glisteningly smooth. The few milliliters of clear, amber-colored serous fluid are secreted by the serosa.

The serous membrane covers both the visceral surface with the visceral layer (*visceral serosa*) and the inner surface of the wall of the body cavity with the parietal layer (*parietal serosa*, Fig. **34**). Visceral and parietal layers converge in cuff-like line (e.g. at the vascular stalk of an organ).

The polymorphism of a serous cavity can be increased by folds which protrude into the interior, or by outpocketings of the parietal layer.

The following *serous membranes* are distinguished according to their *location*:
– in the *pleural cavity* of the thoracic space: the visceral layer is called the *pulmonary pleura*, the parietal layer at the inner surface of the thorax, the *costal pleura*; the parietal layer covers the diaphragm as the *diaphragmatic pleura* and the lateral boundary of the mediastinum as the *mediastinal pleura*;
– in the *pericardial cavity* of the thoracic space: the visceral layer is designated as the *epicardium*, the parietal as the *pericardium*;
– in the *peritoneal cavity* of the abdomnal space: the visceral layer is the *visceral peritoneum*, the parietal layer the *parietal peritoneum*.

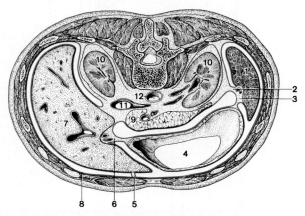

Fig. 34. **Topography of abdominal viscera in peritoneal cavity**
Peritoneum ▬▬▬

1–7 *Organs and "ligaments" situated intraperitoneally*
1 Spleen
2 Lienorenal (splenorenal) ligament
3 Gastrosplenic (gastrolienal) ligament
4 Stomach
5 Falciform ligament of liver
6 Hepatogastric ligament

7 Liver
8 Wall of peritoneal cavity lined by parietal peritoneum
9 *Retroperitoneal organ*: pancreas
10–12 *Extraperitoneal organs*
10 Kidney
11 Inferior vena cava
12 Abdominal aorta

Structure of Serous Membranes

Serous membranes consist of an *epithelial layer* and an underlying *connective tissue layer*.

The **serosal epithelium,** also called *"mesothelium"* because of its origin from the mesoderm, is formed of flat, deformable cells – derivatives of connective tissue cells which have been deformed into epithelial cells. The serosal epithelium permits a strong *fluid transport* into and out of the serous cavities.

The **subserous connective tissue** – depending upon the localization of the serosa – possesses different forms and proportions of connective tissue fibers; elastic networks are developed over deformable viscera. Serous membranes are richly supplied with blood vessels and variably equipped with lymphatic vessels. The parietal serosa possesses a sensory innervation, while the visceral serosa lacks sensory nerve fibers on many organs.

Transsudation and Resorption. The serous membranes are, on the one hand, highly adapted for the secretion (*transsudation*) of fluid into the serous cavities, the serous fluid being renewed constantly. On the other hand, in many places they are able to *resorb* fluids and corpuscular elements from the serous cavities rapidly and in large amounts.

Under diseased conditions, the serous fluid can increase excessively (hydrops); in the case of inflammation the fluid can become clouded by defense cells which issue from the serous membrane and by fibrin.

b) Relation of Viscera to Serous Cavities

The *organs in the thoracic and abdominal spaces* have different *relationships to their respective serous cavities*. The relation of the abdominal and pelvic organs to the *peritoneal* cavity is characterized by special designations (Fig. **34**).

Organs lying in the serous cavities are covered almost completely by the visceral layer of the serosa (e.g. the lungs in the pleural cavity, most of the small intestine in the peritoneal cavity). They are connected with the vascular and nerve trunks coursing in the connective tissue outside of the serous cavity only by way of (frequently ribbonlike) neurovascular routes covered by serosa.

Thin *connective tissue plates* (mesenteries), carrying vessels and nerves and covered over on both sides by *serosa*, connect the organs completely covered by serosa with the connective tissue layers lying outside of the serous cavities. "*Meso-*" is the prefix designation for such organ attachments (e.g. *mesogaster* in the stomach, *mesentery* in the small intestine).

The mesenteries are formed in connection with the development and the segmentation of the embryonic body cavities.

Ligament. When the vessels coursing in the mesentery exhibit a larger caliber and/or connective tissue fiber tracts which enlarge the mesentery, the latter is frequently called a *ligament.* Yet the mesentery obtains mechanical significance only insofar as it limits organ movement like a bridle; the mesentery referred to as a ligament does *not* serve as a suspension apparatus for the viscera.

Abdominal and *pelvic organs* that are covered in this manner, largely by the visceral layer of the peritoneum, lie *intraperitoneally.*

Organs bordering serous cavities are covered only on one surface of their wall by the parietal layer of the serosa (e.g. part of the descending aorta in the thoracic cavity, the pancreas in the abdominal cavity), the remaining walls being attached broadly to the connective tissue layer of the body cavities.

Abdominal and *pelvic organs* that border on the peritoneal cavity, one wall surface of which is covered by the parietal layer of the peritoneum, lie *retroperitoneally.*

Organs lying outside of serous cavities without any relationship to them are given shelter in the *connective tissue layer* of a body cavity (e.g. the esophagus in the mediastinum of the thoracic cavity, the kidney in the retroperitoneal space of the abdominal cavity); they are completely enclosed by connective tissue.

Abdominal and *pelvic organs* which do not exhibit a relationship of any sort to the parietal layer of the peritoneum lie *extraperitoneally.*

5. Glands

In **glands,** *secretory epithelial cells* are collected in large numbers by connective tissue in an organ-like fashion. The *glandular body* can be microscopically small (e.g. small mucosal glands) or have a diameter of several centimeters (e.g. large salivary glands).

A basic distinction between glands concerns the *method of discharge* of their products (Fig. **35**).

Exocrine glands (Fig. **35 a**) possess an *excretory duct* which transports their *secretions* to the external body surface or the inner surface of the viscera. The excretory duct opens at the place on the surface from which the gland has arisen during embryological development; the exocrine gland thus retains its original relationship to the surface.

Exocrine glands are the *sweat, odoriferous* (apocrine) and *sebaceous* glands of the *skin,* as well as the *glands of the digestive, respiratory and reproductive systems.*

The secretions of the exocrine glands of the skin and the mucous membranes of the respiratory system serve chiefly for their protection. Those from the mucosa of the digestive system, among others, serve for the enzymatic decomposition of nutritive substances, wheras the exocrine secretions of the reproductive system function in the preparation for the onset of pregnancy.

Endocrine glands (Fig. **35 b, c**) lack *excretory ducts*; their *secretions (hormones)* are taken up by *blood vessels.* Many endocrine glands also originate by invaginating from a surface, yet this connection, as a rule, disappears.

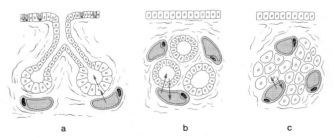

a   b   c

Fig. 35. **Classification of glands according to transport path of secretions**
Arrows indicate the transport direction of secretory building material (from blood vessels) and secretions
a Exocrine glands
b Endocrine glands with follicles
c Endocrine glands without follicles

The *large endocrine glands* are the *hypophysis, thyroid, parathyroid, suprarenal cortex* and *medulla*, the *pancreatic islets*, the *gonads*, the *system of gastro-intestinal endocrine cells*, as well as the small, nodule-like formations, the *paraganglia*, connected to the autonomic nervous system. Moreover, there are cells and cell groups which secrete hormone-like substances in the kidney and in other organs.

Hormones are vitally essential substances which – released into the blood in tiny amounts – regulate processes of metabolism, growth and reproduction by enzyme induction. The "hormonal information" is received only by cells which possess specific receptors in their cell membranes specialized for the hormone in question.

1. Elements and Structural Principles of Exocrine Glands

Exocrine glands are distinguished macroscopically and anatomically by the *shape of their terminal glandular units*, by the *chemical properties of their secretions* (identifiable by stains), and by the *amount and the manner of discharge of their secretions*.

a) Secretory Portion of Glands (Glandular Terminal Units)

Differences in shape. The *terminal units of glands*, i.e. the distal endings of the epithelial tubing arising from the glandular primordium by division, are, as a rule, the *secretory* portions of a gland (Fig. **36**). The remaining, proximal portions of the branches become the *excretory duct system*, which exhibits individual differences in many glands. Depending on the shape of the glandular terminal units, there can be distinguished: *acinar*

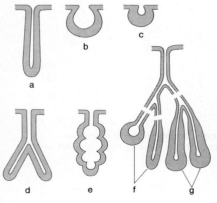

Fig. 36. **Classification of exocrine glands according to shape of terminal secretory units**

a Simple tubular
b Simple alveolar
c Simple acinar
d Branched tubular
e Branched alveolar
f Compound mixed tubular and acinar (also tubulo-acinar)
g Compound tubulo-acinar

end units which resemble a spherical berry, *alveolar terminal units* which form pear-shaped sacs, and *tubular units*, blind-ending units which, at their ends, can be stretched or formed into a glomus (glomus body).

Staining (chemical) differences permit the discrimination of *serous* and *mucous end units* in many glands. A mixed gland contains both types of terminal units.

Differences in the manner of discharge of secretions allow the distinction between *eccrine* (merocrine), *apocrine* and *holocrine terminal units*.

The release of secretions in the (most frequently formed) *eccrine* units takes place without loss of cytoplasm (exocytosis); in the *apocrine* units it involves cytoplasmic constriction; and in the *holocrine* units the entire epithelial cell perishes in the process.

b) Connective Tissue, Muscle Cells of Glandular Terminal Units and Nerves

Connective Tissue. The epithelial cells of the glandular terminal units rest on a basal membrane. Several terminal units are combined into a glandular lobule by connective tissue. A (large) gland consists of numerous lobules which give the surface of the gland a granulated appearance. Large glands are surrounded by a fiber-rich *connective tissue capsule* (*fibrous capsule*).

Muscle Cells. The terminal units of many exocrine glands are surrounded by *smooth muscle cells* which, by contraction, squeeze out the contents of the end units. The muscle cells lie on the epithelial side of the basal membrane; they arise from epithelial cells and are therefore called *myoepithelial cells* (*myoepithelium*).

Nerves. Present morphological knowledge concerning the innervation of secretory epithelium is based chiefly on results obtained from the individual glands of animals. *Cholinergic, aminergic* and *peptidergic axonal endings* are observed in glandular epithelial cells or in their vicinity. On the basis of the glandular influences of autonomic nerves known from physiology, it is established that *exocrine glands are innervated autonomically*.

c) Glandular Excretory Ducts

In *exocrine* glands, the secretion is transported via an excretory duct to a surface (skin or mucosa) (Figs. **35 a** and **36**). Effecting this transport are: *myoepithelial cells* of the terminal units (e.g. sweat glands, large salivary glands), *secretory pressure* (e.g. glands of the digestive tract) and *smooth muscle cells* in the area of the glandular end units (e.g. holocrine glands of hair follicles).

In simple **unbranched glands,** a *single terminal end unit* merges with a *single excretory duct*. This type of opening exists in most tubular glands. At its blind end (= secretory terminal unit), a simple tubule consists of secretory cells, whereas at its outlet they are (mostly) nonsecretory cells with mitoses for the regeneration of the glandular epithelium (e.g. intestinal glands, small sweat glands = glomus bodies).

In **branched glands,** several *glandular terminal units* open directly into a *single, unbranched excretory duct* (e.g. gastric glands, meibomian glands of the eyelids).

In **compound glands,** *numerous glandular terminal units* open into the *branches of a branched excretory duct.* The latter, with its branches, forms an *excretory duct system* (e.g. large salivary glands, mammary glands) in which different – organ-specific – *segments* are (usually) distinguishable.

2. Structural Principles and Organization of Endocrine Glands

The *endocrine system* involves all organs and cell systems which secrete and convey *hormones* to distant target cells via the blood or lymphatic pathways (or to neighboring target cells via intercellular spaces). *Endocrine glands* are exclusively concerned with the production of hormones. Organs which predominantly fulfill other functions (e.g. gastro-intestinal organs), but at the same time, also possess hormone-producing cells systems, can be designated as *endocrine-active organs.* Parts of the central nervous system also belong to the endocrine system. *Hormones* are vital chemical messengers which serve the communication between the cells of an organism. Even small amounts influence the metabolic processes of the target cells. From a chemical point of view hormones can be classified into different groups: *amines* (e.g. adrenalin, noradrenalin, dopamine, melatonin, serotonin), *steroids* (e.g. mineralocorticoids, sexual hormones), *peptides* (e.g. regulatory hormones of the hypothalamus, gastro-enteropancreatic hormones) or *proteins* (e.g. gonadotropins, growth hormone).

Endocrine cells frequently produce more than one hormone (as in the case of peptide hormones). If an endocrine cell secretes different hormones, these can be split off from a common prohormone molecule and form a "family." However, they can also be derived from various forerunners or belong to different groups of substances (as in the case of amines and peptide hormones). Amines and peptides also occur together as active substances in the central and peripheral nervous systems.

APUD cells (*a*mine and/or amine *p*recursor *u*ptake and *d*ecarboxylation cells) comprise those endocrine cells which produce and/or take up not only peptides with hormone properties, but also biogenic amines, or which concentrate precursors of amines, i.e. amino acids, and are able to decarboxylate them into biogenic amines. These cells all appear to be derived from the neural crest.

a) Structural Characteristics of Endocrine Glands

In contrast to exocrine glands, *endocrine* glands have no general features for classifying them according to the shape of their secretory portions or the manner of discharge of their secretions.

The **shape** of the *secretory glandular parts*, i.e. the way in which the epithelial cells are assembled, can, of course, be characteristic for the individual glands. The epithelial cells can be arranged in spheres, cords, or networks or, as an exception, they can also form vesicles (*follicles*) in which the hormone bound to a carrier substance is stored (e.g. thyroid).

The *quantity of hormones*, compared with the secretions from exocrine glands, is slight; the *manner of discharge* takes place (according to present knowledge, in most glands) by *eccrine extrusion.*

Differences in the staining (chemical) behavior of glandular cells are numerous and important for the correlation of individual cell types to hormone production within an endocrine gland. Staining with the methods commonly used, however, does not make possible, a general division of endocrine glands because, in their action, different kinds of hormones can belong chemically to the same group of substances – and only these can be readily demonstrated by staining. On the other hand, specific hormones can be correlated with individual endocrine cells using immunohistochemical methods.

The *function of the excretory ducts* of exocrine glands are taken over in endocrine glands by *capillaries* and *postcapillary veins*; the capillaries are, as a rule, "fenestrated". Endocrine glands are strongly vascularized.

The *connective tissue* of endocrine glands is loose and poor in fibers between the epithelial cells and around the capillaries. The hormones traverse the connective tissue on their way from the secreting cells to the blood vessels. In several endocrine glands, lymphatic vessels have been detected which (probably) also take up hormones and transport them into the blood circulation with the lymph.

Nerves. Endings of efferent *autonomic* (cholinergic, aminergic and peptidergic) axons have been found in several endocrine glands. They terminate with synapse-like formations partly at secretory cells, partly at blood vessels.

b) Organization of Endocrine Glands

The *exocrine* glands directly affect only an adjacent, locally limited area, e.g. within the visceral system to which they belong. The glands are therefore subject to organ-specific regulation. The exocrine glands of the different visceral systems do not influence one another, at least not directly.

The *endocrine* glands (Fig. 37), on the other hand, develop long-distance effects which (usually) involve the entire organism. They work in mutual dependence, regulated by the control centers of the diencephalon.

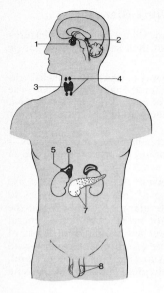

Fig. 37. **Endocrine glands** (disseminated endocrine cell systems not shown)
1 Hypothalamo-hypophysial system
2 Pineal
3 Thyroid
4 Parathyroid
5 Suprarenal cortex
6 Suprarenal medulla
7 Pancreatic islets
8 Endocrine portions of gonads

Diencephalon. The lower part of the diencephalon, the *hypothalamus*, is the control center of the endocrine glands. It consists of the following *order of dependences: Nuclear regions of the diencephalon* (hypothalamic nuclei) dispatch

– *neural efferents*, which – descending in the brainstem to visceromotor nuclear regions – act on endocrine glands via *autonomic nerves*; and
– *hormonal efferents* which regulate the subordinated endocrine glands via the *hypothalamohypophysial system*.

Hypothalamohypophysial system: control hormones (Fig. **38**). Most of the hormones derived from the hypothalamic nuclei act *indirectly* on peripheral endocrine glands by serving as *control hormones*, *releasing factors* and *release inhibiting factors*, which regulate the release of hormones from the anterior lobe of the hypophysis, the *adenohypophysis*. This is a bean-shaped organ situated in the center of the base of the skull beneath the hypothalamus. The adenohypophysis – as the mediator between the hypothalamus and the peripheral endocrine glands – is closely connected with the hypothalamus by blood vessels.

The **adenohypophysis,** induced by control hormones, secretes **glandotropic hormones** which *directly* stimulate growth and the hormone production of the peripheral *endocrine glands* dependent upon the hypothalamohypophysial system (Fig. **38**).

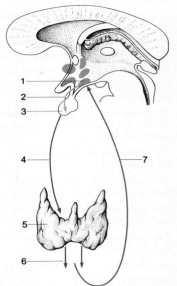

Fig. 38. **Example of arrangement of dependence of endocrine glands,** schematic projection of hypothalamic nuclei of right wall of 3rd ventricle viewed from left side, thyroid gland seen from front

1 Hormone-producing hypothalamic nuclei
2 Control hormones (here: thyrotropin-releasing hormone = thyrotropin-releasing factor = TRF)
3 Adenohypophysis
4 Glandotropic hormone (here: thyroid-stimulating hormone TSH = thyrotropin)
5 Thyroid gland
6 Effector hrmone (here: thyroxine)
7 Feedback via bloodstream to hypothalamus and adenohypophysis

The **peripheral endocrine glands** that depend on the hypothalamohypophysial system produce **effector hormones** which directly intervene in the metabolism of the *target organ.*

The **hypothalamus** and the **adenohypophysis** (growth hormone) intervene directly in the metabolism and management of the target organ through only a few effector hormones, which regulate water retention and initiate the contraction of the smooth musculature of some organs.

Glandotropic hormones of the adenohypophysis act on
– the **ovary,** whose endocrine portions form the cyclic female sex hormones,
– the **testis,** where primarily male sex hormones are produced in the endocrine interstitial cells,
– the **suprarenal cortex,** in which numerous hormones are synthesized, e.g. those which maintain carbohydrate balance, sex hormones, etc., and
– the **thyroid gland,** whose hormones stimulate cellular metabolism, influence body growth and lower the blood calcium level.

The **feedback** from these endocrine organs – directly dependent on the adenohypophysis – is directed partly to the *hypothalamus,* partly to the *adenohypophysis* (Fig. **38**).

The feedback completes the **control system.** *Principle of the control system*: an excessive supply (of a hormone from a peripheral endocrine gland), by feeding back to the control center, leads to a curbing of production; an inadequate supply causes an increase in production.

Influences of the central nervous system (e.g. emotional influence on the hormonally-regulated menstrual cycle) act on the *hypothalamus* and with it on the dependent endocrine glands.

The following **endocrine glands not directly dependent on the hypo-thalamohypophysial system** are partially controlled by the *autonomic nervous system* (i.e. indirectly by *neural efferents of the hypothalamus*) and partially in other organ-specific ways.

The **pineal body** (*epiphysis*), a small organ which is attached posteriorly to the roof of the third ventricle, produces a hormone that (in animal experiments) has inhibitory control over sexual development.

The **suprarenal medulla,** located in the interior of the suprarenal gland that sits on the kidney, produces hormones which, among other things, raise blood pressure.

The **parathyroid gland,** four pea-sized bodies at the posterior side of the thyroid, secretes a hormone which regulates calcium and phosphate metabolism.

The **pancreatic islets,** 0.5–1.5 million microscopically small islands of cells in the pancreas, control the blood sugar level.

The **system of gastro-intestinal endocrine cells** influences the functions of the digestive tract.

Paraganglia, pea-sized bodies at the aorta and in other places, produce – like the suprarenal medulla – hormones affecting the circulation.

The **placenta,** which takes over the transient hormonal *functions of the adenohypophysis* and *ovary* during pregnancy, occupies a *special position* in the organization of endocrine glands. The placenta, as an independent regulatory organ, intervenes in the interaction of numerous other endo-crine glands.

6. Nervous System

By means of the nervous system, the organism is in (passive and active) communication with its environment. The nervous system, as central coordinator, adjusts the performances of the individual organ systems to each other directly (via nerves) or indirectly (via hormones). It controls or regulates the activities of the locomotor apparatus, of the respiratory, circulatory, digestive and urogenital systems, as well as the system of endocrine glands. The nervous system can also intervene indirectly to a slight extent in the performance of the defense system.

The *central nervous system* (CNS) comprises the *brain and spinal cord*; the *peripheral nervous system* (PNS) is the sum of all *nerves and ganglia* (accumulations of nerve cells). The distinction between the CNS and PNS is made for the sake of didactic clarity; both are parts of a continuous system. Knowledge of the structure and organization of the peripheral nervous system is a prerequisite to understanding the functions of the individual parts of the body to be discussed in "Special Anatomy". In the general anatomy of the nervous system, therefore, special emphasis will be placed upon the structural principles of the peripheral nervous system and its connections with the brain and spinal cord.

A. Elements and Structural Principles of the Nervous System

1. Elements of the Nervous System

The specific structural elements of the nervous system develop from the *neural tube*, *neural crest* and *sensory placodes*. *Connective tissue* is involved in the structure of the nervous system through blood vessels and through the development of supporting and connecting structures, the meninges of the brain and spinal cord.

The specific structural elements of the nervous system are the *nerve cells* (*ganglion cells*) and *glial cells*. The nerve cells are the excitatory conducting elements. The glial cells serve partly for the distribution of substances and compartmentation, for mechanical stabilization and for defense, and partly for the isolation of nerve cells. As a structural part of nerve fibers, they are also indirectly involved in the conduction of excitation.

a) Neurons

The *neuron* is the *nerve cell with all of its processes*, the *stimuli-generating* (and *excitation-conducting*) *basic structural element* of the nervous system. As the exclusive carrier of nervous functions, neurons are the *functional units* which communicate with each other by synapses. The metabolism of the usually numerous and long processes of the neuron is controlled by the nucleus-containing perikaryon, the metabolic center of the neuron; the neuron is a *trophic unit*.

Like all cells, the neuron is sensitive. *A stimulus elicits an excitation* (depolarization of the cell membrane), *which is propagated* (as an action potential) *in the cell membrane*. The neuron is distinguished from other cells in that the excitation can be transferred in a cell process up to 1 m long, the axon, over a wide distance and – in the case of myelinated nerve fibers (→ p. 108) very rapidly.

Arrangement of Neurons

Neurons are united with each other usually end to end in the form of circles and chains. Neuronal circles and chains are arranged regularly so that the individual segments of these circles and chains *can be numbered in order*, e.g. the 1st, 2nd, 3rd neuron of a neuron circle (of a neuron chain), etc. At the same time each segment (neuron) of a circle or a chain is represented by a *large number* of parallel-directed nerve cells (neurons). Thus, for example, the 1st neuron of the afferent circuit of a nerve is composed of ten thousand neurons. In *numerical data concerning neurons*, therefore, *order number* and *quantity* must be *distinguished*.

Neurons of the CNS are *intermediate links* of *neuron chains* and *neuron circles*. *Neurons of the PNS*, on the other hand, form *initial* or *terminal links of neuron chains* and are, therefore, specialized – like a necklace (Fig. **39**). But what is said in the following about the arrangement of neurons using the example of an intermediate link is also valid for initial and terminal links.

The neuron is classified into three segments: *dendrite*, *perikaryon* and *axon*, according to the direction of the excitatory sequence (Fig. **40**).

Direction of the excitatory sequence in the neuron: (stimulus →) dendrite → perikaryon → axon (→ effector tissue).

Each of the three parts of the neuron belongs predominantly (not exclusively) to one of the three main functions of the neuron. Dendrites (there are usually several) and axons are branches or processes of the perikaryon.

The **dendrites,** branched like trees with polymorphic processes, receive excitatory-releasing stimuli (in the CNS) via *synapses* from connected

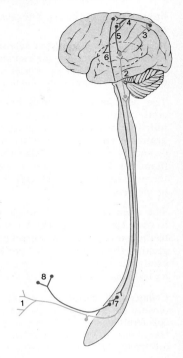

Fig. 39. **Example for organization of nervous system into neuron chains and neuron circuits,** view from left side (each link symbolizes thousands of similarly-directed neurons)
1 *Beginning of neuron chain*: first afferent neuron
2–7 *Links of neuron circuit*
2, 3 Second and third afferent neuron
4, 5 Association neurons
6 Efferent neuron
7 Interneuron
8 *Termination of neuron chain*: last efferent neuron ("final common motor path")

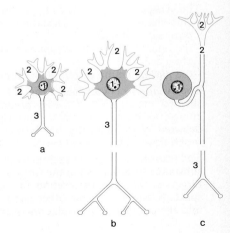

Fig. 40. **Classification of neurons** according to shape
a "Multipolar" neuron with short axon (e.g. interneuron)
b "Multipolar" neuron with long axon (e.g. spinal cord cell of "final common motor path", motor neuron)
c "Pseudo-unipolar" nerve cell (afferent, i.e. sensory cell)
1 Perikaryon (cell body)
2 Dendrites
3 Axon with collaterals

links of neuron chains. *The dendrites are the most important receptor parts of the neuron.*

By means of dendrites the neuron receives, as a rule, excitations from several connected neurons, i.e. the excitations are transmitted from those convergent on the neuron (*convergence principle*). The number of interneuronal synapses of a dendritic tree varies from one to many thousands.

The **perikaryon** (the cell body, or "nerve cell" in colloquial usage) contains the greatest part of the cellular constituents indispensable for nutritive processes and regeneration: cell nuclei (= genetic information), granular endoplasmic reticulum (= protein synthesis), mitochondria (= energy production), also the Golgi apparatus and microtubules and filaments. The greater the dendritic tree or the longer the axon, the larger is the perikaryon. *The cell body is the nutritive structure, the metabolic center of the neuron.*

The **axon** consists of a single process of the neuron, from a millimeter to over 100 cm long, which conducts the excitation to the target organ or to the next link in the neuron chain. The axonal volume can be 100 times greater than that of the perikaryon. The axon usually transmits the excitation to the effector organ chemically with the help of a synapse. *The axon is the effector part of the neuron.*

Collaterals. The axon can give off side branches (collaterals); this regularly occurs directly at the target tissue where it forms an end brush (*telodendron*). The collaterals also end in synapses. By means of collaterals, excitations emanating from a neuron are transmitted to several target cells, i.e. the excitation spreads out divergently (*divergence principles*).

The **synapse** consists basically of three components:
- club-shaped terminal formations of the innervating axon with the *presynaptic membrane*,
- the intercellular cleft (*synaptic cleft*) between the latter and the innervating cell, and
- the plasmalemma of the innervating cell, the *subsynaptic membrane*.

The *synapses* between nerve cells can be seen in the light microscope in silvered preparations ("Golgi preparations") as button-shaped thickenings, as boutons (terminal boutons, Fig. **41**). Synapses can also be detected histochemically by the demonstration of the enzymes which break down the chemical carrier substance, the transmitter.

The transmission of the excitation takes place by the release of a carrier substance (*transmitter*) in the form of a rapidly discharged, short-lasting, target-specific "neurosecretion in quantum" limited to the narrowest space. (Compare, on the other hand, the long-term release of hormones into the circulation by endocrine glands.)

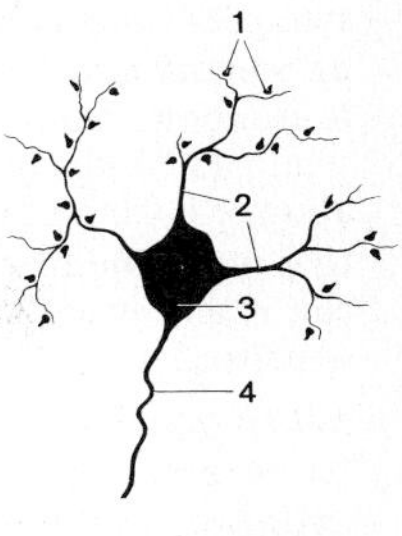

Fig. 41. **Axodendritic synapse,** silver preparation (magnification ca. 200 ×)
1 Button-shaped terminals (boutons) of axons of innervating neurons
2 Dendrites of innervated neuron
3 Cell body
4 Axon

Synapses can be classified on the basis of functional, substrate-specific or localization criteria.

On the basis of *function*, a distinction is made between:
– *excitatory* (stimulating synapses, which stimulate the effector cells (depolarization of the plasmalemma), and
– *inhibitory* synapses, which suppress excitation in the target cells (hyperpolarization of the plasmalemma).

It is possible to contrast synapses with one another according to the different transmitters: *cholinergic, aminergic, peptidergic,* among others, and thus to group together neuronal systems as transmitter systems, i.e. as
– *acetylcholine* systems,
– *amino acid* systems (glycine, glutamate, γ-aminobutyric acid systems),
– systems of *biogenic amines* (dopamine, noradrenalin, adrenalin, serotonin, histamine systems), and
– *peptide* systems (more than 25 known at present).

The *localization* of synapses makes it possible to characterize
– *interneuronal* (neuroneuronal) synapses, by far the most frequent form of synapse, which transfer the transmitter from one neuron to the next,

in the form of:
– *axodendritic* synapses between the innervating axon and the dendrites of the effector cell,
– *axosomatic* synapses between the innervating axon and the cell body of the target cell, and
– *axo-axonal* synapses between the innervating axon and the axon of the target cell, at the cone of origin (initial segment) or at the "presynaptic" end of the axon (before the synapse of the innervating axon);
– *myoneural* synapses, which transfer the transmitter from a neuron to muscle tissue,

in the form of:
– synapses at the *skeletal muscle fiber* ("motor endplate"),

– synapses *"en passant"* (with numerous transmitter-releasing axonal outfoldings) at *smooth muscle cells* and at *cells of the conducting system* of the heart (autonomic nervous system),

synapses *"à distance"*, where the space between the axonal end and the innervating cells (the subsynaptic space) is very wide and the transmitter, which – similar to a hormone from an endocrine gland – is released into the intercellular space, can reach several cells of the target tissue at the same time (autonomic nervous system);

– *neuroglandular* synapses, which transfer the transmitter from a neuron to an exocrine or an endocrine glandular cell;

– synapses between a *sensory cell* and the dendritic process of an *afferent neuron*, as well as between the axonal end of an *efferent neuron* and a sensory cell;

– synapses at cells of the *multiglandular adipose tissue*.

The portions of the initial and terminal segments of the neuron chains situated in the peripheral nervous system exhibit morphological specializations in regard to excitation formation and transmission. Their synapses are different from the previously described synapses of the intermediate segments.

The (sensory) *initial segment* (*the 1st neuron of the afferent circuit*) can be stimulated either by processes at a receptor cell (→ p. 120), or directly by a specific (mechanical, chemical, thermal, electromagnetic) stimulus which the *dendritic process picks up as a receptor* (→ primary receptor, p. 120).

The (motor) *terminal segment* is the *"final common pathway"* to a target tissue, e.g. with a synapse at a skeletal muscle fiber (Fig. **42**), or in other cases at a glandular cell, in the vicinity of smooth muscle cells, or heart muscle cells.

Transmitters discovered so far are: *acetylcholine*, the catecholamines *noradrenalin* and *dopamine*, the indolamine *serotonin* (5-hydroxytryptamine, 5-HT) – noradrenalin, dopamine and serotonin are grouped together as monoamines – and the amino acids *glutamic acid*, *γ-aminobutyric acid* (GABA) and *glycine*. These "classic" transmitters occur in the CNS in approximately half of all synapses. In the other half of the synapses in the CNS, the transmitter substances are (with great probability) *neuropeptides*. In a neuron, both "classic" transmitters (especially monoamines) and peptides can be formed (→ p. 94). The prerequisite for

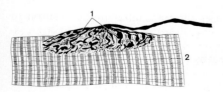

Fig. 42. **Myoneural synapse,** silver preparation (magnification ca. 800x)
1 Button-shaped terminals of collaterals (motor end plates) of innervating neuron
2 Innervated skeletal muscle fiber

transmitter action is, as in the case of hormone action, the presence of *receptor* molecules in the cell membrane of the target cell.

Some transmitters are synthesized in the cell body, others in the end of the axon. Transmitters are stored in the end of the axon, released and partly resorbed. Each of these processes can be influenced by drugs ($\rightarrow$ Physiology). Also many psychopharmacological drugs influence the synapses of certain neuron systems. Synapses are extremely sensitive parts of the neuron chain.

Neuropeptides and peptide hormones. According to recent studies, the "hypothalamic" peptide hormones, which form as neurohormones in the hypothalamus and are released into the blood in the median eminence and neural lobe of the hypophysis, also occur as *active substances in neurons* which project into other parts of the CNS. The same is true for the "adenohypophysial", the "gastro-intestinal" and the peptide hormones occurring in other organs. Conversely, the "hypothalamic" peptide hormones are regularly found in the gastro-entero-pancreatic system. Peptidergic neurons occur in large numbers also in the PNS, where they form, for example, an organ-specific intramural nervous system in the intestinal wall.

Forms of Neurons

The organization of the neuron into dendrites, perikaryon and axon is strongly *modified* in different neurons (Fig. **40**), resulting in characteristic nerve cell shapes which are seen most clearly in the outlines furnished by silvered preparations (Golgi pictures). The different forms of neurons occur regularly in certain recognized connections according to their function. Thus, neurons, whose axons or dendritic processes project into the peripheral nervous system, form a functional unit with the periphery.

Motor neurons (Fig. **40 b**) are usually distinguished by a strongly branched dendritic tree in the direct vicinity of the cell body and by a very long axon (e.g. pyramidal cell of the cerebral cortex, Purkinje cells of the cerebellar cortex). This is also true for the motor end segment of the neuron chain, the multipolar nerve cells of the spinal cord, the axon of which passes to muscle.

Neuromuscular unit. The axon of an individual anterior horn neuron of the spinal cord or a motor neuron of the brain always innervates several muscle fibers via collaterals. About 20 muscle fibers in the eye muscles are innervated in this way, about 300 in the gluteus maximus. The neuron and the muscle fibers dependent on it form a "neuromuscular (motor) unit"

Sensory Neurons (1st neuron of the afferent circuit; Fig. **40 c**) generally have a very long dendritic process which branches off in the periphery as telodendria, whereas the axon in many cases is short (e.g. pseudounipolar nerve cell, bipolar nerve cell).

Sensory unit. The area supplied by the ramifications of a single dendritic process, about $200 \, mm^2$ in the cornea of the eye, together with the neuron to which it belongs, forms a sensory unit. Adjacent supply regions can strongly overlap one another.

The designation "multipolar" or "pseudo-unipolar", customary for certain forms of neurons, characterizes the manner of branching of the nerve cell processes. In principle, each of these cells is bipolar.

b) Nerve Fiber

The *axon* of each nerve cell is covered by a sheath of glial cells (glial sheath) from its exit from the cell body to the target tissue; only the end of the axon remains uncovered.

In the CNS the glial sheath is formed by *central glia* (oligodendroglia), in the PNS by *peripheral glia* (cells of Schwann).

Because of its central position in the glial sheath, the axon is also termed the axis cylinder. *The axon and glial sheath (axon sheath) together form the nerve fiber.* Also the long *dendritic* process of the 1st neuron of the afferent circuit is surrounded by a glial sheath and therefore called *axon*. The glial

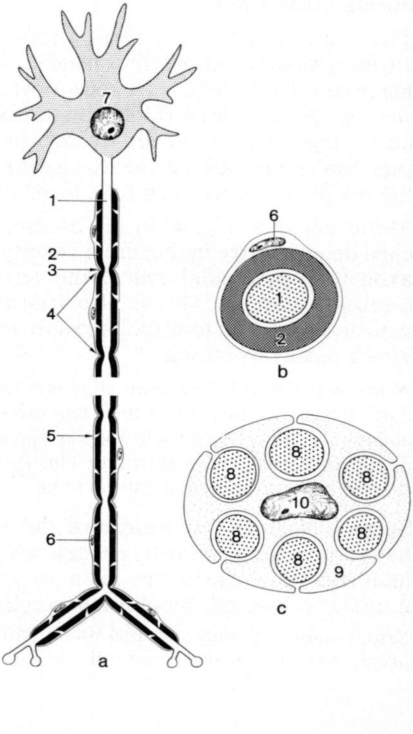

Fig. 43. **Peripheral nerve fiber**
a Longitudinal section
b Cross section through myelinated nerve fiber
c Cross section through nonmyelinated nerve fiber

1 Axon
2 Myelin sheath
3 Node of Ranvier
4 Internode
5 Schmidt-Lanterman's line
6 Cell nucleus of glial sheath (Schwann cell nucleus)
7 Cell body with dendrites
8 Axons
9 Glial sheath which forms no myelin and encloses several axons (only detectable with electron microscope)
10 Cell nucleus of glial sheath

sheath can surround the axon in two ways: as a medullated and as a nonmedullated glial sheath.

Medullated Nerve Fibers

The glial sheath can form a lipid-rich *medullary sheath* (*myelin sheath*) around the individual axon, giving rise to a *medullated* (*myelinated*) *nerve fiber* (Figs. **43 a, b**). The lipids of the sheath give a whitish appearance to the nerve fibers (e.g. white matter in the CNS). Depending on the thickness of the medullary sheath, *myelin-rich* A-nerve fibers and *myelin-poor* B-nerve fibers are distinguished.

The myelin sheath is interrupted at regular 0.2–1 mm long intervals by *nodes of Ranvier* and thus separated into *internodal segments.* The nodes are prerequisites for the saltatory conduction of stimuli (→ Physiology). The ratio of the diameter of the fibers to the length of the internode is about 1:100. The velocity of the conduction of the stimulus (conduction velocity) increases with the fiber diameter. Depending on the fiber diameter and the length of the internode, the conduction velocity amounts to 3–120 m/s.

Myelinated nerve fibers are divided into **fiber groups** of different calibers and conduction velocities (Table 1).

Nonmyelinated Nerve Fibers

The glial sheath in the PNS can enclose several axons at the same time, causing myelin formation to cease. A *myelin-free* (*nonmyelinated*) *nerve*

Table 1. Nerve Fiber Groups

Group	Nerve fiber cross section	Conduction velocity	Example
Myelinated nerve fibers			
Aα	10–20 µm	60–120 m/s	motor nerve fibers to skeletal muscle
β	7–10 µm	40–60 m/s	sensory nerve fibers from skin (touch perception)
γ	4–7 µm	30–40 m/s	motor nerve fibers to muscle spindles
δ	3–4 µm	15–30 m/s	sensory nerve fibers from skin (heat, cold, pain)
B	1–3 µm	3–15 m/s	preganglionic autonomic nerve fibers
Nonmyelinated nerve fibers			
C	0.3–1 µm	0.5–2 m/s	postganglionic autonomic nerve fibers

fiber is thus formed (Fig. **43 c**). In the CNS, nonmyelinated neurons frequently run in bundles between processes of the central glia (astrocytes). The conduction velocity in nonmyelinated nerve fibers amounts to less than 2 m/s Table **1**).

2. Structural Principles of the Nervous System

Knowledge concerning neuronal connections in the nervous system was acquired earlier mainly by investigations involving retrograde (ascending) degeneration, secondary (descending) degeneration and myelogenesis. Today, it is obtained through fluorescence microscopy, immunohistochemistry and the retrograde transport of marker substances in axons.

a) Neuron Chains and Neuron Circuits

Neurons are organized in the central nervous system (brain and spinal cord) and in the peripheral nervous system in *neuron chains* and *circuits* (Figs. **39** and **44**). Each link in a chain or circuit consists of a few up to ten thousands of similarly-directed neurons, whose dendrites and cell bodies are positioned together at a certain place and whose axons course together in the form of nerve fibers in definite pathways. Accumulations of perikarya and bundles of nerve fibers are to a great extent visible macroscopically as gray and white matter. The organization of the approximately one billion neurons determines the shape and inner structure of the nervous system.

Dendrites and axons, by means of which nerve cells contact each other and the target organs, represent an approximate total length of 300,000–400,000 km (the distance from the earth to the moon).

Gray and White Matter

In *sections* through the *brain* or *spinal cord*, reddish or gray-brown regions, the *gray matter*, can be distinguished from glistening white areas, the *white matter* (Fig. **45**).

The **gray matter,** *substantia grisea* (*griseum*), contains the *perikarya* and *dendrites* of (often many million) neurons. The cell bodies of the neurons, which represent the same chain segment within a neuronal chain, frequently lie distinctly separated from the perikarya which belong to another chain segment. Such a delimited accumulation of cell bodies of a definite neuron chain segment is called the *nucleus* (at particular places also *cortex*, *body*, etc.) Since excitations from other chains arrive at the dendrites of the perikarya of a nuclear region and since the axons which leave a nuclear region carry excitations to the perikarya of another chain, the *distribution of gray substance* in the brain section gives insight into the *approximate arrangement of the intermediate place* of the neuron chain.

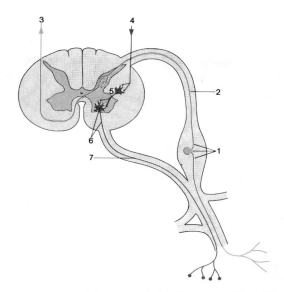

Fig. 44. **Connections of neuron chain in neuron circuit at spinal cord level.** Cross section through spinal cord, left spinal nerve with anterior and posterior roots

1 *Origin of neuron chain:* first afferent neuron
2 Axon of first afferent neuron which enters spinal cord with posterior root of spinal cord
3–5 *Links of neuron chain* in central nervous system
3 Second afferent neuron
4 Efferent neuron
5 Interneuron
6 *End of neuron chain:* last efferent neuron (final common motor path)
7 Axon of last efferent neuron which leaves spinal cord with anterior root of spinal cord

The **white matter,** *substantia alba* (*album*), often consists of many million bundles of *nerve fibers* which pass to and from the nuclear regions. Nerve fibers which have a common origin, course and target, form a *tract* or *fasciculus* (at certain points also called *fibers*, etc.).

The course of fibers of a tract can be demonstrated macroscopically with a spatula, especially after brief freezing to loosen the tissues.

Tracts from different nuclear regions frequently course long distances together. The individual tracts, their origins and their targets then cannot be easily marked off from one another. For this task, special methods of investigating neuronal connections are necessary. Numerous tracts carry antidromic (afferent and efferent) nerve fibers.

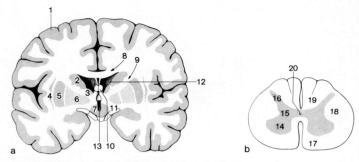

Fig. 45. **Distribution of gray and white matter in central nervous system**
a Frontal section through brain, section surface viewed from behind
b Cross section through spinal cord

1–7 *Gray matter of brain*	11 Optic tract (visual pathway)
1 Cerebrum	12 Lateral ventricle
2–6 *Subcortical nuclei*	13 3rd ventricle
2 Caudate nucleus	14–16 *Gray matter of spinal cord*
3 Thalamus	14 Anterior column (anterior horn)
4 Claustrum	15 Lateral column (lateral horn)
5 Putamen	16 Posterior column (posterior horn)
6 Globus pallidus	17–19 *White matter of spinal cord*
7 Hypothalamic nuclei	17 Anterior funiculus
8–11 *White matter of brain*	18 Lateral funiculus
8 Corpus callosum	19 Posterior funiculus
9 Inner capsule	20 Central canal
10 Fornix	

Ganglia and Nerves

As in the CNS, perikarya and nerve fibers in the *PNS* are also localized differently, but are strictly organized in a neuronal arrangement. Since the peripheral nervous system extends over a wide portion of the body, the distinction between perikarya and nerve fibers – gray and white matter – cannot be provided in a single section. Yet it becomes clear when the entire course of *nerves* and nerve roots is followed; at certain points they show node-like thickenings, *ganglia*.

Ganglia are millimeter- to centimeter-sized thickenings in nerves or nerve roots. *Like the nuclei of the CNS*, they are produced by accumulations of nerve cells (cell bodies) which migrate from the anlage of the nervous system (neural crest) during embryonic development and are colonized at the periphery. The ganglia of the peripheral nervous system are either *sensory ganglia* or *autonomic (motor) ganglia*.

The *sensory ganglia* (Fig. **46**) contain the cell bodies of sensory neurons (→ 1st neuron of the afferent circuit, pp. 105 and 132). *No synapses* are present on the perikarya of these *pseudo-unipolar nerve cells*; afferent

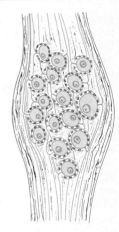

Fig. 46. **Sensory ganglion.** Contains cell bodies of sensory pseudo-unipolar neurons

excitation passes through the sensory ganglion *without synapsing*. Sensory ganglia are the spinal ganglia and the cranial nerve ganglia.

In the *autonomic ganglia* (*organ ganglia*, Fig. **47**), the perikarya and dendrites of autonomic neurons ($\rightarrow$ 2nd neuron of the efferent autonomic circuit, p. 131) are concentrated. At these ganglia, the axons of the 1st neuron of the efferent autonomic circuit ends with *synapses*. The efferent excitation is transferred to the next link in the chain. The autonomic

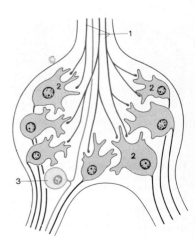

Fig. 47. **Autonomic ganglion**
1 Axons of first neuron of efferent autonomic circuit
2 Cell bodies of second neuron of efferent autonomic circuit
3 Cell body of sensory neuron

ganglia are the paravertebral ganglia of the sympathetic trunk, the prevertebral ganglia, the intramural ganglia and the autonomic ganglia of the cranial nerves.

In comparison with the tracts of the brain and spinal cord, **nerves** are *peripheral tracts.* Together with the blood vessels, they form "peripheral conduction pathways". In the nerves, bundles of nerve fibers are collected together. A nerve which carries sensory and motor nerve fibers or nerve fibers of different fiber groups is called a *mixed nerve. Pure motor* or *pure sensory* nerves contain predominantly motor or sensory nerve fibers. The different fiber portions branch off from the nerve at different places, thus changing the nerve's composition in its course to and from the (different) target organs.

The *nerve fibers* of a nerve are grouped by *connective tissue* (Fig. **48**). It is organized in a characteristic boxed system which – advancing from smaller to larger units – consists of three layers.

The **endoneurium** encloses the nerve fibers as a delicate connective tissue containing collagenous fibers, blood capillaries and lymphatic vessels. The tissue fluid in the endoneurial space comes (very probably) from the cerebrospinal fluid (→ p. 159).

The **perineurium,** as tense connective tissue, groups bundles of a few to several hundred nerve fibers into cables. As the *perineurial sheath,* it forms a barrier between the endoneurial and the epineurial space. Within the cable, the nerve fibers follow a spiral course so that a slight elongation of the nerve is possible without stretching the fibers (reserve length). In the

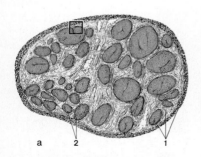
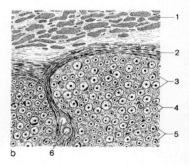

Fig. 48. **Connective tissue investments of peripheral nerves**
a Cross section through peripheral nerve
  Highly magnified section from a

1 Epineurium
2 Perineurium
3 Endoneurium
4 Myelinated nerve fibers

5 Schwann cell nuclei
6 Vein (upper) and artery in
  perineurium

brain and in the spinal cord, on the other hand, where the nerve fibers are not subjected to any stretching, they course in a straight manner.

The **epineurium** connects together the cables of nerve fibers enclosed by perineurium and attaches them to the surrounding tissues with loose, fibrous connective tissue. The individual cables can be isolated macroscopically from the epineurium. In the case of nerve distortion, the epineurium permits a shifting of the nerve fiber cable, but, like the perineurium, acts against any overstretching.

Nerve regeneration. Peripheral nerves can regenerate after severance. The prerequisite for functional recovery is that the connective tissue structures of the proximal and distal stumps are joined by a nerve suture. The axons growing out of the proximal stump reach the target organ in this way. Mitoses by neuroblasts are no longer observed in the human after birth; the number of nerve cells of the CNS no longer increases after birth.

b) Central and Peripheral Nervous System

The *reception of stimuli*, *processing* (*integration*) of excitation generated by the stimulus, and the *response* resulting from the processing play an extensive role in the activity of the nervous system. The reaction can occur on different levels corresponding to the organization of the nervous system.

Central Nervous System

The *site of integration* lies in the brain and spinal cord, in the *central nervous system*. By far the greatest mass of the CNS is involved in the correlation of activities of the locomotor apparatus. The representation of the remaining organ systems in the mass of the CNS, on the other hand, is slight, but vitally necessary.

The average weight of the brain in males (1434 g) is slightly greater than that in females (1306 g). The difference results from sex-specific variation in the development of the locomotor apparatus.

The *processing* of incoming excitations in the brain and spinal cord can occur at the following levels:
– at the lowest level as an *unconditioned (preformed) reflex*,
– at a higher level as a *conditioned (learned) reflex*, and
– at the highest level as a voluntary action.

Motor response is further characterized by *automatism*, *instinctive movements*, and *movements of expression*, which likewise can be caused by incoming excitations, but can also be formed spontaneously.

Unconditioned reflexes are *inborn*, i.e. a functionally preformed reflex arc exists. The unconditioned reflex is caused by an *adequate stimulus*. The functions of an organism are maintained by numerous unconditioned reflexes.

Conditioned reflexes (*those produced by conditioning*) must be learned individually, i.e. the reflex arc must be functionally developed. The conditioned reflex arises by *conditioning*, provided there is repeated *linkage of an adequate with an inadequate stimulus*. Conditioned reflexes play a role in the training and in the adjusting of an organism to its environment.

The function of the CNS is not solely to respond to incoming excitations; it also produces *spontaneous activities* which are determined genetically and which affect, for example, the locomotor apparatus.

Further, the activity of the human brain is capable of *mental accomplishments* (learning, memory, judgment, imagination, speech) which are not, or are not recognizably, connected with correlation and integration performances and which are usually designated as "higher functions" of the CNS. The anatomical bases of these performances are known only to a small degree.

Different inquiries into the functions of the nervous system have led to the development of *various methods* of investigating the nervous system in its widest sense and to *various disciplines*, of which the following are directly connected with the physician's work:

Psychology is concerned with "normal psychic-mental manifestations" in a preliminary "self-perception of a neurological process" (Jodl), although (as yet) the causes of these manifestations have not been adequately related to the structures and functions of the nervous system. *Behavioral research* operates on the basis of psychological and experimental approaches.

Psychiatry is aimed at the diagnosis and therapy of "abnormal psychic-mental manifestations" with the goal of restoring causal connections to (damaged) structures and (disturbed) functions of the nervous system. It succeeds to a limited degree with the help of *neurochemical, neurophysiological* and *neuropharmacological* research.

Neurology (including *neurosurgery*) is based on a largely established foundation of neuroanatomical and neurophysiological knowledge; neurological diagnosis is applied anatomy.

Peripheral Nervous System

Cranial and spinal nerves (Fig. 49). The CNS is connected with the rest of the body via 12 pairs of *cranial nerves* and 31 pairs of *spinal nerves. The sum of all nerves and their node-like ganglia* – accumulations of nerve cells, *ganglion cells* (perikarya) which migrate from the anlage of the nervous system into the periphery during embryonic development – form the *peripheral nervous system* (PNS).

Afferent and efferent nerve fibers (Fig. **50** and **51**). When the *stimulus* is taken up by receptors, it leads to an *excitation* which is conducted via *afferent nerve fibers* of sensory neurons (1st neuron of the afferent circuit) to the spinal cord or the brain. The processing (integration) in the CNS takes place in most cases with the assistance of additional neurons in the CNS.

At *switching stations*, further *circuits* can intervene from higher parts of the CNS. This is especially true for the *motor neurons*, the axons of which leave the CNS in order to pass to the target organs as "final common motor pathways." The neurons also receive, by means of *synapses*, excitations from control systems which influence (accelerate or inhibit) the excitations of the motor neurons.

The *response* is carried via *efferent nerve fibers* (axons of motor neurons) and then transmitted by effector structures (*synapses*) to the target organs (skeletal muscle fibers; through the interposition of autonomic ganglia also smooth muscle cells, cardiac muscle cells, secretory cells). Efferent nerve fibers leave the spinal cord as anterior roots; afferent nerve fibers enter as posterior roots. Both types of fibers, however, course together for long distances bundled as nerves.

Injuries to the excitatory conduction can appear *centrally* or *peripherally*. An injury to the efferent circuit is called (*motor*) *paralysis*; *paresis* is an incomplete *paralysis*. A partial injury of the afferent circuit leads to *hypesthesia*; a complete injury results in *anesthesia* (also called *sensory paresis*).

Somatic and visceral nerve fibers. The distinction between *somatic* and *visceral* nerve fibers (Fig. **52**) corresponds to the structural plan of the vertebrate body, but is *not* completely identical with the functional distinction between carriers of *somatic* and *vegetative functions* (→ somatic and autonomic nervous system, p. 120) which is commonly used in medicine (physiology).

Somatic nerve fibers connect the CNS with the body wall and the limbs, *visceral* nerve fibers (through the interposition of autonomic ganglia) with the viscera in the broadest sense (including smooth musculature and glands in all regions of the body). Whereas all spinal nerves are very similar, composed of somatic and visceral nerve fibers in approximately the same way, the cranial nerves differ greatly in this regard both from spinal nerves and from each other. *Somatic and visceral nerve fibers can be afferent or efferent fibers.*

The spinal nerves carry:
− *somatomotor* (efferent) nerve fibers, which always pass to the striated musculature of the body wall and limbs,

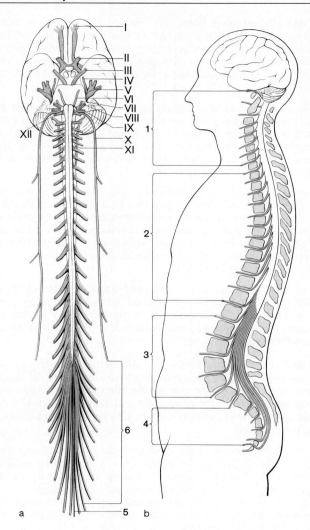

Fig. 49. **Cranial and spinal nerves**
a Ventral view
b View from left side, assignment of spinal nerves to specific segments of vertebral column

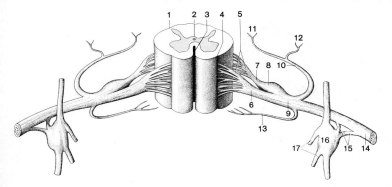

Fig. 50. **Spinal nerve segment, spinal cord segment** with pair of spinal nerves and their connections, ventral view

1 Dorsolateral sulcus (posterior root entrance)
2 Median dorsal sulcus
3 Median ventral fissure
4 Ventrolateral sulcus (anterior root exit)
5 Nerve rootlets
6 Ventral root
7 Dorsal root
8 Spinal ganglion
9 Spinal nerve
10 Dorsal ramus with medial (11) and lateral (12) rami
13 Meningeal ramus
14 Ventral ramus
15 Communicating rami
16 Ganglion of sympathetic trunk
17 Splanchnic nerves

– *somatosensory* (afferent) nerve fibers, which come from the skin or from the musculature (→ muscle and tendon spindles, pp. 136 ff.) of the body wall and limbs,
– *visceromotor* (efferent) nerve fibers, which (through the interposition of autonomic ganglia) pass to the smooth musculature of the viscera, to the blood vessels and glands, and – from the higher thoracic nerves – to the cardiac muscle, and
– *viscerosensory* (afferent) nerve fibers, which come from the viscera.

Concerning the proportions of visceral and somatic nerve fibers in the individual nerves → p. 143 f.

◀ I–XII   *Cranial nerves*
I   Olfactory nerves
II   Optic nerve
III   Oculomotor nerve
IV   Trochlear nerve
V   Trigeminal nerve
VI   Abducens nerve
VII   Facial nerve
VIII   Vestibulocochlear nerve
IX   Glossopharyngeal nerve
X   Vagus nerve
XI   Accessory nerve
XII   Hypoglossal nerve
1–4 *Spinal nerves*
1 Cervical nerves
2 Thoracic nerves
3 Lumbar nerves
4 Sacral nerves and coccygeal nerve
5 Filum terminale
6 Cauda equina = spinal nerve roots and filum terminale caudal to lumbar vertebrae 1–2

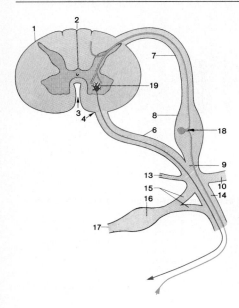

Fig. 51. **Spinal nerve segment,**
cross section through spinal cord,
left spinal nerve with anterior and
posterior roots
Simplest neuron chain between spinal cord and skeletal muscle.
1–17 Explanation of references → Fig. 50
18 Cell body of afferent neuron
19 Cell body of efferent neuron

Reflex Arc

The reflex arc – as an abstract simplification of the integrated activity of
the nerves – consists of the following "connected" structures, organized
as a serial chain and conducting the excitation from the receptor site via
the CNS to the effector tissue:

Receptor → *afferent neuron* (→ *central intermediate neuron*) *efferent
neuron* → *effector tissue.*

Receptor. A sensory cell carrying the receptor structure is called the
primary sensory cell, if it sends out an afferent axon. Thus it is the 1st
order neuron of the afferent circuit (example: sensory cells of the olfactory mucosa, visual cells of the retina). The *secondary sensory cell,* on the
other hand, possesses no axon. It is connected to the 1st neuron of the
afferent circuit, the dendrites of which are stimulated by the secondary
sensory cells (example: sensory cells of taste, balance and hearing organs).

Free nerve endings are the ends of dendrites of the 1st neuron of the
afferent circuit, which in numerous cases lie free and bare (without further
tissue investments) in the epithelium or in the connective tissue of the
inner or the outer body surfaces or in other places in a tissue (receptors
for mechanical, thermal or pain stimuli).

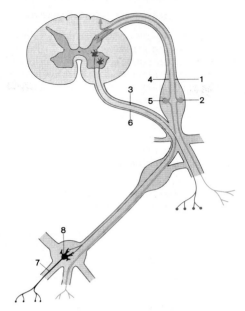

Fig. 52. **Neuronal organization of somatic and visceral nerve fibers in spinal nerves,** cross section through spinal cord, left spinal nerve with anterior and posterior roots, as well as communicating rami and splanchnic nerves

1 Somatosensory neuron (first neuron of afferent circuit)
2 Cell body in spinal ganglion
3 Somatomotor neuron ("motor neuron", "final common motor path")
4 Viscerosensory neuron
5 Cell body in spinal ganglion

6 First visceromotor neuron (preganglionic visceromotor nerve fiber)
7 Second visceromotor neuron (postganglionic visceromotor nerve fiber)
8 Cell body in prevertebral, autonomic ganglion

A *sense organ* is made up of (primary or secondary) sensory cells, or the dendritic endings of the 1st neuron of the afferent circuit, united with other tissue constituents serving for the reception of stimuli (touch corpuscles, muscle and tendon spindles, eye). Secondary sensory cells are always integrated into a sense organ (e.g. hearing and balance organs, taste buds).

Effector. The effector synapses are formed according to the principles described on p. 102. However, they exhibit individual differences (e.g. myoneural synapses, neuroglandular synapses) depending on the type of target tissue.

Muscle reflex → p. 136, visceral reflex → p. 152.

c) Somatic and Autonomic Nervous System

The performance of the nervous system is directed both to the outside and to the inside of the organism. By means of the nervous system, the organism is in (passive and active) communication with its environment. It synchronizes the performances of the individual organ systems with one another, and adjusts them to the changing demands of the organism. In medicine, therefore, a *somatic nervous system* (*environmental nervous system*) and an *autonomic nervous system* (*visceral nervous system*) are generally distinguished. The *somatic nervous system* controls the relations of the organism to its environment; it is an *ecotropic relation system*. The *autonomic nervous system* regulates the internal operation of the organism; it is an *idiotropic regulation system*.

General experience seems to show that the performance of the nervous system in the somatic area extends deeply into consciousness, while those in the autonomic area occur unconsciously. But this viewpoint is a gross generalization which is not tenable.

The concept "autonomic nervous system" is used to varying extents in the narrower definition, it refers to the peripheral nervous system, whereas in the broader one, it also includes the relevant nuclei and tracts of the CNS.

If the concept of somatic and autonomic nervous system in reference to the groups of nerve cells and nerve fibers is firmly established in the structural plan, the following conformities result.

In the **spinal nerves**, the *somatic* nerve fibers represent the *somatic* nervous system, and the *visceral* nerve fibers represent the *autonomic* nervous system.

Afferent somatic (somatosensory) nerve fibers come from the skin and musculature of the body wall and limbs, *afferent autonomic* (viscerosensory) fibers from the viscera. *Efferent somatic* (somatomotor) nerve fibers always pass only to the striated musculature of the body wall and limbs, *efferent autonomic* (visceromotor) fibers to the smooth musculature of the viscera and the blood vessels, as well as to glands and cardiac muscle.

In the **cranial nerves**, on the other hand, the two pairs of concepts are *not identical*. It has been established embryologically that in the head and neck region *derivatives of visceral anlagen* are involved in *communicating with the environment*. Viscerosensory fibers mediate here not only (unconscious) excitations from the viscera, but – in the case of taste fibers – also conscious sensitiveness. And visceromotor fibers convey not only (unconscious) excitations to the smooth musculature of the viscera and to glands, but, in the case of cranial nerves V, VII, IX, X and XI also conscious motor responses (without the interposition of a 2nd efferent neuron) to striated (pharyngeal arch) musculature (→ branchial nerves, p. 141).

Afferent somatic nerve fibers of the cranial nerves come from all "special" (so-called higher) sense organs, *afferent autonomic* fibers form the viscera. *Efferent somatic* nerve fibers pass to (voluntarily innervated) striated muscles of the head and neck organs (extrinsic eye muscles, facial, pharyngeal and laryngeal muscula-ture, trapezius, sternocleidomastoid) whereas *efferent autonomic* fibers (with the interposition of a 2nd efferent neuron) innervate smooth muscle.

The "two nervous systems" are partial aspects of a single nervous system, both "parts" co-operating closely in the periphery, and even more so in the central organ. An exact demarcation is possible only in places. In spite of these considerations, it is expedient for didactic reasons to distinguish between "somatic" and "autonomic" nervous systems at appropriate places.

d) Sense Organs

In *sense organs*, the *receptors*, i.e. the receptor cells or the dendritic endings of the 1st afferent neuron, are assembled *together with portions of other tissues* – auxiliary arrangements which serve for the reception of the stimuli – *to form an organ*.

The *receptors* of individual sense organs are more sensitive toward *certain* stimuli (forms of energy), namely toward *adequate* stimuli, (possessing a lower threshold) than toward other stimuli. But other, inadequate stimuli can also generate an impulse in a receptor. The *perception* arising *is specific*, i.e. of the same type as that produced by an adequate stimulus ($\rightarrow$ Physiology).

This phenomenon, called the "law of specific sensory energy" (Johannes Müller), results not from the receptor, but from the specific region of the brain activated by the afferents. Stimuli of the afferent tracts occurring at any level and of the specific brain region would produce a specific perception. For example, light perception can be elicited by strong pressure on the eye.

Receptors and auxiliary contrivances are specialized for specific stimuli in the individual sense organs, but *a classification of sense organs according to sensory modalities is not combined in like manner with a functional division of receptors contained in them*. For example, cutaneous sense organs (pressure and touch organs) and the ear (organ of hearing) possess mechanoreceptors, whereas taste buds and glomus bodies (for measuring the oxygen partial pressure in the blood) have chemoreceptors. There is, therefore, no entirely satisfactory classification of sense organs.

Cutaneous sense organs perceive pressure and touch, stimuli that come directly from the external environment. Their receptors are therefore called *exteroceptors*. Cutaneous organs are microscopically small, up to a millimeter in size, round or oval bodies. The receptors for cold and heat, on the other hand, are (probably) free nerve endings which also mediate experiences of pain.

Sense organs of deep sensitivities, located in muscles, tendons, and joint capsules, are excited by stretching stimuli from the locomotor apparatus itself, their receptors therefore being designated as *proprioceptors*. Muscle spindles and Golgi tendon organs are classified with these sense organs.

Different types of structures are grouped as **organs of visceral sensitivity**; their receptors are called *interoceptors* (*visceroceptors*) and are differentiated according to their specialization.

Lamellar corpuscles, microscopically small or millimeter-sized, perceive pressure or gravity in the milieu of the viscera and great vessels; they possess *pressoreceptors*, or *baroreceptors*. Plexus-like, *free nerve endings* in the lungs, in the wall of large vessels and in parts of the heart wall have greater significance as pressoreceptors.

Glomus bodies (*carotid body, para-aortic bodies*), pea-sized organs, measure the O_2-partial pressure of the blood; they possess *chemoreceptors*.

Additional *interoceptors*, which measure the blood temperature in the head, the pH of cerebrospinal fluid (brain fluid), the osmotic pressure of the blood plasma and the arteriovenous blood sugar differential, lie, according to physiological studies, *in the brain itself*; the measuring structures are central neurons of specific regions of the brain.

The visual, auditory, olfactory, gustatory and vestibular organs are grouped as **special** or *higher* **sense organs** ($\rightarrow$ vol. 2). Visual, auditory and olfactory organs are called *teleceptors* because they perceive distant processes. Olfactory and gustatory organs possess *chemoreceptors*, whereas the auditory and vestibular organs contain *mechanoreceptors*.

The *eye* is a visual organ, the *ear* a hearing organ, the *nasal mucosa* in the upper region of the nasal cavity an olfactory organ. The *taste buds* in the papillae at the back and base of the tongue together form the gustatory organ. *Semicircular ducts*, *utriculus* and *sacculus* – formations of the labyrinth of the inner ear – are vestibular organs that measure angular or linear acceleration of the head.

B. Structural Plan of the Nervous System

1. Brain and Spinal Cord

The organization of the central nervous system becomes understandable from the embryonic and fetal development of the organ (Fig. **53**). From the expanded *cephalic region* of the neural tube the *forebrain* (*prosencephalon*) and the *hindbrain* (*rhombencephalon*) develop. In their mutual overlapping region the *midbrain* (*mesencephalon*) develops. The *spinal cord* originates from the neural tube in the *trunk region*. The organization of the brain proceeds with a segmentation of the cavity of the brain primordium into the *ventricular system*.

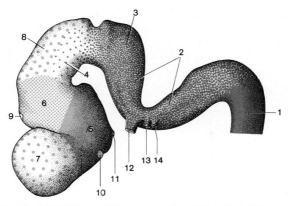

Fig. 53. **Brain anlage in 12.84 mm C.R. human embryo** (after *Hochstetter*)
The primordia of gray matter of individual parts of brain are shown in different colors
(→ Figs. 54–56)

▨ Derivatives of rhombencephalon
▨ Derivatives of prosencephalon

1 Medulla oblongata (myelencephalon)
2 Pons (metencephalon) with cerebellar
  anlage (3)
4 Mesencephalon
5, 6 *Diencephalon*
5 Hypothalamus
6 Thalamus
7 Telencephalon

8 Mesencephalic tectum
9 Anlage of epiphysis
10 Optic stalk
11 Infundibulum
12 Trigeminal nerve
13 Facial nerve
14 Vestibulocochlear nerve

The **spinal cord** (*medulla spinalis*) is the most simply structured part of the
CNS. As a reflex organ, it is connected with the trunk wall and limbs, as
well as with the trunk viscera by means of spinal nerves and, at the same
time, is under the influence of the regulatory parts of the CNS.

The *gray matter* (Fig. **54**) lies centrally in the entire extent of the spinal
cord, surrounds the narrow *central canal* and is organized into *spinal
nuclei*. They contain, among other things, the perikarya of *root cells*,
whose axons form the efferent circuits of the spinal nerves. A cross-
section of the spinal cord has the same form in principle at all levels.
In section, the gray matter has the shape of a letter H or a butterfly in
which anterior, lateral and posterior horns are distinguished on each side.

The *white matter* surrounds the gray matter and contains the connections
to and from higher centers of the CNS: posterior ascending, lateral and
anterior ascending and descending tracts.

The **hindbrain** (*rhombencephalon*, Figs. **54–56**) is the cranial continuation
of the spinal cord and consists of the **medulla oblongata** (*myelencephalon*)

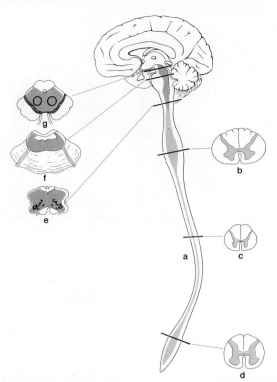

Fig. 54. **Distribution of gray matter in spinal cord ☐ and in tegmentum of brain stem ▦**

a Sagittal section through brain and spinal cord. View from left side
b–g Cross sections through brain stem and
spinal cord
b Cervical enlargement of spinal cord

c Thoracic level of spinal cord
d Lumbosacral swelling
e Medulla oblongata (myelencephalon)
f Pons (metencephalon)
g Mesencephalon

and **pons** (*metencephalon*). Like the spinal cord, it is traversed in its entire length by central gray matter, the *tegmentum* of the rhombencephalon.

The *tegmentum* of the rhombencephalon lies in the *medulla oblongata* and in the *dorsal part of the pons* [*tegmentum pontis*]. It is continued into the tegmentum of the midbrain [*mesencephalic tegmentum*] and contains the *nuclear regions of the cranial nerves* and the greatest part of its *own apparatus*, the *reticular formation*.

The *reticular formation* connects the highly specialized cranial nerve nuclei in a complicated way. By means of the reticular formation, for

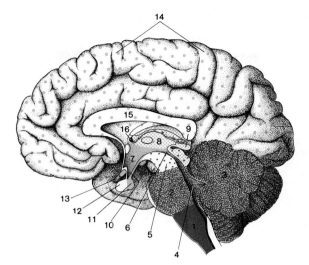

Fig. 55 **Median sagittal section through brain,** view from left side

■ Derivatives of rhombencephalon
▨ Derivatives of prosencephalon
(→ Figs. 53 and 54)

1 Medulla oblongata (myelencephalon)
2 Pons (metencephalon) with cerebellum (3)
4 4th ventricle
5 Mesencephalon
6 Mesencephalic aqueduct
7–11 *Diencephalon*
7 Hypothalamus and thalamus (8) as wall of 3rd ventricle
9 Pineal body (epithalamus)

10 Infundibulum
11 Neurohypophysis
12 Adenohypophysis
13 Optic nerve
14 Telencephalon
15 Corpus callosum
16 Interventricular foramen between 3rd ventricle and lateral ventricle

example, afferent excitations of the largely sensory trigeminal nucleus (→ p. 144) can trigger efferent excitations via purely motor cranial nerve nuclei, e.g. via the nuclei of the nerves to the extrinsic eye muscles (→ p. 141), which possess no afferent circuit themselves. These and many other connections of the reticular formation linking the cranial nerve nuclei make functions involving the entire organism possible.

The individual nuclear regions of the reticular formation, not always exactly distinguishable from one another, coordinate the functions of nerves active in the regulation of respiration, heart frequency and blood pressure, as well as other autonomic activities. Physiologists, therefore, call the parts of the reticular formation: *inspiration center, expiration center, circulatory center,* etc. *Descending* fibers from the reticular formation pass to the *spinal cord* (e.g. for the regulation of respiration, in which the diaphragm and the thoracic and abdominal muscles are

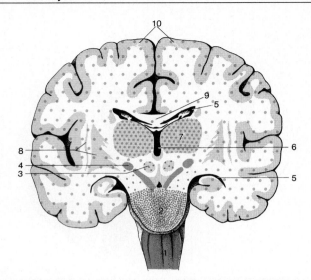

Fig. 56. **Frontal section through brain,** view of section surface from front

▨   Derivatives of rhombencephalon

▨   Derivatives of prosencephalon

(→ Figs 53 and 54)

1 Medulla oblongata (myelencephalon)
2 Pons (metencephalon)
3 Red nucleus
4 Subthalamic nucleus
5 Lateral ventricfe

6 3rd ventricle
7 Thalamus
8 basal ganglia
9 Corpus callosum
10 Cerebral cortex

also active) through a tract coursing downward in the anterior funiculus. *Ascending* fibers connect the reticular formation partly with the higher-placed autonomic nuclear regions in the *hypothalamus,* partly with the *cerebral cortex,* so that impulses caused by sensory impressions can intervene in the performance of the reticular formation and its "centers". On the other hand, fibers ascending to the cerebral cortex from the reticular formation influence the state of consciousness; their excitations increase attentiveness.

In the different parts of the rhombencephalon (medulla oblongata, pons), structures lie on and within the tegmentum which, for the most part, are associated with the strong development of the cerebrum and which give the brain parts their characteristic shape.

Long descending fiber bundles, the *pyramidal tract,* a voluntary motor system pathway, accumulate in front of the *medulla oblongata*; their fibers cross in the medulla oblongata, mostly to the opposite side. Ascending bundles of fibers pass laterally and posteriorly. The medulla oblongata extends up to the level of the lower part of the *4th ventricle.*

The *pons* encloses the rostral part of the rhomboid-shaped *4th ventricle.* The tegmentum is covered ventrally in the region of the pons by the *pontine fiber bundles* and dorsally by the *cerebellum.*

As *pontine fiber bundles* (*pars ventralis pontis*), the thick bundles form a bulge and connect the cerebrum with the cerebellum via nuclear regions within these bundles.

The *cerebellum* is an important *coordination organ of the motor system.* It receives on both sides three cerebellar peduncles, the thickest of which comes from the ventral part of the pons, which provide continuous *advance information* from different regions of the brain concerning coordinated movements. The cerebellum "compares" these regularly with *previous information* from the locomotor apparatus and vestibular organs and intervenes as a stabilizing regulatory system correcting and adjusting the coordinated movements. It influences muscle tonus and the temporal sequence of movements. In cooperation with the labyrinth organ of the inner ear, it provides for the maintenance of equilibrium.

The **midbrain** (*mesencephalon*) is located in the border region between the hindbrain and forebrain (diencephalon). It contains, as part of the ventricle, a thin tube, the *aqueduct* (*mesencephalic aqueduct*), which connects the 3rd and 4th ventricles. In the *mesencephalic tegmentum,* the rostral continuation of the pontine tegmentum, lies the cylindrical *red nucleus,* in which numerous excitations converge which influence motor response and which progress ultimately to the spinal cord in descending tracts.

Thick descending tracts lie basally close to the tegmentum of the midbrain as cerebral peduncles. One part of them, the pyramidal tract, becomes visible again after traversing the pons at the anterior side of the medulla oblongata; another part passes to the cerebellum. Between the cerebral peduncles and the tegmentum, on both sides, the dark-colored *black nucleus* (*substantia nigra*) is inserted in a cup-shaped fashion, a nuclear region of the involuntary motor system (→ p. 128) that is connected with the cerebral cortex. Laterally, in the tegmentum of the midbrain, thick ascending tracts are present, whereas posterior to it the roof of the midbrain is spread out as the lamina quadrigemina – reflex centers of the auditory and visual pathways that influence motor responses.

Anatomical nomenclature groups the rhombencephalon and mesencephalon as the **brain stem** (*encephalic trunk*). Because of their close functional connection, however, the basal ganglia, and often also the diencephalon, the telencephalon and the basal part of the rhinencephalon, are included in the brain stem in clinical colloquial usage.

The **forebrain** (*prosencephalon*, Figs. **55** and **56**), which follows the rhombencephalon rostrally, consists of the *diencephalon* and *telencephalon*. No cranial nerve nuclei reside in the forebrain (on the special position of the 1st and 2nd cranial nerves, → pp. 140 and 141).

The **diencephalon** encloses the *3rd ventricle*. It consists of the following parts of the brain, some of which are powerfully developed: the *thalamus*, an upper group of nuclei, contains *synapses* for long antidromic (ascending and descending) tracts to the cerebral cortex and to other nuclear regions of the telencephalon, as well as to the hypothalamus. With the exception of a portion of the temporal lobe, all areas of the cerebral cortex connect antidromically with thalamic nuclei.

The *epithalamus* with the *pineal body* (epiphysis), an endocrine gland, is attached to the thalamus posterosuperiorly.

The *hypothalamus*, the lower group of nuclei, contains *higher-order nuclear regions for autonomic functions*.

Vitally important *visceral motor* (autonomic) functions, connected with the intake of food, secretion, reproduction and affective defense, are coupled functionally with somatic motor performance through the posterior hypothalamic nuclei; the hypothalamus contains centers for sleep, hunger and sexual functions. Special hypothalamic cell groups indirectly regulate the activity of most lower-order glands (→ Vol. 2, Hypothalamus) by *influencing the higher-order endocrine gland*, the adenohypophysis. Another group of nuclei of the hypothalamus *directly releases hormones* which regulate water balance and stimulate the smooth musculature of some organs.

The *optic nerve*, the 2nd cranial "nerve", also belongs to the diencephalon in terms of its origin. The optic nerve is, in reality, not a peripheral nerve, but a part of the visual pathway displaced to the periphery (receptors → Vol. 2, Retina); in the posterior part of the group of thalamic nuclei, in the *metathalamus*, it possesses a nuclear region from which a thick fasciculus of fibers ascends to the cerebral cortex.

The *globus pallidus*, a lateral nucleus of the diencephalon, lies in the vicinity of, and in functional relation to, the extensive "subcortical" areas, i.e. nuclear regions of the *telencephalon* lying below the cerebral cortex which proceed from the ganglionic hillock of the telencephalon. In this way the strongly developed *basal ganglia* originate – synapses of voluminous neuron chains, in which parts of the cerebral cortex are also included and which serve the motor system.

By means of the basal ganglia, voluntary movements are organized into coordinated movement sequences, adjusted in time and space to the total situation and provided with accessory movements, including expressive movements (facial expression). In the execution of learned movements, the decisive task is probably carried out by the basal ganglia.

Injuries to one of the neuron circuits in which the basal ganglia participate always leads to a disturbance of the total motor system – including the movements (facial expression, speech) controlled by cranial nerves. The injury frequently involves the inhibiting neuron circuit, resulting in uncoordinated, exaggerated movements, e.g. St. Vitus's dance (chorea).

The **end-brain** (*telencephalon*) consists of right and left *cerebral hemispheres* and unpaired, connecting parts. Each hemisphere contains a *lateral ventricle*. Its gray matter is organized into the *pallium* and into the *basal ganglia* (*basal nuclei*) located in the interior. At the base of the cerebral hemispheres lie parts of the *smell-brain* (rhinencephalon), which is rudimentary in humans.

The *olfactory nerves*, together called the "1st cranial nerve", are bundled axons of the primary sensory cells of the olfactory mucosa (organ of smell). They pass to the primary olfactory center at the base of the cerebral hemisphere and enter the *olfactory bulb* as nonmyelinated nerve fibers.

The **cerebrum** includes the *cerebral cortex*, which is very strongly developed in humans, and its connections; it covers the entire brain stem. The mass of fibers communicating with the cerebral cortex also lend a typically "human" appearance to other parts of the brain, e.g. the pons.

Cerebral cortex (*telencephalic cortex*). In the cerebrum and cerebellum, nerve cells which migrate to the surface of the brain during embryonic development form a closed covering of gray matter, a *"cortex"*. The surface of the cerebrum, greatly enlarged by gyri and sulci, is occupied by the cerebral cortex. Its differentiation is completed only after birth.

The cerebrum is the higher *organ of integration* for the brain stem and spinal cord. The performance of the cerebrum, however, depends upon a close cooperation with all parts of the nervous system.

An intact structure of the cerebral cortex is a prerequisite, on the one hand, for stimuli received by sense organs to enter *consciousness*, be recorded in *memory*, and to be *recalled*; on the other hand, it makes a *conscious motor response* in the broadest sense possible. In neuropathological experience, the sensory qualities taken up by the individual sense organs can be associated with individual cortical regions. Within such regions, distinction is made between *projection fields*, which primarily receive afferents, and *association fields*, the efferents of which arrive at other cortical regions and/or deeper nuclear regions. Large areas of the cortex are concerned with speech and writing comprehension and with speaking and writing; these abilities are localized in the left cerebral hemisphere. There is insufficient knowledge about the function of numerous regions of the cerebral cortex.

Many *disturbances of communication* have been registered in neurology, which are caused by injury to individual fields in the cerebral cortex and which can be grouped under three headings. In *aphasia*, the significance of the spoken or written word is no longer recognized, although the functioning of the sense organs is maintained. *Agnosia* refers to a condition in which the person affected is unable to recognize an object from the stimuli (touch, vision) transmitted to him by a sense organ. In *apraxia*, there is an inability to carry out significant purposeful movements, although the motor system is fully intact. The disturbances subsumed under these headings are interrelated in many ways, and an abundance of symptoms results from them.

2. Connections between the Central Nervous System and the Peripheral Nervous System

a) Organization of the Peripheral Nervous System connected to the Spinal Cord

The spinal cord and spinal nerves are closely related to the segments of the vertebral column and the trunk wall (Fig. **49**). *Spinal cord segments* are therefore distinguishable and are divided into the *cervical, thoracic, lumbar* and *sacral* regions of the spinal cord. However, spinal cord segments and vertebral segments do not correspond in level (Fig. **49 b**).

For the *identification of a spinal nerve* and the spinal cord segment belonging to it, abbreviations of the vertebral segment in which the spinal nerve exits through the intervertebral foramen and the number of the nerve are employed, e.g. C1, T2, L3, etc. For approximate orientation, the designations *cervical, thoracic, lumbar* and *sacral nerves* are used.

The *spinal cord* is connected with the trunk wall, upper and lower limbs and with the thoracic, abdominal and pelvic viscera (→ sympathetic trunk, p. 146ff.) by 31 pairs of *spinal nerves*. Each spinal nerve originates in the intervertebral foramen from an *anterior (motor)* and a *posterior (sensory) root;* the posterior root contains the rice-grain-sized, sensory *spinal ganglion* close to the spinal nerve (Figs. **50** and **51**).

Anterior Root of the Spinal Nerve

The *anterior (ventral) root* is formed by the axons of the **root cells** which are the efferent neurons of the spinal nerves. Somatomotor and visceromotor (autonomic) root cells are distinguishable (Fig. **52**).

The *somatomotor root cells* (multipolar cells) are the largest cells of the spinal cord; they lie in groups in the anterior horn. Each nerve cell group corresponds to specific muscles of the locomotor apparatus.

The spinal cord possesses about 1/2 million somatomotor root cells (*motor neurons*). This relatively small number of nerve cells is acted upon by many millions of higher-order neuron chains of the CNS ($\rightarrow$ convergence principle, p. 102). The *axons* of the somatomotor root cells therefore form the *"final common motor pathway"* for all excitations entering the relevant posterior root from higher nuclear regions. The "final common motor path" – the *efferent segment of the somatic nervous system* – consists, therefore, with regard to its neuronal organization of *a single neuron*.

Visceromotor (autonomic) root cells. In the autonomic root cells, two groups are distinguished: *sympathetic* and *parasympathetic root cells* (Fig. **64**), designations based on colloquial usage derived from the neurons in the autonomic ganglion innervated by them.

The *efferent pathway of the autonomic nervous system,* in contrast to that of the somatic system, is formed by *two neurons*. The visceromotor (autonomic) root cells are the 1st neuron; the perikaryon of the 2nd neuron lies in the autonomic ganglion (*organ ganglion*) at the periphery. The nerve fibers of the 1st neuron, therefore, are also called *preganglionic fibers*.

The *sympathetic root cells* (multipolar nerve cells) lie in the lateral horn of the thoracic and lumbar segments of the spinal cord (C8–L2, 3). In these segments the lateral horn is strongly developed. The axons of the sympathetic cells pass to the spinal nerves with the *anterior root*. In the *rami communicantes,* which connect the spinal nerve with the sympathetic trunk, they arrive at the segmental *sympathetic trunk ganglia* on both sides of the vertebral column in front of the heads of the ribs. For the further course of these fibers $\rightarrow$ postganglionic nerve fibers, p. 148.

The *parasympathetic root cells* lie in the sacral (S2–4) region of the spinal cord medial to the lateral horn. The cells are multipolar; their axons leave the spinal cord with the ventral root. They form the *pelvic splanchnic nerves* and innervate the pelvic viscera at the junction of the innervation region of the parasympathetic vagus nerve.

The remaining spinal cord segments also contain root cells, which are counted as parasympathetics by some authors in view of the behavior of the 2nd neuron (cholinergic neuron) innervated by them, although they and their 2nd neuron are contained in the fiber mass and the ganglia of the sympathetic trunk. The autonomic efferents reach the trunk wall and the extremities. This part of the autonomic nervous system is also called the *"system of segmental autonomic fibers"* because of its strictly segmental extension. For the further course of these fibers $\rightarrow$ segmental autonomic nerve fibers, p. 150.

In contrast to the root cells, the axons of the **interneurons** (intercalated, internuncial, and cells of the *intrinsic apparatus*) remain in the CNS. Interneurons are the second neuron of the afferent circuit. The perikarya of these cells lie in the nucleus of the posterior horn; their bundled axons course in the spinal cord funiculi as ascending conduction tracts.

Posterior Root of the Spinal Nerve

The *posterior* (*dorsal*) *root* consists, for the most part, of the bundled axons of *sensory pseudo-unipolar nerve cells*, the perikarya of which comprise the *spinal ganglion*. Among them are *somatosensory* and *viscerosensory* nerve cells – the *first neuron of the afferent circuit* (Figs. **51** and **52**).

The *somatosensory nerve cells* carry excitations from the skin and the receptors of the musculature (→ muscle spindles, tendon spindles, p. 136 f.) of the body wall and limbs to the perikarya of the 2nd neuron in the spinal cord and medulla oblongata. With respect to its neuronal arrangement, the *afferent segment of the somatic nervous system* consists, like the efferent, of a *single neuron*. Altogether about 2 million nerve fibers enter the spinal cord through the posterior roots of the spinal nerves.

The *viscerosensory nerve cells* carry excitations from receptors in the viscera and blood vessels. The *afferent segment of the autonomic nervous system* – in contrast to the efferent – is also formed from a *single neuron*. The afferent nerve fibers course in the sympathetic branches to the spinal nerves, the perikarya lying (usually) in the spinal ganglion, the axons likewise passing via the posterior root to the 2nd neuron in the spinal cord.

The *spinal ganglion*, a sensory ganglion, is part of the posterior root of each spinal nerve shortly before its junction with the anterior root. It is enclosed by a meningeal sheath rich in collagenous fibers (→ spinal cord meninges, pp. 153 ff.).

Spinal Nerve

The *spinal nerve formed in the intervertebral foramen from the union of dorsal and ventral roots* is mixed (sensory-motor) and about 1 cm long. Immediately after passing through the foramen, the short nerve trunk divides into four unequally thick *branches* (*rami*, Figs. **50–52**).

The sensory *meningeal ramus*, a small branch, courses back into the vertebral canal to the spinal meninges.

The mixed *posterior branch* (*dorsal ramus*) supplies the skin for about a hand's breadth alongside the vertebral column, as well as the autochthonous trunk musculature.

The mixed *anterior branch* (*ventral ramus*) innervates the remaining skin and the musculature of the trunk wall or, by means of a plexus, the limbs, as well as the skin and several muscles of the neck.

The *rami communicantes*, postganglionic and sensory sympathetic fibers, in segments C8-L2, 3 also preganglionic sympathetic fibers (→ p. 131), connect the spinal nerve with the sympathetic trunk. The preganglionic sympathetic fibers pass from the spinal nerve into the sympathetic trunk, the postganglionic fibers pass back into the spinal nerve from the sympathetic trunk.

Segmental Innervation

The human body wall, like that of all vertebrates, is constructed *segmentally* (→ metamerism of the body wall, p. 12), the original *metamerism* being still partially preserved by the autochthonous muscles of the trunk and thorax (intercostal muscles). The *dorsal branches of all spinal nerves* and the *ventral branches of thoracic spinal nerves* (T2–12) likewise retain the segmental form of innervation and within these regions of innervation, the musculature and adjacent skin have the same segmental relationship – with the reservation that the areas of cutaneous innervation overlap.

Segmental innervation of the skin (Fig. 57). The course of a (uni)segmental cutaneous nerve can only be followed in dissection up to the subcutaneous connective tissue. Clinical experience provides information concerning the structure in the skin itself. According to this, *adjacent*

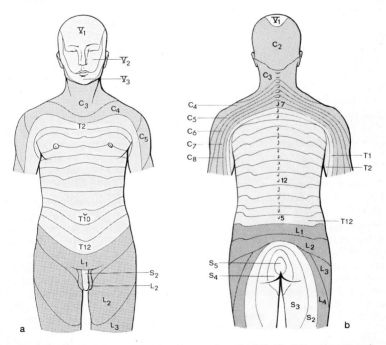

Fig. 57. **Segmental relations of fields of innervation of adult skin** (after *Hansen* and *Schliack*)
a Anterior view
b Posterior view

segments (following one another craniocaudad) overlap. One segment overlaps up to one-half of the neighboring segment – a cutaneous segment is thus always innervated by three adjacent nerves, of which the middle one provides the greatest number of nerve fibers for "its" segment. Only touch and temperature fibers take part in this overlapping, however, not the pain fibers. "Head's zones" (→ p. 153) are therefore also confined to one segment. Moreover, the spread of a segmental nerve rarely shows a purely belt-like form. On the contrary, it is characterized by variable wave-like processes on both sides.

The *demarcation* of cutaneous segments (*dermatomes*) and their relation to specific spinal nerves cannot be sufficiently clarified in anatomically-dissected preparations. This is due to the overlapping of adjacent segments in the region of the finest ramifications, in which the various sensory qualities participate to different degrees. Divergent data concerning the boundaries of dermatomes are based on *clinical observations* (disturbed functions after transverse lesions of the spinal cord, herniae of intervertebral discs, shingles, segmental nevi, etc.) which are not completely uniform. This is true, above all, of the *hiatus* between the cervical and thoracic segments.

The failure of a single sensory root, a *"monoradicular disturbance"*, is diagnosed by *examination of the sense of pain* (pinching), since the pain zones do not overlap adjacent segments. Loss of the sensation of touch in a segment is always based upon a disturbance in more than one segment, due to the overlapping of the touch zones.

Shingles (herpes zoster), produced by a virus-induced inflammation of a spinal ganglion, clearly displays a cutaneous segment through the painful reddening of the skin and the formation of blisters.

Plexus Formation

During embryonic development – chiefly in the region of the anlage of the limbs – segmental muscle primordia are newly organized in localized regions of the ventrolateral body wall by division and polymerization; new individual muscles arise. At the same time, the parts of the nerve fibers of spnal nerves connected at an early point with the muscle anlagen are accordingly redistributed. The original metamerism is thereby lost. A newly formed individual muscle collects nerve fibers from several segments, one segment giving nerve fibers to several individual muscles. The combined interlacing of nerve fibers from several segments and their composition into individual peripheral nerves is called *plexus formation* (Fig. 58). Since the limbs originate in the ventrolateral region of the body wall, *only the ventral branches* of the spinal nerves lying in the area of the limbs are involved, not the dorsal. In the region of the plexus innervation, the segmental relationships of the musculature and covering skin no longer coincide.

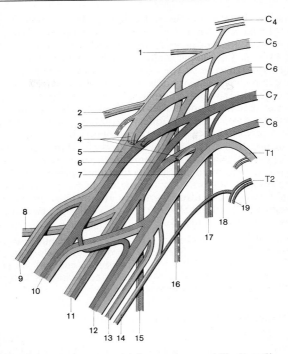

Fig. 58. **Plexus formation** (brachial plexus) (after *von Lanz* and *Wachsmuth*).
The distribution of individual spinal nerves in the composition of a nerve plexus is made
evident by color-coding the nerves

1, 2 *Short dorsal branches of plexus*
1 Dorsal scapular nerve
2 Suprascapular nerve
3, 4 *Short ventral branches of plexus*
3 Nerve to subclavius
4 Pectoral nerves
5 Lateral cord
6 Posterior cord
7 Medial cord
8 Axillary nerve
9 Musculocutaneous nerve
10 Median nerve

11 Radial nerve
12 Ulnar nerve
13 Medial antebrachial cutaneous nerve
14 Medial brachial cutaneous nerve
15–17 *Short dorsal branches of plexus*
15 Thoracodorsal nerve
16 Subscapular nerve
17 Long thoracic nerve
18 Intercostobrachial nerve
19 Intercostal nerves

The *cervical plexus* (C1–4) and *brachial plexus* (C5–T1) are formed with
the *upper limb* (and with the diaphragm arising from primordia of the
cervical region), whereas the *lumbar plexus* (T12–L4) and *sacral plexus*
(L4–S4) arise with the *lower limb*.

Innervation of the skin in the plexus region. The segmental relations of the skin of the limbs are not demonstrable by dissection, since each nerve of the limb gives afferent fibers to several segments – the segmental relations of the skin in the plexus region can only be ascertained from clinical findings. Interruption of the dorsal root of a spinal nerve in the plexus region can result in sensory deficiencies in several nerves of the plexus. As in the case of segmental cutaneous nerves, the innervation regions also overlap in the cutaneous nerves of the plexus. The *autonomic region* of a cutaneous nerve, which it innervates alone, is distinguished from its *maximal region*, where adjacent cutaneous nerves are involved in the innervation. If a single cutaneous nerve is damaged peripherally, the deficiency is specific and total only in the autonomic region. If a single cutaneous nerve remains intact, its maximal region can be demonstrated. The autonomic region of a cutaneous nerve is usually small; in exceptional cases it can also be entirely absent. Also in the overlapping of (plurisegmental) cutaneous nerves of a plexus, the different sensory qualities are variably involved.

Peripheral interchange of fibers. Aside from the redistribution of fibers of ventral branches of spinal nerves in the formation of a plexus, which always occurs close to the spinal nerve trunk (i.e. near the vertebral column), fibers are still interchanged between individual nerves far in the periphery, both in the case of segmental nerves and plexus nerves.

Elements of Muscle Proprioceptive Reflex

Muscle reflexes can occur via both *spinal nerves* and *cutaneous nerves* (→ reflex arcs, p. 118). In the case of muscle reflexes (reflex activities of the striated musculature), the receptor lies *in the muscle* or *tendon = proprioceptive reflex* or *in the skin* or *mucosa = exteroceptive reflex*. The *receptors of the proprioceptive reflex* are the *proprioceptors* in the sense organs (muscle spindle or Golgi tendon organs). The *effectors* form myoneural synapses (motor end plates, Fig. **59**).

Muscle spindles lie in the midst of striated muscle. The muscle spindle is up to 20 mm long and about 0.2 mm thick. It is separated from, and anchored to the muscle by a connective tissue capsule which contains elastic networks.

The *muscle spindle* contains 4–10 striated muscle fibers ("intrafusal fibers"), each of which communicates with an afferent and an efferent nerve fiber. The intrafusal fibers are *nuclear-bag fibers* (cell nuclei in the middle region, only the end fibers being contractile) or *nuclear-chain fibers* (cell nuclei distributed uniformly, the entire fiber being contractile). Both types of fibers lie adjacent not only to *receptor structures* (sensory axonal endings), but also to *myoneural synapses* (motor axonal endings). The receptor structure is either an *annulospiral* (dendritic) ending of an $A\alpha = nerve\ fiber$, which wraps around the middle, noncontractile part of the intrafusal fiber, or an *"umbelliform"* (flower-spray) ending of an $A\beta$-*nerve fiber*, which lies

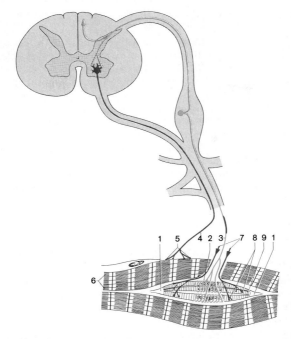

Fig. 59. **Elements of muscle proprioceptive reflex,** cross section through spinal cord, left spinal nerve with anterior and posterior roots, muscle spindle and muscle fibers

1 Muscle spindle
2 Annulospiral ending of afferent α-neuron (3)
4 Efferent α-motor neuron with myoneural synapse (5) at (working) muscle fibers (6)
7 Efferent γ-motor neuron with myoneural synapses (8) at (intrafusal) muscle fibers (9)

predominantly at the nuclear-chain fibers. The annulospiral receptors register stretching and velocity of stretch, the umbelliform only constant stretching.

Muscular traction and contraction lead to the deformation of receptors and to different excitatory formations. At the contractile ends of the intrafusal muscle fibers, the *efferent Aγ-nerve fibers* from the anterior horn of the spinal cord give rise to the *effector* in the form of *motor end plates* which can adjust the sensitiveness of intrafusal fibers to the different states of muscular contraction. Both arrangements serve as a feedback mechanism by which the muscle length is controlled ($\rightarrow$ Physiology).

The absolute and relative number of muscle spindles fluctuates. In the latissimus dorsi, 368 muscle spindles have been counted, but only 1.4 per g of muscle weight. In the abductor pollicis brevis, on the other hand, there were 80 altogether, but

29.3 per g of muscle weight. Likewise, in the ocular and laryngeal musculature there is a relative abundance of spindles.

The **Golgi tendon organs** (neurotendinous endings) lie in the collagenous fiber bundles of tendons at their site of origin near the muscle. There is one organ for every 5–25 muscle fiber insertions. In the region of the organ, the fiber bundle is insignificantly swollen ("tendon spindle").

The dendritic branches of *afferent β-neurons* end between the collagenous fibers. The receptor endings are deformed and stimulated both by stretching and contraction. The Golgi tendon organs are *receptors* serving as a feedback mechanism for the regulation of muscular tension (→ Physiology).

The *afferent neuron* of the proprioceptive reflex begins (with the annulospiral ending) in the muscle spindle or (with ramifications) in the Golgi tendon organ. The perikaryon lies in the spinal ganglion. The axon arrives at the spinal cord through the posterior root of the spinal nerve; it gives collaterals (*reflex collaterals*) to α-motor neurons in the anterior horn of the spinal cord. Interneurons are absent as a rule: the *proprioceptive reflex* is (preponderantly) monosynaptic.

The *reflex collaterals* of the afferent neuron from the muscle spindle stimulate the α-motor neurons of the muscle in question and thus cause the contraction of the muscle (starter function → Physiology).

The reflex collaterals of the afferent neuron from the Golgi tendon organs inhibit the α-motor neurons of the muscle in question and by this means limit the increase in stretching (autogenous inhibition → Physiology).

An **efferent neuron** is an α-motor neuron or a γ-neuron. Its axon leaves the spinal cord in the anterior root of the spinal nerve and terminates with myoneural synapses in the working muscle (α-motor neuron) or in the muscle spindle (γ-neuron).

The **myoneural synapse** forms the *effector structure* of the axon terminals.

Examples of proprioceptive reflexes: patellar tendon reflex, Achilles tendon reflex, biceps tendon reflex. Striking any of the above-mentioned tendons leads to rapid stretching of the muscle, which produces a prompt contraction.

Golgi-Mazzoni corpuscles are lamellated corpuscles with a structure similar to the Vater-Pacini corpuscles. They occur as *stretch receptors* at sites of tendinous attachments. Similar corpuscles in joint capsules bring about *perception of position*.

Elements of Muscular Exteroceptive Reflex

The *receptors through which the exteroceptive reflex* is released reside outside of the muscle. They are *cutaneous receptors*: pain, temperature and touch receptors of the skin (cutaneous sense) or mucosal receptors (Fig. **60**).

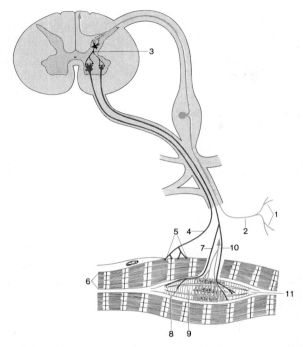

Fig. 60. **Elements of muscle exteroceptive reflex,** cross section through spinal cord, left spinal nerve with anterior and posterior roots, muscle spindle and muscle fibers

1 Free nerve endings as cutaneous receptors of afferent neuron (2)
3 Interneuron
4 Efferent α-motor neuron with myoneural synapse (5) at (working) muscle fibers (6)

7 Efferent γ-motor neuron with myoneural synapses (8) at (intrafusal) muscle fibers (9)
10 Afferent α-neuron with annulospiral ending of muscle spindle (11)

The afferent neurons, A-, B- or C-fibers, do not end directly at motor neurons; on the contrary, varying numbers of *interneurons* are inserted between collaterals and motor neurons, the *exteroceptive reflex* being *polysynaptic*. The interneurons possess collaterals, by means of which they reach the motor neurons of *several spinal cord segments*, the exteroceptive reflex being able to activate several muscles. In contrast to the proprioceptive reflex, the interneurons (in which stimuli can accumulate) make the exteroceptive reflex very variable in its effect.

The **efferent neuron,** as in the proprioceptive reflex, is an α-neuron or γ-neuron of the anterior horn. It terminates with a myoneural synapse.

Examples of exteroceptive reflexes: cremasteric reflex, abdominal wall reflex, plantar reflex. When the skin on the inner side of the thigh (or the abdominal skin or the skin on the sole of the foot) is stroked, a contraction is elicited from the cremaster muscle (or the abdominal wall musculature or the short flexors of the foot). Exteroceptive reflexes play an important role as *protective reflexes* (cough and sneezing reflexes, corneal reflex; lacrimal reflexes are also exteroceptive).

b) Organization of the Peripheral Nervous System Connected to the Brain

The *brain stem* contains vitally important nuclear regions, coordinating e.g. respiration, circulation, and endocrine glands. All parts are in close functional and morphological relationship to one another. The brain stem contains the nuclei of the cranial nerves.

Cranial Nerve Nuclei

The *nuclei* of cranial nerves III-XI lie in the tegmentum of the brain stem (Fig. **54**).

Cranial nerve I: the nerves of smell (*olfactory nerves*) enter an advanced basal part of the telencephalon, the *olfactory bulb*, directly, the only nerves to do so.

Cranial nerve II: the nerve of sight (*optic nerve*) is an advanced tract of the diencephalon and consists of the axons of the 3rd neuron of the visual pathway. (The receptor cells of the retina are counted as the 1st neuron).

Cranial nerve XII: the nerve of the tongue musculature (*hypoglossal nerve*) is, by origin, the *motor root* of a receded superior *spinal nerve* (occipital nerve), whose nuclear region marks the transition from the gray matter of the spinal cord to the tegmentum of the rhombencephalon.

The cranial nerve nuclei are called **nuclei of origin** (*motor nuclei*), and comprise the perikarya of the efferent (motor) *somatic portion* of the cranial nerves. The motor neurons of the cranial nerves, like the somatomotor root cells of the spinal cord, form a *"final common motor pathway"*, their nerve fibers terminating in myoneural synapses at striated muscle fibers.

Autonomic nuclei are formed by the perikarya of the efferent, *vegetative parts* of the cranial nerves. The autonomic nuclei of the cranial nerves all belong to the parasympathetics. In cranial nerves the *efferent segment of the autonomic nervous system* is also arranged in *two neurons*. The perikarya of the 1st neuron, comparable to the visceromotor root cells of the spinal cord, lie in the autonomic cranial nerve nucleus; the perikarya of the 2nd neuron are in a parasympathetic ganglion supported by the cranial nerve.

In the **terminal nuclei** (*sensory nuclei*) begins the *2nd neuron of the afferent circuit* of a cranial nerve, comparable to the funicular cells of the spinal cord. The axons of the *1st neuron of the afferent circuit* terminate at the perikarya of the terminal nuclei. The perikarya of this first afferent neuron are collected into *sensory ganglia* of the cranial nerve, except for the afferent fibers from the masticatory muscles. Whereas the sensory spinal ganglia are all of approximately the same size, the sensory ganglia of cranial nerves differ considerably both in size and in histology.

Efferent and afferent fibrous components of a cranial nerve, in distinction to the spinal nerves, leave or enter the brain stem together.

Characteristic Features of Cranial Nerve Organization

The peripheral nervous system attached to the brain consists of 12 pairs of *cranial nerves* that are distinguished both from the spinal nerves and also from one another. The individual nerves are *not equivalent* with regard to their origin, connections and functions; their special behavior is determined by the characteristic formation of the head, whose anlage and development cannot be compared with the segmental primordia of the trunk and limbs.

The *numbering* of the cranial nerves from I to XII reflects the *sequence of their exit from the brain* from rostral to caudal (Fig. **61**). When the cranial nerves are organized according to *fiber components* and *peripheral association* (Table **2**), some nerves lying far apart must be grouped together (Fig. **62**).

The *olfactory nerves* (I), the *optic nerve* (II) and the *vestibulocochlear* nerve (VIII) are **pure sensory nerves** from "special sense organs." They are also classified by many authors into somatosensitivities in the broader sense. On the other hand, the cranial nerves carrying taste fibers from the gustatory organ, a "special sense organ", are mixed visceromotor-viscerosensory nerves.

The *olfactory* and *optic nerves* cannot be compared to the remaining afferent circuits of peripheral nerves; the olfactory nerves consist of axons of primary sensory cells, and the optic nerve is a part of the visual pathway.

Nerves of the extrinsic eye muscles. A special group of pure motor nerves that serve the ocular motor system (visual adjustment) are the *oculomotor* (III), *trochlear* (IV) and *abducens* (VI). Many authors consider them to be somatomotor nerves. Yet, the oculomotor also carries visceromotor (autonomic) nerve fibers, which (via an intermediate autonomic ganglion) supply the intrinsic eye muscles.

Branchial nerves. Another group of cranial nerves are the branchial nerves (nerves of the branchial arches) associated with the branchial (pharyngeal) arches: *trigeminal* (V, 1st branchial arch), *facial* (VII, 2nd branchial arch), *glossopharyngeal* (IX, 3rd branchial arch), as well as the *vagus* (X, 4th branchial arch) and the *accessory nerve* (XI) segmented off from it.

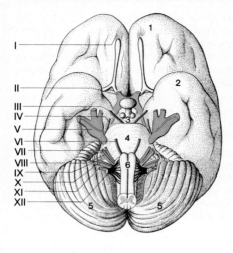

Fig. 61. **Cranial nerves,** basal view

☐ Pure sensory nerves
■ Nerves for extrinsic eye muscles
☐ branchial nerves
■ Nerve to tongue musculature (as ventral root of first spinal nerve)

I   Olfactory nerves
II   Optic nerve
III   Oculomotor nerve
IV   Trochlear nerve
V   Trigeminal nerve
VI   Abducens nerve
VII   Facial nerve
VIII   Vestibulocochlear nerve
IX   Glossopharyngeal nerve
X   Vagus nerve
XI   Accessory nerve
XII   Hypoglossal nerve

1, 2 *Cerebrum*
1 Frontal lobe
2 Temporal lobe
3–6 *Brain stem*
3 Infundibulum with hypophysis
4 Pons
5 Cerebellar hemispheres
6 Medulla oblongata

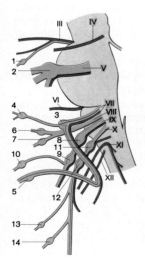

Fig. 62. **Nerve fiber components and ganglia of cranial nerves III–XII and their first branchings,** view from left side

■ Voluntary motor fibers
☐ Sensory fibers and ganglia
☐ Parasympathetic fibers and ganglia

Numerals III–XII designate cranial nerves

1 Ciliary ganglion (III)
2 Trigeminal ganglion (V)
3 Geniculate ganglion (VII)
4 Pterygopalatine ganglion (VII)
5 Submandibular ganglion (VII)
6 Vestibular ganglion (VIII)
7 Cochlear ganglion (VIII)
8 Superior ganglion (IX)
9 Inferior ganglion (IX)
10 Otic ganglion (IX)
11 Superior ganglion (X)
12 Inferior ganglion (X)
13, 14 Autonomic ganglia in thorax and abdomen

Table 2. Fiber components and peripheral organization of cranial nerves

Sequence and Designation	SS	VS	VM	Spec. VM	SM	Peripheral Organization
I. Olfactory	(+)					Olfactory epithelium (nerve of smell)
II Optic	(+)					Retina (nerve of sight)
III Oculomotor					(+)	Extrinsic eye muscles
			+			Intrinsic eye muscles
IV Trochlear					(+)	Extrinsic eye muscles
V Trigeminal	+	+				Face and head up to crown, nasal, eye, oral cavities
				+		Mandibular arch muscles
VI Abducens					(+)	Extrinsic eye muscles
VII Facial		+				Taste fibers (anterior half of tongue)
				+		Hyoid arch muscles
			+			Salivary, lacrimal glands
VIII Vestibulocochlear	(+)					Labryrinth organ (nerve of hearing and balance
IX Glossopharyngeal		+				Taste fibers (posterior half of tongue, pharynx)
				+		Pharynx
			+			Parotid gland
X Vagus	+					Part of external acoustic meatus
		+				Laryngeal taste buds
				+		Larynx
			+			Intestinal canal up to transverse colon, lungs, bronchial tubes, heart
XI Accessory				+		Trapezius, sternocleidomastoid
XII Hypoglossal					+	Tongue musculature

Abbreviations: SS somatosensory, VS viscerosensory, VM visceromotor, Spec. VM special visceromotor, SM somatomotor

The *afferents* of the branchial nerves come from the external skin of the head (general cutaneous sensitivity, classified by many authors under somatic sensitivities) and from the viscera (visceral sensitivities, including taste). The *efferents* arrive at the muscle derivatives of the pharyngeal arches in the head-neck region, as well as at the autonomic ganglia of the viscera (visceromotor, including secretomotor). Yet, the visceromotor nerves which pass to the musculature of the face, pharynx and larynx, to the trapezius and sternocleidomastoid muscles – muscles formed from visceral anlagen which serve for communication with the environment – possess a *"special visceromotor"* component; they carry fast-conducting nerve fibers of the somatomotor nerve type. Their "final common motor pathway" is represented by a single neuron.

In higher vertebrates, these fiber components are distributed unequally in the strongly specialized branchial nerves. *All* fiber constituents of the branchial nerves – in contrast to the spinal nerves – leave or enter the brain *laterally*.

The *trigeminal nerve*, the branchial nerve component (V2, 3) of which is enlarged by annexation of a sensory cranial nerve anlage (V1) for the embryonic frontal process, mainly carries fibers of general cutaneous and mucosal sensitivities from the head. In addition, the trigeminal nerve contains "special visceromotor" fibers for the masticatory muscles.

The *facial nerve* possesses visceromotor (secretomotor) fibers, as well as "special visceromotor" fibers for the facial musculature and viscerosensory (taste) fibers.

The *glossopharyngeal* and *vagus nerves* are composed in a way similar to the facial nerve; their "special visceromotor" fibers innervate the striated musculature of the pharynx, esophagus and larynx.

The *vagus* also possesses a large portion of general visceromotor fibers for the heart, bronchi and the digestive tract, as well as a small portion of fibers of general cutaneous sensitivity from the external acoustic meatus.

The *accessory nerve* is an independent motor portion of the vagus nerve with an extensive nuclear region which reaches far into the cervical portion of the spinal cord; the nerve – as part of a branchial nerve – exits laterally from the spinal cord. The accessory nerve carries only "special visceromotor" fibers which innervate the trapezius and sternocleidomastoid muscles.

The **nerve to the musculature of the tongue**, the *hypoglossal* (XII), is distinguished from all other cranial nerves in that it is established as a spinal nerve, the sensory root of which degenerates in the course of embryonic development. As the *"motor root"*, the hypoglossal leaves the brain ventrolaterally at the superior end of a ventrolateral furrow, in which all the following motor roots of the spinal nerves leave the spinal cord.

c) Organization of the Peripheral Autonomic (Vegetative) Nervous System

The *autonomic nervous system* supplies the smooth musculature in the viscera, the blood vessels, glands, hair muscles, heart and sexual organs. The perikarya, which innervate these organs and tissues, lie in *autonomic ganglia*.

Autonomic Ganglia

The *neurons* residing in the *autonomic ganglia* – the second neuron of the efferent vegetative circuit – form, together with the organs innervated by them, a *functional unit* (comparable perhaps to the neuromuscular unit of motor neurons and skeletal muscle fibers → p. 105). The autonomic ganglia, therefore, can also be considered as "*organ ganglia*" (Fig. **63**). In view of the postganglionic course of their axons (and in analogy to the designation "preganglionic neurons"), these neurons are also grouped as "postganglionic neurons".

The autonomic ganglion cells, in their embryological migration, establish themselves at different *distances* from their organs. Topographically, therefore, autonomic ganglia can be divided into:
– *intramural ganglia* (residing within the organ; parasympathetic neurons),

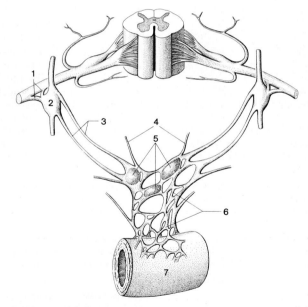

Fig. 63. **Autonomic ganglia (organ ganglia) and plexuses** (neuronal organization → Fig. 65)

1 Communicating rami of spinal nerves (→ Figs. 50 and 51))
2 Sympathetic trunk ganglia
3 Splanchnic nerves of sympathetic trunk
4 Parasympathetic branches
5 Autonomic ganglia
6 Autonomic plexus
7 Target organ

—*prevertebral* ganglia (situated in front of the vertebral column, halfway between the spinal cord and the organs; predominantly sympathetic, but also parasympathetic neurons), and
—*paravertebral ganglia* (located beside the vertebral column near the spinal cord; sympathetic neurons).

These autonomic ganglia contain the perikarya of the *2nd neuron of the efferent vegetative circuit*. The *1st neuron of this pathway* is established with its perikarya *in the CNS* (→ sympathetic and parasympathetic root cells, p. 131).

Sympathetic Nervous System

The ganglia of the sympathetic nervous system form a more or less uniform cord, the **sympathetic trunk** (Fig. **64**; cf Fig. **63**), which borders the vertebral column on both sides and extends from the base of the skull to the coccyx. It consists on both sides of a series of ganglia which are combined into a chain by bundles of nerve fibers (*interganglionic rami*). The trunk lies in front of the transverse processes of the cervical vertebrae and the heads of the ribs, lateral to the bodies of the lumbar vertebrae and, in the sacral region, medial to the anterior sacral foramina.

The **ganglia of the sympathetic trunk** are, with slight variability, developed segmentally in the *thoracic, lumbar* and *sacral regions*. The lowermost pair of sacral ganglia fuse into an unpaired ganglion. In the *cervical region*, on the other hand, the ganglia are reduced to three (more rarely two) ganglia. The largest of these is the spindle-shaped *superior cervical ganglion* below the base of the skull, which is approximately 2 cm long. The small *middle cervical ganglion*, which is occasionally absent, is located at the level of the 5th cervical vertebra. The *inferior cervical ganglion* generally fuses with the 1st thoracic ganglion to form the *cervicothoracic ganglion* (*stellate ganglion*).

The **superior cervical ganglion** has a special position, inasmuch as the perikarya of the 2nd neuron of the entire *cervical sympathetics* (eye, salivary glands and blood vessels), as well as some of the perikarya of the 2nd neuron passing to the heart are located in it.

There are *no* sympathetic ganglia in the *head* itself (except for isolated small groups of perikarya of the 2nd sympathetic neurons); autonomic ganglia in the head region contain perikarya of the 2nd neuron of the parasympathetics.

---

1 Ciliary ganglion
2 Pterygopalatine ganglion
3 Otic ganglion
4 Submandibular ganglion
5 Superior cervical ganglion
6 Cervicothoracic (stellate) ganglion
7 Cardiac ganglia
8 Celiac ganglion
9 Superior mesenteric ganglion
10 Aorticorenal ganglia
11 Inferior mesenteric ganglion
12 Pelvic splanchnic nerves
13 Pelvic ganglia
14 Nerve fibers for vasodilators and sweat glands
    (segmental autonomic nerve fibers)

▶

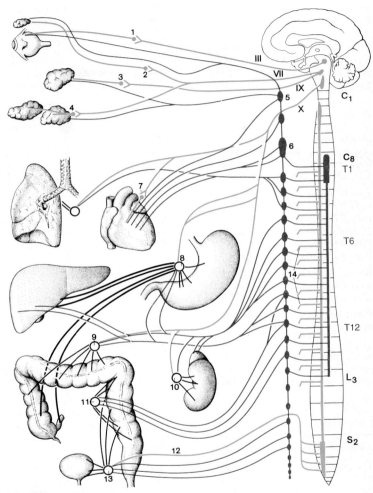

Fig. 64. **Scheme of autonomic nervous system**
■ Sympathetic
■ Parasympathetic
III   Oculomotor nerve
VII   Facial nerve
IX   Glossopharyngeal nerve
X   Vagus nerve

Rami communicantes connect the sympathetic trunk ganglia with the spinal nerves. In *segments C8-L2,3,* in which the perikarya of preganglionic neurons of the entire sympathetic trunk lie in the lateral horn of the spinal cord, the *rami communicantes* carry *pre-* and *postganglionic nerve fibers.* The preganglionic fibers synapse with their postganglionic neuron not only in the same segment, but ascend or descend in the sympathetic trunk with *collaterals* and innervate additional postganglionic neurons in other trunk ganglia or in the prevertebral ganglia.

Each preganglionic neuron innervates an average of 8–10 postganglionic neurons. By this means, the excitation of the preganglionic neurons, conducted in a thin fiber bundle from the spinal cord, is transmitted to a large number of postganglionic neurons, the excitation spreading out diffusely. The ascending collaterals of the preganglionic neurons dominate up to T7; in the cervical sympathetic trunk only ascending efferent fibers are found. The descending collaterals synapse below T11; lumbar and sacral sympathetic trunks carry only descending efferent fibers.

The **interganglionic rami** consist of about 50% ascending and descending *collaterals of the preganglionic rami communicantes.* The remaining fibers are *afferent fibers,* primarily "pain fibers" from the viscera. The perikarya of these fibers lie mostly in the spinal ganglia, but also partly in the sympathetic trunk ganglia. These "pain fibers" enter the spinal cord in the "sympathetic segments" C8-L2,3.

Before this, the pain fibers can still course for varying distances in the interganglionic rami as a *"paramedullary"* (because they are located next to the spinal cord) *afferent circuit.*

Postganglionic nerve fibers exit from the sympathetic trunk to all spinal nerves.

The postganglionic nerve fibers *from the superior cervical ganglion* travel into the head, for the most part, as plexuses with the arteries of the head (e.g. *external carotid plexus, internal carotid plexus*). The preganglionic fibers for the superior cervical ganglion arise in segments C8-T3 of the spinal cord.

An injury to spinal cord segments C8-T3 or to the cervical sympathetic trunk results in the loss of the sympathetics to the head, which is evident in the eye of the affected side. The smooth musculature of the orbit and the iris innervated by the sympathetics loses its tonus; the pupil is small, the eye recedes into the orbit, the palpebral fissure narrows (Horner's syndrome).

The postganglionic nerve fibers from the *middle* and the *inferior cervical ganglia,* pass to the heart and bronchi; in addition, the inferior ganglion gives postganglionic fibers to the upper limb. The preganglionic fibers of these ganglia originate from segments T3-7. The postganglionic nerve fibers *from the remaining sympathetic trunk ganglia* return to the spinal nerve in the rami communicantes and pass peripherally with the nerve to the trunk wall or limbs.

Visceral nerves (*splanchnic nerves*) pass to the abdominal and pelvic viscera. The sympathetic fibers are, for the most part, not connected with the sympathetic trunk ganglia by the 2nd neuron. Their *preganglionic* nerve fibers travelling to the sympathetic trunk in the rami communicantes course through the sympathetic trunk ganglia into the body cavities as *splanchnic nerves.* The perikarya of the 2nd neuron of the splanchnic nerves lie in the *prevertebral ganglia* of the visceral cavity.

Prevertebral ganglia are large, macroscopically-visible accumulations of *perikarya of the 2nd autonomic neuron*; they frequently lie at blood vessels (examples: *celiac, superior mesenteric, inferior mesenteric arteries*). The postganglionic nerve fibers exiting from the prevertebral ganglia pass to the viscera in dense plexuses of fibers (*autonomic plexuses*) which are situated on the wall of the large arteries.

Variability of prevertebral ganglia. During colonization of the ganglia by the perikarya of the autonomic 2nd neuron, some of them do not quite reach the site of colonization and occasionally form smaller accumulations situated proximally. This leads to a great *variability* of ganglia and explains why perikarya of postganglionic neurons are also found outside of ganglia, e.g. in the entire course of the splanchnic nerves, and why *intermediate ganglia* occur between the sympathetic trunk and prevertebral ganglia.

Since the perikarya of the 2nd neuron of the parasympathetics for the thoracic, abdominal and pelvic viscera are also not always entirely displaced into the periphery, *prevertebral ganglia* also contain *perikarya of the parasympathetic 2nd neuron* in great number. Therefore, parasympathetic postganglionic nerve fibers can also course in the postganglionic fiber plexuses.

Parasympathetic Nervous System

The *"parasympathetic nervous system"* is not a uniform structure. It consists of two parts, *cranial* and *sacral*, both of which supply the *viscera* (Figs. **62** and **64**).

The *perikarya of the 1st efferent neuron* of these two systems lie in the *nuclear regions* of the cranial nerves affected and in the *base of the lateral horn* of spinal cord segments S2–4. The *perikarya of the 2nd neuron* are found in the *peripheral autonomic ganglia.*

The *perikarya of the 2nd efferent neuron of the parasympathetics*, the "parasympathetic ganglia", lie (in the thoracic and abdominal cavities) usually near to, or in, the target organ (→ intramural ganglia, p. 145), whereas the *perikarya of the 2nd neuron of the sympathetic nervous system*, the "sympathetic ganglia", reside near the vertebral column. *The preganglionic, parasympathetic nerve fibers are, therefore, as a rule, longer than the sympathetic.*

Cranial Part (*mesencephalo-rhombencephalic parasympathetics*). A portion of the parasympathetic fibers passing to the viscera course with *cranial nerves III, VII, IX and X.* The parasympathetic area of distribution of the vagus adjoins that of the sacral parasympathetics near the left colonic flexure.

Sacral Part (*sacral parasympathetics*). The sacral part leaves the spinal cord with *spinal nerves S2–4* and supplies the viscera of the small pelvis via the *pelvic splanchnic nerves.*

The *craniosacral parasympathetics* supply the viscera of the head, as well as the viscera of the thoracic, abdominal and pelvic cavities, but not the body wall. The body wall and limbs receive the following nerve fibers antagonistic to the sympathetics.

Segmental autonomic nerve fibers are components of the autonomic preganglionic neurons, whose perikarya lie *in all segments of the spinal cord* in the region of the base of the lateral horn. The segmental autonomic fibers leave by the anterior root and synapse (probably) in the sympathetic trunk ganglia at its 2nd neuron. The axons of the perikarya of the 2nd neuron reach the trunk wall and limbs with the spinal nerves as postganglionic nerve fibers. These segmental autonomic nerve fibers innervate (cholinergically) the cutaneous glands. The fibers are grouped by some authors with the parasympathetics because of the cholinergic synapses, by others with the sympathetics because of the location of their perikarya in the sympathetic trunk.

In distinction to the sympathetic fibers, which are not segmentally distributed to the body wall, the *segmental autonomic nerve fibers* strongly adhere to the *segmental boundaries* marked off by the "pain fibers."

Since the segmental autonomic fibers innervate, among other things, the sweat glands, the failure of innervation of a cutaneous segment can also be demonstrated with the help of a (chemical) skin-sweat test.

Autonomic Plexus

The *postganglionic autonomic nerve fibers* which pass to the viscera from the prevertebral ganglia usually carry both *sympathetic and parasympathetic components.* The nerve fibers form a *plexus (autonomic plexus)* at the wall of the aorta and the large arteries, with which they reach the organs. Sympathetic and parasympathetic fiber components cannot be separately dissected in the plexus itself, but can be partially demonstrated immunohistochemically or with the fluorescent microscope. Although the autonomic plexuses communicate to a great extent, portions of them are specially named – mostly after the arteries which support them, or after the organs to which they pass, e.g. *celiac plexus, renal plexus.*

Intramural Nervous System

The *perikarya of autonomic neurons* and the extensive *plexuses of the autonomic nerve fibers* lie in the *wall of internal organs* (gastro-intestinal tract, urinary bladder, prostate and bronchi, among others). They form the intramural nervous system of each organ (Fig. **65**; cf. Fig. **64**).

In several organs (e.g. in the urinary bladder), the intramural perikarya, as far as is known at present, represent the 2nd efferent neuron of the parasympathetics (= *intramural ganglion*). In the wall of the gastro-intestinal tract, on the other hand, the intramural nervous system possesses an independent neuronal organization (as yet not described here) with afferent and efferent neurons that are localized partly in the intestinal wall, partly in the prevertebral ganglia. It can still stimulate

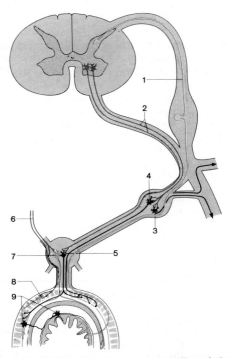

Fig. 65. **Neuronal organization in autonomic nerves, ganglia and plexuses** (→ Fig 63), cross section through spinal cord, left spinal nerve with anterior and posterior roots, communicating rami and splanchnic nerves

1 Viscerosensory neuron
2 First visceromotor sympathetic neuron
3 Second sympathetic neuron in sympathetic ganglion to body wall
4 Second sympathetic neuron in sympathetic ganglion to viscera
5 Second sympathetic neuron in prevertebral ganglion (organ ganglion) to viscera
6 First visceromotor parasympathetic neuron
7 Second parasympathetic neuron in prevertebral ganglion (organ ganglion) to viscera
8 Second parasympathetic neuron in viscera
9 Neuron of intramural nervous system

the activity of the isolated organ, but it is subordinate to the higher-order, regulating influence of the sympathetics and parasympathetics.

Elements of Visceral Reflex

The peripheral autonomic nervous system possesses, like the somatic, *afferent circuits, central integration sites* and *efferent circuits*, i.e. the anatomical basis for visceral reflexes in the broadest sense. These can occur at the level of the brain stem or the spinal cord, as visceral reflexes of the intramural nervous system of the intestine, as well as at the level of the organ ganglia (concerning *receptors* in the viscera → organs of visceral sensitivities, p. 122).

The **visceral reflexes at the level of the brain stem** play an important role in the regulatory mechanism by which the internal conditions of the organism are held constant; they operate as a feedback mechanism (→ physiology).

Receptors measure the *arterial blood pressure* (in the wall of the carotid sinus and the aorta), the *central venous pressure* (in the wall of the large veins), the *expansion of the lung* (in the lungs), the *oxygen partial pressure* (carotid body, para-aortic bodies), among others. Their *afferent neurons* course in the cranial nerves (*facial, glossopharyngeal, vagus*); the *perikarya* lie in the sensory ganglia of the cranial nerves in question. The axons of the afferent neurons lead to the *control centers* in the brain stem (circulatory and respiratory centers, etc. → reticular formation, p. 124). "*Central interoceptors*" lie in the brain itself (receptors for the pH of cerebrospinal fluid, the osmotic pressure of the blood plasma, the arteriovenous blood sugar differential, etc.).

Visceral reflexes at the level of the spinal cord (Fig. **65**) are known in the lumbar and sacral regions. Their *afferent* segment can – as in the case of defecation and micturition reflexes – come *from the viscera* or – exceptionally, as in the case of erection and ejaculation reflexes – emanate from *cutaneous receptors*. Yet no somatomotor reflexes exist comparable to the strictly segmental reflex arcs in all segments of the spinal cord.

In the **viscerovisceral reflex**, afferents from the viscera stimulate efferent autonomic root cells, frequently in several segments. Thus, the expansion of the urinary bladder wall leads to a reflex contraction of the musculature of the bladder wall and to a relaxation of the bladder sphincter (micturition reflex).

Afferents from the intestinal wall can influence the intestinal motor response at the level of the prevertebral ganglia.

A **viscerocutaneous reflex** occurs when the axon of an efferent autonomic root cell, which is stimulated by afferents from the viscera (on passing through the sympathetic trunk), gives off collaterals to the 2nd neuron supplying the body wall. When inflammatory diseases of the inner organs occur, the body wall, for example, can be reddened (increased blood supply) on the affected side.

In the **visceromotor reflex**, afferents from the viscera are conveyed to the somato-motor neurons by collaterals via intermediate cells. This reflex arc is effective in the case of an "abdominal defense reflex", a muscle spasm of the abdominal wall owing to (inflammatory) diseased abdominal organs.

In the **cutaneovisceral reflex**, collaterals from axons of somatosensory neurons transfer the excitation from the skin to autonomic root cells in the spinal cord via intermediate cells. Through these reflex arcs, influence on the inner organs from the skin is said to be possible (e.g. by warmth).

Vasodilatory axon reflex ("*antidromic vasodilation*"). It is known from physiological investigations that the stimulation of afferent nerve fibers from the skin can lead to a dilation of the blood vessels of the skin segment concerned. The effect also occurs if the spinal nerve is severed distal to the spinal ganglion.

The process is supported by the stimulation of afferent nerve fibers ("pain fibers") which possess the strongly vaso-active peptide, *substance P*, as the transmitter. The peptide can be released from the fibers not only at the central end of the process in the spinal cord, but also at the peripheral end in the skin, and thus can produce a vasodilation. These neurons can therefore display an afferent and an efferent action at the same time – an unusual feature. In some individuals, the stroking of the skin alone can cause a localized reddening or pallor of the skin (dermatography).

Radiated Pain (Head's Zones)

The *phenomenon of radiated pain* is evident in diseases of the inner organs when specific cutaneous zones (*Head's zones*) become painfully hyper-sensitive. Head's zones correspond with the area of distribution of pain fibers from spinal nerves; in the trunk region the zones are belt-shaped.

This phenomenon is not to be understood as a reflex – *reflex arcs are absent*. It indicates, however, that autonomic and somatic afferents can communicate with one another at the segmental level. The phenomenon is based on the fact that both the 1st afferent neurons coming from the viscera and those coming from the skin synapse in the spinal cord with a *common 2nd neuron*, whereby a localization of pain is impossible. Since the higher central nuclear regions have "learned", however, that pain usually comes from the body surface, the affected skin segment becomes "painful" (*convergence theory of Head's zones*).

C. Membranes of the Brain and Spinal Cord

The central nervous system possesses three connective tissue coverings, which are designated in the region of the brain as *cranial meninges* and in the region of the spinal cord as *spinal meninges*. In sequence from the outside inward, they are the:

– tough cranial and spinal membrane, dura mater (pachymeninx),
– spider-webbed membrane, arachnoid, and
– delicate cranial and spinal membrane, pia mater.

The arachnoid and pia together form the *leptomeninx* (delicate cranial and spinal membranes in the broader sense); they enclose the *subarachnoid cavity*, which is filled with *cerebrospinal fluid* (Fig. **67**).

a) Tough Cranial and Spinal Membrane

The *tough cranial* and *spinal membrane, dura mater* (Figs. **66** and **67**), is a strong membrane woven from connective tissue fibers. Its structure in the cranial cavity differs from that in the vertebral canal.

In the **cranial cavity,** the external surface of the *cephalic dura mater* is firmly *coalescent* with the *periosteum* of the bones bordering the cavity, in the child more firmly than in the adult – except for a few places at which both layers, periosteal and meningeal, withdraw from each other in order

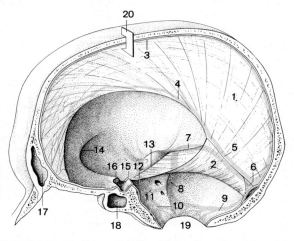

Fig. 66. **Dura mater**, paramedian section through cranium, viewed from left side

 1 Falx cerebri
 2 Tentorium cerebelli
 3–14 *Venous sinuses*
 3 Superior sagittal sinus
 4 Inferior sagittal sinus
 5 Straight sinus
 6 Confluens of sinuses
 7 Transverse sinus
 8 Sigmoid sinus
 9 Occipital sinus
10 Basilar plexus
11 Inferior petrosal sinus

12 Cavernous sinus
13 Superior petrosal sinus
14 Sphenoparietal sinus
15 Internal carotid artery
16 Optic nerve
17, 18 *Paranasal sinuses*
17 Frontal sinus
18 Sphenoidal sinus
19 Foramen magnum
20 Magnified section → Fig. **237**

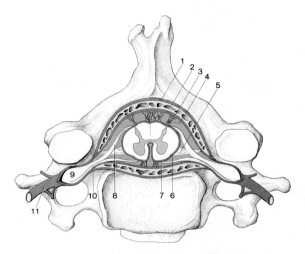

Fig. 67. **Membranes of spinal cord and contents of vertebral canal**. 3rd cervical vertebra, cranial view

1 Periosteum
2 Epidural space, contains internal vertebral venous plexus and fat
3 Dura mater
4 Arachnoid
5 Denticulate ligament
6 Pia mater
7 Subarachnoid space
8 Dorsal root of spinal nerve with spinal ganglion (9)
10 Ventral root of spinal nerve
11 Spinal nerve

to provide space for venous sinuses, arteries or nerves. An epidural space surrounding the dura is absent in the cranial cavity.

The *conduction pathways*–apart from the cranial nerves leaving the cranial cavity–supply regions on both sides, toward the dura, as well as toward the cranial bones. The *inner side* of the dura is smooth and glistening.

Dural Septa. The cranial dura mater penetrates into the large fissures between the brain parts with *septa-like formations*–longitudinal and transverse partitions of the skull roof according to the organization and course of the fibers. The *falx cerebri* separates the two cerebral hemispheres. The *tentorium cerebelli* roofs over the cerebellum; the *falx cerebelli* is inserted against the vermis of the cerebellum.

The **venous sinuses** of the tough dura (*dural sinuses*, Fig. **66**) are tubular or cleft-shaped blood spaces between the meningeal and periosteal layers of the dura or between the two layers from which the dural septa arise. The wall of the sinus is formed of connective tissue fibers and lined by endothelium; in contrast to the wall of veins, it is rigid and lacks a muscular layer.

In the **vertebral canal,** the *spinal dura mater* and *periosteum* are *separated* from one another (Fig. **67**); an epidural space (*epidural cavity*) filled with adipose tissue is formed, which receives the veins, arteries, and sensory nerves of the dura.

b) Spider-Webbed Membrane

The *spider-webbed membrane* (*arachnoid*, Fig. **67** and **68**), situated between the dura and pia mater, forms a collagenous trabecular network

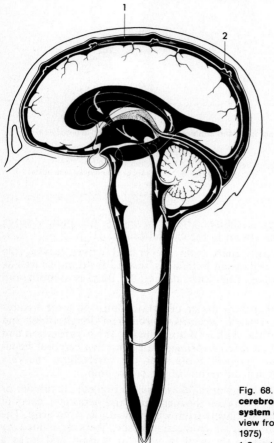

Fig. 68. **Circulation of cerebrospinal fluid in ventricular system and sub-arachnoid space** view from left side (after *Gardner*, 1975)
1 Superior sagittal sinus
2 Arachnoid granulations

which is covered by flat, epithelial-like cells (*meningeal cells*). The external (subdural) arachnoid layer facing the dura consists of several layers of meningeal cells. Its outermost layer, bordering on the connective tissue cells of the dura, appears as a continuous union of cells (*neurothelium*) and forms a very active barrier between the *fluid milieu of the leptomeninx* and the *blood milieu of the dura* (→ blood and fluid milieu, p. 159). The fiber-poor connective tissue of the pia mater is also covered by meningeal cells, so that the interstitial spaces of the arachnoid, which together form the subarachnoid space, are completely surrounded by meningeal cells.

The subdural arachnoid layer lies directly on the dura. It is held in this position by the pressure of the cerebrospinal fluid which fills up the subarachnoid space. When there is a diminution of fluid pressure in the cadaver, an artificial space (*subdural space*) arises between the arachnoid layer and the dura. Near the nerve passages and at the entry and exit sites of the cranial and spinal blood vessels from the cranial cavity and the vertebral canal, the subdural arachnoid layer is continued into the *perineural sheath* (and into the *perivascular connective tissue*). Fluid can flow off into the endoneurial space – enclosed by the perineurial sheath. When the brain is removed, the arachnoid layer, as a rule, remains on the brain.

Arachnoid granulations (*Pacchionian bodies*), avascular, small tufts of leptomeninges, project from the (external) arachnoid layer into dilations of the dural sinuses (and in a similar fashion also into the veins of the intervertebral foramina). They are of value as excretory passages for cerebrospinal fluid.

Subarachnoid space (Fig. **68**). Numerous fine spider-web trabeculae pass from the (external) arachnoid layer through the *subarachnoid space* (*subarachnoid cavity*), which is filled with cerebrospinal fluid, to the outer surface of the delicate cranial and spinal meninges, which, for their part, lie close to the surfaces of the brain and spinal cord. The subarachnoid space of the cranial cavity is in continuous contact with that of the vertebral canal.

Cisterns. Since the inner surface of the cranial cavity lined by the dura and the (external) arachnoid layer is separated from the surface of the brain in places, circumscribed *enlargements of the subarachnoid space* (*subarachnoid cisternae*) arise in the cranial cavity.

c) Delicate Cranial and Spinal Membrane

The *delicate cranial* and *spinal membrane* (in the narrow sense; → p. 154), or pia mater, clings closely to the surface of the brain and spinal cord as loose connective tissue, entering into all fissures (Fig. **67**). The pia covers the branches of the cranial vessels and penetrates with them a short distance into the brain (spinal cord) substance in the shape of a funnel (pial funnel, in which the vessel is slightly movable). When removed from the cranial cavity, the brain and spinal cord are covered by the arachnoid and pia.

d) Cerebrospinal Fluid

Cerebrospinal fluid fills the ventricles of the brain as "inner fluid", the subarachnoid space as "outer fluid". The inner and outer fluids of the cranial cavity communicate with each other by three openings of the 4th ventricle (Fig. **68**). The fluid of the cranial cavity is continuous with that of the vertebral canal. The total amount of cerebrospinal fluid in the adult amounts to about 140 ml.

Cerebrospinal fluid protects the brain and spinal cord against *mechanical* influences (pressure distribution, e.g. when centrifugal forces occur, and, in cooperation with the bony capsule and its venous circuits, also against *thermal* influences. The fluid plays a role in the *equalization of volume fluctuations* of the cranial arteries. The role of the fluid as a pathway for metabolic products, hormones, etc. is still little known; but the fluid in the brain and spinal cord, as an *intercellular*, interstitial *fluid*, must take over the tasks carried out by lymph in other organs. The brain and spinal cord do not possess lymphatic vessels.

Fluid dynamics. About 55% of cerebrospinal fluid is secreted in the *cerebral ventricles*, about 45% in the *subarachnoid space*, and altogether about 700 ml in 24 hours. The *inner* fluid is secreted from blood vessels about equally by tuft-like, vascular-rich formations of the brain wall (*choroid plexuses*) and by the *walls of the ventricle*. The origin of the outer fluid is not precisely known.

The **choroid plexuses** (Fig. **69**), which project into all four cerebral ventricles, are covered on their ventricular surface by a simple cuboidal *epithelium*, which shows signs of secretion. By origin, the epithelium is a receded part of the brain wall. It protrudes villous-like from the exterior into the ventricular lumen by means of many *vascular tufts*. The distinct vascular pulsations of the choroid plexus are transferred to the cerebrospinal fluid.

A **flow of fluid** occurs between the formative and resorptive sites of the fluid. It is superimposed by oscillating movements caused by the pulsation of the cranial vessels and by respiratory and compression movements.

The arachnoid villi, among others, are regarded as the *resorption sites* of cerebrospinal fluid. The fluid also drains away (in lymphatic tracts of the periphery), however, via the endoneurial space, which is surrounded by processes of the meninges that accompany the cranial and spinal nerves as perineurial sheaths.

e) Blood-Brain Barrier, Blood Milieu and Fluid Milieu

Blood-brain barrier. The brain has a unique position among all the organs with regard to exchange processes involving substances of particular

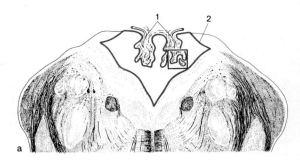

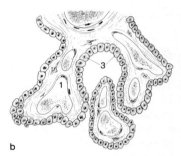

Fig. 69. **Choroid plexus**
a Cross section through 4th ventricle
b Higher magnified section of choroid
  plexus from a
1 Blood vessel in tela choroidea
2 Ependymal cells as ventricular lining
3 Ependymal cells as plexal epithelium

molecular sizes and properties. The brain capillaries generally form a *blood-brain barrier*. (In *parts of other organs* comparable barriers are formed, e.g. *blood-retina, blood-thymus, blood-testis barriers*.) Only in a few, very narrowly restricted places in the brain, the *neurohemal regions of the circumventricular organ* ($\rightarrow$ Vol. 2) is a blood-brain barrier absent. In these, neurohormones are given off into the blood. "Impenetrable" substances, which are usually held back by the blood-brain barrier, leave the blood vessels and enter the perivascular space.

Blood and fluid milieus. The blood-brain barrier separates the *blood milieu* in the blood vessels from the *fluid milieu* of the intercellular space of the brain which contains the intramural fluid. The latter communicates with the *ventricular fluid* via the permeable intercellular clefts of the ependymal cells (and is controlled by means of them). The *intercellular space of the brain* communicates with the *intercellular space of the leptomeninx* via the perivascular fissures of the cerebral vessels.

The blood-brain barrier is supplemented by a *blood-fluid barrier* which is formed at the borders of the neurohemal regions of the circumventricular organs and between the tough and the delicate meninges.

7. Skin and Integumentary Appendages

Skin is designated as the covering of the external surface of the body. It is developed differently over the various parts of the body. Specific formations of the skin are the cutaneous sense organs, as well as the "integumentary appendages" – cutaneous glands, hairs and nails.

In contrast to skin, the mucosae cover the inner surfaces of organs – except the conjunctiva, which is frequently grouped with mucous membranes. At the body openings – lips, nares, urethral orifices, vaginal entrance and anus – as well as at the margins of the eyelids, the skin is continuous with the mucosa.

A. Skin

The skin, about 1.6 m^2 in the adult, is an organ with many functions.

Protective function. The skin protects the body from mechanical, thermal and chemical injuries, as well as from the penetration of numerous pathogenic agents owing to the cornification of its epithelium and the secretion of its glands.

Numerous substances (e.g. ointments, medications dissolved in them) can penetrate, however, into the skin.

Temperature regulation. By dilation or constriction of the cutaneous blood vessels and by fluid excretion from the cutaneous glands, the skin contributes to the regulation of body temperature.

If inappropriate clothing hinders the dissipation of heat, an accumulation of heat can occur (with slight rise in temperature).

Water balance. The skin protects the body, on the one hand, from the loss of fluid; on the other hand, it gives off fluid and salts in controlled amounts via glands.

The loss of skin (e.g. from burns) from about 9% of the body surface (approximately the skin from an arm) leads to a life-threatening situation through the loss of salt and water, among others things.

Sensory function. The large number of receptors (cutaneous sense organs) transforms the entire skin into a sense organ which can perceive mechanical and thermal, as well as pain stimuli.

Through the loss of these sensory functions by disease, we are vulnerable to mechanical, thermal or chemical influences.

Communication. The skin is transformed into an "organ for the communication of the autonomic nervous system", i.e. a communication organ, through phenomena – controlled by efferent fibers of autonomic nerves – such as turning red, turning pale, "hair-erection" and others.

Also the electrical resistance of the skin is influenced, among others, by the autonomic nervous system via glandular secretions (the basis for "lie detectors").

Immune function. The skin possesses a considerable number of cells of the specific defense system and participates in characteristic ways in immunobiological defense reactions.

Generally-known, specific modes of reaction of the skin are, for example, the cutaneous changes appearing in scarlet fever, measles, and rubella.

Most of these different functions are the collective achievement of structures of all the layers comprising the skin.

The skin is more directly accessible to the physician for observation and study than any other organ. Since it also involved in the symptomatology of numerous general disorders (e.g. cyanosis in the case of heart disease, localized reddening in the case of infectious diseases, changes due to nutritional disturbances, hormonal disorders, etc.), it deserves special interest. The skin is considered in the differential diagnosis of almost every internal illness.

1. Layers of Skin

The skin consists of two components. The superficial layer of the skin arises from the surface ectoderm, the deeper layers from the mesenchyme lying beneath it. The differentiations of both components are sharply delimited in all formations of the skin by a basement membrane.

The **integument** is comprised of *skin* and *subcutaneous connective tissue* (Fig. **70**) and extends up to the general fascia of the body.

The **skin** consists of two layers:
– the *epidermis*, a stratified, cornified, squamous epithelium, and
– the *dermis* (*corium*), a narrow plexus of collagenous fibers and elastic networks, which interdigitates with the epidermis.

Epidermis and dermis are divided into further layers.

The **subcutaneous connective tissue**, a connective tissue layer containing adipose tissue lobulated by fiber tracts, is closely attached to the dermis, but is displaceable against the general body fascia.

The histological structure and thickness of the layers of the skin vary considerably over the different parts of the body.

a) Epidermis

As the **superficial layer**, the *epidermis* forms the outer covering of the skin and thus the cutaneous surface (Fig. **70**)

Surface of the Skin

The *surface of the skin* possesses a variable gross pattern (relief) and a constant fine pattern.

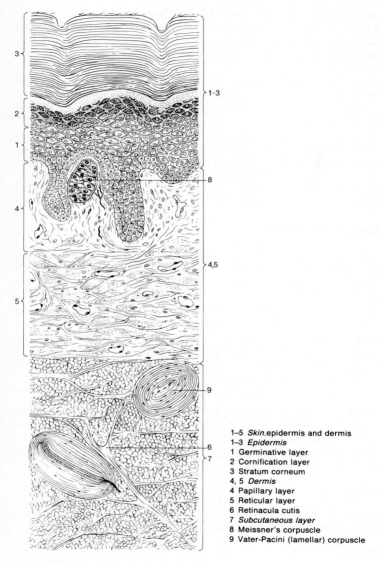

1–5 *Skin*.epidermis and dermis
1–3 *Epidermis*
1 Germinative layer
2 Cornification layer
3 Stratum corneum
4, 5 *Dermis*
4 Papillary layer
5 Reticular layer
6 Retinacula cutis
7 *Subcutaneous layer*
8 Meissner's corpuscle
9 Vater-Pacini (lamellar) corpuscle

Fig. 70. **Skin and subcutaneous tissue (integument)**
(from *Feneis*, 1982)

The *gross pattern* comes about by the *formation of creases* – in the well-nourished youngster by *reserve creases*. These are strongly developed over joints, especially over those extensor surfaces which stretch during flexion. With increasing age, *creases* normally also appear over other body parts. They are caused chiefly by changes in the connective tissue ground substance, combined with a decrease in water content and a decrease in the elasticity of the elastic networks in the cutaneous connective tissue.

With respect to the *fine surface pattern*, skin appears in the form of *fields* or *ridges*.

By far the largest portion of the skin is subdivided by fine, groove-shaped furrows into rhombic **fields**. Depending on the locally different mechanical requirements, the interdigitation between the epidermis and dermis varies locally. The skin over the knee and elbow, for example, is characterized by numerous, deep interdigitations, whereas that of the cheek is distinguished by less numerous, flat interdigitations.

Sweat glands open at the height of the fields: in circumscribed areas there are also odoriferous glands. Hairs with sebaceous glands occupy the furrows.

Ridged skin, which covers the *palms of the hands* and *soles of the feet*, displays parallel ridges and furrows, whose arrangement is traced back to the character of the dermis (→ papillary layer, p. 165). In ridged skin, the epidermis and dermis are very strongly interdigitated. The design of the ridges is genetically determined and, thus, characteristic for the individual person; in the case of regeneration after removal of the uppermost layers of skin, e.g. after burns, it returns to its original form.

Four types of ridge patterns – variable within themselves – are distinguishable on the fingertips: arches, loops, double loops, whorls. The genetically determined, individually specific formation of ridge patterns on the fingertips forms the basis for the use of fingerprints (dactylograms) for identification purposes.

Ridge skin possesses neither hairs nor sebaceous or odoriferous glands. The sweat glands open at the height of the ridges.

Layers of Epidermis

The **epidermis,** a stratified and cornified squamous epithelium, is 0.04 mm thick, at most 0.2 mm. thick, over most of the body. On the palm of the hand and sole of the foot (ridge skin), the epidermis measures 0.75–1.2 mm, on calluses 2 mm and more.

The epidermis regenerates constantly from a basal epithelial layer. From two daughter cells of one of numerous mitoses, one always migrates to the surface in the course of about 30 days, whereby the cells – gradually cornifying – change in appearance and stainability and are finally cast off as horny scales. The process leads to the formation of microscopically visible epidermal layers, which, of course, are universally developed only in ridge skin: the *regenerative layer* (stratum basale), the *differentiation layer* (cornification layer: stratum granulosum and stratum lucidum) and the *horny layer* (stratum corneum).

The *regenerative layer* contains, besides the cornifying cells (keratocytes), also pigment cells (melanocytes), cells of the immune system (Langerhans' cells) and Merkel's tactile discs ($\rightarrow$ p. 169).

The *melanocytes* produce after birth the brownish-black pigment, *melanin*, and release it into epithelial cells – in finely granular form in light-skinned races, in coarsely granular form in dark-skinned races. The melanin pigment protects the basal layer of the epidermis from ultraviolet rays, which are injurious to mitoses. Intensified irradiation can provoke melanin formation (suntan).

Langerhans' cells are branched and not connected with the epithelial cells by cell contact. As *accessory cells of the immune system*, they are capable of taking up antigens ($\rightarrow$ p. 78).

In the cells of the *differentiation layer* arise *lamellated granules* (*keratohyaline granules*) and *bundles of filaments*. The lamellated granules contain lipids which – excreted into the intercellular spaces – spread out and form a barrier that prevents the body fluids from being lost in the intercellular space. Lipids can spread into it, however, also from the surface of the skin (e.g. ointments).

The keratohyaline granules fuse with the filaments into *horny scales*. These are resistant against acids, but alkalis release the desmosomes and with them the epithelial cells. Cornification is controlled by vitamin A; vitamin-A deficiency leads to excessive cornification (hyperkeratosis).

Skin Color

The color of skin is determined by two factors: by the *color of the blood of the cutaneous vessels* and by the *melanocytes*; a further color component arises by infiltration of *carotene* into the epidermis. Skin color in light-skinned races exhibits the following local differences.

The red *color of arterial blood* determines the skin color of the face, palms of the hand, soles of the feet, upper half of the trunk and the buttocks. The bluish *color of venous blood* dominates in the lower half of the trunk and on the dorsum of the hands and feet.

The brown *melanin pigmentation* is concentrated in the skin of the axilla, the external genitalia, the inner side of the thigh, and in the peri-anal skin. Provoked by the action of light, facial skin and the skin of other parts of the body exposed to light also show concentrated melanin pigmentation.

Carotene generates a yellowish color chiefly in the face, palms of the hand and soles of the feet, which can be intensified by food rich in carotene.

An increased bluish discoloration in the parts of the skin supplied by arterial blood (cyanosis) indicates an oxygen deficiency of arterial blood, e.g. in heart disease.

b) Dermis

The **dermis** (*corium*, Fig. **70**), is a dense plexus of collagenous fibers interspersed with elastic networks. It gives the skin tensile strength and reversible deformability; from the dermis of animal skins, leather is obtained by tanning. The dermis possesses numerous blood and lymphatic vessels, nerves and receptors; it contains the roots of the hairs and their root sheaths, as well as the cutaneous glands. In the meshwork of the dermis lie connective tissue cells and cells of the defense system. On the basis of its fibrous organization, two layers can be distinguished: *papillary* and *reticular*.

Layers of Dermis

The **papillary layer** of the dermis borders directly on the epidermis and interdigitates with it by means of conelike projections of collagenous fibers, the *connective tissue papillae*; these project into corresponding indentations of the epidermis, thereby counteracting a shearing off of the epidermis. The loose connective tissue which accompanies the collagenous fibers contains loops of blood capillaries, as well as lymphatic capillaries, nerve branches, sense organs ($\rightarrow$ Meissner's corpuscles, p. 170), and connective tissue cells (fibroblasts and cells of the defense system).

The **reticular layer** separates the papillary layer from the subcutaneous connective tissue. It contains interwoven bundles of thick collagenous fibers which provide for the tensile strength of the skin. The extensibility of the skin can be traced back chiefly to the angular placement of the bundles of collagenous fibers; elastic networks produce the interweaving of the fiber plexus.

The collagenous fiber plexus is differently oriented locally. Pricking the skin with a needle leaves a slit, not a round hole; the direction of the cleavage line corresponds to the tension differences in the skin (Fig. **71**).

If a cut is made perpendicular to the course of the cleavage line, the skin gapes. The surgeon places the skin incision in the direction of the cleavage lines, thus accelerating healing and improving the cosmetic results.

In the case of considerable overdistention of the skin, e.g. abdominal skin during pregnancy, lacerations arise in the texture of the dermis which become visible as light stripes (striae distensae).

c) Subcutaneous Connective Tissue

The **subcutaneous connective tissue** (Fig. **70**), a loose connective tissue rich in adipose tissue lobulated by fibrous connective tissue trabeculae, represents the connection between the skin and the superficial fascia and makes possible the mobility of the skin. The subcutaneous connective

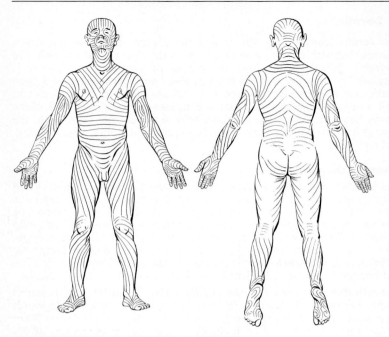

Fig. 71. **Cleavage lines of skin** (after *Benninghoff*)

tissue is an important fat depot and insulator. The adipose tissue occurs as "structural fat" – subdivided like quilted cushions into compression chambers by rigid fibrous connective tissue trabeculae (e.g. in the sole of the foot). More frequently, adipose tissue appears as "fat depots" (e.g. as a fat pad, panniculus adiposus, beneath the skin of the trunk). At the border of the skin and subcutanous connective tissue and in the latter itself there are additional sense organs (→ Vater-Pacini corpuscles, p. 170).

The development of "fat depots" is also genetically determined and, among other things, hormonally controlled. In males the abdominal skin, in females the skin of the breast, hips and buttocks is favored for subcutaneous fat deposition.

Taut connections of the skin with the underlying tissues are afforded by stout connective tissue trabeculae (*retinacula cutis*, e.g. palm of the hand, sole of the foot). In the regions of the face, scalp and anus, the skin is solidly united with the underlying musculature or tendons (in the face: the basis for facial expressions).

Loose connections of the skin with the underlying tissue permit a strong mobility of the skin which is augmented over several body parts (e.g. eyelids, lips, penis, scrotum) by the lack of subcutaneous adipose tissue.

In parts of the skin connected loosely with the underlying tissue, increased tissue fluid can be deposited very easily (edema formation).

2. Vessels and Nerves of the Skin and Subcutaneous Connective Tissue

a) Blood Vessels and Lymphatic Vessels

The blood vessels of richly vascularized skin serve both for the nourishment of the skin and for the regulation of the temperature of the body.

Temperature regulation. The heat generated chiefly in the muscles and the liver is carried into the skin with the blood. A temperature gradient arises which is regulated, among others, by arterioles and arteriovenous anastomoses of the skin. Stronger blood flow leads to an increased loss of heat, and the temperature of the "body covering" (trunk skin, distal portions of the arms and legs) rises. With a decrease in circulation, the heat loss and temperature of the "body covering" falls. The "body nucleus" (central part of the trunk and head) remains constant in temperature.

Measurements of body temperature in the region of the "body covering", therefore, can only then be directly compared when they are taken at the same place and with the same environmental temperature. The temperature of the "body nucleus" can be measured orally and rectally.

The **arteries** of the skin (Fig. **72**) form a plexus between the dermis and the subcutaneous connective tissue, from which branches descend to the roots of the hairs and sweat glands and ascend to the papillary layer of the dermis. The ascending branches form the subpapillary plexus, which sends out capillary loops to the connective tissue papillae of the dermis.

By means of *arteriovenous anastomoses* – small arteriovenous organs at the distal parts of the limbs (finger tips) – the flow velocity in the arteries and veins can be influenced considerably for temperature regulation by bypassing of the capillary loops.

The density of the capillary loops fluctuates, amounting to 20–60 capillary loops per mm^2. Since the tissue pressure normally lies below the blood pressure in the capillaries, these remain open.

In the case of an external pressure of 60–80 mm Hg and more, e.g. when bedridden, the cutaneous capillaries are slowed down. Brief slowing down of the circulation has no consequence but in the case of long-lasting reduction, the skin undergoes nutritional disturbances which lead to ulcers, giving rise to a decubitus.

The **veins** likewise form networks in the dermis, especially beneath the

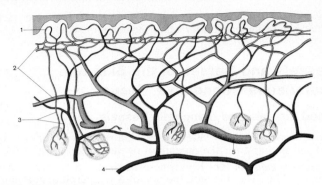

Fig. 72. **Blood vessels of the skin** (after *Horstmann*)
1 Capillary loops in dermal papillae
2 Cutaneous venous plexus
3 Branches to hair roots and sweat glands
4 Subcutaneous arteries
5 Subcutaneous veins

papillae, and in the subcutaneous connective tissue (cutaneous venous plexus, Fig. **72**).

Lymphatic vessels, arranged net-like in the layers of the skin, receive inflow from the capillaries of the papillary layer of the dermis. The lymph flows off mostly via subcutaneous lymphatic tracts. Connections to subfascial lymphatic pathways exist in numbers varying locally.

b) Nerves

The skin is richly innervated by sensory, as well as autonomic efferent nerve fibers.

The *autonomic efferent nerve fibers* supply blood vessels, glands and hair muscles of the skin.

On the one hand, the *sensory cutaneous nerves* comprise a warning system for the protection of the body; on the other hand, they perform important regulatory processes, e.g. heat regulation. The sensory cutaneous nerves mediate numerous different sensory sensations – among others, touch, pressure, vibration, tickling, pain, warmth, heat, cold.

According to physiological studies, the identification of definite nervous structures of the skin as specific receptors of these cutaneous sensory sensations is possible only to a limited degree. In the case of some sensory sensations, the central processing of afferents coming from the skin probably also plays a role.

The *dendritic processes of sensory cutaneous nerves* end either in *terminal corpuscles of nerves* or as *free nerve endings*.

Terminal Corpuscles of Nerves

The *terminal corpuscles of nerves* of the skin (Figs. **70** and **73**) are considered as *mechanoreceptors*. Mechanical deformations of the terminal corpuscles lead to the formation of excitations in the afferent nerve fiber. In the terminal corpuscles of the nerves, the nerve fiber endings are each built up in a special way with other cellular tissue elements to form small sense organs, which are surrounded by a connective tissue capsule.

The afferent nerve fiber from the terminal corpuscles (= dendritic processes of pseudo-unipolar ganglion cells of the spinal ganglion) are myelinated of Type Aβ (diameter 10–15 μm, conduction velocity 30–60 m/s). A nerve fiber can be connected with several corpuscles by collaterals.

Among the numerous well-known forms which occur regularly at definite places in the skin are *Merkel's tactile discs*, *Meissner's tactile corpuscles*, *Vater-Pacini lamellated corpuscles*, and the *genital corpuscles*.

Merkel's tactile discs are light cells in the basal layers of the epidermis, to which endings of peripheral processes of sensory neurones are attached.

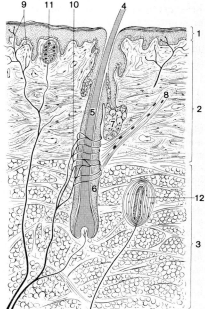

Fig. 73. **Hair and nerve endings in the skin**

1 Epidermis
2 Dermis
3 Subcutaneous connective tissue
4 Hair shaft
5 Hair root
6 Hair root sheath
7 Sebaceous gland
8 Arrector pili muscle
9 Free nerve endings in epidermis and dermis
10 Free nerve endings at hair root sheath
11 Meissner's corpuscles
12 Vater-Pacini corpuscles

Meissner's tactile corpuscles lie in the connective tissue papillae of the dermis, mainly the finger pads. The oval corpuscles about 0.1 mm long and 0.04 mm wide are formed from 5 to 10 wedge-shaped cells layered over one another.

Vater-Pacini lamellated (*Pacinian*) **corpuscles** lie in the dermis, where they are especially abundant in the palms of the hand and the soles of the feet (they occur also in the vicinity of fascia, periosteum, tendons, and blood vessels, as well as in mesenteries and in retroperitoneal organs, e.g. pancreas). The 2–4 mm long, macroscopically visible, pear-shaped corpuscles which are as firm as cartilage consist of 50 and more lamellated cells layered over one another like the skin of an onion.

Free Nerve Endings

"Free nerve endings" are considered as *receptors for pain, pressure, hot and cold sensations*, as well as for *itching*. Free nerve endings are frequently found at *hair follicles, blood vessels* and *free in the connective tissue*.

Free nerve endings at hair follicles form a *nerve cuff*. They enter the root sheath, course centrally in a longitudinal direction, peripherally in a more circular organization – especially pronounced in tactile hairs (Fig. **73**). Touching of the hairs produces lever-like effects which are perceived by the nerve cuff as a type of *mechanoreceptor*.

Free nerve endings at blood vessels and in connective tissue are partly *nociceptors* (*pain receptors* and *receptors for itching*) – i.e. they are stimulated by substances which are liberated by tissue damage. These nerve endings are also considered partly as *mechanoreceptors* (touch sensation, itching) and as *thermoreceptors* (hot and cold sensations).

3. Wound Healing and Aging of Skin

Wound Healing. After an injury to the skin, epithelial tissue from the wound margin grows over the regenerating connective tissue of the wound, forming a scar. Because of the strong vascularization of the regenerating connective tissue, the scar is initially colored reddish. With an increase in collagenous fibers in the dermis, the scar becomes silver white. Cutaneous appendages in the region of the scar are not formed again.

Aging of the skin proceeds with alterations which are mainly an expression of the *general aging of connective tissue*. The papillary layer of the dermis atrophies with a diminishing in the height of the connective tissue papillae. The decrease in elasticity of the elastic network results in a retardation in the resiliency of skin folds. Changes in the chemical composition of the connective tissue ground substance leads to water depletion and to a decrease in skin turgor. Melanocytes perish or lose their contact with the epidermis, the pigmentation of the skin becoming "spotted".

Ultraviolet light (ultraviolet lamp) hastens the loss of elasticity of the skin.

B. Appendages of Skin

The skin appendages – *glands*, *hairs*, *nails* – grow into the connective tissue in a formally homogeneous manner as solid epithelial cords and are differentiated secondarily. The surrounding connective tissue participates in their construction. In hairs, nails and sebaceous glands, a *stratification* appears which can be compared with the layering of the cornified, stratified squamous epithelium of the epidermis.

1. Skin Glands

Three types of *cutaneous glands* can be distinguished, each of which produces a specific secretion: *sweat glands*, *odoriferous glands*, and *sebaceous glands* (Fig. **74**).

The **sweat glands** (*sudoriferous glands*), altogether about 2 million, occur almost everywhere in the skin, being most abundant in the skin of the forehead, palms of the hands and soles of the feet. The acid secretion of these glands (pH 4.5) hinders bacterial growth on the skin by forming an "acidic protective mantle" (mainly of lactic acid) and supports heat regulation through evaporation. In addition, substances are also excreted (salt content about 0.4%, decreasing to 0.03%).

The **odoriferous glands** (*apocrine sweat glands*) lie in the form of larger glandular units in the skin of the axilla, mons pubis, labia majora, and as *circumanal glands* in the peri-anal skin. Smaller glands of the same type are present in the eyelids (*ciliary glands*), in the skin of the external

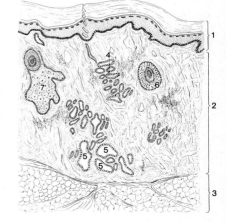

Fig. 74. Integumentary glands, axillary skin
1 Epidermis
2 Dermis
3 Subcutaneous connective tissue
4 Sweat gland
5 Apocrine sweat gland
6 Hair root sheath
7 Sebaceous gland with hair root sheath

acoustic meatus (*ceruminous glands*), and in the nasal vestibule. The *mammary glands* and the *areolar glands* of the nipple are also classified as odoriferous glands. All of these glands produce a fatty, alkaline secretion. In the female, cyclically-determined fluctuations are observed in the production of these secretions.

Since the acidic protective mantle is absent in the region of the odoriferous glands, these glands are often infected by skin bacteria (so-called sudoriparous abscess).

With few exceptions, the **sebaceous glands** occur only in hairy skin as hair glands. Their secretion (*sebum*), 1–2 gm of which are produced daily, is antiseptic due to its content of fatty acids; it makes the skin supple and resistant to water – especially in the mixture with sweat – and contributes to the luster of hair.

A blackhead (comedo) arises by the blockage of an excretory duct of a sebaceous gland.

2. Hairs

Hairs function in heat protection and the sense of touch. They are absent only in a few places on the surface of the body (palms of the hands, soles of the feet, parts of the external genitalia). *Lanugo* and *terminal hairs* are distinguishable, with intermediate forms of these customary divisions not included.

Lanugo hairs develop in the fetus. They are single, short, thin, fair and rooted in the dermis. They disappear postnatally and are superseded in the child by an *intermediate hair coat* which, for the most part, is replaced by terminal hairs, a process intensified at puberty.

Terminal hairs (Fig. 73) are longer and thicker than lanugo hairs and pigmented. They arise in different intervals of postnatal life, but their development increases and becomes sexually differentiated at puberty. Terminal hairiness exhibits varying degrees of local development and especially in the male, can cover almost the entire skin. Individual differences of hairiness are numerous. According to location, the following can be distinguished in the *head region*: *capilli* (hairs of the head, *barbae* (hairs of the beard), *tragi* (hairs of the external acoustic meatus), *vibrissi* (hairs of the nasal vestibule); in the *trunk region*: *hirci* (axilla hairs) and *pubes* (pubic hairs).

The *sexually-specific distribution* of terminal hairiness is hormonally determined. The pubic hairiness ascending to the navel, the hairiness of the chest and the inner surface of the thigh, and the beard growth are typical for *males* – with great individual variability. Typically masculine is the tendency to baldness. For *females,* pubic hairiness marked by a horizontal border at the top and an absence of terminal hairiness on the trunk are characteristic.

Endocrine disturbances in females which lead to masculinization (e.g. diseases of the suprarenal cortex) can bring about the formation of a masculine hair coat (hypertrichosis) and baldness (virilism, hirsutism). Male castrates, on the other hand, lack the typical masculine hair coat.

Terminal hairs are fixed obliquely to the surface in the cylindrical *root sheath*. By means of the collective obliquity of larger hair regions, *hair lines* and *whorls* arise. *Sebaceous glands* open into the root sheath. Above the opening of the sebaceous gland, the root sheath widens into an *infundibulum*. Below the opening of the sebaceous gland, a bundle of smooth muscle cells (*arrector pili muscle*) arises on the side of the bending of the hair and passes obliquely upward into the dermis. The muscle can raise the hair (pilo-erection) and compress the sebaceous gland, which causes the epidermis to be drawn in at the site of the muscle insertion, forming little pits ("goose flesh").

A hair consists of a *shaft*, which protrudes from the surface of the skin, and a *root*, the *bulb* of which rests on the connective tissue *papilla of the hair*. The bulb, papilla and surrounding connective tissue constitute the *hair follicle*.

Molting. Hair grows cyclically in three phases: *growth*, *involution* and *resting*, then falls out. Approximately 80% of the hairs are in the growth phase, 15% in the resting phase. About 50 hairs are lost daily. The hair bulb separates from the papilla and is displaced outward as a *club hair*. From the epithelial remains of the bulb, a new hair grows again above the cord-like extracted papilla. Terminal hairs grow about 1 cm per month; they can survive for months or years.

3. Nails

Nails protect the tips of the fingers and toes. At the same time, they serve for the sensations of touch as they form an abutment for the pressure which is exerted on the tactile elevations; when lost, the tactile sensation of the affected finger tip is reduced.

The **nail** (Fig. **75**), like a hair, is a localized, modified cornification of the epidermis – a cornified plate about 0.5 mm thick which is anchored to the nail bed (in particular, to its epithelium, the *hyponychium*). The nail consists of polygonal, tile-like, stacked horny scales.

The **body of the nail** (*nail plate*) has a distal, free margin, whereas the lateral margins and the proximally-situated nail root are covered by a fold of skin, the *nail wall* (proximal nail fold). In the region of the nail, this fold forms the *nail sac*, which is about 0.5 cm deep. An epithelial cuticle (*eponychium*) extends over the nail plate from the proximal nail fold. The lateral margins of the nail are inserted into the *nail groove* of the nail bed.

The **nail bed** is the epithelial tissue underlying the nail plate, from which the nail grows constantly, 0.14 – 0.4 mm daily. The proximal part of the nail bed (nail

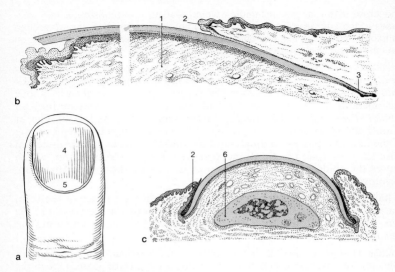

Fig. 75. **Fingernail** (after *Rauber-Kopsch*)
a Exterior
b Longitudinal section through nail bed
c Cross section through nail bed
1 Nail bed
2 Eponychium
3 Nail root
4 Nail body
5 Lunula
6 Phalanx

matrix) lies hidden in the nail sac. The distal part glistens light pink through the nail and near the proximal nail wall forms a distally convex *lunula*. Distal to the lunula, the nail bed continues into the *hyponychium*, shining dark pink through the nail. The nail is pushed forward distally by this epithelial layer. The connective tissue, which corresponds to the papillary layer of the skin and lies beneath the epithelium of the nail bed and the hyponychium, is arranged in longitudinally-coursing ridges. The blood of the capillaries in these connective tissue ridges cause the pink coloration of the nails.

When the nail body is surgically removed, the nail bed is preserved, and a new nail grows again. If the nail bed is destroyed, however, nail growth ceases. In some diseases, the nail reveals diagnostically important changes in size, shape, surface and color.

Special Human Anatomy

8. Upper Limb

The errect posture of the human and the development of the typical bipedalism (two-footedness) have resulted in a division of labor and the specialization of both pairs of limbs. The *lower limbs* have remained an *organ of locomotion*, although under somewhat different mechanical conditions than in quadripeds (four-footed animals) since they alone carry the body weight. Owing to bipedalism the *upper limb* has become free for other duties. Its distal segment, the hand, has developed into a highly specialized *grasping* and *touching organ*, which possesses a differentiated motor system and a rich sensory innervation. The hand has become an important expressive organ (gestures) and has taken on creative functions. The instruments of the hand are the fingers, whereby the thumb has a special status. It can be placed opposite the other fingers (*opposition* of the thumb) so that the hand can act as a grasping pincer.

When its specific human functions are considered, the upper limb shows an advantageous construction in its connection with the trunk that permits the hand to have as large a range of movement as possible. The base of the upper limb, the shoulder girdle – in contrast to the pelvic girdle – is not firmly anchored to the trunk, but has an extremely movable connection with the thorax. The shoulder girdle hangs in a muscular sling, and the single skeletal connection with the trunk is functionally a ball and socket joint (medial clavicular joint).

The structure and organization of both limbs are nonetheless largely congruent. Upper and lower limbs always consist of a *limb girdle* and the *free limb*. Apart from the *clavicle*, which together with the *shoulder blade* forms the *shoulder girdle* of the upper limb, all skeletal elements of both limbs are cartilage bones.

The girdle of the lower limb, the *pelvic girdle*, is formed in the adult from the *hip bone*; this arises from the synostotic fusion (18–20 years of age) of three bones which developed in a homogeneous, cartilaginous pelvic plate: *ilium, ischium* and *pubis*.

The *organization of the free limbs* and the skeletal elements belonging to the individual segments are noted in Table 3.

In primitive four-footed vertebrates (e.g. lizards), the upper arm and thigh are spread out from the body laterally and can be lifted off the ground only with a great expenditure of energy. The forearm and leg are angled away toward the ground. "Elbows" and "knees" face laterally. In mammalian ancestors among the reptiles, the limbs were placed parallel to the body and brought close to or under the body, which then could be carried freely by the limbs. The posterior (lower) limb was thereby rotated forward (the "knee" being directed craniad), and the anterior (upper) limb brought backward to the body (the "elbow" facing back-

Table 3. Organization of the Limbs and Pertinent Skeletal Elements

Pertinent Skeletal Elements	*Limb Segments*		Pertinent Skeletal Elements
Upper Limb			**Lower Limb**
Humerus	**Upper Arm**	**Thigh**	Femur
	Elbow	Knee	
Radius Ulna	**Forearm**	Leg	Tibia Fibula
	Hand	**Foot**	
	organized	into:	
Carpal bones	Wrist	Ankle	Tarsal bones
Metacarpal bones	Metacarpus	Metatarsus	Metatrsal bones
Phalanges	Fingers	Toes	Phalanges

ward). The trunk was thus braced spring-like. In the case of anterior limbs which were flexed backwards, the "hand surface" could rest on the ground, the "finger tips" pointing craniad, with the forearm bones crossed (pronation position). Since the posterior limb was turned forward (craniad), the former dorsal side of this limb was directed ventrally in the case of the upright standing man. The extensors in the thigh and leg (genetically dorsal muscles) were located on the anterior side, i.e. in front of the corresponding limb bones, whereas the extensors in the arm and forearm had preserved their original dorsal position.

A. Shoulder and Axilla

1. Shoulder Girdle

a) Skeletal Elements of the Shoulder Girdle

The **skeleton of the shoulder girdle** consists of the *shoulder blade* (*scapula*) and the *collar bone* (*clavicle*).

The **scapula** (Figs. **76** and **77**) forms a thin triangular bony plate which is reinforced frame-like and lies on the dorsolateral wall of the thorax. The surface turned toward the thorax (*costal surface*) is slightly hollowed out (*subscapular fossa*) and serves as the surface of origin of the subscapularis muscle. On the *posterior surface*, the palpable *spine of the scapula* elevates the skin. It ascends obliquely lateral and craniad from the *medial margin* of the scapula, which lies parallel to the vertebral column and terminates with a flat, well-developed process, the *acromion*, that overlaps the shoulder joint from behind and above.

The apex of the angle formed by the lateral margin of the acromion with the spine of the scapula is designated as the *acromial angle*. At its anterior margin the acromion bears the oval, almost level *acromial articular surface* for articulation with the clavicle.

The spine of the scapula subdivides the dorsal surface of the scapula into the smaller, cranial, *supraspinous fossa* (for the origin of the supraspinatus muscle) and into the *infraspinous fossa*, the extensive field of origin for the infraspinatus muscle.

The medial margin of the scapula is often slightly convex, the pad-like thickened *lateral margin* straight or insignificantly concave. Both margins meet to form the *inferior angle*, the dorsal surface of which gives origin to the teres major muscle. The medial upper angle of the scapula (*superior*

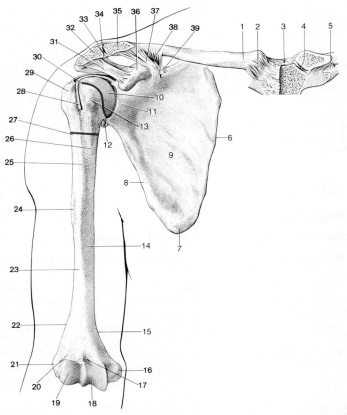

Fig. 76. **Skeletal elements and connections of shoulder girdle, humerus and shoulder joint** (opened), ventral view (right lateral and left medial clavicular joints opened by frontal section)

angle) serves as the insertion surface for the levator scapulae muscle. In the cranial margin (*superior margin*) is the *scapular notch*. It is closed off cranially by the *superior transverse scapular ligament*, which is often ossified. The suprascapular nerve passes through the notch beneath the ligament, the suprascapular vessels course above it.

The hook-shaped *coracoid process* projects from the superior margin of the scapula lateral to the scapular notch. Directed ventrolaterally, it serves as an attachment surface for the pectoralis minor, coracobrachialis and short head of the biceps brachii muscles. A broad band, the *coraco-acromial ligament*, passes from this process to the acromion and forms the ligamentous roof of the shoulder joint (Figs. **76, 82** and **83**). Occasionally the central region of the ligament is reduced or absent so that it appears V-shaped or in two parts. The coraco-acromial ligament functions as a tension girdle for the acromion.

At the *lateral angle* the scapula is thickened and bears the laterally-directed, oval articular cavity (*glenoid cavity*) for the head of the humerus. A small bony prominence, the *supraglenoid tubercle*, projects at the superior margin of this socket and serves for the attachment of the tendon of the long head of the biceps. An *infraglenoid tubercle* situated below the cartilage-covered joint surface gives origin to a part of the tendon of the long head of the triceps. Medial to the glenoid cavity, the scapula is constricted to form the neck (*collum scapulae*).

The **clavicle** (Fig. **76**), a bony rod bent slightly S-shaped, is curved convex ventrally in its medial portion and is thickened at its triangular *sternal extremity*. It possesses a fibrocartilaginous, generally saddle-shaped *sternal articular surface* at its joint union with the articular disc of the

1 Sternal end of clavicle
2 Anterior sternoclavicular ligament
3 Interclavicular ligament
4 Articular disc in sternoclavicular joint
5 Costoclavicular ligament
6 Medial margin of scapula
7 Inferior angle of scapula
8 Lateral margin of scapula
9 Subscapular fossa
10 Head of humerus
11 Lateral angle of scapula
12 Articular capsule of shoulder joint (folded)
13 Lesser tubercle of humerus
14 Anterior medial surface of humerus
15 Medial margin of humerus
16 Medial epicondyle of humerus
17 – 20 Humeral condyle
17 Coronoid fossa
18 Trochlea of humerus
19 Capitulum of humerus
20 Radial fossa
21 Lateral epicondyle of humerus
22 Lateral margin of humerus
23 Anterior lateral surface of humerus
24 Deltoid tuberosity
25 Crest of greater tubercle
26 Crest of lesser tubercle
27 Surgical neck of humerus
28 Tendon of long head of biceps
29 Greater tubercle of humerus
30 Anatomical neck of humerus
31 Coraco-acromial ligament
32 Acromion
33 Articular disc in acromioclavicular joint
34 Acromioclavicular ligament
35 Acromial end of clavicle
36 Coracoid process
37 Trapezoid ligament ⎫ Coracoclavicular
38 Conoid ligament   ⎬ ligament
39 Superior transverse scapular ligament

sternoclavicular joint. The *acromial end* is concave ventrally, strongly flattened and widened at its extremity. The slightly arched *acromial articular surface* is directed dorsolaterally.

The costoclavicular ligament is anchored at a deepened, rough bony area on the undersurface of the sternal extremity. On the caudal surface of the acromial extremity close to the posterior margin lie the *conoid tubercle* and (lateral to it) the *trapezoid line*. Attached here are the two parts of the coracoclavicular ligament, the conoid and trapezoid ligaments.

The clavicle can be partially or totally absent so that the patients can move their shoulders forward until they touch each other (cleidocranial dysostosis,

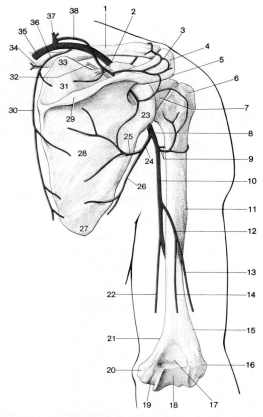

Fig. 77. **Skeletal elements of shoulder girdle and humerus, branches of subclavian and brachial arteries**, dorsal view.

dominant hereditary disease with an ossification disturbance, principally of the membrane bones).

Fractures of the clavicle are relatively frequent (about 16% of all bone fractures) and usually involve the middle third. The medial end of the fracture is pulled upward by the clavicular head of the sternocleidomastoid muscle, the lateral fractured piece downward by the deltoid muscle. The shoulder drops (weight of the arm), the arm is adducted and rotated inward (the bony brace against the action of adduction and internal rotation is absent). In the case of the rare fracture lateral to the attachment of the coracoclavicular ligament, the trapezius muscle pulls the bone fragment upward.

The **ossification** of the *scapula* (Fig. **78**) begins in the region of its neck in the 8th embryonic week. Independent ossific centers appear postnatally at the concavity of the coracoid process (1st year), at its root (10–12th year) and in the acromion (15–18th year). In addition, ossifications occur (between ages 15 and 19) within its processes in the region of the glenoid cavity, at the apex and base of the coracoid process, at the medial margin of the scapula and at its inferior angle. The cartilaginous joints sometimes do not disappear until around the 21st year.

The intramembranous ossification of the *clavicle* (Fig. **78**) begins in the 7th embryonic week (first bone formation of the skeleton). In the 18–20th year, a center of ossification appears in the sternal cartilaginous growth zone which often does not fuse with the "body" of the clavicle until the 24th year (risk of misinterpretation in radiograms).

b) Connections of the Shoulder Girdle

The clavicle articulates with the sternum at the medial (sternal) clavicular joint, the only articular contact between the shoulder girdle and the

---

1 Clavicle
2 Superior transverse scapular ligament
3 Acromial network
4 Acromion
5 Acromial angle
6 Greater tubercle of humerus
7 Head of humerus
8 Axillary artery
9 Anterior and posterior circumflex humeral arteries
10 Brachial artery
11 Deltoid tuberosity
12 Profunda brachii artery in groove for radial nerve
13 Radial collateral artery
14 Middle collateral artery
15 Lateral margin of humerus
16 Lateral epicondyle of humerus
17 Olecranon fossa
18 Trochlea of humerus
19 Groove for ulnar nerve
20 Medial epicondyle of humerus
21 Medial margin of humerus
22 Superior ulnar collateral artery
23 Neck of scapula
24 Subscapular artery
25 Circumflex scapular artery
26 Thoracodorsal artery
27 Inferior angle of scapula
28 Infraspinous fossa
29 Spine of scapula
30 Deep branch of transverse cervical artery (dorsal scapular artery)
31 Supraspinous fossa
32 Suprascapular nerve
33 Superior angle of scapula
34 Superficial branch of transverse cervical artery
35 Subclavian artery
36 Transverse cervical artery
37 Thyrocervical trunk
38 Suprascapular artery

trunk. The clavicle and scapula communicate with one another by an *articulation* at the lateral (acromial) clavicular joint (in clinical practice usually designated as acromial joint) and *ligamentously* by the coraco-clavicular ligament. The scapula is movably fixed to the thorax by a muscular sling and moves on the thorax (especially on the serratus anterior muscle) by means of a loose movable layer (subcapsular gliding layer) with the subscapularis muscle originating at the costal surface.

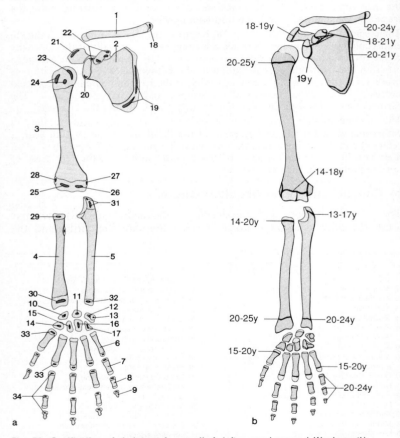

Fig. 78. **Ossification of skeleton of upper limb** (after *von Lanz* and *Wachsmuth*)
a Appearance of ossific centers
b Closure of epiphysial and apophysial synchondroses
(EW = embryonic weeks, M = postnatal months, Y = postnatal years)

The **medial clavicular joint** (Fig. **76**) is two-chambered. A fibrocartilagi-nous, thick *articular disc* (which is derived from the intramembranous episternum of lower vertebrates) is inserted between the incongruent, fibrocartilaginous articular surfaces of the sternal end of the clavicle and the clavicular notch.

The thickened end of the sternal extremity clearly projects over the superior margin of the sternum and deepens the jugular notch. The interarticular disc decreases the incongruities of the joint surfaces and permits more extensive joint movements.

Ligaments. The flaccid joint capsule is strengthened on the anterior and posterior surfaces by the *anterior* and *posterior sternoclavicular ligaments.* The fiber tracts of both ligaments restrict the possibilities of forward or backward movement of the clavicle. The flaccid *interclavicular ligament* unites the sternal ends of both clavicles and is attached firmly to the jugular notch at the superior margin of the sternum. It prevents the lowering of both clavicles. If a clavicle becomes distinctly lower, the other clavicle must be placed obliquely with the acromial end higher, otherwise the short, horizontal fiber tract of the interclavicular ligament would be overstretched or might tear. The *costoclavicular ligament* passes from the cartilage-bone border of the 1st rib to the costoclavicular impression at the undersurface of the sternal end of the clavicle. It is stretched by extreme lifting and forward movement of the clavicle.

In the **lateral clavicular joint** (*acromioclavicular articulation*, Fig. **76**), the joint surfaces are not proportionately different. The superior wall of the capsule is strengthened by the *acromioclavicular ligament* (Fig. **82**).

◀

1 – 9 *Beginning of diaphysial ossification*
1 Clavicle, 7 EW
2 Scapula, 8 EW
3 Humerus, 7–8 EW
4 Radius, 7 EW
5 Ulna, 7 EW
6 Metacarpals I–V, 9 EW
7 Proximal phalanges, 9 EW
8 Middle phalanges, 11–12 EW
9 Distal phalanges, 7–8 EW
10 –17 *Appearance of ossific centers in carpal bones*
10 Scaphoid, 5–6 Y
11 Lunate, 4–5 Y
12 Triquetrum, 2–3 Y
13 Pisiform, 8–12 Y
14 Trapezium, 4–7 Y
15 Trapezoid, 4–6 Y
16 Capitate, 1–6 M
17 Hamate, 1–7 M
18 – 32 *Appearance of epiphysial and apophysial ossific centers*

18 Sternal end of clavicle, 18–20 Y
19 Medial margin and inferior angle of Scapula, 15–19 Y
20 Glenoid cavity, 15–19 Y
21 Acromion, 15–18 Y
22 Coracoid process: chief nucleus in concave curvature, 11–12 M; base, 10–12 Y; convex curvature and apex, 15–19 Y
23 Head of humerus, 1–2 Y
24 Greater and lesser tubercles of humerus, 2–4 Y
25 Trochlea of humerus, 10–12 Y
26 Capitulum of humerus, 1–2 Y
27 Medial epicondyle of humerus, 5–6 Y
28 Lateral epicondyle of humerus, 8–13 Y
29 Head of radius, 15–7 Y
30 Distal epiphysis of radius, 1–2 Y
31 Olecranon, 8–12 Y
32 Head of ulna, 5–7 Y

The articular surface of the acromion is flat or forms a shallow, oval fossa, whereas the acromial articular surface on the clavicle can be insignificantly arched. Frequently, a fibrocartilaginous *articular disc* is present, but the articular cavity is rarely completely doubled.

Dislocations (luxations) of the clavicular joints are rare on account of the ligamentous reinforcement of the articular capsules. They are somewhat more frequent in the acromioclavicular joint than in the medial clavicular joint. During this process, usually the lateral end of the clavicle is pushed out over the acromion.

The **ligamentous union of clavicle and scapula,** the strong *coracoclavicular ligament* (Figs. **76** and **82**), is bipartite. It relieves the lateral clavicular joint by transferring the weight of the arm from the coracoid process to the clavicle. The quadrangular *trapezoid ligament* lies laterally and ventrally. Its surfaces are almost transverse to the longitudinal axis of the clavicle, i.e. in the rest position almost sagittal to the clavicle. The weaker, triangular *conoid ligament* lies medial and posterior. The base of the triangle is fixed at the clavicle, the apex directed toward the coracoid process. Into the recess between the two ligaments, a broad laterally inserting subclavius muscle can be moved; it is usually filled up by fat tissue or a mucous bursa.

Movement possibilities of the shoulder girdle. The two clavicular joints are functionally ball and socket joints. The direction and extent of the movements in the acromioclavicular joint are determined essentially by the range of joint motion possible for the scapula, which is fixed at the thoracic wall by muscular slings. The range of movement is further restricted by the coracoclavicular ligament, the trapezoid ligament preventing shoulder movement forward, the conoid ligament backward.

Both clavicular joints participate in the movements – in different proportions. Movements at the sternoclavicular joint alone – without participation of the acromioclavicular joint – are not possible since the clavicle and scapula are not connected by muscles which can fix the joint. By a movement exclusively at the acromioclavicular joint, a change in position of only the scapula could (theoretically) result.

The connections of the shoulder girdle permit:
– *elevation* or *depression of the shoulder* (= vertical displacement of the scapula),
– *forward* or *backward movement of the shoulder* (= horizontal displacement of the scapula ventrolaterally or dorsomedially), or
– *rotation of the scapula* around the *longitudinal axis* of the clavicle, whereby 2/3 of the movement take place in the lateral, 1/3 in the medial clavicular joints (total circumference of rotatory movement about 60%).

In the sternoclavicular joint the depression of the clavicle from the resting position is possible to a slight degree, elevation in a more pronounced degree (at the acromial end up to 10 cm). In extreme utilization of the movement range at the sternoclavicular joint, the acromial extremity describes a transversely-placed ellipse. In the process, the clavicle is necessarily rotated around its longitudinal axis.

If the straps of a heavy backpack pull the clavicle backwards for a long time, the venous reflux from the arm can be greatly hindered, and the lower "root" branches of the brachial plexus can be irritated. In the case of extreme back loads and depression of the clavicle, the subclavian artery can be pressed against the 1st rib and pinched off so that the radial pulse disappears.

Movements in which chiefly the *lateral clavicular joint* is involved exist in:
– *turning movements of the lower angle of the scapula* around a *horizontal* axis through the acromioclavicular joint and
– *wing movements of the scapula* around a *vertical* axis coursing through the lateral clavicular joint.

Turning movements of the inferior scapular angle are the prerequisites for the elevation of the arm above the horizontal plane (the glenoid cavity is thereby directed obliquely upward). In the case of high forward elevation of the arm, they take place around a frontal axis, in the case of high lateral elevation, around a sagittal axis and in the case of the exclusive participation of the acromioclavicular joint, they are possible to about 40°(otherwise 60°).

In the case of *wing movements*, the medial margin of the scapula is lifted away from the thorax (angel wing position) or pressed against the thoracic wall. The circumference of movement amounts to about 50°.

c) Arrangement and Innervation of the Shoulder Girdle Musculature

The muscles which connect the skeletal elements of the shoulder girdle with the trunk and move them originate from different sources. The trapezius, which forms the superficial layer in the cranial segment of the back, is a branchiomeric muscle that has been mixed to a slight extent with material from the upper cervical somites. The muscle layer located beneath the trapezius, the levator scapulae and rhomboids, and the serratus anterior represents – in reference to the limbs – a dorsal muscle group in the transition region from trunk to limbs. The subclavius and pectoralis minor can be considered as their ventral counterparts. All of these muscles are derivatives of the ventrolateral trunk musculature and are innervated by ventral branches of the lower cervical nerves (brachial plexus).

The levator scapulae, rhomboids, and serratus anterior are usually grouped together with the latissimus dorsi and teres major as *spinohumeral muscles*, the subclavius and pectoralis muscles as the *thoracohumeral muscle group*. They are regarded as derivatives of the dorsal (extensor) or ventral (flexor) groups of limb musculature which have pushed forward secondarily on the thorax again and have spread out superficially to the autochthonous dorsal and ventrolateral trunk musculature.

The trapezius, levator scapulae, rhomboids and latissimus dorsi which have migrated into the back region are also grouped with the serratus posterior muscles as *superficial back muscles* as opposed to the *deep* back muscles (= autochthonous back musculature → p. 481).

Dorsally Situated Muscles of the Shoulder Girdle

The **trapezius** (Fig. 79) arises from the supreme (or superior) nuchal line and the external occipital protuberance of the occipital bone, from the ligamentum nuchae, from the spinous processes of the thoracic vertebrae and from the supraspinous ligament of the thoracic region. The insertion takes place at the lateral third of the clavicle, at the acromion and at the spine of the scapula.

The cranial fibers pass from their origin obliquely downwards as the *descending part*, the middle fibers course horizontal as the *transverse part*, and the caudal bundles ascend upward as the *ascending part*.

The triangular tendinous level in the region of origin of the transverse part (Fig. 188), together with the tendinous level of the opposite side, takes the shape of a rhomboid. The tendinous rhomboid frequently appears as a deepening on the external skin. The marginal contour of the muscle of both sides likewise represents a rhombus.

The right and left trapezius muscle are frequently asymmetrical. In a right-handed person the origin of the left ascending part reaches caudally usually only up to the 10th or 11th thoracic spinous process.

Innervation: The accessory nerve, as well as the ventral branches of cervical nerves (2), 3 and 4 for the cranial segment.

The accessory nerve courses through the lateral triangle of the neck down to the ventral surface of the muscle approximately parallel to the lateral margin of the levator scapulae.

The **levator scapulae** (Fig. 79) arises from the posterior tubercles of the transverse processes of the first four cervical vertebrae between the scalene muscles and the splenius. The original portion is visible in slender, very muscular individuals in the lateral triangle of the neck. The muscle, covered by the trapezius, passes obliquely downward to the superior angle and to the medial margin of the scapula above its spine.

Innervation: dorsal scapular nerve (with additional fibers from the cervical plexus).

The **rhomboids** (Fig. 79) form a strong, rhomboid-shaped muscular plate, whose fibers originate in the spinous processes of the 5th (6th) cervical vertebrae up to the 4th thoracic vertebra and in the corresponding

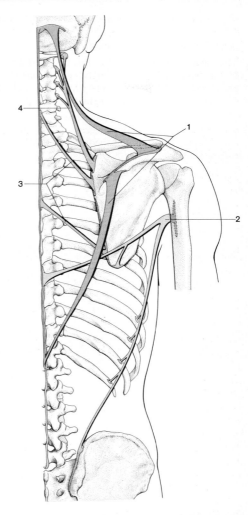

Fig. 79. **Muscles of shoulder
girdle and latissimus dorsi**,
dorsal view
1 Trapezius
2 Latissimus dorsi
3 Rhomboideus major and minor
4 Levator scapulae
Innervation:
▨ Accessory nerve and ventral rami
of cervical nerves (II) III and IV
☐ Dorsal scapular nerve
☐ Thoracodorsal nerve

segments of the ligamentum nuchae and supraspinous ligament. They
insert at the medial margin of the scapula, caudal to the insertion of the
levator scapulae.

A narrow, cranial part of the muscle is separated off by a branch of the deep ramus
of the transverse cervical artery (or by the dorsal scapular artery). It represents the

rhomboideus minor as opposed to the larger, caudal segment, the *rhomboideus major*.

Innervation: dorsal scapular nerve.

The **serratus anterior** (Fig. **80**) has shifted its origin to the ventrolateral trunk wall only secondarily – demonstrable in human ontogenesis. It arises by 9 (10) slips from ribs I–VIII (IX) and inserts at the inferior surface of the medial margin of the scapula (Fig. **85**).

The strong, large-surfaced muscle spreads out on the ventrolateral thoracic wall between pectoralis major, latissimus dorsi and the origin of the external abdominal oblique. It forms the medial wall of the axilla. The slips of origin of the superior part come from ribs 1 and 2 and course almost horizontally to the

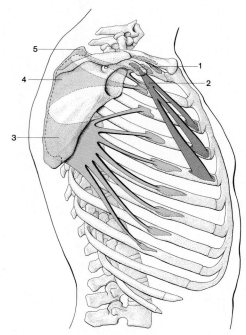

Fig. 80. **Serratus anterior and ventral muscles of shoulder girdle**
1 Subclavius
2 Pectoralis minor
3 Inferior part ⎫
4 Middle part ⎬ Serratus anterior
5 Superior part ⎭
Innervation:
▢ Long thoracic nerve
▢ Subclavian nerve
▨ Medial and Lateral pectoral nerves

superior angle of the scapula. The *middle part* is rather thin and frequently exits only from the 2nd rib. The muscle bundles diverge to insert at the medial margin of the scapula. The *inferior part* arises with 6–7 slips from ribs 3–8 (9). It forms the largest segment of the muscle and possesses the longest bundles of fibres. These converge toward the scapula and insert in the caudal region of the medial margin of the scapula, above all, at the inferior angle.

Innervation: Long thoracic nerve, the main trunk of which passes downward in the axillary line to the serratus anterior.

Ventrally Situated Muscles of the Shoulder Girdle

The subclavius and pectoralis minor extend from the anterior trunk wall to the ventral segment of the shoulder girdle. The pectoralis minor, however, due to its close genetic and topographical relations to the pectoralis major, is discussed with the muscles of the shoulder girdle (→ p. 205).

The **subclavius** (Figs. **80** and **197**) is a small, strong, pennate muscle which passes from the ventral margin of the 1st rib (cartilage-bone border) to the inferior surface of the clavicle.

It courses almost parallel to the clavicle, whose medial end it presses against the articular disc of the sternoclavicular joint, thus providing resistance to an externally directed traction acting on the shoulder girdle. Due to obliquely coursing fibers, it can only insignificantly depress the non-elevated clavicle.

Innervation: Nerve to the subclavius.

d) Action of Muscles and Muscle Groups on the Shoulder Girdle

The medial margin of the scapula presents a bony line for the attachment of the muscular plate formed by the levator scapulae, rhomboids and serratus anterior. By the graduated interplay of these muscles, the scapula can move on the thorax and be brought in each case into the most favorable starting position for the movements of the arm. Since the tendon fibers of the descending part of the trapezius are attached more laterally on the shoulder girdle than the tendon fibers of the ascending part, a contraction of both parts of the muscle, or of the total muscle, leads to a rotation of the scapula (aided decisively by the serratus anterior) so that the glenoid cavity faces upward (a prerequisite for raising the arm above the horizontal plane).

The combined movements of the shoulder girdle are executed in muscle slings whereby the extent of shortening of the respective antagonists at the moment of tension equilibrium determines the position of the clavicle or scapula.

The *acromial end of the clavicle is* (Fig. **16**)
- *elevated* or *depressed* by the longitudinal muscle sling: levator scapulae – ascending part of the trapezius, descending part of the trapezius – pectoralis minor,

> whereby the rhomboids, pectoralis major (clavicular part) and sternocleidomastoid (clavicular head) can support the elevation of the shoulder, while the caudal pulling of the pectoralis major and latissimus dorsi, together with the subclavius, can assist in its depression;

- *carried ventrolaterally* or *dorsomedially* by the transverse muscle sling: superior and middle parts of the serratus anterior – transverse part of the trapezius,
  whereby the rhomboids, ascending and descending tracts of the trapezius, and the cranial fibers of the latissimus dorsi retract the shoulder, while the pectoralis minor and pectoralis major help to carry it forward.

The *inferior angle of the scapula* is
- *turned anteriorly* or *posteriorly* (thus directing the glenoid cavity upward or downward) by the obliquely arranged muscle sling:
  inferior part of serratus anterior – rhomboids,
  whereby the anterior turning is effected substantially by the cooperation of the descending and ascending parts of the trapezius, and the posterior turning can be supported by the levator scapulae and pectoralis minor.

The *trapezius* with its descending part counteracts the pull directed downwards, which attempts to depress the shoulder girdle (e.g. when carrying luggage). The *levator scapulae* can extend the cervical vertebral column when the shoulder girdle is fixed. By means of the rhomboids-serratus sling, the scapula is pressed against the thorax.

Paralyses. In a complete paralysis of the *trapezius* (simultaneous injury to the accessory nerve and the upper cervical nerves), the shoulder lies deeper than on the healthy side. The nuchal-shoulder line no longer follows the form of an arch, but is broken. The scapula is further removed from the midline, the glenoid cavity facing forward and downward. The shoulder can only be raised with weak energy (levator scapulae) and carried backwards only slightly (rhomboids). Lateral elevation of the arm is greatly reduced; the arm usually cannot be abducted to the horizontal plane. Forward elevation of the arm is negligibly restricted (rotation of the scapula by the serratus anterior), whereas elevation in the sagittal plane is strongly impeded.

If only the accessory nerve is severed, the function of the descending part of the trapezius is preserved in varying degrees (concomitant innervation by upper cervical nerves). The positional changes of the scapula are not so conspicuous. The elevation of the arm toward the side or backward, however, is just as much restricted.

When the *serratus anterior* is paralyzed, the medial margin of the scapula lies closer to the vertebral column and somewhat away from the thorax (angel-wing position, winged scapula). The forward movement of the shoulder is executed feebly (pectoralis major). The arm cannot be lifted forward above the horizontal plane, the scapula being levered down wing-like.

In the case of injury to the dorsal scapular nerve with a paralysis of the *levator scapulae* and *rhomboids,* the medial margin of the scapula stands somewhat away from the thorax. When the shoulder is lifted (descending part of the trapezius), the inferior angle of the scapula is turned ventrolaterally since the medial margin of the scapula can no longer be held fast by the paralyzed rhomboids.

Clavicle and subclavian vessels. The subclavius muscle and clavipectoral fascia, which encloses the muscle at the inferior surface of the clavicle, cover the subclavian vessels and the "root" branches of the brachial plexus like a protective cushion so that they are not, as a rule, endangered by a splintered fracture of the clavicle. Since the subclavian vein is attached at the periosteum of the 1st rib and the clavipectoral fascia, it is always kept open. Every movement in which the clavicle is withdrawn from the 1st rib enlarges the lumen of the vein by traction on the fascia and expedites the venous return of blood. Since the subclavian vein does not collapse when injured, air can be drawn in at the injury site (danger of an air embolism).

2. Shoulder Joint

a) Skeletal Elements of the Upper Arm

The *scapula* and the *upper arm bone*, the *humerus*, articulate in the shoulder joint.

The *humerus* (Figs. **76** and **77**) presents a shaft (diaphysis) and the proximal and distal end pieces (proximal and distal epiphyses).

At the *proximal end* the large, hemispherical *head of the humerus* (*caput humeri*) is directed *mediocranially* and forms an angle of about 130° with the axis of the shaft. Its cartilage-covered surface articulates with the glenoid cavity of the scapula. The massive *greater tubercle* faces *laterally*, the *lesser tubercle ventrally*. A bony ridge passes distally from both prominences: *crest of the greater tubercle and crest of the lesser tubercle*. Both tubercles and both crests border a groove, the *intertubercular sulcus*, which contains the tendon of the long head of the biceps (Fig. **82**).

The tendons of the teres minor, infraspinatus and supraspinatus muscles insert from dorsal to ventral at the three fields of the greater tubercle. The subscapularis tendon is attached to the lesser tubercle.

In the humerus varus (as a result of growth disturbances, cretinism, rickets, etc.), the angle between the diaphysial axis and the axis of the humeral head decreases to almost 90°. The greater tubercle is situated relatively high.

The annular constriction of the proximal end of the humerus between the head and both tubercles, the *anatomical neck*, inclines obliquely medialward (Fig. **76**). In contrast, the *surgical neck*, a slight constriction of the humeral shaft distal to the tubercles, lies in a horizontal plane.

Fractures of the humerus occur more frequently at the surgical neck than at the anatomical neck or at the thicker segments of the shaft.

The *diaphysis of the humerus* presents *anteromedial* and *anterolateral surfaces* which are bordered by the *medial* and *lateral margins* of the posterior surface. On the anterolateral surface in the middle of the shaft is a roughness, the *deltoid tuberosity*, for the insertion of the deltoid muscle.

In the middle of the humeral diaphysis, somewhat distal to the deltoid tuberosity, the *sulcus for the radial nerve* passes in a steep spiral direction from the posterior surface around the lateral margin to the anterolateral surface. In this sulcus – close to bone and therefore at risk in fractures – the radial nerve courses, together with the profunda brachii artery and vein.

The *distal epiphysis* of the humerus (Fig. **90**) is widened and flattened dorsoventrally. The sharp medial margin runs into the distinctly protruding *medial epicondyle*, the sharp lateral margin into the less prominent *lateral epicondyle*. Both bony projections serve as sites of origin for the forearm musculature. The ulnar nerve courses close to the skin on the dorsal surface of the medial epicondyle in the *sulcus for the ulnar nerve* (funny bone). Between both epicondyles and distal to them, there is the segment of the humerus known as the *condyle of the humerus*. Medially it bears the *trochlea*, a pulley that articulates with the trochlear notch of the ulna. Laterally, the *capitulum*, well defined by a bony ridge, forms a hemispherical prominence on the anterior surface of the condyle.

Above the capitulum there is a flat cavity, the *radial fossa*, into which the head of the radius slides during maximum flexion of the elbow joint. Proximal to the trochlea there is another cavity, the *coronoid fossa*, for the coronoid process of the ulna. It can communicate by a small opening with the deep *olecranon fossa* on the dorsal side of the condyle, into which the olecranon is pushed during extreme extension of the elbow joint.

About 5–6 cm above the medial epicondyle there occasionally appears (in about 1% of Europeans) a small osseous process, the *supracondylar process*, from which a ligamentous band passes to the epicondyle. Through the opening bounded in this way, the median nerve and the brachial artery pass. In many mammals the *supracondyloid foramen* is completely surrounded by bone.

Torsion of the humerus. In the adult, a frontal axis drawn through the elbow joint intersects the line of projection of the axis of the head of the humerus from the

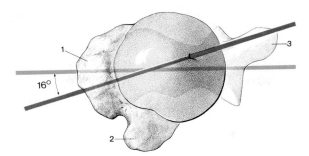

Fig. 81. **Torsion of humerus in adults** (proximal end of right humerus projected on the humeral condyle, dorsal side above)
Projection line of axis of head of humerus ▬
Frontally-placed flexion-extension axis of elbow joint ▬
 1 Greater tubercle of humerus
 2 Lesser tubercle of humerus
 3 Medial epicondyle of humerus

greater tubercle to the middle of the humeral head at an acute angle (Fig. **81**). The humerus is slightly torqued (14–20°). In the newborn child, the torsion of the humerus amounts to nearly 60°; in the young fetus, the two axes form approximately a right angle. The decrease in torsion is correlated with the postnatal positional changes of the scapula resulting from the change in shape of the thorax. In the newborn with its barrel-shaped thorax, the glenoid cavity faces more ventrally, whereas in the adult with a transversely oval thorax, it faces more laterally. The torsion of the humerus must be adapted to the position of the scapula if the range of movement of the hands is to be in the field of vision.

The **ossification** of the *diaphysis of the humerus* (Fig. **78**) begins in weeks 7–8 of the embryonic period. In the first years of life, ossific centers appear in the head and both tubercles, which fuse in the 5th year. By this means, a uniform, secondary cartilaginous joint arises, which is formed in front by the two apophysial joints and behind by the original epiphysial joint. It lies dorsal and medial within the capsule of the shoulder joint, ventral and lateral extracapsularly, and is several millimeters wide. The (secondary) *proximal* epiphysial joint of the humerus closes relatively late; the longitudinal growth of the humerus is concluded in about the 25th year of life.

The (secondary) *distal* epiphysial joint of the humerus ossifies very early, usually in the 14–16th year. It originates at about the 13–15th year when the separate ossific centers appearing at different times at the distal end of the humerus (capitulum very early, 1st postnatal year; trochlea very late, 12th year of life; lateral epicondyle, ages 8–13) become fused into a uniform secondary epiphysial complex. The apophysial center in the medial epicondyle (from the 5th year of life) remains independent until its fusion with the diaphysis (14–18th year).

Epiphysial fractures in the region of the proximal epiphysial joint as a childbirth trauma can involve the primary joint (in the region of the anatomical neck).

More frequent is an epiphysial fracture in the broad secondary cartilaginous joint. With correct treatment of an epiphysial fracture, the risk of growth disturbance is slight.

b) Capsule and Ligamentous Apparatus of the Shoulder Joint

In the **shoulder joint** the glenoid cavity of the scapula articulates with the head of the humerus (Figs. **76**, **82** and **83**). The surface of the hemispherical joint head is 3–4 times as large as the pear-shaped, flat joint socket, whose greatest sagittal diameter amounts to only two thirds of the vertical. Its surface is enlarged by a *socket* (or joint) *lip* (*glenoid lip*) about

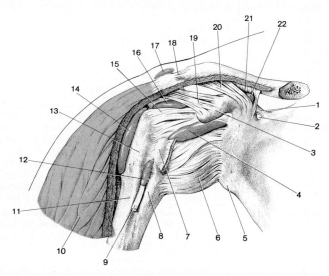

Fig. 82. **Synovial bursae in region of shoulder joint**, ventral view

1 Superior transverse scapular ligament
2 Scapular notch
3 Coracoid process
4 Subscapular bursa
5 Infraglenoid tubercle
6 Articular capsule of humerus
7 Lesser tubercle of humerus with attachment of subscapularis muscle (severed)
8 Crest of lesser tubercle
9 Tendon of long head of biceps in intertubercular groove
10 Deltoid (clavicular origin omitted)
11 Crest of greater tubercle
12 Intertubercular synovial sheath
13 Greater tubercle of humerus
14 Subdeltoid bursa
15 Coracohumeral ligament
16 Subacromial bursa
17 Subcutaneous acromial bursa
18 Acromioclavicular ligament
19 Coraco-acromial ligament
20 Trapezoid ligament ⎫ Coracoclavicular
21 Conoid ligament   ⎬ ligament
22 Synovial bursa between coracoid process and clavicle

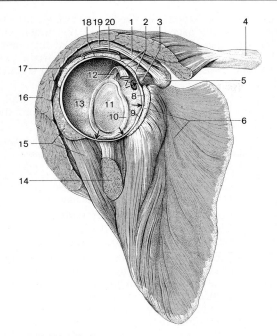

Fig. 83. **Shoulder joint**, lateral view
Articular capsule opened, humerus removed

1 Coraco-acromial ligament
2 Coracohumeral ligament + superior glenohumeral ligament
3 Subscapular bursa
4 Clavicle
5 Coracoid process
6 Subscapularis
7 Communication of subscapular bursa with articular cavity
8 Middle glenohumeral ligament
9 Inferior glenohumeral ligament
10 Glenoid lip
11 Glenoid cavity

12 Tendon of long head of biceps
13 Articular capsule, inner surface
14 Long head of triceps brachii
15 Teres minor
16 Deltoid
17 Infraspinatus
18 Supraspinatus
19 Acromion
20 Subacromial bursa, opened
→ weak sites of articular capsule

5 mm broad, which is attached to the margin of the socket. Tendon fibers of the long head of the biceps radiate into it above, those of the long head of the triceps below. The difference in size between the joint head and the socket gives the joint its extreme mobility, which makes it the most movable, but also the most vulnerable ball-and-socket joint of the human body.

The *articular capsule* is broad and flaccid. It slackens into folds in the lower portion when the arm is adducted, in the upper portion when abducted. The capsule is attached to the scapula at the outer margin of the glenoid lip. Above, however, it encloses the origin of the biceps tendon in the joint cavity. At the humerus the capsule is attached to the anatomical neck.

Ligaments (Figs. **82** and **83**). The anterior, upper capsular wall is strengthened by the *coracohumeral ligament*, which passes from the coracoid process to the greater tubercle.

Beneath it, the *superior glenohumeral ligament* courses in the direction of the protuberances of the humerus. The *middle glenohumeral ligament* (to the lesser tubercle) strengthens the anterior wall of the capsule, and the *inferior glenohumeral ligament* reinforces the capsule between the tendon of the subscapularis and the origin of the long head of the triceps. The glenohumeral ligaments radiate out from the joint lip and can be recognized only on the inner surface of the capsule.

All strengthening ligaments of the shoulder joint prevent an excessive external rotation. The coracohumeral and superior glenohumeral ligaments are also stretched during adduction of the arm.

The funnel-shaped muscle-covering which encloses the joint is more important in strengthening the joint capsule than the ligamentous traction. It is formed on the cranial and dorsal sides of the joint capsule by the supraspinatus, infraspinatus and teres minor, the *rotatory cuff* of the orthopedic surgeon, and on the anterior side by the subscapularis. Fibers radiate into the capsule wall from the tendons of these muscles and, as a *capsule tenser*, prevent a pinching of the capsular folds.

The deltoid forms a second, superficial muscle covering of the shoulder joint. It likewise strengthens the joint closure and counteracts a sliding of the head from the socket.

The tendon of the long head of the biceps coursing within the joint cavity can be regarded as an intracapsular "reinforcement", adjustable in its length and tension. It lies on the weak portion of the capsule between the anterior margin of the cranial part of the muscle mantle and the coracohumeral ligament and is covered in the intertubercular groove by an extension of the joint inner membrane, the *intertubercular synovial sheath*.

Other weak places in the capsular wall are found above and below the middle glenohumeral ligament and in the lower segment of the capsule that is not covered over by muscles, in front or behind the origin of the tendon of the long head of the triceps.

The *innervation of the joint capsule* is effected by branches of the subscapular and musculocutaneous nerves (ventral), suprascapular nerve (dorsal and above) and axillary nerve (dorsal and below).

The *relaxation position* of the shoulder joint during joint effusion, in which all parts of the capsule are stretched as little as possible, consists in an abduction of about 45° (with 0° rotation). The arm is placed against the body (force of gravity), the abduction at the shoulder joint is hidden by the simultaneous medial turning of the inferior angle of the scapula.

Luxations of the upper arm at the shoulder joint are not rare (most frequent dislocation) in view of the asymmetry of the head and socket. Depending on the type and direction of the traumatic force, the head of the humerus usually dislocates forward (subscapular fossa), rarely backward. Tears in the capsule occur, as a rule, at the weak sites (between the glenohumeral ligaments, in front of and behind the origin of the long head of the triceps). In very rare cases, the head of the humerus can dislocate upward and destroy the roof of the shoulder. Luxations of the shoulder can be accompanied by paralysis of the axillary nerve.

Detachments of tendons of the muscles inserting at the greater tubercle (partly in connection with luxations of the shoulder) usually lead to extensive capsular tears.

Movement possibilities in the shoulder joint exist, as in all ball and socket joints, around many axes. They result from the combination of movements around three main axes:
- *anteversion* or *retroversion* (lifting the arm forward or backward) around a *transverse* axis,
- *abduction* or *adduction* around a *sagittal* axis, and
- *inner* or *outer rotation* around the *longitudinal axis* of the humerus.

From the rest position, the arm, when hanging down, can antevert in the shoulder joint about 60° in the sagittal plane and can be lifted forward and outward to about 105°. Retroversion is possible to about 37° in the sagittal plane. An abduction can be carried out to about 90°, an adduction to about 10°. A greater lateral elevation of the arm is prevented by the roof of the shoulder, which is formed by the acromion, coracoacromial ligament and coracoid process.

The extent of rotation and the ratio between potential external and internal rotation are dependent on the position of the humerus. Conversely, inner and, above all, outer rotation restrict the extent of possible abduction, anterversion and retroversion. An arrest of movement in extreme positions takes place chiefly by the tension of the musculature covering the shoulder girdle, as well as by the tension of the ligaments strengthening the joint capsule. When all the given movement possibilities of the shoulder joint are utilized, the distal end of the humerus describes an elliptical path. A forced rotation ensues owing to the tension and contortion of the joint capsule.

The inclusion of movement possibilities of the shoulder girdle decisively increases the range of motion of the upper arm. It takes place early before the range of movement of the shoulder joint is exhausted. The scapula is moved and rotated on the thorax in such a way that the glenoid cavity is brought into the most favorable initial position for the movements of the arm. Through the outward rotation of the inferior angle of the scapula and the cranial rotation of the glenoid cavity linked with it, it becomes possible to raise the arm above the horizontal plane. Collateral movements of the vertebral column and thorax are necessary for elevating the arm to the vertical plane.

Mucous bursae in the region of the shoulder joint (Figs. **82** and **83**). The *subtendinous bursa of the subscapularis muscle* usually communicates with the joint cavity. This mucous bursa is located behind the upper margin of the tendon of the subscapularis and extends forward up to the root of the coracoid process. It communicates with the joint cavity between the superior and middle glenohumeral ligaments.

Between the tendon of the supraspinatus and the joint capsule on the one side and the acromion and deltoid muscle on the other side, the *subacromial* and *subdeltoid bursae* are situated; these latter usually communicate with each other, but not with the articular cavity. They form an important sliding space for movements in the shoulder joint and are designated as *subacromial accessory joints*.

Small mucous bursae, which do not communicate with the shoulder joint, often lie between the margin of the socket and the tendons of the shoulder muscles.

c) Arrangement and Innervation of the Shoulder Musculature

The muscles that act on the shoulder joint can be divided into a *dorsal* and a *ventral* group. Of the dorsal muscle group, the supraspinatus, infraspinatus, and teres minor insert at the greater tubercle, while the deltoid inserts distal to this at the deltoid tuberosity. The subscapularis, teres major and latissimus dorsi attach at the lesser tubercle and the crest extending from this prominence. Included in the ventral group are the pectoralis major, pectoralis minor and coracobrachialis.

Dorsal Group

The **supraspinatus** (Figs. **83** and **84**) arises in the supraspinous fossa of the scapula (laterally up to the neck of the scapula) and at the overlying fascia which is attached at the margin and spine of the scapula. The tendon courses beneath the acromion, sends out fibers into the capsule of the shoulder joint and attaches at the anterior facet of the greater tubercle.

Innervation: Suprascapular nerve.

The nerve passes into the supraspinous fossa beneath the superior transverse scapular ligament.

The **infraspinatus** (Figs. **83** and **84**) comes from the infraspinous fossa (the portion bordering at the neck of the scapula remains free) and attaches at the joint capsule and the middle facet of the greater tubercle. Together with the teres minor, it is covered by a fascia which is fixed to the margins of the scapula.

Innervation: Suprascapular nerve.

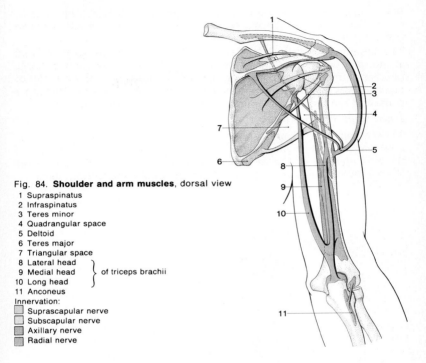

Fig. 84. **Shoulder and arm muscles**, dorsal view
 1 Supraspinatus
 2 Infraspinatus
 3 Teres minor
 4 Quadrangular space
 5 Deltoid
 6 Teres major
 7 Triangular space
 8 Lateral head ⎫
 9 Medial head ⎬ of triceps brachii
10 Long head ⎭
11 Anconeus
Innervation:
 ☐ Suprascapular nerve
 ☐ Subscapular nerve
 ☐ Axillary nerve
 ☐ Radial nerve

The nerve proceeds from the supraspinous fossa around the neck of the scapula into the infraspinous fossa.

The **teres minor** (Figs. **83**, **84** and **86**) originates at the lateral margin of the scapula and passes to the posterior facet of the greater tubercle.

The muscle is frequently attached so closely to the infraspinatus that its demarcation is only possible on the basis of its different innervation.

Innervation: Axillary nerve.

The branch to the teres minor leaves the axillary nerve immediately after passing through the lateral axillary space and courses to the muscle on the posterior surface of the tendon of origin of the long head of the triceps.

The **deltoid** (Figs. **82** and **86**) is a thick muscular mantle, embracing the proximal end of the humerus from above, from the front, the side and from behind. It contours the curvature of the shoulder, which is caused, however, not by the muscle tissue itself, but by the bony form, especially by the greater tubercle.

When spread out, the muscle resembles a large, inverted Greek delta since its origin at the shoulder joint is very extended, whereas the insertion at the humerus is very narrow.

The deltoid arises at the lateral third of the clavicle, at the acromion and at the spine of the scapula. The acromial part is complex pennate (large number of fibers – large physiological cross section). The thick bundles of muscle fibers converge toward the tendon which is situated on the inner surface of the muscle and which is inserted at the deltoid tuberosity.

Innervation: Axillary nerve.

The **subscapularis** (Figs. **83** and **85**) pads the subscapular fossa as a strong muscular plate. It originates from tendinous bands, which are attached at the muscular line of the costal surface of the scapula, and inserts at the lesser tubercle and also at the joint capsule with some tendon fibers.

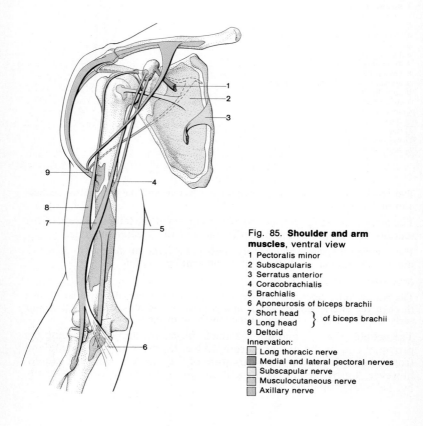

Fig. 85. **Shoulder and arm muscles**, ventral view
1 Pectoralis minor
2 Subscapularis
3 Serratus anterior
4 Coracobrachialis
5 Brachialis
6 Aponeurosis of biceps brachii
7 Short head ⎱ of biceps brachii
8 Long head ⎰
9 Deltoid
Innervation:
☐ Long thoracic nerve
■ Medial and lateral pectoral nerves
☐ Subscapular nerve
☐ Musculocutaneous nerve
☐ Axillary nerve

Innervation: Subscapular nerve.

The **teres major** (Figs. **84** and **86**) arises on the dorsal surface of the inferior angle of the scapula, winds around the long head of the triceps and inserts at the crest of the lesser tubercle dorsal to the terminal tendon of the latissimus dorsi (grown together with it at the lower margin).

The teres major is an offshoot of the subscapularis. Moreover, it is closely related genetically to the latissimus dorsi, which arises from the same anlage.

Innervation: Subscapular nerve.

Axillary spaces (Figs. **84** and **86**). The triangle bordered by the teres minor, teres major, and the humerus is subdivided by the long head of the triceps brachii into a *lateral quadrangular* and a *medial triangular* axillary space. The circumflex scapular artery with its accompanying veins courses through the *medial axillary space*, which is bordered by the teres minor, teres major and the long head of the triceps brachii. The axillary nerve, posterior circumflex humeral artery and accompanying veins pass through the *lateral axillary space* (bounded by the teres minor, teres major, triceps and humerus).

The **latissimus dorsi** (Figs. **79** and **87**) spreads broadly on the back surface. It arises from the spinous processes of the lower 6 thoracic vertebrae and the accompanying segments of the supraspinal ligament, from the spinous processes of all lumbar vertebrae and the sacrum via the thoracolumbar fascia, from the iliac crest and from the (9th) 10–12th ribs, frequently also from the inferior angle of the scapula. The muscle fibers course obliquely upward, converge toward the attachment at the humerus, wind themselves around the teres major and insert at the crest of the lesser tubercle (grown together at the lower margin with the terminal tendon of the teres major, but otherwise separated by a mucous bursa).

The fibers that originate farthest cranially attach at the distal portion of the bony ridge, whereas the fiber bundles arising from the ribs attach farthest proximally. The part of the muscle close to the humerus is therefore twisted. This rotation is offset by elevation of the arm. It prevents the individual muscle portions from being stretched too unequally when the arm is elevated; for, on the elevated humerus, the distal part of the crest lies furthest cranially.

Innervation: Thoracodorsal nerve.

Ventral Group

The **pectoralis major** (Fig. **86**), a derivative of the flexor group of the upper limb, spreads out from the shoulder girdle (clavicle) to the ventral thoracic wall. It arises from the sternal half of the clavicle, from the sternum and from the cartilages of the (1st) 2nd–7th ribs, as well as from the anterior layer of the rectus sheath. The fibers of the *sternocostal* and *abdominal parts* cross under the fiber bundle of the *clavicular part* and attach proximally at the crest of the greater tubercle, the clavicular

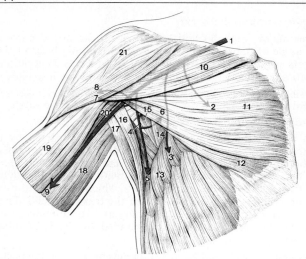

Fig. 86. Connective tissue pathways from axilla, ventral and somewhat caudal view

To the neck:
1 Subclavian artery

To the anterior and lateral thoracic wall:
2 Pectoral branch of thoraco-acromial artery
3 Lateral thoracic artery
4 Subscapular artery
5 Thoracodorsal artery
6 Circumflex scapular artery through triangular space

In the deltoid region:
7 Posterior circumflex humeral artery through quadrangular space
8 Anterior circumflex humeral artery

To the arm:
9 Brachial artery

10 Clavicular part ⎫
11 Sternocostal part ⎬ of pectoralis major
12 Abdominal part ⎭
13 Serratus anterior (slips of origin alternate with origins of external oblique muscle)
14 Subscapularis
15 Teres minor
16 Latissimus dorsi
17 Teres major
18 Triceps brachii
19 Biceps brachii
20 Coracobrachialis
21 Deltoid

portion inserting distally. As in the case of the latissimus dorsi, a muscle pocket thus arises that is open cranially and revealed during abduction and anteversion of the arm.

When the arm is hanging down, the pectoralis major has a quadrangular form, but when the humerus is abducted, it is triangular in shape. Its lateral margin forms the anterior fold of the axilla. The posterior axillary fold is created by the lateral margin of the latissimus dorsi.

In the depth between the clavicular parts of the pectoralis major and the deltoid there is a connective tissue space through which the cephalic vein passes. The space is very narrow in strong, muscular individuals; but when the clavicular part of the pectoralis major is weakly developed, it broadens out toward the clavicle so that it resembles a triangle standing on the apex. It then justifies the name *clavipectoral triangle*. The skin is depressed here to form the *infraclavicular fossa* (Mohrenheim's fossa).

Innervation: medial and lateral pectoral nerves (from the medial and lateral cords of the brachial plexus).

A **sternalis muscle** of variable form and size can be developed on the pectoralis fascia and extend along the sternal margin on one or both sides (in about 5% of Europeans). If this muscle is innervated by branches of the pectoral nerves, it is regarded as the rudiment of a mammalian cutaneous muscle (panniculus carnosus). It frequently communicates with the sternocleidomastoid and may be innervated by branches of intercostal nerves.

The **pectoralis minor** (Figs. **80**, **87**, and **197**), covered completely by the pectoralis major, arises from the ventral end of the bony (2nd) 3–5th ribs and inserts at the coracoid process of the scapula.

The muscle has developed from the same blastema that gave rise to the pectoralis major. Normally, it connects only the shoulder girdle with the thoracic wall, but occasional variants of the muscle which insert at the crest of the greater tubercle point to an origin from the limb musculature.

Innervation: medial and lateral pectoral nerves.

The **coracobrachialis** (Fig. **85**) belongs genetically to the ventral muscle group of the upper arm (flexors) and – like the biceps brachii and brachialis – is innervated by the musculocutaneous nerve. However, it acts only on the shoulder joint and is therefore described here.

The muscle originates at the coracoid process together with the short head of the biceps and inserts at the inner surface of the humerus, distal to the crest of the lesser tubercle.

With the arm hanging down, the coracobrachialis lies concealed in the axilla. It serves as the conducting muscle for the neurovascular trunk of the arm.

Innervation: musculocutaneous nerve.

d) Action of Muscles and Muscle Groups on the Shoulder Joint

In movements of the shoulder joint, parts of several muscles always work together, whereby the antagonists have a decisive voice in the direction, extent and velocity of a movement. The action of a muscle or its parts depends on the given position of the joint (ball-and-socket joint); the muscle function can be transformed into its opposite action under altered initial circumstances. Apart from rotatory movements of the arm when it is hanging down, normal movements of the shoulder joint (almost) always involve a phase of complex movement, in which primarily the shoulder muscles, but also the arm muscles, work together.

During a physician's examination of the movement possibilities of the shoulder joint, the scapula must be fixed to the thorax in order to eliminate collateral movements of the shoulder girdle as far as possible.

An approximate homogeneous *relaxation of the shoulder muscles* (e.g. when immobilizing the arm in an upper-arm fracture) is attained by an abduction of the upper-arm (in the frontal plane) up to the horizontal plane with a simultaneous right-angled flexion of the horizontally-placed forearm.

In the shoulder joint the arm is:

- *anteverted* (raised ventrally) through the combined action of the acromial and clavicular parts of the deltoid, the two heads of the biceps brachii, the coracobrachialis, the clavicular (and sternocostal) portions of the pectoralis major and the supraspinatus,

  whereby the subscapularis, infraspinatus and teres minor help to a slight degree in flexion;

- *retroverted* (carried dorsally) through the combined effort of the spinous parts of the deltoid, teres major and latissimus dorsi, and – when returning the anteverted arm to its normal position – by the long head of the triceps brachii;

- *abducted* by the acromial part of the deltoid, by the supraspinatus and the long head of the biceps,

  whereby with increasing abduction, parts of the infraspinatus, the clavicular and spinous parts of the deltoid, and – to a slight degree – also parts of the subscapularis and teres minor support the movement;

- *adducted* by the pectoralis major, teres major and latissimus dorsi, as well as by the long head of the triceps,

  whereby the subscapularis, coracobrachialis and the short head of the biceps cooperate and, in advanced adduction, are supported slightly by the infraspinatus, teres minor, as well as the portions of the deltoid originating at the clavicle and spine of the scapula;

- *rotated inward* by the subscapularis, pectoralis major and biceps,

  assisted by the action of the teres major, latissimus dorsi and the clavicular portion of the deltoid;

- *rotated outward* primarily by the infraspinatus, but also by the teres minor and the spinous part of the deltoid,

  whereby the long head of the triceps and the supraspinatus support the external rotation.

Through the cooperation of muscles or muscle parts with different functions, mixed movements can be realized. For example, by the contraction of the spinous parts of the deltoid, the teres major and the latissimus dorsi, the arm can be placed on the back. An especially powerful movement results in throwing, produced by the combination of the adduction, anteversion and inner rotation.

The subscapularis, supraspinatus, infraspinatus and teres minor act as *tensors of the capsule*.

In the fixed arm, the *pectoralis major* and *latissimus dorsi* can adduct the trunk to the arm (pulling up the body for ascending stairs or climbing). When luggage is carried, the *deltoid* and *coracobrachialis* secure the shoulder joint, whereby the descending part of the *trapezius* seeks to prevent the descent of the scapula.

The *latissimus dorsi* compresses the scapula at the thorax. With the arm fixed, the *teres major* can turn the inferior angle of the scapula laterally and forward. The *pectoralis minor* is capable of so tilting the scapula that the inferior angle is lifted off of the thoracic wall. The *coracobrachialis* assists in carrying the arm from the different positions to its normal position.

In patients with a chronic cough, the lateral parts of the margin of the latissimus dorsi can be painful or, in the case of impeded exhalation over a longer period, they can hypertrophy. These findings can be interpreted as follows: when the arm is supported, the lateral muscular portions strengthen the thoracic kyphosis and thus can effect exhaling.

Paralyses. In a paralysis of the *supra-* and *infraspinatus muscles* after severance of the suprascapular nerve, the distinct atrophy of these muscles on the dorsal side of the scapula is striking. The humerus is strongly rotated inwards. Indeed, considerable, but feeble, external rotation is still possible (teres minor). In the abduction of the arm, there is risk of a downward subluxation of the head of the humerus.

Especially the *deltoid* is affected by a paralysis of the axillary nerve. A powerful abduction is impossible without the participation of the acromial portion of the deltoid.

When the *subscapularis* and *teres major* are paralyzed (e.g. as a result of a severance of the subscapular nerve), the arm becomes rotated externally. Only a diminished inward rotation is possible; the patient can no longer reach the lower segment of the back with his hand.

With the loss of the *latissimus dorsi* (severance of the thoracodorsal nerve), the arm can still be brought up to the body in the frontal plane (pectoralis major, teres major). The patient, however, has difficulty adducting the retroverted arm vigorously.

A complete paralysis of the *pectoralis major* and *pectoralis minor* occurs (as a rule) only when both the medial and the lateral cords of the brachial plexus, or the pectoralis nerves coming from them, are paralyzed. The shoulder can then be lowered only slightly (loss of the pectoralis minor and the caudal fibers of the large thoracic muscles arising caudally). Power for the adduction of the arm is reduced, and the arm deviates laterally during anteversion.

3. Axilla

The **axilla** is the connective tissue space bordered (largely) by muscles between the lateral thoracic wall and the upper arm. Through the axilla, blood vessels and nerves are conducted from the lateral triangle of the neck to the arm as a *neurovascular trunk* so that, on the one hand, they do not restrict the movements of the shoulder girdle and the arm and, on the other hand, are not injured by these movements (stretched, strained, pinched, or clamped). From the taut fibrous connective tissue covering of the neurovascular bundle, tracts and lamellae of loose connective tissue extend to the walls of the axilla. They effect a careful displacement of the neurovascular cord during changes in the size and shape of the axilla (as a result of movements of the shoulder girdle and upper arm).

Fat tissue provides a deformable filling material between the connective tissue cords and plates (storage fat, for the most part)

If there is an increased fluid accumulation (e.g. as a result of an inflammation) leading to a strong filling of the interstices or to a shrinking of the connective tissue meshwork, the mobility of the shoulder joint is restricted.

a) Walls of the Axilla

When the arm is abducted, the axilla (Fig. **86**) resembles a four-sided *pyramid*, whose *apex* lies behind the middle of the clavicle. The *base* faces laterally and caudally and is formed by the axillary fascia.

The *ventral wall* of the axilla is composed of the pectoralis major and pectoralis minor muscles (as well as the clavipectoral fascia). The lateral margin of the large thoracic muscles builds the *anterior axillary fold*. It corresponds to the *anterior axillary line* ($\rightarrow$ p. 550).

The *dorsal wall* is formed medially by the subscapularis, laterally by the teres major and the lateral marginal portion of the latissimus dorsi, which builds at the same time the *posterior axillary fold*. It corresponds to the *posterior axillary line* ($\rightarrow$ p. 550).

The *medial wall* is formed by the slips of origin of the serratus anterior.

The *lateral wall* is narrow. The proximal end of the humerus, coracobrachialis and short head of the biceps participate in its composition.

The anterior wall of the axilla on the body surface corresponds to the *infraclavicular fossa* and the lateral part of the *mammary region*, which follows it caudally without a sharp boundary.

The area of the body over the base of the axilla is designated as the *axillary region*. It comprises the two axillary folds and the cutaneous zone situated between them, which is deepened into the *axillary fossa* (hairy in the adult).

b) Fascia of the Axilla and Thoracic Wall

The **axillary fascia,** a connective tissue plate, borders the axilla laterally and caudally when the arm is abducted. At the anterior axillary fold it merges into the pectoral fascia and at the posterior axillary fold into the fascia of the back. Toward the arm it continues as the brachial fascia. In the depth the axillary fascia communicates with the fasciae of the muscles bordering the axilla and with the clavipectoral fascia. In the area which underlies the hair and sweat gland regions of the axillary skin, the axillary fascia is thin and abundantly perforated (lamina cribrosa axillaris). Numerous lymphatic vessels, small arteries, veins and nerve branches pass through the fascia in this oval field. The strengthened connective tissue tracts which enclose this loosened and perforated area are called *fascial axillary arches* (medial margin of the lamina cribrosa axillaris) and *arm arches* (lateral margin).

Muscle bundles can radiate into the axillary fascia and pass along the fascial axillary arch over the neurovascular cord and the coracobrachialis. They can connect the tendons of the latissimus dorsi and pectoralis muscles: *muscular axillary arches*. (The muscular material can come not only from the panniculus carnosus or the pectoralis major, but also from the blastema of the latissimus dorsi).

The axillary fascia is stretched and the skin taut when the arm is abducted. The coracobrachialis, the conducting muscle for the neurovascular trunk, bulges distinctly in front (position of the arm for examination of the axilla or for operative treatment). When the arm is adducted, the fascia is relaxed (position of the arm for digital examination of the contents of the axilla). When the arm is kept in the resting position for a long period of time, both the axillary fascia and the capsule shrink so that the mobility of the shoulder joint is reduced.

Sebaceous and sweat (eccrine and odoriferous) glands of the axilla lie in the dermis of the axillary skin, *superficial* to the fat-poor subcutaneous connective tissue and the axillary fascia. The fascia, therefore, must not be cut open during the incision of a sweat gland abscess. Of course, the axillary fascia offers only limited resistance to the spread of inflammation into (or from) the deep tissues.

The **thoracic fasciae** (Figs. **210** and **211**) are not fasciae of the autochthonous thoracic musculature, the intercostals, but communicate with the shoulder girdle and shoulder muscles pushed forward on the thoracic wall. The "superficial" thoracic fascia separates the subcutaneous connective tissue from this muscle layer; it possesses close topographical and functional relations to the mammary glands. The "deep" thoracic fascia encloses the ventral muscles of the shoulder girdle.

The (superficial) thoracic fascia (**pectoralis fascia**) covers the pectoralis major and continues cranially into the superficial layer of the cervical fascia, laterally into the axillary fascia and caudally into the superficial fascia of the abdomen. The pectoralis fascia is fixed at the clavicle and sternum and firmly connected with the external perimysium at the anterior surface of the large thoracic muscles. A loose connective tissue layer between the thoracic fascia and breast permits the displacement of the mammary glands against the fascia and thoracic muscles.

The displaceability of the breast is terminated by a carcinoma of the mammary glands if the tumor has infiltrated the thoracic wall.

The "deep" thoracic fascia (**clavipectoral fascia**) encloses the pectoralis minor and subclavius. It is attached cranially at the clavicle and at the coracoid process. It communicates with the pectoral fascia at the lateral margin of the pectoralis major. The clavipectoral fascia is very well developed cranial to the pectoralis minor. Here, it spreads over the subclavian vein, growing together with its wall, and also covers the subclavian artery and brachial plexus. The fascia can be stretched by the pectoralis minor and can exert traction on the wall of the vein, which keeps the lumen of the vein open and accelerates the drainage of blood to the superior vena cava. The clavipectoral fascia is separated from the lower surface of the pectoralis major by a loose displaceable layer (interpectoral fissure).

c) Connective Tissue Body of the Axilla

The deformable connective tissue body of the axilla is penetrated by the neurovascular trunk for the free upper limb, by vessels and nerves of the shoulder and shoulder girdle musculature, and by an extensive system of lymphatic tracts. Moreover, it harbors the different groups of axillary lymph nodes. In a well nourished individual, the conduction pathways occupy about half of the axilla.

With regard to the spread of inflammation, the connective tissue body of the axilla represents a uniform space in which the delicate connective tissue lamellae do not stop the advancement of pus formation or the effusion of blood.

The axilla communicates with the connective tissue spaces of adjacent regions. The axillary connective tissue continues (Fig. **86**):

– to the *neck* along the subclavian vessels and the trunks of the brachial plexus into the inferior segment of the lateral triangle of the neck,
– to the *arm* along the neurovascular trunk of the upper limb into the medial bicipital sulcus,
– into the *deltoid region* (region above the deltoid) along the anterior circumflex humeral vessels or through the lateral axillary space along the posterior circumflex humeral vessels,
– into the *scapular region* (region above the scapula) through the medial axillary space along the circumflex scapular vessels,
– to the *lateral thoracic wall* beneath the pectoralis muscles (ventral) and beneath the latissimus dorsi (dorsocaudal), and
– into the *infraclavicular region* along the vessels and nerves penetrating the clavipectoral fascia (thoraco-acromial vessels, cephalic vein, pectoral nerves).

Along these connective tissue routes, inflammatory processes can spread fairly rapidly into the depth of the axillary connective tissue

body. From the connective tissue and adipose tissue in the interpectoral and subpectoral regions, subpectoral phlegmons (phlegmon =
inflammation brought about by pus producers with the tendency to
spread into connective tissue spaces) advance along the intercostal
vessels penetrating the thoracic wall (lateral through the serratus
anterior) into the subpleural connective tissue or (ventral) into the
mediastinum.

d) Axillary Lymph Nodes and their Drainage

In the region of the axilla there are about 30 lymph nodes (*axillary lymph
nodes*, Figs. **112** and **210**) which communicate with one another via the
axillary lymphatic network.

The three *superficial groups of lymph nodes* (*superficial axillary lymph
nodes*) consist of *regional* lymph nodes that lie partly in the fibrous
lamellae of the axillary fascia, partly directly beneath the axillary fascia.
The following nodes are distinguished:
– *lateral axillary lymph nodes* (at the medial and dorsal periphery of the
   distal two thirds of the axillary vein), which receive the superficial
   (epifascial) and deep lymphatic vessels of the arm;
– the *pectoral axillary lymph nodes* (at the lower margin of the pectoralis
   minor, on the serratus anterior along the lateral thoracic vessels), the
   drainage of which includes the anterior and lateral thoracic wall,
   the mammary glands (partly via the *paramammary lymph nodes* at the
   lateral margin of the breast) and the anterior abdominal wall above
   the navel; and
– the *subscapular axillary lymph nodes* (between the subscapularis and
   teres major, around the subscapular vessels), to which lymphatic vessels
   pass from the lower nuchal region, from the dorsal region of the
   shoulder and from the posterior thoracic wall.

Nominally classified with the axillary lymph nodes are three *regional*
groups of nodes that do not directly lie in the area of the axilla:
– the (1–2) *cubital axillary lymph nodes* medial to the basilic vein and
   above the elbow joint, which receive lymph from the ulnar regions of the
   fingers, hand and arm;
– the (1–2) *brachial axillary lymph nodes* along the cephalic vein in the
   clavipectoral triangle, to which lymph flows from the radial side of
   the arm; and
– the *interpectoral axillary lymph nodes* between the two thoracic muscles,
   which conduct lymph from the breast to the central and apical axillary
   lymph nodes.

The *deep axillary lymph nodes*, the second and third filter stations, form a
chain on the medial side of the neurovascular trunk which reaches to just
below the clavicle. They are usually difficult to palpate in the connective

tissue body of the axilla even when enlarged. The following deep axillary lymph nodes can be distinguished:

– the *central axillary lymph nodes* (behind the pectoralis minor) with inflow from the superficial axillary lymph nodes, and

– the *apical axillary lymph nodes* (cranial to the pectoralis minor, below the clavicle, along the subclavian vein). They receive lymph from the central lymph nodes, as well as direct inflow from the lymphatic vessels of the arm coursing with the cephalic vein and from a marginal cranial zone of the mammary gland.

From the apical lymph nodes, lymph from the entire arm and the thoracic wall discharges into the subclavian trunk (Figs. **112** and **210**), which usually empties independently into the venous angle.

The right subclavian trunk occasionally forms a *right lymphatic duct* with the right jugular trunk; the left subclavian trunk can enter the thoracic duct.

Since the superficial axillary lymph nodes communicate with one another, diseases can be transmitted from one group of nodes to another (important, for example, with metastases). From the close proximity of the intercostobrachial nerve to the superficial axillary lymph nodes, but also to the central axillary lymph nodes, pain radiating to the thoracic wall and inner side of the upper arm, which appears when these nodes are diseased becomes understandable (many times the first indication of a mammary carcinoma).

e) Neurovascular Trunk in the Axilla

In the axilla, the *neurovascular trunk of the arm* (Fig. **87**) consists of the *axillary artery* and *axillary vein*, together with the accompanying *lymphatic tracts* and the *infraclavicular part of the brachial plexus*. When the upper arm is moderately abducted, the neurovascular bundle passes from the middle of the clavicle to the proximal end of the medial groove of the upper arm, at which site the coracobrachialis (located somewhat ventrolaterally) serves as the conducting structure.

The neurovascular trunk courses near the anterior wall of the axilla. It becomes more closely related with the dorsal wall only in the lateral region of the axilla, where it crosses muscular attachments passing to the lesser tubercle (subscapularis) and the crest of the lesser tubercle (latissiumus dorsi, teres major). During adduction of the arm, the trunk is adjacent to the serratus anterior.

When the arm is extremely abducted, the neurovascular trunk comes into close contact with the head of the humerus and is stretched. Through continued pressure of the humeral head (e.g. during narcosis with the arm elevated), the medial bundle of the brachial plexus can be accidentally injured. The typical "narcotic paralysis" caused by wrong positioning involves, however, the upper "roots" of the brachial plexus (C5, 6, Erb's palsy); when the arm is raised and pulled backward, the clavicle is pressed against the transverse process of the cervical vertebral column, crushing these nerve branches in their exit from the scalene gaps. Crutches, which used to be standard, created axillary pressure againt the upper arm and, if used for an extended period, led to "crutch paralysis", which affected primarily the radial nerve.

The path of the neurovascular trunk through the axilla can be divided into three segments in which the positional relationships between the artery and nerve plexus vary strikingly, whereas the axillary vein follows a constant course ventromedial to the axillary artery.

In the *proximal axillary segment* (between the subclavius and pectoralis minor), the primary bundle (*trunk*) of the brachial plexus at first retains its dorsocranial position to the artery. They then draw closer together, however, and begin to be organized into three nerve cords (*fasciculi*).

In the *middle axillary segment* (behind the pectoralis minor), the regrouping of the trunks continues. Three cords arise which adjoin the axillary artery on three sides. The *lateral cord* passes directly on the lateral side of the artery. The *medial cord* curves around it dorsally and lies on its dorsomedial side. The *posterior cord* joins the axillary artery dorsally.

In the *distal segment of the course* (between the pectoralis minor and the lower margin of the pectoralis major), the fascicular formation is completed. A separation of the medial cord curves around the axillary artery ventrally as the medial root and forms, with the lateral root from the lateral cord, the *median nerve*.

From the three nerve bundles originating in the axilla a total of 7 "long" nerves proceed to the musculature and skin of the free limb. Moreover, in the axilla the *infraclavicular part* of the brachial plexus sends out 4 "short" nerves to the shoulder musculature. In addition, there are two other nerves which pass through the axilla: the *intercostobrachial nerve*, which joins the medial brachial cutaneous nerve from the medial cord, and the *long thoracic nerve* (from the supraclavicular part of the brachial plexus), which passes downwards relatively protected in the compact fascia of the serratus anterior and innervates the muscle.

Axillary Vessels

Axillary artery. The main artery to the arm, the subclavian artery, is designated as the *axillary artery* at the lateral margin of the 1st rib. At the lower margin of the pectoralis major (anterior axillary fold), it continues as the *brachial artery*.

The branches of the axillary artery exhibit considerable variability with regard to their mode and level of origin. The following description provides a basic model of their vascular organization.

The proximal **branches of the axillary artery** (Fig. **87**), the variable, usually weak *superior thoracic artery* and the strong *thorao-acromial artery* (which occasionally arises in common, but is 70% independent), pass chiefly to the ventral wall of the axilla; individual small *subscapular branches* course directly to the subscapularis.

The *superior thoracic artery* sends branches to the subclavius, 1st and 2nd intercostals, pectoralis major and minor and the seratus anterior (superior slips).

In the opposite direction, the *thoraco-acromial artery* penetrates the clavipectoral fascia jointly with the cephalic vein and divides at the upper margin of the pectoralis minor into *pectoral branches* to both thoracic muscles, a *clavicular branch* to the subclavius and clavicle, an *acromial branch* to the acromial plexus, an arterial network on the summit of the shoulder, and *deltoid branches* to both muscular margins of the clavipectoral triangle.

The *lateral thoracic artery*, in the middle segmental part behind (rarely lateral to) the pectoralis minor, courses downward usually clearly ventral to the long thoracic nerve and supplies the medial wall of the axilla (middle slips of the serratus anterior). It also supplies the large thoracic muscle and sends *lateral mammary branches* to the breast.

The *subscapular artery*, a short vascular trunk (with small branches to the subscapularis), and its anterior terminal branch, the *thoracodorsal artery*, pass caudally in the connective tissue body of the axilla along the posterior axillary fold. The thoracodorsal artery gives off branches to the subscapularis, latissimus dorsi, teres major and the caudal slips of the serratus anterior. The dorsal terminal branch, the *circumflex scapular artery*, reaches the infraspinous fossa through the medial axillary space.

1 Phrenic nerve
2–7 *Brachial plexus*
2 Superior trunk
3 Middle trunk
4 Inferior trunk
5 Posterior cord
6 Lateral cord
7 Medial cord
8 Scalenus anterior, in the depth – at back wall of subclavian artery – origin of costocervical trunk (not illustrated)
9 Subclavian artery
10 Thyrocervical trunk
11 Vertebral artery
12 Internal thoracic artery
13 Common carotid artery
14 Axillary artery
15 Superior thoracic artery
16 Pectoral branch of thoraco-acromial artery
17 First intercostal nerve
18 Second intercostal nerve
19 Intercostobrachial nerve
20 Pectoralis minor
21 Lateral thoracic artery
22 Long thoracic nerve
23 Circumflex scapular artery
24 Subscapular artery
25 Thoracodorsal artery and nerve
26 Medial brachial cutaneous nerve
27 Medial antebrachial cutaneous nerve
28 Latissimus dorsi
29 Long head of triceps brachii
30 Ulnar nerve
31 Superior ulnar collateral artery
32 Median nerve
33 Musculocutaneous nerve
34 Middle collateral artery
35 Radial nerve
36 Radial collateral artery
37 Profunda brachii artery
38 Brachial artery
39 Anterior circumflex humeral artery
40 Axillary nerve
41 Posterior circumflex humeral artery
42 Deltoid branch of thoraco-acromial artery
43 Acromial branch of thoraco-acromial artery
44 Clavicular branch of thoraco-acromial artery
45 Acromial network
46 Acromial branch of suprascapular artery
47 Suprascapular artery
48 Suprascapular nerve

►

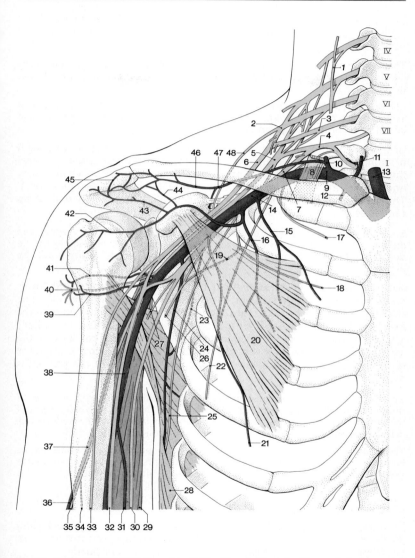

Fig. 87. **Arteries and nerves in region of shoulder girdle and axilla**, ventral view
(Short branches of brachial plexus shown, but for reasons of clarity not labelled,
→ Fig. 58)

The *anterior* and *posterior circumflex humeral arteries* (from the distal axillary segment) curve around the humerus at the level of the surgical neck.

The *anterior circumflex humeral artery* passes under the coracobrachialis to the intertubercular groove of the humerus and supplies the deltoid and the capsule of the shoulder joint.

The well-developed *posterior circumflex humeral artery* courses through the lateral axillary space (together with the axillary nerve) to the deltoid, to the long and lateral heads of the triceps, and to the joint capsule.

Branches of the axillary artery to the shoulder anastomose with branches of the cervical arteries of the subclavian artery (lateral thoracic artery ↔ descending ramus of transverse cervical artery and, above all, circumflex scapular artery ↔ suprascapular artery). Therefore, when the axillary artery is ligated before the exit of its branches, a sufficient collateral circulation can be formed.

Since no anastomoses exist between the branches of the axillary artery and the artery of the arm in over 75% of the cases, a ligature between the exit of the posterior circumflex humeral artery and the profunda brachii artery should be avoided.

Axillary vein (Fig. **111 a**). The ulnar brachial vein proximal to the lower margin of the pectoralis major is designated as the *axillary vein*. The radial accompanying vein of the brachial artery empties into it high in the axilla, after it has crossed ventral to the brachial plexus and axillary artery. In addition to the accompanying veins of the branches of the axillary artery, the axillary vein receives the *thoraco-epigastric veins* in the distal axillary segment and the *cephalic vein* proximal to the pectoralis minor.

The *thoraco-epigastric veins* anastomose at the abdominal wall with branches of the superficial epigastric vein (Fig. **209**). Cutaneous and accompanying veins of the thoraco-acromial and supreme thoracic arteries empty into the *cephalic vein* before its passage through the clavipectoral fascia (in Mohrenheim's fossa).

The axillary vein is so stretched in the axilla by connective tissue tracts that its lumen is widened by appropriate arm movements. In open injuries of the vessel or a larger branch, there is the danger of an air embolism.

Brachial Plexus

Two parts of the brachial plexus can be distnguished: the *supraclavicular part* (with branches to the rhomboids, levator scapulae, serratus anterior, supraspinatus and infraspinatus) and the *infraclavicular part*.

The **cord formation of the infraclavicular part** of the brachial plexus (Figs. **58** and **87**) takes place in principle in the following way.

Each of the three primary *trunks* (→ p. 745) are divided (already above the clavicle) into anterior and posterior "branches" (for the genetic flexors and extensors of the arm).

The division can be displaced so far proximally that the detachment of the "dorsal branch" already takes place at the ventral rami of spinal nerves C5-T1, which form the brachial plexus (i.e. at the plexus "roots"). In this case the trunks consist only of ventral twigs of plexus "roots".

All "dorsal branches" of trunks (or plexus "roots") are united into the *posterior cord* (C5-T1). The "ventral branches" from the *superior trunk* (C5, 6) and *middle trunk* (C7) join together to form the *lateral cord*. The "ventral branches" of the *inferior trunk* (C8, T1) form the *medial cord*.

Short Branches of the Infraclavicular Part of the Brachial Plexus

The short branches of the infraclavicular part of the brachial plexus can also be arranged in ventral (flexors) and dorsal (extensor) branches (Fig. **58**).

Ventral Branches to the Shoulder Musculature

The **medial pectoral nerve** (from the medial cord or from the inferior trunk [C8, T1]) and the **lateral pectoral nerve** (from the lateral cord or 2 branches from the superior and middle trunks [C5–7]) pass downward in front of the axillary artery, supply the pectoralis minor, pass through the clavipectoral fascia (one branch with the cephalic vein), and ramify in the pectoralis major.

Dorsal Branches to the Shoulder Musculature

The **subscapular nerve** (usually 2 branches from the posterior cord [C5, 6(7)] reaches the subscapularis after a short distance. The lateral branch generally supplies the teres major.

The **thoracodorsal nerve** (Fig. **87**, from the posterior cord [C6–8]) passes with the vessels of the same name between the dorsal wall of the axilla and the trunk wall through the axillary connective tissue (endangered by curettage of the axilla) to the latissimus dorsi. Occasionally, it also carries branches for the teres major.

Long Branches of the Infraclavicular Part of the Brachial Plexus

The *musculocutaneous nerve* and the *lateral root of the median nerve* arise from the *lateral cord* (Fig. **87**).

The **musculocutaneous nerve** (C5–7) lies most laterally in the neuro-vascular trunk of the axilla, gives off a branch to the coracobrachialis, penetrates the muscle in its middle third, courses between the biceps brachii and brachialis distally, and passes through the fascia with its sensory terminal branch, the *lateral antebrachial cutaneous nerve*, at the distal end of the lateral bicipital groove. It innervates all flexors at the upper arm and, as a cutaneous nerve, the radial side of the forearm.

The **lateral root of the median nerve** (C6,7) winds itself laterally around the axillary artery to the ventral side of the vessel and unites with the medial root from the medial cord to form the median nerve.

In addition to the *medial root of the median nerve*, the *medial cord* provides two cutaneous nerves, the *medial brachial cutaneous* and the *medial antebrachial cutaneous nerves*, as well as the *ulnar nerve* (Fig. **87**).

The **medial brachial cutaneous nerve** ([T1, 2], occasionally divided into two nerves) is united with the intercostobrachial nerve in the axilla (or in the upper arm). At the level of the anterior axillary fold it courses through the fascia and ramifies on the medial side of the upper arm (from the axilla to the elbow).

The **medial antebrachial cutaneous nerve** (C8, T1) courses ventrally between the axillary artery and vein at the end of the distal axillary segment, penetrates the fascia of the upper arm together with the basilic vein and innervates the skin on the medial side of the forearm (between the elbow and wrist) via *anterior* and *posterior rami*.

The **ulnar nerve** (C6–8, T1), upon leaving the axilla, is displaced from dorsal to lie between the axillary artery and vein. It passes behind the medial intermuscular septum in the upper arm, distally in the ulnar route in the forearm, whereby the flexor carpi ulnaris serves as its conducting muscle. Thus, at the level of the elbow joint the nerve still lies on the extensor side. It supplies the ulnar flexors in the forearm and hand, as well as the skin on the ulnar side of the hand and ulnar fingers.

The **medial root of the median nerve** passes from medial to the ventral side of the axillary artery to arrive at the site of union with the lateral root.

The **median nerve** passes in the upper arm to the cubital fossa in the medial bicipital groove, during which it winds itself in a long-drawn spiral from lateral to ventral to the medial side of the brachial artery. In the forearm it lies between the superficial and deep flexors of the fingers as far as the wrist. It innervates a large part of the flexors in the forearm and in the hand, as well as the skin of the wrist, thenar eminence, palm of the hand and the flexor side of 3 1/2 radial fingers.

The median nerve exhibits considerable variation. It can shift distally in the upper arm, possess doubled medial or lateral roots and, in close to 5% of the cases, can be absent. (In this last case all nerve fibers for the flexors and the skin on the flexor side of the arm course in the axilla first in the "lateral" cord. The branches of the medial cord are segmented off only after the exit of the musculocutaneous nerve and cross ventrally from the axillary artery toward the medial side). It is not unusual for communicating branches to go from the musculocutaneous to the median nerve.

Two mixed nerves arise from the *posteior cord*: the *axillary* and the *radial nerves* (Fig. **87**).

The **axillary nerve** (C5, 6) passes through the lateral axillary space around the surgical neck close to the attachment of the capsule. It sends a main branch, the *superior lateral brachial cutaneous nerve*, to the lateral shoulder region and to the dorsolateral side of the upper arm and supplies the deltoid and teres minor.

The **radial nerve** (C6–8, T1) courses in the axilla dorsal to the axillary artery and arrives at the dorsal side of the humerus with the profunda brachii artery. In the groove for the radial nerve, it winds itself near the bone around the lateral margin of the humerus, perforates the lateral intermuscular septum, and passes on the flexor side above the elbow joint. Directly distal to the joint, it divides into the sensory *superficial branch*, which in the forearm uses the brachioradialis as the conducting muscle, and into the larger motor *deep branch*, which passes into the supinator muscle and with a spiral turn descends on the extensor side of the forearm. The radial nerve innervates all extensors in the arm; three cutaneous branches, the *inferior lateral brachial cutaneous, posterior brachial cutaneous*, and the *posterior antebrachial cutaneous nerves*, innervate the skin on the extensor side of the arm (except the deltoid region) and hand (except the ulnar margin, the 4th and 5th fingers, and the terminal segment of the 2nd and 3rd fingers).

Owing to their close relationships to the head of the humerus and the surgical neck, the axillary nerve and the posterior circumflex humeral vessels are especially at risk in the case of fractures at the proximal end of the humerus, luxations of the shoulder joint and repositioning attempts. The suspicion of a traumatic injury of the axillary nerve can be easily determined by examining the cutaneous sensitivity in the deltoid region (superior lateral bachial cutaneous nerve).

B. Upper Arm and Elbow Region

1. Upper Arm

a) Organization and Innervation of the Upper Arm Musculature

The upper arm musculature is organized into the *ventral* group of muscles (*flexor group*) situated on the anterior surface of the humerus and the *dorsal* group (*extensor group*) located on the posterior surface of the humerus. The brachialis and biceps brachii, both of which are innervated by the musculocutaneous nerve, belong to the flexor group. The extensor group consists of the triceps brachii and the anconeus, which are innervated by the radial nerve.

The **brachial fascia** (Fig. **88**) encloses the flexors and extensors in the upper arm. *Intermuscular brachial septa*, which extend on both sides between bones and fascia and at the same time serve as surfaces for

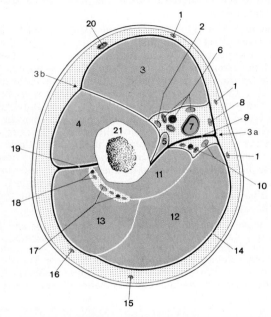

Fig. 88. **Cross section of middle third of arm**, section surface viewed from distal side

1 Branch of medial brachial cutaneous nerve
2 Musculocutaneous nerve
3 Biceps brachii
3a Medial bicipital groove
3b Lateral bicipital groove
4 Brachialis
5 Coracobrachialis
6 Median nerve, brachial artery, brachial veins
7 Basilic vein
8 Medial antebrachial cutaneous nerve
9 Medial brachial intermuscular septum
10 Ulanr nerve and superior ulnar collateral artery with accompanying veins
11 Medial head ⎞
12 Long head ⎬ of triceps brachii
13 Lateral head ⎠
14 Brachial fascia
15 Posterior brachial cutaneous nerve
16 Inferior lateral brachial cutaneous nerve
17 Radial nerve and middle collateral artery with accompanying veins
18 Radial collateral artery and vein
19 Lateral brachial intermuscular septum
20 Cephalic vein
21 Humerus

muscle origins, separate the two groups of muscles and circumscribe, together with the brachial fascia, the *anterior* and *posterior* muscle compartments.

The brachial fascia communicates proximally with the axillary fascia (on the flexor side) and with the fascia of the deltoid (on the extensor side). Distally it continues into the antebrachial fascia. At the humerus, the brachial fascia is fixed directly at the epicondyles, indirectly at the medial and lateral margins of the humerus by the medial and lateral brachial intermuscular septa, which extend proximally up to the insertion of the coracobrachialis and up to the deltoid tuberosity. At the ulna the brachial fascia is attached at the olecranon.

Brachial sulci. The biceps brachii lies ventral to the brachialis and uses the latter as a sliding tract. Along both biceps margins *medial* and *lateral brachial furrows* pass to the cubital fossa. In strongly-muscled, thin individuals, the medial furrow, the *medial bicipital sulcus* (Fig. **88**), is usually distinctly marked in the contour of the skin. The neurovascular bundle of the arm courses in its depth. Close to the lateral groove, more rarely in the *lateral bicipital sulcus*, the cephalic vein, a cutaneous vein, traverses toward the shoulder.

Extensor Groups (Dorsal Muscles)

The **triceps brachii muscle** (Figs. **84**, **86** and **87**) is distinguished by a deeper-situated *medial head* and two superficial heads, the *lateral head* and the bijointed *long head.*

The *medial head* arises at the posterior surface of the humerus medial and distal to the sulcus of the radial nerve and at both intermuscular septa (above all, at the medial). The *lateral head*, which proceeds from a narrow, band-shaped field of origin proximal and lateral to the sulcus of the radial nerve, covers a large part of the medial head. The medial head, however, also reaches the lateral surface in a narrow field above the lateral epicondyle. The *long head* comes from the infraglenoid tubercle of the scapula and from the adjacent segment of the lateral scapular margin. The muscle inserts at the olecranon by means of a rather extensive superficial tendinous plate. Lateral bundles of tendinous fibers enter into the antebrachial fascia and act as a reserve extensor apparatus if the olecranon is broken. Deep tracts of fibers attach at the capsule of the elbow joint. They can be defined as the *articularis cubiti muscle.*

The sulcus of the radial nerve is converted to a "radial canal" by the fibers of the medial head of the triceps originating distal to the bony groove and by the lateral head of the triceps brachii passing over the sulcus. Within the canal, the radial nerve, with its accompanying blood vessels, winds around the dorsolateral surface of the humerus near the bone.

Innervation: Radial nerve.

The branches to the triceps brachii and anconeus already leave the radial nerve in front of and at the entrance into the "radial canal".

The **anconeus** (Fig. **84**) forms the distal continuation of the lateral portion of the medial head of the triceps brachii. Its fibers spread out fan-like from the narrow field of origin at the lateral epicondyle of the humerus, at the joint capsule, and at the radial collateral ligament to the dorsal surface at the proximal end of the shaft of the ulna.

Innervation: Radial nerve.

Flexor Group (Ventral Muscles)

The **biceps brachii** (Figs. **85** and **86**) arises with the *long head* at the supraglenoid tubercle, with the *short head* at the coracoid process. The long head of the biceps (only the tendon of origin is long) passes over the head of the humerus and – enclosed in the intertubercular synovial sheath – enters the intertubercular groove (Figs. **76** and **82**). The terminal tendon of the common muscle belly inserts at the radial tuberosity in the depth of the cubital fossa. A tendinous band, the *aponeurosis of the biceps brachii*, splits off from the terminal tendon and radiates ulnarward into the antebrachial fascia.

During flexion at the elbow joint, the biceps brachii is especially prominent because it is lifted off the joint and is pushed forward by the brachialis muscle.

Innervation: Musculocutaneous nerve

After penetrating the coracobrachialis, the musculocutaneous nerve sends muscular branches to both heads of the biceps and, rather more distal, the branch to the brachialis muscle.

The **brachialis** (Fig. **85**) arises at the anterior surface of the humerus, distal to the deltoid tuberosity (which can be regarded as an osseous inscription of a uniform deltoid-brachialis muscular tract), and inserts at the ulnar tuberosity.

Innervation: Musculocutaneous nerve. The lateral muscular bundles (almost) regularly receive nerve fibers via the radial nerve.

Since the brachialis rests directly on the humerus, it can easily be damaged if a force exerted from the outside squeezes the muscle against the bone or if the muscle is pierced by the ends of fractures in the case of a (supracondylar) hyperextension fracture (extension fracture) of the humerus. The connective tissue scar, which arises at the site of destroyed muscular tissue, shrinks and can bring about a shortening of the brachialis. The arm can then no longer be completely extended at the elbow joint.

b) Neurovascular Routes in the Upper Arm

The anterior of the two muscle compartments – bordered by fascia, septa and the humerus – receives the flexors of the upper arm and the neurovascular bundle (Fig. **87**), which consists of the median nerve, the brachial artery with its accompanying veins, and the deep lymphatic trunks. The neurovascular route leads from the axilla over the *medial brachial groove* (*medial bicipital sulcus*) into the *cubital fossa*. The dorsal muscle compartment, on the other hand, is closed distally. From this compartment inflammatory processes of the upper arm cannot spread easily beyond the olecranon to the forearm. Besides the extensors, the dorsal compartment harbors two neurovascular routes (for the radial nerve + profunda brachii vessels and for the ulnar nerve + superior ulnar collateral vessels).

Neurovascular Trunk of the Arm

The guiding structure for the neurovascular trunk in the arm is for a short proximal distance the coracobrachialis muscle, otherwise the biceps brachii (Fig. **88**). The *brachial artery* passes to the cubital fossa along (and below) the medial margin of the muscle. The lateral accompanying vein is weaker than the *ulnar brachial vein*, which receives the basilic vein at about the middle of the upper arm. Between both accompanying veins there are numerous cross connections. The *median nerve*, which gives off no branches in the upper arm, is wound in an elongated helix from the ventrolateral side of the artery (at the level of the anterior axillary fold) across the ventral surface (middle of upper arm) to the dorsomedial side (near the cubital fossa, Fig. **87**). *Deep lymphatic tracts* course in the connective tissue sheath of the neurovascular trunk – closely adjacent to the arm veins – so that inflammation of the deep lymphatic vessels can spread to the wall of the veins.

The following nerves pass proximally in the neurovascular trunk:
- the *medial antebrachial cutaneous nerve*, which usually perforates the brachial fascia with the basilic vein;
- the *ulnar nerve*, which leaves the brachial artery at the upper arm and arrives at the extensor compartment through the medial brachial intermuscular septum; and
- the radial nerve, which, beneath the tendon of the teres major, enters the "radial canal" situated between the lateral head of the triceps and the shaft of the humerus and bordered distally by the medial head of the triceps brachii.

The median nerve can be overstretched by a supracondylar hyperextension fracture of the humerus (falling on the hand when the elbow is extended, a relatively frequent occurrence in children).

The **brachial artery** (Figs. **77** and **87**) is the main artery of the upper limb from the lower margin of the pectoralis major (anterior axillary fold) to its division in the cubital fossa.

Variants of the brachial artery and its branches are not very rare. Thus, for example, a *superficial brachial artery* can be preserved. It branches off in the axilla from the true brachial artery and courses in the upper arm ventral to the median nerve. The brachial artery then usually sends branches to the shoulder region and to the upper arm, whereas the superficial brachial artery continues into the radial artery and occasionally also into the ulnar artery. Another variant found now and again in the upper arm is a "high origin" of the radial artery, more rarely the ulnar artery. If a supracondylar process is present, the brachial artery can course behind the bony process with the median nerve.

The *brachial artery* emits (in addition to branches to the musculature of the upper arm) the *profunda brachii artery*, which divides into the *middle collateral artery* to the medial head of the triceps and into the *radial collateral artery* to the articular plexus of the elbow, and the *superior* and *inferior ulnar collateral arteries*, which likewise supply the articular network of the elbow (Figs. **87** and **92**).

The *profunda brachii* originates at the lower margin of the teres major, courses together with the radial nerve between the long head of the triceps and the humerus (sulcus of the radial nerve), and gives off the *deltoid branch* to the muscle of the same name and *nutrient arteries* to the humerus.

The *superior ulnar collateral artery* proceeds from the brachial artery at the border of its proximal to middle third, occasionally also together with the profunda brachii, joins the ulnar nerve, and courses toward the elbow dorsal to the medial brachial intermuscular septum (Fig. **88**).

The *inferior ulnar collateral artery* leaves the brachial artery near the bend of the elbow, winds itself over the brachialis toward the ulna, and anastomoses with the anterior branch of the ulnar recurrent artery via an anterior branch and with the articular network of the elbow via a branch passing through the medial septum.

The brachial artery can be ligated distal to the exit of the profunda brachii artery with little risk since an adequate collateral circulation can be established via the articular network of the elbow.

The pulse of the brachial artery can be felt along a straight line which connects the medial margin of the bulge produced by the coracobrachialis muscle with the middle of the bend of the elbow (in the supinated forearm). The guiding structure in the operative search for the artery is the ulnar margin of the biceps.

Radial Nerve and Profunda Brachii Vessels

The *radial nerve*, the *profunda brachii artery* and its *accompanying veins* pass dorsally around the middle third of the shaft of the humerus – in the sulcus of the radial nerve laying directly on the bone (Fig. **87**). The neurovascular route begins proximally above the medial intermuscular septum and courses downward – along the proximal margin of the surface of origin of the medial head of the triceps – between the long head and humeral shaft in a descending half-spiral to the lateral brachial intermuscular septum. The radial nerve and a ventral branch of the radial collateral artery (terminal branch of the profunda brachii) pass through the septum from the extensor compartment into the flexor compartment in the elbow region between the brachialis and brachioradialis muscles (Fig. **92**).

At about the middle of the "radial canal" the **profunda brachii artery** (Figs. **88** and

92) dispatches the *middle collateral artery*, which branches in the medial head of the triceps brachii and connects with the articular network of the elbow. The main branch of the *radial collateral artery*, which penetrates the lateral intermuscular septum together with the radial nerve, anastomoses with the radial recurrent artery; the dorsal branch courses to the articular network of the elbow.

Before entering into the "radial canal," the **radial nerve** gives off the *inferior lateral brachial cutaneous nerve* to the skin on the dorsolateral side of the upper arm, as well as muscular branches to the three heads of the triceps and to the anconeus. In the "radial canal" the *posterior brachial cutaneous nerve* (to the skin on the distal half of the dorsal side of the upper arm) and the *posterior antebrachial cutaneous nerve* (to the skin in the elbow region and on the dorsal side of the forearm) leave the neurovascular trunk.

Both cutaneous nerves pass between the lateral head of the triceps and the brachialis to the brachial fascia which is perforated by the posterior brachial cutaneous nerve at the boundary to the distal third of the upper arm and by the posterior antebrachial cutaneous at the distal end of the lateral brachial sulcus.

Because of its course adjacent to bone, the radial nerve can be easily damaged when continuous external pressure is applied (when the arm hangs down over a sharp edge for a long period of time). Quite frequently, a radial paralysis occurs when the shaft of the humerus is fractured, owing to stretching or crushing of the nerve at the moment of fracture, scar contraction or excessive callus formation. Because of the high exit of the branches to the triceps brachii, this muscle is usually not affected by such a paralysis.

Ulnar Nerve and Superior Ulnar Collateral Vessels

The *superior ulnar collateral artery* with its *accompanying veins* lies on the *ulnar nerve*, which courses dorsomedial to the brachial artery; together with the nerve, it runs from the flexor into the extensor compartment through the brachial intermuscular septum (Fig. **92**). The neurovascular route courses in the medial head of the triceps brachii.

The **ulnar nerve,** which lacks branches to the upper arm, passes into the elbow region in the sulcus of the ulnar nerve.

The **superior ulnar collateral artery** sends muscular branches to the brachialis and medial head of the triceps before it joins the articular network of the elbow.

Whereas the ulnar nerve can avoid impact or pressure in the upper arm region, it lies directly on the bone in the sulcus of the ulnar nerve behind the medial epicondyle of the humerus and can easily be crushed there. The nerve is especially endangered by fractures of the distal end of the humerus, particularly the medial epicondyle. The ulnar nerve can also be dislocated from the bony sulcus by the appropriate direction of a traumatic force.

2. Elbow Joint

a) Skeletal Elements of the Forearm

In the elbow joint the *humerus* articulates with both bones of the forearm (*ulna* and *radius*).

The *ulna* assumes the lead in the articulation of the forearm bones with the humerus; the *radius* articulates with the carpals. The radius and ulna are connected by an *interosseous membrane* (*antebrachial interosseous membrane*, Fig. **89**). With the arm hanging down and the palmar surface of the hand facing ventrally, the radius (on the thumb side) and ulna (on the little finger side) lie parallel to one another: *supination* position. They cross when the hand is inverted so that the radius comes to lie in front of the ulna: *pronation* position (Fig. **97**).

The axis of the shaft of the humerus and the longitudinal axis of the ulna form a laterally open, obtuse angle of close to 170° (mean variation 164–174°, Fig. **110 a**). In females this physiological abduction position of the forearm is somewhat more

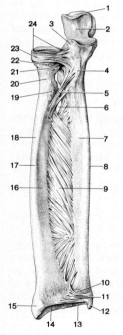

Fig. 89. **Skeletal elements of forearm and antebrachial interosseous membrane**, ventral view
1 Olecranon
2 Trochlear notch
3 Coronoid process
4 Tuberosity of ulna
5 Oblique ligament
6 Opening for posterior interosseous vessles
7 Anterior surface of ulna
8 Anterior margin of ulna
9 Antebrachial interosseous membrane
10 Articular circumference of ulna
11 Thickened capsule of distal radio-ulnar joint
12 Styloid process of ulna
13 Articular disc
14 Carpal articular surface
15 Styloid process of radius
16 Anterior surface of radius
17 Anterior margin of radius
18 Lateral surface of radius
19 Tuberosity of radius
20 Neck of radius
21 Quadrate ligament
22 Sacciform recess
23 Anular ligament of radius
24 Head of radius

pronounced, the angle being about 2° smaller. The axis of the humero-ulnar joint bisects, in general, the abduction angle so that the ulna is congruent with the humerus when flexed.

The **radius** (Fig. **89**) is a slender bony rod, whose distal end is broader and stronger than the proximal end, the *head of the radius*. The proximal surface of the head forms a flat, cartilage-covered fossa (*articular fovea of the radius*), which articulates with the capitulum of the humerus. Another cartilaginous, narrow joint surface (the *articular circumference of the radius*) runs like a band around the head of the radius; it rotates against the radial notch of the ulna and the anular ligament of the radius during pronation and supination movements.

The head of the radius is connected with the middle piece, or *body of the radius*, by the narrower *neck*, which is slightly bent against the shaft of the radius dorsolaterally. The body of the radius is triangular in cross section. At its proximal end, the *radial tuberosity*, which serves for the attachment of the tendon of the biceps brachii, projects medially.

The sharp *interosseous margin* of the radius is turned toward the ulna. The *anterior* and *posterior margins* are somewhat more rounded. The *anterior surface* (in the supinated forearm) faces ventromedially, the *posterior surface* dorsomedially. The *lateral surface* is bordered by the anterior and posterior margins.

The broad, well-developed distal end of the radius (Fig. **98**) supports the cartilage-covered *carpal articular surface*, which articulates with the scaphoid and lunate of the wrist. On the medial side there is an *ulnar notch*, which moves on the articular circumference of the ulna. The distal end of the radius runs laterally into the *styloid process*.

The palmar surface of the distal endpiece is smooth; on the posterior side – separated by the *dorsal tubercle* – the tendons of the extensor pollicis longus (medial) and the extensores carpi radiales (lateral) glide in shallow grooves.

The **ulna** (Fig. **89**) – in contrast to the radius – is much better developed proximally than distally. Its proximal end, whose diameter clearly exceeds the thickness of the head of the radius, curves around the trochlea of the humerus forceps-like. The hook-shaped, dorsal bony process (*olecranon*) lies close to the skin. The tendon of the triceps brachii is attached to it. The anterior *coronoid process* is weaker. Shaped like a half-moon, the *trochlear notch*, which receives the trochlea of the humerus, lies between it and the olecranon. The cartilage-covered articular surface of the trochlear notch merges at the lateral margin into the likewise cartilage-covered *radial notch*, with which the articular circumference of the radius articulates. Immediately distal to the coronoid process there is a rough bony surface, the *ulnar tuberosity*, which serves for the insertion of the tendon of the brachialis muscle.

At the triangular *shaft of the ulna*, the sharp *interosseous margin* separates the *anterior* and *posterior surfaces* from one another. The *anterior* and *posterior margins* border the *medial surface*. A bony ridge, the *supinator crest*, is more or less distinctly prominent on the posterior surface distal to the radial notch; it gives origin to the supinator muscle.

The ulna ends distally in the weak *head of the ulna*. Its slightly convex, cartilage-covered end surface, which is separated from the proximal row of carpal bones by an articular disc, continues into the *articular circumference of the ulna* at the lateral margin (Fig. **98**). It corresponds to the articular circumference of the radius at the proximal end of the radius and articulates with the ulnar notch of the radius. Medially, the *styloid process of the ulna* projects over the distal end surface of the head of the ulna.

In general, the styloid process of the radius reaches further distally than the styloid process of the ulna (in the adult about 8–10 mm, Fig. **89**). If both styloid processes are at the same height after an accident, a compression fracture of the radius should be suspected. The ulna, of course, can also be just as long as the radius or longer.

A *radiogram* of the distal epiphysial joint of the radius and ulna is frequently consulted in assessing growth disturbances (rickets) or lead poisoning.

Diaphysial **ossification** begins in the *radius* in the 7th embryonic week, in the *ulna* only a few days later (Fig. **78**). The ossific center of the distal epiphysis appears in both forearm bones earlier than the proximal (distal epiphysis of radius 1–2 years of age; head of radius 5–7th year; head of ulna 5–7th year; olecranon 1–2 centers in 8–12th year [the proximal end of the ulna with the trochlear notch ossifies, for the most part, from the diaphysis]). The proximal cartilaginous epiphysial joint closes earlier in the radius (14–20th year) and in the ulna (13–17th year) than the distal growth plates (20–25th year).

b) Capsule and Ligamentous Apparatus of the Elbow Joint

The **elbow joint** is a complex joint. In it the humerus articulates with the two forearm bones in the *humero-ulnar* and *humeroradial joints*; the proximal end pieces of the radius and ulna articulate with each other in the *proximal radio-ulnar joint*. All three joints possess a common recess-rich joint cavity, which is enclosed by a uniform capsule.

The *humero-ulnar articulation* is a hinge joint. The trochlea of the humerus articulates with the trochlear notch of the ulna. In so doing, a spine-like guiding ridge of the ulna glides in the grooved cavity of the trochlea.

The bending of the guiding groove from the circular plane is so insignificant that the resultant deviation of flexion or extension movements from a hinge movement is practically meaningless. The guidance of movement – as in all human joints – is not completely rigid. The contact of the articular surfaces is greatest in a position of slight flexion.

In the *humeroradial joint* the capitulum of the humerus articulates with the plate-shaped, deepened articular fovea of the radius. According to the shape of the articular surfaces, the joint is a ball and socket joint. The radius, however, is bound to the ulna by the interosseous membrane and the ligamentous bands of the radio-ulnar joint so that a degree of freedom is lost and only flexion or extension movements, as well as pronation or supination are still possible.

In the *radio-ulnar articulation* the articular circumference of the radius rotates in the ring formed by the radial notch of the ulna and the anular ligament (Fig. **89**). The joint is a pivot joint.

In rotation the beveled proximal margin of the circumference glides on a ridge which sets off the trochlea from the capitulum and serves as a guiding ridge not only for pronation or supination, but also for flexion or extension movements.

The *capsule* of the elbow joint (Fig. **90**) is attached at the humerus on the ventral side proximal to the radial and coronoid fossae and passes distal to the epicondyles on the dorsal surface, where it encloses the olecranon fossa. At the radius the capsule extends to the neck. This part of the capsule is expanded into a thin-walled *recessus sacciformis* and can be twisted so that the rotation of the head of the radius is not hindered. At the ulna the capsule is attached at the cartilage-bone border; only at the

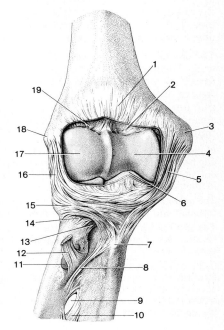

Fig. 90. **Elbow joint**, ventral view
 1 Articular capsule of elbow (opened on the ventral side)
 2 Coronoid fossa
 3 Medial epicondyle of humerus
 4 Trochlea of humerus
 5 Ulnar collateral ligament
 6 Coronoid process of ulna
 7 Tuberosity of ulna
 8 Oblique cord
 9 Opening for posterior interosseous vessels
10 Antebrachial interosseous membrane
11 Bicipitoradial bursa
12 Tendon of biceps brachii
13 Quadrate ligament
14 Sacciform recess
15 Anular ligament of the radius
16 Radial collateral ligament
17 Capitulum of humerus
18 Lateral epicondyle of humerus
19 Radial fossa

olecranon and the coracoid process is it fixed to the bone at some distance from it.

The anterior and posterior walls of the capsule are relatively thin. Deformable folds of fat over the capitulum of the humerus, the coronoid fossa and, above all, over the olecranon fossa fill up the spaces made by the bony projections during movements of the elbow joint. The anterior wall becomes folded during flexion, the posterior wall during extension. Tendon fibers of the brachialis and triceps muscles, which radiate into the capsule as an *articularis cubiti muscle*, counteract a squeezing.

Ligaments (Fig. **90**). Collateral ligaments which hinder an abduction in the elbow joint are woven into the lateral part of the capsule.

The *ulnar collateral ligament* forms a triangular plate. Its fibers originate in front of and behind the axis of rotation at the medial epicondyle of the humerus and pass fan-shaped into the medial margin of the trochlear notch. A part of the fiber bundle is thus stretched in every position of the joint. The ligamentous segment lying close to its attachment is collected proximal to the trochlear notch by superficial, transverse fiber tracts (transverse part).

The *radial collateral ligament* radiates from the lateral epicondyle into the anular ligament of the radius where its fibers course around the head of the radius to the anterior and posterior margins of the radial notch of the ulna. It therefore does not restrict rotatory movements of the radius, but does hinder the abduction of the forearm medially.

The *anular ligament of the radius* is inserted completely into the capsular wall. Together with the cartilage-covered radial notch of the ulna, it forms an osteofibrous ring which curves around the articular circumference of the radius. The head of the radius can rotate unhindered in the ring during pronation or supination, but, at the same time, is so firmly enclosed (in the adult) that it can only be dislocated by a very great traumatic force.

In the child the anular ligament is weaker and broader. The head of the radius can be detached from the osteofibrous ring by a sudden jerk or by a prolonged pull on the hand of a reluctant child and subluxated or luxated (subluxation = incomplete dislocation).

The *quadrate ligament* consists of fibrous tracts which attach distal to the anular ligament and pass from the radial notch of the ulna to the neck of the radius.

The *innervation* of the joint capsule is by branches of the musculocutaneous (ventral and medial), ulnar (medial and dorsal), and radial (dorsal, lateral and ventral) nerves.

In the case of effusion, the *relaxed position* of the joint is a slight flexion of the forearm. Prolonged immobilization of the elbow requires an elbow joint flexed at a right angle and an intermediate position of the radio-ulnar joint since the elbow joint is prone to stiffen and, therefore, this position is functionally most favorable if rigidity should occur.

Fractures in the region of the condyles of the humerus, the supracondylar fossa, the head of the radius and proximal segment of the neck of the radius, coronoid process of the ulna and the olecranon (exclusive of the dorsal corner of the elbow), as well as loosening of the epiphyses near the joints always involve the elbow joint. In fractures of the epicondyles of the humerus, the fracture line can run outside of the capsule.

Luxations almost always involve the humero-ulnar joint and (especially in women and juveniles, who can often overextend at the elbow joint) are very frequent despite the pronounced bony guidance of the joint. In the case of a fall on the outstretched arm, the apex of the olecranon presses into the olecranon fossa and can lever the trochlear notch above the trochlea of the humerus, which causes the anterior wall of the capsule to rupture.

Since the epicondyles of the humerus and the olecranon can be palpated through the skin, it can be easily established whether normal positional relationships exist at the elbow joint (Fig. **91**). When inspected dorsally in the extending position, both condyles and the palpable bony points are in a straight line with the olecranon.

When flexed at a right angle, the three bony points define an isoceles triangle, the elbow triangle.

It can be recognized in lateral view that the elbow triangle in the right-angled, flexed joint lies in the plane of the axis of the shaft of the humerus, from which it is tilted ventrally by acute-angled flexion, dorsally by increasing extension.

Movement possibilities in the elbow joint are:
– *flexion* or *extension* in the humero-ulnar and humeroradial joints around a *transverse* axis (below the epicondyles, through the capitulum and trochlea of the humerus), whereby the movement is carried on exclusively in the humero-ulnar joint;

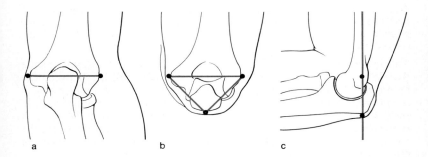

Fig. 91. **Positional relations of epicondyles of humerus to olecranon**
a Extension position of forearm, dorsal view
b Right-angled flexion of forearm, dorsal view
c Right-angled flexion of forearm, medial view

–*pronation* and *supination* in the proximal (and distal) radio-ulnar joints around an *oblique* axis which courses from the middle of the head of the radius through the neck of the radius and interosseous membrane to the head of the ulna near the base of the styloid process (Fig. **97 a**).

During *flexion* and *extension movements*, the circumference of movement amounts altogether to about 120–140° (maximal flexion up to 40°, maximal extension up to an arm-forearm angle of 175° and more; an extension of more than 180° is not rare, especially in women and children).

The impairment of flexion is a soft tissue impediment. Only in the strongest flexion is the coronoid process driven into the coronoid fossa. The impairment of extension results from the resistance of the stretched flexor muscles and the lateral ligaments (anterior tracts), which are stretched to the maximum, but the olecranon is also often pushed into the olecranon fossa.

During *pronation* and *supination* (= turning movements of the hand) the circumference of movement also amounts to about 120–140° in the living. In general, the radius (and with it the hand) rotates around the ulna. With the hand fixed, however, the ulna can also be carried around the radius, if the upper arm or the entire body (e.g. in gymnastics) is moved correspondingly.

The axis of rotation extends from the central point of curvature of the head of the humerus, to the ring finger (hand and arm in stretched position). Pronation or supination of the forearm and inner or outer rotation of the humerus take place, therefore, (in the stretched elbow joint) around the same axis and together achieve a total movement circumference of about 230°. By additional movements of the shoulder girdle and the trunk, a complete rotary movement of the hand (360°) can be attained.

Pronation or supination of the forearm is slowed, above all, by the tension of the stretched supinators or pronators (muscle inhibition). Moreover, in extreme pronation, the soft tissues (deep flexors of the forearm) squeezed in between the crossed forearm bones do the inhibiting (soft tissue inhibition).

The *mucous bursae* in the vicinity of the elbow joint do not communicate with the joint cavity. The *bicipitoradial bursa* (Fig. **90**) lies between the tendon of the biceps and the radial tuberosity. The *subcutaneous olecranon bursa* between the olecranon and skin is normally present and, in the case of persisting irritation (miners), is often chronically inflamed. A *subtendinous bursa of the triceps brachii tendon* can be formed between the triceps tendon and the joint capsule and an *intratendinous olecranon bursa* may exist within the fiber tracts of the triceps tendon.

Occasionally, a subcutaneous mucous bursa lies between the lateral or medial epicondyle and the skin. An *interosseous cubital bursa*, which can be extended up to the oblique cord, is formed in about 20% of the cases between the end of the biceps tendon, the tendon of the brachialis and the ulna.

c) Action of Muscles and Muscle Groups on the Elbow Joint

In the elbow joint:
- all muscles *flex* which pass *ventral* to the frontal axis (through capitulum and trochlea);
- all muscles *extend* which course *dorsal* to the axis.

Main flexors are the biceps brachii and brachialis.

The brachioradialis, pronator teres and – from a flexion position – the extensor carpi radialis longus function in support.

The *brachialis* is a pure flexor. The *biceps brachii* always tries to supinate at first. Its torque as a flexor decreases during pronation (chin-ups easier with underhand grip), whereas it increases for the brachioradialis and pronator teres. The torque of all flexors increases until somewhat beyond the right-angled flexion and becomes less with increasing acute-angled flexion.

The contributions of the flexor carpi radialis, palmaris longus, and the extensor carpi radialis brevis are insignificant in flexion of the elbow.

The *main extensor* is the triceps brachii, especially its two heads originating from the humerus.

The *anconeus* functions primarily as a *capsule tensor* and prevents the pinching of parts of the joint capsule during extension.

Excluding the force of gravity that replaces or (in the case of extension against resistance) complements the action of the extensors when the upper arm is hanging down, the torque of the extensors is somewhat less than that of all flexors of the elbow joint (about two-thirds). The two main flexors, the biceps brachii and the brachialis, together have approximately the same torque as the extensors.

Paralyses. By a severance of the musculocutaneous nerve, the *biceps brachii* and *brachialis muscles* become paralyzed. Provided no double innervation of the brachialis muscle (more rarely the biceps brachii) is present via the radial nerve, the torque of the flexors is reduced by almost one third. If an extensive collateral innervation of the upper arm exists via the radial nerve, an injury of the musculocutaneous nerve can remain largely hidden.

In a paralysis of the *triceps and anconeus muscles* (injury of the radial nerve before entering the "radial canal"), an extension of the elbow joint is only possible with the help of gravity (and/or centrifugal force).

In the radio-ulnar joint:
- all muscles *pronate* which cross the axis of rotation (through the head of the radius and head of the ulna) on the *ventral side;*
- all muscles *supinate* which pass over this axis on the *dorsal* side.

Since all muscles for the rotatory movements of the hand – except the biceps brachii – belong to the forearm muscles, their effect on the radio-ulnar joint will be discussed later (→ p. 253).

3. Cubital Fossa

The **cubital fossa** is a Y-shaped connective tissue space on the flexor side of the elbow region. On the extensor side there is the elbow joint.

The muscular *border* of the cubital fossa is formed proximally by the biceps brachii, which bulges in the middle of the brachialis between the two brachial furrows. (In the flexed elbow the biceps tendon juts out and can be easily palpated through the skin). The superficial flexors of the forearm which arise at the medial epicondyle form the boundary of the connective tissue space on the ulnar side, and the muscles of the radial group which take their origin from the lateral margin of the humerus and from the lateral epicondyle form the lateral side. In the distal segment at the base of the fossa, the humeral head of the pronator teres lies medially, the supinator laterally. The closure of the cubital fossa toward the subcutaneous connective tissue is effected by the brachial and antebrachial fasciae, strengthened medially by the bicipital aponeurosis.

When the elbow is extended, it stretches the fascia and bulges the cutaneous vein (intermediate cubital vein), which courses epifascially. The bicipital aponeurosis is likewise stretched and protects the brachial artery coursing in the cubital fossa during extraction of blood or intravenous injections.

Depending on the formation of subcutaneous fat tissue, the thin, hairless skin over the cubital fossa is somewhat depressed. This anterior segment of the elbow region is designated as the *bend of the elbow (anterior cubital region)*. (According to many authors, the bend of the elbow is also synonymous with cubital fossa.)

The transverse skin furrow appearing at the bend usually lies 1–2 cm proximal to the elbow joint.

Vessels and Nerves in the Cubital Fossa

In the cubital fossa vessels and nerves are rearranged.

Brachial Artery and Median Nerve

The *neurovascular trunk* passes from the medial furrow of the upper arm into the cubital fossa, where the *brachial artery* with its *accompanying veins* – along the deep biceps tendon – is oriented more toward the middle, whereas the *median nerve* stays more ulnarwards and enters the middle route of the forearm through the cleft between the humeral and ulnar head of the pronator teres (Fig. **92**). The brachial artery divides into the *radial* and *ulnar arteries* under the bicipital aponeurosis somewhat distal to the joint fissure.

During flexion of the elbow joint, the brachial artery cannot be lifted off the brachialis muscle. With maximal flexion it is compressed (possibility of temporary control of hemorrhage, danger of ischemia with longer duration).

The **radial artery** (Fig. **92**) courses in the radial route (between the brachioradialis and flexor carpi radialis) superficial to the tendon of insertion of the pronator teres. It supplies the radial muscle group of the forearm (the radially situated flexors), the back of the hand, the thenar eminence and, via the deep palmar arch, the middle of the hand and the fingers.

In the cubital fossa the *radial artery* gives off (besides muscle branches) the *recurrent radial artery*, which – medial to the radial nerve – courses proximally between the brachialis and brachioradialis, supplies the neighboring muscles, anastomoses with the radial collateral artery and sends variable twigs through the lateral brachial intermuscular septum to the articular network of the elbow.

The **ulnar artery** (Fig. **92**) crosses under the pronator teres and reaches the ulnar route (along the radial margin of the flexor carpi ulnaris) on the flexor digitorum profundus. It supplies the ulnar part of the superficial flexors, the deep flexors via the *anterior interosseous artery*, the extensor muscles of the forearm via the *posterior interosseous artery*, further, the hypothenar eminence and – via the superficial palmar arch – the metacarpals and fingers.

The *ulnar artery* gives off in the cubital fossa (besides muscular branches) the *ulnar recurrent artery* and the *common interosseous artery* (about 4 – 5 cm distal to the joint cavity).

The *ulnar recurrent artery* passes proximally toward the ulna between the pronator teres and brachialis. After a short distance, it divides into an *anterior branch* (in front of the medial epicondyle of the humerus) and a *posterior branch*, which goes behind the medial epicondyle.

The *anterior branch* crosses the brachialis and anastomoses with the inferior ulnar collateral artery. The *posterior branch* turns back and accompanies the ulnar nerve, giving off branches to neighboring muscles and anastomosing with the superior ulnar collateral artery.

The *common interosseous artery* leaves the ulnar artery at the upper margin of the pronator teres and divides shortly after its origin into the *anterior* and *posterior interosseous arteries*. The anterior interosseous artery passes distally on the interosseous membrane in the palmar interosseous route and communicates with the palmar carpal network. The posterior interosseous artery courses distally together with the radial nerve in the dorsal forearm route and reaches the dorsal carpal network with its terminal branch.

The *anterior interosseous artery* supplies the deep flexors of the forearm and, in addition, sends a branch to the dorsal carpal network. The *posterior interosseous artery* gives off numerous branches to the superficial and deep extensors. Immediately after passing through the interosseous membrane, the *recurrent interosseous artery* branches off and arrives at the articular network of the elbow by turning back beneath the anconeus.

The (usually) weak *companion artery of the median nerve*, which accompanies the median nerve and ramifies on the musculature and both forearm bones, usually arises from the anterior interosseous artery, occasionally from the vascular trunk, rarely from the ulnar artery or very rarely from the brachial artery. During ontogenesis it replaced the interosseous artery as the main artery of the forearm. In the definitive condition, the radial and ulnar arteries have taken over its role.

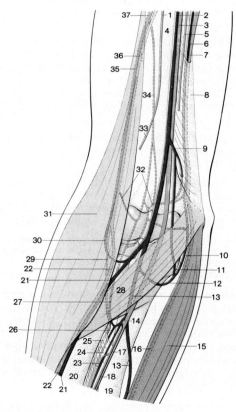

Fig. 92. **Arteries and nerves in region of elbow**, ventral view

Articular network of the elbow (Fig. **92**). Numerous anastomoses exist at the elbow joint between descending branches of the brachial artery and recurrent branches from the radial, ulnar and posterior interosseous arteries. The extensive *arterial network of the elbow*, which is formed mainly on the dorsal side of the joint, is fed by these vessels. On account of the expansible anastomoses, an extensive collateral circulation can be developed – if the brachial artery is ligated distal to the exit of the profunda brachii artery.

The *articular network of the elbow* receives tributaries from

descending branches of arteries of upper arm:
radial collateral artery
middle collateral artery
superior ulnar collateral artery
inferior ulnar collateral artery

recurrent branches of arteries of forearm:
radial recurrent artery
ulnar recurrent artery
interosseous recurrent artery

Brachial veins. The deep veins accompany the brachial artery and its branches. In the elbow a connection exists between the epifascial and the deep veins by one (or several) valveless intermediate deep cubital veins.

Deep lymphatic vessels discharge lymph from the deep layers of the forearm along the brachial vessels. Occasionally, some *deep cubital lymph nodes* are inserted in the deep lymph pathways within the cubital fossa.

In the cubital fossa the **median nerve** gives off muscular branches to the superficial flexors (except the flexor carpi ulnaris).

1 Musculocutaneous nerve
2 Brachial artery ⎫ in neurovascular
3 Median nerve ⎭ bundle of arm
4 Humerus
5 Medial antebrachial cutaneous nerve
6 Superior ulnar collateral artery
7 Ulnar nerve
8 Medial brachial intermuscular septum
9 Inferior ulnar collateral artery
10 Posterior branch of ulnar recurrent artery
11 Anterior branch of ulnar recurrent artery
12 Ulnar recurrent artery
13 Ulnar artery
14 Common interosseous artery
15 Flexor carpi ulnaris
16 Ulnar nerve in ulnar route
17 Median nerve
18 Companion artery ⎫ in forearm
  to median nerve ⎭ median route
19 Ulna
20 Radius
21 Radial artery ⎫
22 Superficial branch ⎬ in radial route
  of radial nerve ⎭

23 Anterior interosseous artery ⎫ in palmar
  Anterior [antebrachial] ⎬ interosseous
  interosseous nerve ⎭ route
24 Antebrachial interosseous membrane
25 Posterior [antebrachial] ⎫ in dorsal
  interosseous nerve ⎬ forearm route
26 Posterior interosseous artery ⎭
27 Recurrent interosseous artery
28 Pronator teres
29 Deep branch of radial nerve
30 Recurrent radial artery
31 Brachioradialis
32 Articular network of elbow
33 Lateral antebrachial cutaneous nerve
34 Middle collateral artery
35 Radial collateral artery
36 Radial nerve (at penetration of lateral brachial intermuscular septum)
37 Profunda brachii artery

Radial Nerve and Accompanying Vessels

The **radial nerve** and the ventral branch of the *radial collateral artery* (together with the accompanying veins) pass from the depth of the lateral bicipital sulcus into the cubital fossa. The *lateral antebrachial cutaneous nerve*, which courses in the forearm between the biceps brachii and the brachialis, passes at the distal end of the lateral forearm furrow through the brachial fascia to the radial side of the forearm.

The *radial nerve* (Fig. **92**) in the cubital fossa gives off branches to the radial muscle group, generally also to the lateral fiber tracts of the brachialis (more rarely to the biceps brachii) and divides somewhat proximal to the joint cavity into *superficial* (sensory) and *deep* (motor) *rami*.

The *superficial branch of the radial nerve* – covered by the brachioradialis muscle – passes distally on the supinator. It courses into the radial route on the lateral side of the radial vessels.

The *deep branch of the radial nerve* within the supinator winds around the proximal end of the radius and arrives at the dorsal forearm route between the superficial and the deep layer of the extensors.

Since the deep ramus of the radial nerve is carried in the supinator near the proximal end of the radius and cannot be displaced, it is endangered in fractures of the neck of the radius or dislocations of the head of the radius. In the supinated position, it travels especially close to the articular cavity of the elbow joint.

Ulnar Nerve and Accompanying Vessels

The **ulnar nerve** (Fig. **92**) passes on the dorsal side of the elbow joint over the articular cavity. From the sulcus of the ulnar nerve at the dorsal surface of the medial epicondyle of the humerus, where it is covered by a reinforced antebrachial fascia, it passes under the tendinous arch that unites the humeral and ulnar heads of the flexor carpi ulnaris. The branches for the flexor carpi ulnaris and the ulnar head of the deep flexors of the fingers are usually given off here. By means of an anastomosis, the median and ulnar nerves can exchange fibers. The ulnar nerve passes distally below the ulnar carpal flexor in the ulnar route and joins the ulnar vessels medially.

In the region of the elbow, the ulnar nerve is accompanied proximally by the *superior ulnar collateral artery*, distally by the *posterior ramus* of the *ulnar recurrent artery*. Since it courses close to the axis of rotation of the elbow joint, it is scarcely stretched during flexion movements.

C. Forearm and Hand

1. Forearm

a) Organization and Innervation of the Forearm Musculature

The forearm musculature is divided genetically into a *ventral* group of muscles (*flexor group*) situated on the palmar side and a *dorsal* muscle group (*extensor group*) located on the dorsal side. This arrangement, however, oversimplifies, as several muscles of the dorsal group have been shifted around the radius on the palmar side of the forearm and thus – in reference to the elbow joint – have become flexor muscles (*radial muscle group*).

The **antebrachial fascia** (Fig. **96**) encloses the forearm musculature and – strengthened by tendon fibers – serves simultaneously in the elbow region as a surface of origin for the superficial flexors and extensors. The fascia is attached to bone at both humeral epicondyles, at the olecranon and at the dorsal border of the ulna. From the undersurface of the fascia, connective tissue septa penetrate between the muscle groups of the forearm. In this way three *compartments* are formed: *ventral* (*flexors*), *dorsal* (*extensors*, in the narrow sense) and *radial* (for the *radial* muscle group); they are bordered by the antebrachial fascia (the fascia of the groups), the two forearm bones, and the interosseous membrane.

Ventral and dorsal compartments are organized proximally by intermuscular septa, distally by layers of loose connective tissue that separate the superficial and deep flexors or extensors.

The connective tissue spaces permit inflammation and bleeding to spread in a longitudinal direction. Forearm phlegmons frequently emanate from inflammatory tendon sheaths (tendovaginitis) in the carpal canal and, therefore, usually appear in the flexor compartment.

At the level of the radiocarpal joint, the antebrachial fascia is strengthened on the dorsal side by transverse fiber tracts which form the *extensor retinaculum* (Fig. **94**). Distally, it is continued into the *dorsal fascia of the hand*, which covers the extensor tendons and is connected with the dorsal aponeurosis of the fingers.

On the palmar side, transverse fiber tracts attached at the radius and ulna likewise strengthen the portion of antebrachial fascia near the wrist joint which continues into the fascia of the palmar surface at the wrist. In the palmar region this superficial fascia is strengthened into the *palmar aponeurosis* (Fig. **106**). Distally and more deeply, the transverse fascial tracts communicate with a firm ligament, the *flexor retinaculum* (Figs. **102** and **107**), over which the palmar aponeurosis passes. The flexor retinaculum bridges the groove formed by the carpal bones and converts it into an osteofibrous canal (*carpal canal*), through which the tendons of the long flexors of the fingers course.

The **antebrachial interosseous membrane** (Figs. **89** and **96**) extends between the radius and ulna. Its fibers take a predominantly oblique course from proximolateral to distomedial; in the distal part they also run in the opposite direction. The membrane secures the two forearm bones against longitudinal shifting, prevents excessive supination and, at the same time, serves as a surface of origin for the deep extensors and flexors of the forearm.

The earlier belief that pressure on the radius via the hand is transferred to the ulna by the membrane as a pulling force, is not supported by experimental studies in which the membrane was severed longitudinally.

In the proximal segment of the interosseous space, a gap is left for the radial tuberosity and the biceps tendon, which are rotated medially during pronation. This gap is bordered distally by a tense fiber tract, the *oblique cord*, whose bundles of fibers go out from the ulnar tuberosity and course – in opposition to the majority of fibers of the interosseous membrane – from proximal on the ulnar side to distal on the radial. Together with the proximal margin of the interosseous membrane, the oblique cord borders the point of passage for the posterior interosseous vessels.

The forearm is tapered distally since the muscular tissue of the long forearm muscles lies proximally. Thus, the forearm is lighter distally and more movable, especially since the origin of the forearm muscles has advanced proximally on the humerus. The superficial flexors arise from the medial epicondyle of the humerus and the superficial extensors from the lateral epicondyle.

On the basis of their insertions the *forearm muscles* can be *grouped* into:
– muscles which insert on the radius: brachioradialis, supinator, pronator teres, pronator quadratus. Acting across the radio-ulnar joint, they are thus pronators or supinators. The brachioradialis and pronator teres, moreover, assist in flexion at the elbow joint;
– muscles which attach to the metacarpal bones (or at the pisiform): extensor carpi radialis longus, extensor carpi radialis brevis, extensor carpi ulnaris, abductor pollicis longus, flexor carpi radialis, flexor carpi ulnaris, palmaris longus. Above all, they move the wrist (abductor pollicis longus, of course, only when the thumb is adducted to the index finger);
– muscles which pass to the phalanges and implement (both hand and) finger movements.

The long extensor and flexor muscles of the fingers pass over the phalangeal joints and the wrist joints; the flexor digitorum superficialis additionally flexes at the elbow joint; at the same time, the fibers of these muscles are relatively short. As a result, their contractability is not sufficient to produce a maximal extension or flexion in all joints: *active insufficiency*. By the same token, the muscle fibers cannot be stretched so far that all joints over which the muscle passes can be brought into a maximal extension or flexion opposite to the muscle action: *passive insufficiency*.

Extensor Group (Dorsal Muscles)

Radial Muscle Group

The radial muscle group has been separated from the superficial layer of the dorsal muscles of the forearm; their origin at the lateral epicondyle of the humerus has been expanded proximally and pushed between the triceps brachii and brachialis. The muscles of this group pass distally *in front of* the axis of flexion of the elbow joint. Thus, they are flexors of the elbow joint and course in an oblique helical line at the lateral side of the radius so that they obtain a pronator component.

The **brachioradialis** (Figs. **93 a** and **96**) lies at the lateral border of the radius and originates at the lateral surface of the humerus, above the lateral epicondyle, and from the lateral brachial intermuscular septum. It inserts at the root of the styloid process of the radius.

Innervation: radial nerve.

After the radial nerve has entered the lateral sulcus of the upper arm through the lateral intermuscular septum, it dispatches branches to the muscles of the radial group and usually also fine twigs to the lateral bundles of the brachialis muscle.

The **extensor carpi radialis longus** (Figs. **93 a** and **96**) arises from the lateral margin of the humerus – distal to the origin of the brachioradialis – and from the lateral brachial intermuscular septum. It inserts at the base of the second metacarpal bone.

The upper margin of the muscle belly is covered over by the brachioradialis, whereas it bulges laterally over the lateral epicondyle and covers the proximal segment of the extensor carpi radialis brevis.

Innervation: radial nerve.

The **extensor carpi radialis brevis** (Figs. **93 a** and **96**) takes its origin from the lateral epicondyle, from the annular ligament of the radius and from the connective tissue septum which separates the muscle from the extensor digitorum muscle. The brevis tendon inserts at the styloid process of the third metacarpal.

The tendons of the extensor carpi radialis longus and brevis travel distally at the lateral margin of the radius, are crossed by the muscle bellies of the abductor pollicis longus and extensor pollic brevis, and course through the 2nd tendon compartment below the extensor retinaculum (Fig. **94**).

Innervation: deep ramus of the radial nerve.

The muscular branch leaves the deep ramus of the radial nerve before the latter passes into the supinator. However, it does not penetrate into the muscle until it passes further distally.

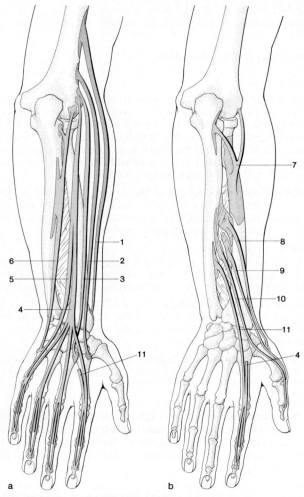

Fig. 93. **Extensor group of forearm muscles**, dorsal view
a Radial muscle group (1–3) and superficial layer of extensors (4–6)
b Deep layer of extensors (7–11)

1 Brachioradialis
2 Extensor carpi radialis longus
3 Extensor carpi radialis brevis
4 Extensor digitorum
5 Extensor digiti minimi
6 Extensor carpi ulnaris
7 Supinator

8 Abductor pollicis longus
9 Extensor pollicis brevis
10 Extensor pollicis longus
11 Extensor indicis

Innervation:
☐ Radial Nerve ☐ Deep ramus of radial
nerve

Superficial Layer of Extensors

The **extensor carpi ulnaris** (Figs. **93 a** and **96**) forms the medial, marginal contour of this muscle group. Its *humeral head* arises from the lateral epicondyle of the humerus between the fields of origin of the anconeus and extensor digitorum. Its *ulnar head* originates from the antebrachial fascia and from the dorsal edge of the ulna. It inserts at the base of the 5th metacarpal.

The bipennate muscle lies on the dorsal surface of the ulna. Its tendon glides above the head of the ulna in a groove bordered medially by the styloid process of the ulna and passes through the 6th tendon compartment below the extensor retinaculum (Fig. 94).

Innervation: deep ramus of the radial nerve.

The **extensor digitorum** (Figs. **93 a** and **96**) lies in the middle of the forearm on the radial side of the extensor carpi ulnaris. It originates from the lateral ligamentous tracts of the elbow joint, the antebrachial fascia and from the connective tissue septum separating it from the extensor carpi radialis brevis. It inserts at the dorsal aponeurosis of fingers $2-5$.

The 4 tendons of the muscle lie in the same layer and pass together through the 4th tendon compartment below the extensor retinaculum. In the region of the metacarpals, the tendons communicate closely with one another by transverse ligamentous bands (*intertendinous connections*); on the backs of the fingers, they form the *dorsal aponeurosis* (Figs. 94 and 105). The middle tendinous band of each tendon ends at the base of the middle phalanx; the lateral cords pass over the middle joint, are united distally from it on the dorsal side of the middle phalanx and attach at the base of terminal segments II–V.

Innervation: deep ramus of the radial nerve.

After exiting from the "supinator canal", the deep ramus of the radial nerve gives off a branch, which ramifies at the extensor digitorum and extensor digiti minimi muscles, and directly after that sends another branch to the extensor carpi ulnaris. All three muscular branches can also arise from a short, common trunk.

The **extensor digit minimi** (Figs. **93 a** and **96**) has split off from the extensor digitorum and is separated from this muscle at the origin only by a tendinous sheet. Its tendon occupies a single tendon compartment (the 5th) and inserts at the dorsal aponeurosis of the 5th finger (Fig. **94**).

Innervation: deep ramus of the radial nerve.

The innervation of the extensor digit minimi by the same nerve branch which supplies the extensor digitorum is indicative of the very close genetic relationship between these two muscles.

Deep Layer of Extensors

The **supinator** (Fig. **93 b**) arises from the lateral epicondyle of the humerus, the lateral tendinous tracts of the elbow joint and from the supinator crest of the ulna. The thin muscular plate curves around

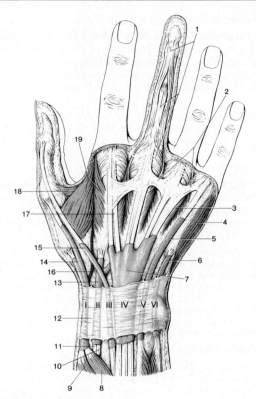

Fig. 94. Tendon sheaths at back of hand

1 Dorsal aponeurosis of middle finger
2 Intertendinous connection
3 Dorsal interosseus IV
4 Abductor digiti minimi
5 Synovial sheath of extensor digiti minimi
6 Synovial sheath of extensor carpi ulnaris
7 Sypovial sheath of extensor digitorum and extensor indicis
8 Extensor pollicis brevis
9 Abductor pollicis longus
10 Tendon of extensor carpi radialis longus
11 Tendon of extensor carpi radialis brevis

12 Extensor retinaculum
13 Synovial sheath of extensor carpi radialis
14 Synovial sheath of abductor longus and extensor pollicis brevis
15 Synovial sheath of extensor pollicis longus
16 Radial artery in "anatomical snuff-box"
17 Tendon of extensor indicis
18 Adductor pollicis
19 Dorsal interosseus I
I-VI Synovial sheaths beneath extensor retinaculum

the radius laterally and from behind and attaches at the anterior surface of the radius between the radial tuberosity and the field of insertion of the pronator teres.

The deep ramus of the radial nerve enters the muscle in the vicinity of the proximal margin and passes through the muscle distally in the "supinator canal", which courses in the shape of a helix.

Innervation: deep ramus of the radial nerve.

The muscular branch leaves the deep ramus before the latter penetrates the supinator. Fine branches can be given off by the deep ramus during its course through the "supinator canal".

The **abductor pollicis longus** and **extensor pollicis brevis** form a genetic and functional unit; the muscle bellies frequently also form a morphological one (Figs. **93 b**, **96** and **105**). They originate from the dorsal surface of the radius (2nd and 3rd quarter) and from the antebrachial interosseous membrane. The bipennate abductor pollicis longus originates distal to the origin of the supinator and also has a field of origin on the ulna. The abductor pollicis longus attaches at the base of the 1st metacarpal and the extensor pollicis brevis at the base of the proximal phalanx of the thumb. Tendon fibers of the short thumb extensor fuse with the terminal tendon of the extensor pollicis longus and form a weak dorsal aponeurosis.

Both muscles cross the tendons of the extensor carpi radialis longus and brevis at an acute angle, and their tendons course in the radial groove on the dorsal side of the distal end of the radius and pass through the 1st tendon compartment (palmar to the axis of flexion of the wrist).

Innervation: deep ramus of the radial nerve.

The muscular branches for both muscles usually proceed from a common trunk, which leaves the deep ramus distal to the supinator and divides after a short distance.

The **extensor pollicis longus** (Figs. **93 b** and **96**) arises from the interosseous membrane and from a narrow band on the dorsal surface of the ulna, which adjoins the field of origin of the abductor pollicis longus and extensor pollicis brevis distally and toward the ulnar side. Its tendon, which courses through the 3rd tendon compartment, inserts at the base of the distal phalanx of the thumb (Fig. **94**).

The tendon of insertion of the muscle is bordered on the ulnar side by a fossa designated as "snuff-box", in whose depth the radial artery and its companion veins course toward the extensor side of the wrist. The osseous floor of the fossa is formed by the trapezium and scaphoid, and its radial boundary by the tendons of the extensor pollicis brevis and abductor pollicus longus. When these muscles are contracted, their tendons – located close to the skin – jut out so that the fossa becomes distinctly visible.

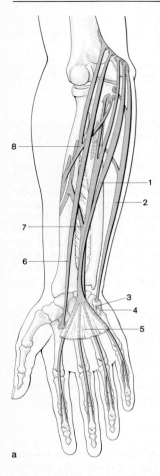

a

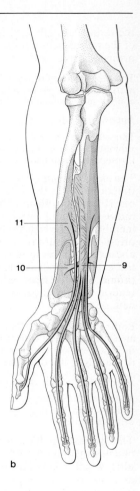

b

Fig. 95. **Flexor groups of forearm muscles,** palmar view.
a Superficial layer of flexors
b Deep layer of flexors

1 Palmaris longus
2 Flexor carpi ulnaris
3 Pisohamate ligament
4 Pisometacarpal ligament
5 Palmar aponeurosis
6 Flexor carpi radialis
7 Flexor digitorum superficialis
8 Pronator teres
9 Flexor digitorum profundus

10 Pronator quadratus
11 Flexor pollicis longus
Innervation:
▢ Median nerve
▢ Anterior interosseous (antebrachial)
  nerve
▢ Ulnar nerve

Innervation: deep ramus of the radial nerve.

The **extensor indicis** (Fig. **93 b**) lies furthest distally and medially of all deep extensors. It arises exclusively from the ulna (distal third of the dorsal fascia). Its tendon, together with the tendons of the extensor digitorum, passes through the 4th tendon compartment and attaches to the dorsal aponeurosis of the index finger (Figs. **94** and **105**).

Innervation: deep ramus of the radial nerve.

The long muscular branch already exits from the deep ramus in the middle third of the forearm or arises from a common trunk, the proximal branch of which supplies the long extensor of the thumb.

Dorsal Tendon Sheaths

The dorsal surfaces of the radius and ulna, together with the extensor retinaculum, delimit an osteofibrous canal which is divided by connective tissue septa into 6 compartments. Generally, a *tendon sheath* occupies each compartment (Fig. **94**). Proximally, the tendon sheaths begin about 1 cm above the extensor retinaculum; distally, they end at the level of the metacarpals. The tendon sheaths of the extensor carpi radialis and ulnaris extend only to the distal row of carpal bones.

Tendon compartments. Through the *first* compartment, which is also situated furthest radially, the tendons of the abductor pollicis longus and extensor pollicis brevis pass in a common tendon sheath. The *second* compartment harbors the tendons of the extensors carpi radialis longus and brevis in a uniform tendon sheath that bifurcates distal to the retinaculum. Through the *third* compartment the tendon of the extensor pollicis longus passes, and through the *fourth*, the tendons of the extensor digitorum and extensor indicis. Through the *fifth* compartment the tendon of the extensor digiti minimi courses, while the tendon of the extensor carpi ulnaris passes through the *sixth*, which is situated furthest on the ulnar side.

Flexor Group (Ventral Muscles)

A superficial and a deep muscle layer is customarily distinguished in the flexor group. In the connective tissue septum which separates both layers, the median nerve (forearm middle route) is located. The muscles of the superficial layer originate from the medial epicondyle of the humerus; the deep flexors take their origin at the radius, ulna and interosseous membrane.

Superficial Layer of Flexors

The **pronator teres** (Figs. **92**, **95 a** and **96**) arises with its *humeral head* from the medial epicondyle of the humerus and from the medial brachial intermuscular septum, together with the superficial flexors of the forearm.

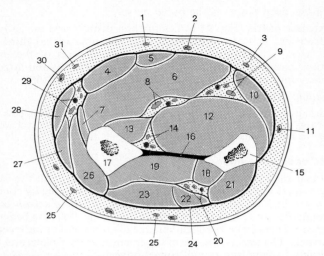

Fig. 96. Cross section in middle third of forearm, distal view of section surface

1 Medial antebrachial cutaneous nerve, anterior branch
2 Intermediate antebrachial vein
3 Medial antebrachial cutaneous nerve, posterior branch
4 Flexor carpi radialis
5 Palmaris longus
6 Flexor digitorum superficialis
7 Pronator teres
8 Median nerve, companion artery of median nerve } in middle route of forearm
9 Ulnar artery and nerve with accompanying veins } in ulnar route
10 Flexor carpi ulnaris
11 Basilic vein
12 Flexor digitorum profundus
13 Flexor pollicis longus
14 Anterior [antebrachial] interosseous nerve, anterior interosseous artery } in palmar interosseous route
15 Ulna
16 Antebrachial interosseous membrane
17 Radius
18 Extensor pollicis longus
19 Abductor pollicis longus and extensor pollicis brevis
20 Posterior [antebrachial] interosseous nerve, posterior interosseous artery } in dorsal route of forearm
21 Extensor carpi ulnaris
22 Extensor digiti minimi
23 Extensor digitorum
24 Antebrachial fascia
25 Posterior antebrachial cutaneous nerve
26 Extensor carpi radialis brevis
27 Extensor carpi radialis longus
28 Brachioradialis
29 Superficial ramus of radial nerve, radial artery with accompanying veins } in radial route
30 Cephalic vein
31 Lateral antebrachial cutaneous nerve

The irregularly developed *ulnar head* comes from the medial surface of the ulna between the coronoid process and the ulnar tuberosity. The muscle passes obliquely over the ulna and radius, curves around the anterior margin of the radius and attaches to the lateral surface of the radius distal to the insertion of the supinator.

The muscle, together with the brachioradialis, borders the cubital fossa distally. The median nerve passes between the humeral and ulnar heads.

Innervation: median nerve, occasionally also the musculocutaneous nerve.

In the cubital fossa, a superior branch of the median nerve passes to the proximal part of the humeral head, and a distal ramus supplies both heads of the pronator teres.

The **flexor carpi radialis** (Figs. **95 a** and **96**) originates from the common field of origin of the superficial flexors at the medial epicondyle of the humerus, as well as from the antebrachial fascia and the connective tissue septum separating it from the adjacent muscles. It inserts at the base of the 2nd (and often also the 3rd) metacarpal bone.

The long tendon of the bipennate muscle passes obliquely downward and to the ulnar side of the radial artery and radial veins on the distal third of the radius and travels in its own canal under the flexor retinaculum (Fig. **102**).

Innervation: median nerve.

The **flexor carpi ulnaris** (Figs. **92**, **95 a** and **96**) forms the ulnar marginal contour of the flexor group. The *humeral head* comes from the medial epicondyle of the humerus and from the medial brachial intermuscular septum; the *ulnar head* arises from the olecranon, from the proximal two-thirds of the posterior margin of the ulna and the antebrachial fascia. The two heads communicate by a tendinous band, beneath which the ulnar nerve passes to the flexor side of the forearm. The tendon of the muscle borders the ulnar forearm route (ulnar nerve and artery, ulnar veins) medially. It does not course through the carpal canal, but is affixed at the pisiform bone and is continued to the hamate and fifth metacarpal bones in the *pisohamate* and *pisometacarpal ligaments* (Figs. **95 a** and **100**).

Owing to the insertion of the pisiform bone as a sesamoid bone in the tendon of the muscle, the distance from the axis of rotation is increased, and the flexor carpi ulnaris obtains a favorable torque for palmar flexion.

Innervation: ulnar nerve.

After the ulnar nerve has traveled from the sulcus behind the medial epicondyle and beneath the tendinous arch of the flexor carpi ulnaris, it sends a branch to the ulnar carpal flexor and usually two branches to the ulnar part of the deep flexors of the fingers ([3rd,] 4th and 5th fingers). Distal to the elbow joint an additional second branch can be given off to the flexor carpi ulnaris.

The **palmaris longus** (Figs. **95 a** and **96**) lies between the flexor carpi radialis and flexor carpi ulnaris. The short muscle belly goes over into a long tendon, which passes to the palm of the hand medial to the tendon of the flexor carpi radialis and superficial to the flexor digitorum superficialis. It is visible through the skin in the flexed hand, passing over the flexor retinaculum (Fig. **107**) and radiating into the palmar aponeurosis, which it can stretch. The muscle can be absent (in about 20%), double-headed or can be doubly developed.

Innervation: median nerve.

The **flexor digitorum superficialis** (Figs. **95 a** and **96**) is two-headed and lies somewhat deeper than the previously named muscles, which partially cover it. Its *humero-ulnar head* originates from the field of origin of the superficial flexors at the medial epicondyle of the humerus and from the coronoid process; its *radial head* springs from a narrow strip on the anterior surface of the radius, distal to the attachment of the pronator teres. Its terminal tendon inserts at middle phalanges II – IV.

The muscular tissue extends nearly to the flexor retinaculum and is incompletely organized into 2 superficial bellies (for the middle and ring fingers) and 2 deep muscle bellies (index and little finger). Their tendons pass through the carpal canal, and each divides above the proximal phalanges into 2 slips, between which the tendons of the flexor digitorum profundus pass through to the distal phalanx (hence, the designations "perforated flexors" for the superficial flexors of the fingers and "perforating flexors" for the deep flexors of the digits, Figs. **103** and **104**). The tendinous slips attach at both lateral margins of middle phalanges II – V. The deep tendon fibers of the flexor digitorum superficialis separate first (*proximally*). They reunite immediately after the passage of the deep flexor tendons – lying directly on the bone, cross each other (*tendinous chiasma*), and form the dorsal part of a sliding collar. The lateral wall of this tube is formed by the longitudinally-coursing slips of the split tendons of the superficial flexors; the incomplete, short palmar partition is composed of the proximal, superficial, still-undivided section of tendon.

Innervation: median nerve.

A proximal branch, which also innervates the palmaris longus muscle with a lateral twig, passes into the superficial flexor of the fingers (muscle belly for the 2nd finger) at the level of the elbow. Somewhat distal to it, a second branch is ramified at the muscle bellies for the 3rd – 5th fingers. A distal branch for the muscle belly of the 2nd finger divides off from the anterior [antebrachial] interosseous nerve.

Deep Layer of Flexors

The **flexor digitorum profundus** (Figs. **95 b** and **96**) arises in a great expanse from the anterior and inner surface of the ulna (proximal two-thirds), from the interosseous membrane and the antebrachial fascia. The large muscle belly, which embraces the ulna in front and medially, serves as a sliding surface for the superficial flexor of the fingers. The 4 tendons lie next to one another in the carpal canal (Fig. **106**), penetrate the tendons of the flexor digitorum superficialis (Figs. **102**, **103** and **104**), and reach the base of the distal phalanges of fingers 2 – 5.

Innervation: radial portion by the anterior [antebrachial] interosseous nerve of the median nerve, ulnar portion by the ulnar nerve.

The muscle belly to the index finger is supplied only by the median nerve. The remaining muscle bellies can be doubly innervated in exceptional cases.

The **flexor pollicis longus** (Figs. **95b** and **96**) is a part of the flexor digitorum profundus that has become phylogenetically independent. Its field of origin extends on the anterior surface of the radius from the radial tuberosity to the proximal margin of the pronator quadratus and can be expanded onto the interosseous membrane. Its tendon courses through the carpal canal (Fig. **102**), lies embedded between the two heads of the flexor pollicis brevis at the thumb (Fig. **106**), and is attached at the base of the terminal segment of the thumb (Fig. **104**).

Innervation: anterior [antebrachial] interosseous nerve of the median nerve.

The **pronator quadratus** (Fig. **95b**) connects the anterior surfaces of the ulna and radius in their distal fourth, whereby the field of origin at the ulna touches on the medial surface somewhat around the anterior margin.

Innervation: anterior [antebrachial] interosseous nerve of the median nerve.

b) Neurovascular Routes in the Forearm

Radial Route

The *superficial ramus of the radial nerve* (lateral), the *radial artery* with 2 *accompanying veins* and the *deep lymphatic vessels* course in the radial route (Figs. **92** and **96**) – covered by the muscle belly of the brachioradialis.

The **superficial ramus of the radial nerve** leaves the radial route in the middle of the forearm. It turns under the tendon of the brachioradialis on the extensor side, passes through the antebrachial fascia into the subcutaneous connective tissue, and innervates the skin of the back of the hand, as well as that of $2\frac{1}{2}$ radial fingers (at the 2nd and 3rd fingers only up to the middle phalanx).

The **radial artery** follows the conducting muscle on a line from the middle of the elbow to the base of the styloid process of the radius and from there travels on the dorsal side of the wrist (Figs. **102** and **107**). In the distal half of the forearm it is covered only by the fascia medial to the tendon of the brachioradialis so that the pulse can be felt at this point particularly well. The artery gives off only small branches in the forearm.

At the termination of the radial route, it dispatches the *palmar carpal branch* to the palmar network of the wrist, a fine vascular plexus on the palmar side of the wrist.

Ulnar Route

The conducting muscle of the ulnar route (Figs. **92**, **96** and **107**) is the flexor carpi ulnaris, which the **ulnar nerve** follows for the entire distance of the forearm until it arrives at the flexor retinaculum on the radial side of the pisiform bone and divides into the *deep ramus* (for lumbricals III, IV, the palmar and dorsal interossei, the adductor pollicis, the deep head of the flexor pollicis brevis, the muscles of the hypothenar eminence) and the *superficial ramus* (for the palmaris brevis and the skin over $1\frac{1}{2}$ ulnar fingers).

The *ulnar nerve* in the forearm gives off (proximally) *muscular branches* to the flexor carpi ulnaris and to the ulnar portion of the deep flexors of the fingers. It then dispatches (at about the middle) the *dorsal ramus* to the skin of the back of the hand and the dorsal side of $2\frac{1}{2}$ ulnar fingers, as well as (at a variable level) the *palmar ramus* to the skin of the hypothenar eminence.

The dorsal ramus of the ulnar nerve passes beneath the tendon of the flexor carpi ulnaris and around the ulna on the extensor side; it is therefore vulnerable in fractures at the distal third of the ulna.

The **ulnar artery**, with companion veins and deep lymphatic vessels, comes from the cubital fossa, joins the nerve in the middle of the forearm on the radial side, and courses with it to the wrist – covered by the muscle belly and tendon of the flexor carpi ulnaris (Figs. **96** and **107**). Only for a short distance proximal to the pisiform bone does the artery appear from beneath the tendon on the radial side and lies here on the underside of the reinforced antebrachial fascia.

At the distal margin of the pronator quadratus, the *palmar carpal branch* passes to the palmar network of the wrist, while the *dorsal carpal branch* runs under the tendon of the flexor carpi ulnaris to the back of the hand (Fig. **107**).

Forearm Middle Route

In the forearm middle route (Figs. **92** and **96**), the **median nerve** begins between the humeral and ulnar heads of the pronator teres and passes distally between the superficial and deep flexors. It is embedded in the connective tissue at the undersurface of the flexor digitorum superficialis and is accompanied proximally by the *companion artery of the median nerve*, distally by a thin branch of the *anterior interosseous artery*. Near the wrist joint the nerve lies close to the surface (Figs. **102** and **107**), firmly under the strengthened antebrachial fascia. It usually passes between the tendons of the flexor carpi radialis and palmaris longus, or occasionally on the ulnar side of the palmaris tendon, to the carpal canal.

Owing to its superficial position proximal to the wrist joint, the nerve is very exposed to injury e.g. through cuts.

At the forearm the *median nerve* dispatches *muscular rami* to the superficial flexors (except the flexor carpi ulnaris at the level of, or distal to, the pronator teres), the *anterior [antebrachial] interosseous nerve* to the deep flexors in the palmar inerosseous route, and (in the distal third) the *palmar ramus* to the skin of the thenar eminence and the lateral palm of the hand.

Palmar Interosseous Route

In this neurovascular route the *anterior [antebrachial] interosseous nerve* (from the median), the *anterior interosseous vessels*, and the deep lymphatic vessels course distally on the ventral surface of the interosseous membrane, in the depth between the flexor pollicis longus and the flexor digitorum profundus (Figs. **92** and **96**).

The **anterior [antebrachial] interosseous nerve** innervates the flexor pollicis longus, the flexor digitorum profundus and, with its terminal branch, the pronator quadratus.

The **anterior interosseous artery** (from the common interosseous artery) supplies the deep flexors with muscular branches and reaches the palmar carpal network with weak terminal branches. A stronger branch perforates the interosseous membrane at the upper margin of the pronator quadratus and passes to the dorsal carpal network.

Dorsal Forearm Route

In the connective tissue layer the *deep ramus of the radial nerve* and the *posterior interosseous vessels* (accompanied by deep lymphatic vessels) course between the superficial and deep extensors without forming a uniform neurovascular bundle (Figs. **92** and **96**).

The **deep ramus of the radial nerve**, which winds around the proximal end of the radius in the supinator, innervates all extensors *per se* of the forearm. Its terminal branch, the *posterior [antebrachial] interosseous nerve*, gives off branches for the extensor pollicis longus and extensor indicis. It passes to the capsule of the wrist joint on the dorsal side of the interosseous membrane.

The **posterior interosseous artery** (from the common interosseous artery) passes into the extensor compartment at the superior margin of the interosseous membrane, distal to the oblique cord, and ramifies at the extensors. It communicates with the dorsal carpal network.

2. Distal Radio-ulnar Joint and Wrist Joint

a) Distal Radio-ulnar Joint

In the **distal radio-ulnar articulation** (Fig. **99**), the radius with its ulnar notch moves around the articular circumference of the ulna, thereby moving also the hand (*turning movements* of the hand). In the supination position the two forearm bones are parallel to each other; in the pronation position they are crossed (Fig. **97**). Proximal and distal radio-ulnar

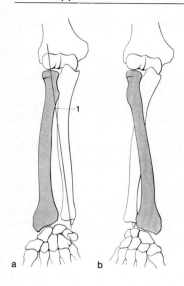

Fig. 97. **Turning movements of right hand**
Forearm bones in supine position (supination)
(a) and in prone position (pronation) (b)
1 Axis of rotary movements of hand

joints always act in tandem to execute pronation or supination movements. They represent two spatially separated divisions of a functionally uniform articulation.

The triangular *articular disc* (Figs. **89** and **99**) that separates the ulna from the carpal bones is attached to the radius with its broad base, to the styloid process of the ulna with its apex. It rotates against the cartilage-covered distal surface of the head of the ulna during pronation and supination.

The fibrocartilage plate is thicker at the margin than in the center, where it can be perforated – especially in older people.

The *joint capsule* is flaccid and wide and is evaginated proximally to form the *recessus sacciformis*. Distally, it is attached to the articular disc so that the joint cavity resembles an L in longitudinal section.

Luxations of the distal radio-ulnar joint usually appear in connection with a classic fracture of the radius. The fracture line runs transversely through the distal end of the radius, sloping somewhat distally toward the ulna, and lies outside of the joint capsule. In epiphysial fractures (separation of the epiphysis), the joint can be affected. Since the synovial membrane in the region of the recessus sacciformis lies only loosely, it can be detached from the joint capsule without the joint cavity being opened.

b) Action of Muscles and Muscle Groups on the Radio-ulnar Joint

In the *extended* elbow joint, the torque of all pronators is distinctly greater than that of the supinators since the force of the inner rotators of the shoulder joint, which here cooperate, clearly exceeds that of the outer rotators. In the *flexed* forearm the strength of the supinators predominates since the torque of the biceps brachii for supination increases in the elbow joint during flexion. For right-handed people, tools for drilling or screwing are so fashioned that they utilize supination movements (e.g. corkscrew).

In the radio-ulnar joint the following muscles:

– *supinate*: biceps brachii and supinator,
    whereby the abductor pollicis longus and the extensor pollicis longus can assist slightly, as well as the brachioradialis when the arm is extended and in pronation position;

– *pronate*: pronator teres, pronator quadratus and flexor carpi radialis,
    whereby the brachioradialis (with increasing flexion of the elbow joint from the supine position) and extensor carpi radialis longus (when the forearm is flexed and extremely supinated) can support the movement slightly.

The *supinator* can supinate, in contrast to the *biceps brachii*, in each position of the elbow joint, and its torque remains constant. Like the biceps tendon, it is unwound from the radius in supination, while the pronator teres is wound around the anterior surface of the radius. When the arm is flexed at a right angle, its torque amounts to about a fourth; when the arm is extended, it amounts to half of the torque of the biceps, which decreases with increasing extension at the elbow joint.

The *pronator teres* is a powerful pronator in the flexed arm. When extension of the elbow joint is increased, its pronation action is less. Independent of the position of the elbow joint, the *pronator quadratus* can pronate the supinated forearm,whereby it is somewhat unwound from the ulna. It brings the joint surfaces of the radius and ulna closer together and secures the articular contact at the distal radio-ulnar joint.

The *brachioradialis* is, first of all, a flexor muscle of the elbow joint. In the weakly flexed arm, it can supinate slightly; in the forearm flexed at a right angle, it can supinate only about 20° from the maximal pronation position. Its ability to pronate the supinated arm is much greater and increases with the degree of flexion at the elbow joint.

When both forearm bones are fractured proximal to the insertion of the pronator teres, the proximal fragments are supinated (supinator, biceps brachii). If the site of the fracture is in the middle of the shaft, they are in the mid-position.

A **paralysis** of the individual *supinators* or *pronators* is barely evident in the extended arm since the external and internal rotators of the upper arm turn around the same axis. In the flexed elbow joint, supination is still possible in

the case of a radial paralysis with the help of the biceps brachii (musculocutaneous) or with the help of the supinator muscle in the case of a biceps paralysis.
In a paralysis of the median nerve, pronation is still weakly possible when there
is a double innervation of the pronator teres by the musculocutaneous nerve;
otherwise, the flexed forearm can be pronated only up to the mid-position.

c) Skeletal Elements of the Wrist and Middle of the Hand

In the **hand,** three segments can be distinguished in a sequence from
proximal to distal: *wrist (carpus), metacarpus* and *fingers (digits).* The
skeletal elements comprising these segments are: the *wrist bones (carpals),*
the *metacarpals* and the *finger bones (phalanges*: two in the thumb, three
in the other fingers, Fig. **98**). The *ventral surface of the hand* is termed the
palm, the *dorsal surface,* the *dorsum.* The lateral margin represents the
radial or thumb margin; the medial margin is either the ulnar or little
finger margin.

Topographically, the hand is marked off proximally by a line which connects the
base of the styloid process of the radius with the apex of the styloid process of the
ulna. It corresponds approximately to the distal flexion crease of the palm (which,
of course, extends partly into the region of the wrist, Fig. **98 a**). The distal
boundary of the hand is marked on the palmar side by the interdigital folds, at the
back of the hand by the heads of the metacarpals ("knuckles").

The **carpal bones** are arranged in two rows (Figs. **98** and **99**). The *proximal*
row consists of three bones: *scaphoid* (on the radial side), *lunate* (in the
middle) and *triquetrum* (on the ulnar side). The *pisiform* is inserted as a
small sesamoid in the tendon of the flexor carpi ulnaris. It lies on the
triquetrum.

The *distal* series of carpals contain four skeletal elements, which are from
radial to ulnar: *trapezium, trapezoid, capitate* and *hamate.*

The cartilage-covered proximal surfaces of the first carpal row form an
ovoid joint head for articulation with the radius and the articular disc.
The distal contour of the proximal series of bones resembles a wavy line
which, on the radial and ulnar sides, exhibits a wavy crest formed by the
scaphoid and triquetrum. In the troughs of the waves the capitate and the
pointed proximal end of the hamate are inserted distally.

Distally, the trapezium possesses a saddle-shaped articular surface for metacarpal
I and a small cartilage-covered area for metacarpal II, the groove-shaped base of
which articulates mainly with the trapezoid. The capitate bears metacarpal III; the
hamate exhibits distally a subdivided articular surface for metacarpals IV and V.

The surfaces of the carpal bones of each row facing each other are covered with
cartilage just like their proximal and distal surfaces and articulate with one
another: intercarpal joints.

The carpal bones do not lie in a horizontal plane. The trapezium is clearly
angled off (about 70°) toward the palmar surface. The smooth, contoured

dorsal surface of both rows of carpals is curved convexly in a transverse direction, giving rise on the palmar side to a longitudinal carpal groove (*sulcus carpi*). The radial margin of this groove is formed by the *tubercles* of the *scaphoid* and of the *trapezium*, both of which are palpable through the skin. The *pisiform*, which can also be palpated beneath the skin, and the hook of the hamate (*hamulus*) project on the ulnar side. The protuberances of both sides (*carpal eminences*) are united by a transverse band, the *flexor retinaculum* (Figs. **102**, **106** and **107**), which closes the groove, thus converting it into a *carpal canal* for the passage of the tendons of the flexors of the fingers.

The 5 **metacarpals** (Figs. **98** and **99**) are typical small tubular bones. The body (*corpus*) corresponds to the shaft; the proximal end is designated as the *base*, the distal end as the *head*.

Proximally, the *base* has a joint surface (of varying shape in the individual metacarpals) for articulation with the distal carpal bones. In metacarpals 2 – 5, it is continued on the lateral surfaces of the base facing each other. In metacarpal 1, the carpal articular surface is saddle-shaped. On the dorsal, radial side, the base of metacarpal 3 becomes a *styloid process*, at which the extensor carpi radialis brevis is attached.

The *body* resembles a prism. The palmar margin has a slightly concave form in the longitudinal direction, whereas the dorsal surface is weakly convex.

The *head* is spherical in shape, somewhat broader on the palmar side than on the dorsal, and articulates with the proximal phalanx. On each side there is a small pit for attachment of the collateral ligament.

The *metacarpus* is curved transversely and is narrower proximally than distally since the metacarpal bones diverge somewhat on the distal side. Metacarpal 1 is the shortest and strongest, metacarpal 2 the longest of these bones.

Radiograms of the carpal bones provide various diagnostic information. From the time at which ossific centers appear, for example, conclusions can be drawn about the degree of skeletal development at a given age. Occasionally, accessory carpal bones appear, which can be confused in the radiogram with bone chips.

The **ossification** of the *carpal bones* (Fig. **78**) begins only after birth. Whereas the ossific nuclei in the hamate (0 – 7th month) and capitate (1st – 6th month) appear relatively early within a definite time span, the remaining carpal bones (in their sequence: triquetrum, lunate, trapezium, trapezoid, scaphoid, pisiform) usually ossify much later and at widely varying times (the pisiform, for example, between the 8th and 12th year).

In the *metacarpals*, diaphysial ossification begins at the end of the 2nd embryonic month. An epiphysial center of ossification appears in metacarpal 1 in the *proximal* epiphysis and in the remaining metacarpals in the *distal* epiphyses between the 2nd and 4th year of life. The epiphysial joints disappear between the 15th and 20th year.

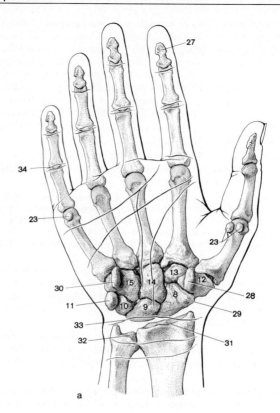

Fig. 98a

Additional epiphysial centers (pseudo-epiphyses) can appear in isolated cases even in normally-developed children at metacarpal 1 (distal), 2 and 5 (proximal), which fuse relatively soon with the diaphysis (by the 6th year).

d) Capsules and Ligamentous Apparatus of the Joints of the Hand

Joints of the hand (in the broader sense) are those joints in the carpal region which act together in the movements of the hand. They are:
– the *proximal joint of the hand* (*radiocarpal articulation*).
– the *distal joint of the hand* (*midcarpal articulation*),

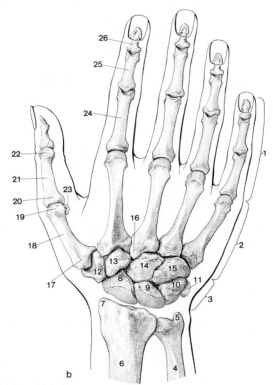

Fig. 98. Skeleton of hand
a Palmar view, relative positions of flexure lines of palm
b Dorsal view

 1 Bones of the digits (phalanges)
 2 Metacarpal bones
 3 Carpal bones
 4 Ulna
 5 Styloid process of ulna
 6 Radius
 7 Styloid process of radius
 8 Scaphoid
 9 Lunate
10 Triquetrum
11 Pisiform
12 Trapezium
13 Trapezoid
14 Capitate
15 Hamate
16 Styloid process of third metacarpal
17 Base of metacarpal bone
18 Body of metacarpal bone

19 Head of metacarpal bone
20 Base of phalanx
21 Body of phalanx
22 Head of phalanx
23 Sesamoid bone
24 Proximal phalanx
25 Middle phalanx
26 Distal phalanx
27 Tuberosity of distal phalanx
28 Tubercle of trapezium
29 Tubercle of scaphoid
30 Hook of hamate
31 Carpal articular surface of radius
32 Articular circumference of ulnar head
33 Distal flexure crease proximal to palm
   of hand (rasceta)
34 Flexure crease at proximal interphalangeal
   joint of finger

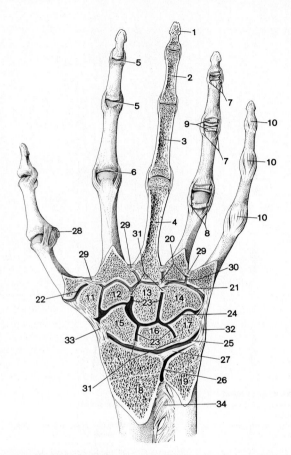

Fig. 99. **Coronal section of hand: joints of hand and fingers** dorsal view (showing collateral ligaments at joints of thumb and index finger, joint capsules and collateral ligaments at the fifth finger, joint capsules at fourth finger cut open and retracted)

■ Articular cavity of distal radio-ulnar joint
☐ Articular cavity of radiocarpal joint
▓ Articular cavities of midcarpal and intercarpal joints
☐ Articular cavities of carpometacarpal and intermetacarpal joints
☐ Articular cavity of carpometacarpal joint of thumb

1 Distal phalanx
2 Middle phalanx
3 Proximal phalanx
4 Metacarpal III
5 Interphalangeal joints II
6 Metacarpophalangeal joint II
7 Collateral ligaments of distal and middle
  joints of fourth finger
8 Collateral ligaments of metacarpophalangeal
  joint of fourth finger

- the articular connections between the proximal and distal carpal bones (the *intercarpal articulations*),
- the carpometacarpal joints (the *carpometacarpal articulations*), and
- the joints between the bases of the metacarpal bones (the *intermetacarpal articulations 2–5*).

Proximal Joint of the Hand

In the *radiocarpal articulation* (Fig. **99**), the joint cavity is formed by the articular carpal surface of the radius and the triangular surface of the articular disc lying distal to the head of the ulna. The cartilage-covered surfaces of the three proximal carpal bones (scaphoid, lunate, triquetrum) and the interosseous ligaments connecting them form the ovoid articular head, which is considerably larger.

The *joint capsule* is attached at the cartilage border of the articulating bones and at the disc. In principle, the articular cavity is closed on all sides, yet in almost 40% of the cases a communication exists with the pisiform joint.

Frequently (about 25%), the proximal joint of the hand is in communication with the distal radio-ulnar joint (by a slit at the basal attachment of the articular disc at the radius), more rarely with the distal hand joint (by gaps between the lunate and scaphoid or triquetrum).

These connections of joint cavities are not important for the mechanics of movement, but they do permit a rapid spread of inflammation.

On the basis of the shape of its articular surface, the proximal joint of the hand is a pure *ovoid joint*. It permits flexion (palmar flexion) or extension (dorsal flexion) of the hand (around the large transverse axis) and radial or ulnar abduction (around the small, dorsopalmar-directed joint axis). In a dorsally-flexed hand, the most proximally-situated, transverse skin crease, which arises at the wrist, indicates the location of the joint line.

◀ 9 Articular capsule, cut open and retracted
10 Articular capsule of metacarpophalangeal joint
11 Trapezium
12 Trapezoid
13 Capitate
14 Hamate
15 Scaphoid
16 Lunate
17 Triquetrum
18 Radius
19 Ulna
20 Intermetacarpal joints
21 Carpometacarpal joints

22 Carpometacarpal joint
23 Intercarpal joint
24 Midcarpal joint
25 Radiocarpal joint
26 Distal radio-ulnar joint
27 Articular disc
28 Ulnar sesamoid at metacarpophalangeal joint of thumb
29 Metacarpal interosseous ligaments
30 Metacarpophalangeal interosseous ligament
31 Intercarpal interosseous ligaments
32 Ulnar collateral ligament
33 Radial collateral ligament
34 Antebrachial interosseous membrane

Distal Joint of the Hand

The *midcarpal articulation* (Fig. **99**) possesses a complex undulating articular space (→ p. 254), which is bordered by the distal surfaces of the proximal carpals and the proximal surfaces of the distal carpal bones.

The *capsule* of the midcarpal joint is tense on the palmar side, flaccid on the dorsal. It is attached in each case at the border of the cartilage-covered surfaces. The multi-recessed joint cavities communicate with the articular cavities of the inter-carpal joints.

Articular Connections within the Carpal Rows

The articular connection of the carpal bones within a row occurs in the *intercarpal articulations* (Fig. **99**). In the *proximal* row, the carpals are fixed by tense *interosseous intercarpal ligaments*, but not held immovably. These ligaments form the proximal border of the articular cavity of the intercarpal joints, which are continued distally into the joint cavities of the midcarpal joint. The *distal* carpals are firmly fixed to one another by interosseous ligaments and can be displaced only insignificantly in respect to each other. Of course, the interosseous intercarpal ligaments do not completely close off the joint cavity, so that the intercarpal joints of the distal row communicate proximally with the midcarpal joint and distally with carpometacarpal joints 2 – 5. Only between the capitate and hamate can the interosseous ligament be so strong that it completely closes the joint cavity distally.

The **pisiform joint** forms the articular connection between the pisiform and the triquetrum.

The pisiform is inserted as a sesamoid bone in the tendon of the flexor carpi ulnaris which is continued distally to the hamate bone as the pisohamate ligament and to the base of metacarpals 4 and 5 as the pisometacarpal ligament. The articular surface of the pisiform is weakly concave, the ovoid joint surface of the triquetrum slightly curved. The flaccid capsule permits extensive displacements of the pisiform.

Carpometacarpal joints

The *carpometacarpal joint of the thumb* (Fig. **99**) is an independent joint. On the basis of the shape of the joint surfaces of the trapezium and metacarpal 1, it is a pure saddle joint. The wide, flaccid capsule and the cartilage covering of the joint surface, which is up to 1 mm thick and slightly deformable, passively allow a turning, however, and with the opposition of the thumb a slight rotation of metacarpal 1 is also combined. A voluntary rotation is not possible since the necessary muscles are absent.

Carpometacarpal articulations 2 – 5 (Fig. **99**) are rigid amphiarthroses without noteworthy mobility. The joint cavity is usually uniform for all joints, but can be subdivided by an especially strong *carpometacarpal interosseous ligament*, which passes from the capitate to the base of metacarpals 3 and 4. Proximally, it communicates with the intercarpal joints, distally it continues into the short joint cavity of the three intermetacarpal joints (between the bases of metacarpals 2 – 5).

Ligaments of the Joints of the Hand

Ligaments (Figs. **100** and **101**) enclose the carpus like a rather closed collar and influence to a high degree the mechanics of the hand joints. The fiber tracts are not sharply defined and can be represented individually only in diagrams. The ligaments of the proximal joints of the hand usually also pass over the midcarpal joint and are closely allied with the ligaments of the intercarpal and carpometacarpal joints. The ligaments emanating from the radius are stronger than the ligamentous tracts on the ulnar side, just as the palmar ligaments are stronger than the dorsal.

The *palmar radiocarpal ligament* courses obliquely toward the ulna from the styloid process and the adjacent distal margin of the radius. Its strong bundles of fibers, which are arranged like a fan, attach at the lunate, triquetrum and capitate. A deep ligamentous tract courses to the scaphoid. The weaker *dorsal radiocarpal ligament* passes from the radius primarily to the triquetrum and capitate. Both ligaments course with the greater part of their fibers proximal to the axis of abduction (middle of the capitate). They are, therefore, stretched during radial abduction.

The weak *palmar ulnocarpal ligament* radiates from the styloid process of the ulna and from the distal margin of the head of the ulna to the lunate, triquetrum and capitate. It is stretched during abduction of the ulna. Together with the palmar radiocarpal ligament, its fibers form a bow-shaped ligamentous band, which embraces the heads of the capitate and lunate and restricts dorsal flexion in the proximal hand joint. The palmar ligaments are stretched during supination, and the dorsal fiber tracts during pronation.

The short, strong *radial collateral carpal ligament* (from the styloid process of the radius to the scaphoid) is stretched during ulnar abduction, the weak *ulnar collateral carpal ligament* (from the styloid process of the ulna to the triquetrum and pisiform) during radial abduction (of the hand).

The long fiber tracts of the *palmar intercarpal ligaments*, which radiate out from the capitate and unite it with the adjacent carpals (except for the lunate), are called the *radiate ligament of the wrist*.

The superficial, long *dorsal* bundles of fibers (*dorsal intercarpal ligaments*) form an arched band coursing from the scaphoid to the triquetrum, which covers the joint heads of the distal carpal row formed by the capitate and hamate and prevents their bulging during palmar flexion. The short-fibered *palmar* and *dorsal intercarpal ligaments* and the *interosseous intercarpal ligaments* bridge over the joint cavity between two adjacent carpal bones of a row, on the palmar side also between the proximal and distal rows of bones. They convert the carpal bones into a solid structure which only permits displacements of the carpal bones (and then chiefly of the proximal row) along the lateral surfaces.

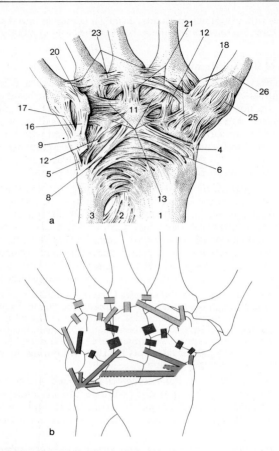

Fig. 100. **Ligaments of wrist joint**, palmar view
a Ligaments in dissected preparation
b Scheme of ligaments
Color code for Figs. 100 and 101
▨ Ligaments between bones of forearm and wrist
▨ Ligaments between bones of wrist
▨ Ligaments between bones of wrist and metacarpals
▨ Ligaments between metacarpals

1 Radius
2 Antebrachial interosseous membrane
3 Ulna
4 Radial collateral ligament
5 Ulnar collateral ligament
6 Palmar radiocarpal ligament

7 Dorsal radiocarpal ligament
8 Palmar ulnocarpal ligament
9 Pisiform
10 Triquetrum
11 Capitate
12 Palmar intercarpal ligaments

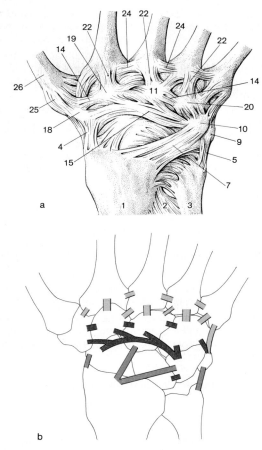

Fig. 101. **Ligaments of wrist joint,** dorsal view
a Ligaments in dissected preparation
b Scheme of ligaments

13 Radiate ligament of wrist
14 Short bands of dorsal intercarpal ligaments
15 Arched ligament formed by superficial long
   bands of dorsal intercarpal ligaments
16 Pisohamate ligament
17 Pisometacarpal ligament
18 Trapezium
19 Trapezoid

20 Hamate
21 Palmar carpometacarpal ligaments
22 Dorsal carpometacarpal ligaments
23 Palmar metacarpal ligaments
24 Dorsal metacarpal ligaments
25 Articular capsule of carpometacarpal
   joint of thumb
26 First metacarpal

By means of the *palmar, dorsal* and *interosseous carpometacarpal ligaments*, as well as the *palmar, dorsal* and *interosseous metacarpal ligaments*, carpometacarpal joints 2–5 are strengthened into rigid amphiarthroses.

The *deep transverse metacarpal ligament* unites the heads of the metacarpals (on the palmar side), the palmar ligaments and the fibrous sheaths of the flexor tendons with one another. It renders a separation of the metacarpals impossible.

The *innervation of the joint capsule* of the hand joints takes place on the palmar side by branches from the ulnar and median nerves, on the dorsal side by the dorsal ramus of the ulnar nerve and branches of the radial nerve (posterior antebrachial cutaneous, posterior [antebrachial] interosseous nerves), whereas branches of the lateral antebrachial cutaneous nerve and the supeficial ramus of the radial nerve are ramified on the radial side of the hand joints both on the dorsal and on the palmar sides.

The capsule of the 1st carpometacarpal joint is innervated by branches of the median (palmar), lateral antebrachial cutaneous and radial (dorsal) nerves.

The *relaxation position* of the joints of the hand is the "normal posture" of the hand, that is, when the hand joints are extended and the longitudinal axes of the forearm, capitate and the third finger lie in a straight line. The joints of the hand are also stiffened in this position or in slight dorsal flexion if necessary. A long-term immobilization of the joints of the hand should be carried out in a middle dorsal flexion. Since the palmar flexing muslces are more powerful than the extensors, they could otherwise gradually bring about or strengthen a palmar flexion that does not permit a strong closure of the fist.

Among the *fractures* of the carpal bones, those of the scaphoid are critical (e.g. falling on the outstretched hand, recoiling of a crank against the palm) since this bone sometimes heals slowly (danger of pseduo-arthrosis).

Movement Possibilities in the Joints of the Hand

Movements which can be actively carried out are:
– *palmar* or *dorsal flexion* (in each case close to 90°) around transverse axes, and
– *radial* or *ulnar abduction* (altogether close to 60°) around a sagittal axis.

Movements around sagittal and transverse axes can be combined, whereby the extent of possible flexion is not diminished by a simultaneous abduction.

Palmar flexion occurs predominantly in the proximal wrist joint (the articular socket of the radius faces toward the palm), dorsiflexion for the most part in the distal wrist joint (the palmar check ligaments are stronger in the proximal wrist joint than in the distal). The transverse axis of flexion courses through the lunate in the proximal carpal joint and through the capitate in the distal joint. The dorsopalmar-directed abduction axis goes through the middle of the capitate.

From the normal position, in which the hand is already abducted radially about 12° to the forearm, the hand can be abducted around 40° toward the ulnar side and about 15° toward the radial. Ulnar and radial abduction, therefore, are possible to a rather equal extent (close to 30°) from the standard position.

In abduction, the body of the joint formed by the proximal row of carpal bones is rotated around the axis of abduction, and the distal row of carpals is moved in the opposite direction toward the ulnar or radial sides. In ulnar abduction the wrist is compressed and shortened on the ulnar side, whereas in radial abduction this occurs on the radial side.

In ulnar abduction, the triquetrum can be brought so close to the pliable articular disc that sufficient space is freed for the distal row of carpals (especially the hamate) to be pushed toward the ulnar side. In radial abduction, a shortening at the radial margin of the wrist is only possible when the scaphoid is tipped toward the palm. It can then be distinctly palpated through the skin on the palmar side. The trapezium glides proximally on the dorsal side of the scaphoid.

Slight inevitable rotations occur in the radiocarpal joint during intermediate movements (combinations of flexion and abduction movements). Passive rotations are possible to a limited extent but cannot be voluntarily carried out since there is no innervation pattern for these movements.

There are **movement possibilities in the carpometacarpal joint 1** for:
– *abduction* or *adduction* of the thumb (35–40°) around an *oblique* axis coursing from dorsal and radial to palmar and ulnar, and
– *flexion* or *extension* of the thumb (altogether 60°) around a likewise *oblique* axis (perpendicular to the abduction axis) coursing from palmar and radial to dorsal and ulnar.

Opposition is the forceps-like grasping movement in which the thumb is placed opposite the flexed index or middle finger, for example, and is brought into contact with them (e.g. holding a needle). Depending on the execution, this mixed movement can be considered as a combination of abduction, flexion, adduction and slight inevitable inner rotation of the thumb. The opposite movement, *reposition*, returns the thumb to its normal position.

Flexion and opposition, as well as extension and reposition are used by many authors as synonyms.

e) Action of Muscles and Muscle Groups on the Wrist Joint

Palmar or dorsal flexion can be carried out in the wrist joint with considerably more power than radial or ulnar abduction. The torque of the palmar flexing muscles is more than twice as great as that of the dorsal flexors (extensors). Each of the long flexors of the fingers has a greater torque than both marginal flexors together. The effect of the long flexors of the fingers on the wrist joint is the stronger, the more the fingers are extended. The more the fingers are flexed, the higher the tendon strength of the extensor digitorum for the dorsal flexion of the hand.

In the *wrist joint*, the hand:

- *palmar flexes* by means of the flexor digitorum superficialis, flexor digitorum profundus, flexor carpi ulnaris, flexor carpi radialis (relatively slight) and the flexor pollicis longus,

  whereas the flexing action of the abductor pollicis longus is insignificant and that of the palmaris longus is variable;

- *dorsiflexes* by means of the extensor digitorum, extensor carpi ulnaris, extensor carpi radialis longus and brevis,

  whereby the extensor indicis and extensor pollicis longus support these movements;

- *abducts radiad*, especially by the extensor carpi radialis longus, whose torque is as great as that of the remaining radiad abductors together: extensor carpi radialis brevis, abductor and extensor pollicis longus, extensor indicis and flexor carpi radialis; and

- *abducts ulnad* by means of the extensor and flexor carpi ulnaris.

Mixed movements can be carried out in the wrist joint by a combination of muscle action.

The muscles of the forearm, which attach at the 1st metacarpal bone (abductor pollicis longus), at the proximal phalanx of the thumb (extensor pollicis brevis), or at the distal phalanx (extensor or flexor pollicis longus), do not act alone at the *1st carpometacarpal joint*. Movements in the "saddle joint of the thumb" are decisively fashioned by means of the muscles of the thenar eminence and the 1st dorsal interosseus (origin at metacarpal 1). The action of all of these muscles, therefore, shall be discussed later (→ p. 278).

In a **paralysis** of the *median nerve*, palmar flexion is only weakly possible (by the ulnar part of the flexor digitorum profundus and the flexor carpi ulnaris); in radial abduction, the hand is then simultaneously dorsiflexed. Likewise, in a *paralysis of the ulnar nerve*, the hand can be palmar flexed and abducted toward the ulnar side only with reduced strength. In a *paralysis of the radial nerve* proximal to its division into superficial and deep rami, the hand hangs down in the flexed position (*wrist-drop*). If the injury involves only the deep branch of the radial nerve, the hand can still be extended straight, but deviates toward the radial side (extensor carpi radialis longus).

f) Carpal Canal and Palmar Tendon Sheaths

Through the *carpal canal* bordered by the carpal bones and the flexor retinaculum, the median nerve and the tendons of the superficial and deep flexors of the fingers pass into the middle chamber (chamber of the flexors of the fingers) of the palm. Likewise covered by the flexor retinaculum, but separated from the true carpal canal by a connective tissue septum, the tendon of the flexor carpi radialis courses to the base of the 2nd metacarpal in a short, radially-situated canal. The carpal canal unites the forearm with the deep palmar region and facilitates the spread of inflammations, blood clots, etc. between the two regions.

In the narrow canal, designated by surgeons also as the carpal tunnel, the median nerve can be injured by compression from various sources, which results in sensibility disturbances, later also in motor deficiencies of the thenar muscles innervated by the median nerve: *carpal tunnel syndrome*.

Carpal tendon sheaths (Fig. **102**). In the region of the wrist, the tendons of the flexor carpi radialis, of the long flexors of the thumb and of the flexors of the fingers are each enveloped in *tendon sheaths*. The short *synovial sheath of the flexor carpi radialis* passes outside of the true carpal canal up to the base of the 2nd metacarpal. The narrow *synovial sheath of the flexor pollicis longus* lies on the radial side of the carpal canal, and the broad *common synovial sheath of the flexor muscles* on the ulnar side. Both synovial sacs extend proximally somewhat beyond the radiocarpal joint.

The tendon sheath of the flexor pollicis longus ends distally at the base of the distal phalanx of the thumb. The carpal and digital part of this sheath consequently form a unit. Likewise, the digital tendon sheath of the flexor tendon to the 5th finger (generally) communicates with the common carpal sheath. On the tendons to the 2nd – 4th fingers, however, the sheaths terminate at the level of the bases of the metacarpal bones.

Digital tendon sheaths (Fig. **15** and **102**) enclose the tendons of both long flexors with a double covering on the palmar surface. The *fibrous sheaths* determine the course direction of the tendons on the bones; the *synovial sheaths* facilitate the undisturbed gliding of the tendons within the ligamentous covering.

Together with the palmar surfaces of the phalanges in each finger, the fibrous sheaths of the digits of the hand form an osteofibrous canal, which possesses a well-developed connective tissue wall in the region of the body of the phalanx, whereas it is thin-walled in the vicinity of the joints. The oblique fiber tracts of the fibrous sheath are designated as the *cruciform part of the fibrous sheath*, and the slender, transverse fibrous rings as the *anular part*.

The synovial tendon sheaths of fingers 2 – 4 extend from the heads of the middle phalanges up to the heads of the metacarpals. External and internal layers are connected by tendinous connective tissue mesotendons (*vincula*) proximal to the insertion of the tendons (Fig. **103**).

In the case of an inflammation of the tendon sheaths of the thumb or the little finger, the process can be spread proximally into the carpal segment of the tendon sheath. The pathogens can pass through the thin septum between the two synovial sacs and wander distally into the tendon sheath of the tendons of the little finger or the sheaths of the flexor pollicis longus. Finally, the typical symptoms of the V-shaped phlegmon can develop.

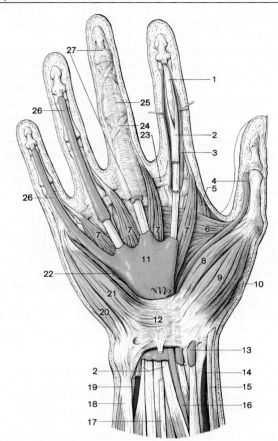

Fig. 102. **Carpal and digital tendon sheaths of flexors of fingers**

1 Tendon of flexor digitorum profundus
2 Tendon(s) of flexor digitorum superficialis
3 Synovial sheath of flexor tendons of index finger, opened
4 Synovial tendon sheath of flexor pollicis longus
5 Dorsal interosseus 1
6 Adductor pollicis
7 Lumbricals 1–4
8 Flexor pollicis brevis
9 Abductor pollicis brevis
10 Opponens pollicis
11 Common synovial sheath of flexor muscles
12 Flexor retinaculum
13 Synovial tendon sheath of flexor carpi radialis
14 Radial artery
15 Tendons of abductor pollicis longus and extensor pollicis brevis
16 Median nerve
17 Tendon of palmaris longus, severed
18 Flexor carpi ulnaris
19 Ulnar artery and nerve, transected
20 Abductor digiti minimi
21 Flexor digiti minimi brevis
22 Opponens digiti minimi
23 Deep transverse metacarpal ligament
24 Cruciate part of fibrous sheath
25 Annular part of fibrous sheath
26 Synovial sheaths of tendons of digits of hand
27 Fibrous sheath of middle finger

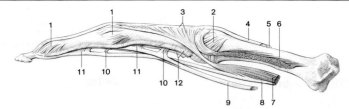

Fig. 103. **Joints of finger, tendons of long flexors of finger, lumbricals and dorsal interossei**, view of index finger from radial side

1 Collateral ligaments of middle and
  distal joints
2 Collateral ligament of proximal
  (metacarpophalangeal) joint
3 Dorsal aponeurosis
4 Tendon of extensor digitorum
5 Tendon of extensor indicis
6 First dorsal interosseus muscle (ulnar head)
7 First lumbrical muscle

8 Tendon of flexor digitorum profundus
  ("perforating flexor")
9 Tendon of flexor digitorum superficialis
  ("perforated flexor")
10, 11 Vincula of tendons
10 Long vinculum
11 Short vinculum
12 Fibrous sheath, opened

The development of tendon sheaths can vary from the pattern previously described. In the newborn, the digital tendon sheaths are still separated from the carpal tendon sheaths. The fusion can be omitted on the little finger side (5%), occasionally also at the tendons of the long flexors of the thumb. In these cases no V-shaped phlegmon can form. Also, the development of the carpal synovial sacs can vary. For example, the radial sac may also enclose the flexor tendons to the 2nd finger, or a third intermediate sac may be present.

3. Hand and Finger

a) Skeletal Elements of the Finger

The **bones of the finger** are short tubular bones. Fingers 2–5 each possesses a *proximal, middle* and *distal segment* (*proximal, middle* and *distal phalanx*, Figs. **98** and **99**). At the *thumb* (*pollex*) only two phalanges are developed.

The proximal end of each phalanx is designated as the *base*, the middle piece as the *body* (*diaphysis*) and the distal end as the *head*. The base of each proximal phalanx contains the articular socket for the head of the corresponding metacarpal. In the proximal and middle phalanges, the head is formed as a trochlea. The ridges of the base of the middle or terminal phalanx glide in the guiding grooves of the trochlea.

The diaphysis of each phalanx is flat on the palmar side (appositional surface for the tendons of the flexors of the fingers) and rounded on the dorsal surface. The head of the terminal phalanx is flattened. The rough surface on the palmar side is the *distal tuberosity*, which gives attachment to the tense connective tissue tracts emanating from the tactile elevations of the fingers.

The **ossification** of the *phalanges* (Fig. **78**) begins in the diaphyses in the 3rd embryonic month (sequence: distal, proximal, middle phalanx). The *proximal* epiphysial centers appear 1 – 3 years after birth. The cartilaginous epiphysial joints disappear between the ages of 20 – 24.

b) Capsules and Ligaments of the Joints of the Fingers

The **proximal joint of the finger** (*metacarpophalangeal joints 2 – 5*) is a ball and socket joint (Fig. **99**).

The articular head formed by the metacarpal bone corresponds to a section from a spherical casing which is broadened on its palmar side and projects out into 2 tubercles, between which the tendon sheath of the flexor of the finger is attached. The moderately concave articular socket at the base of the proximal phalanx has its greatest diameter in the radio-ulnar direction.

The *joint capsule* is wide and flaccid; with a strong pull of the extended finger, the joint socket can be drawn away from the head. In the wall of the capsule on the palmar side the *palmar ligament* is embedded, a fibrocartilaginous plate which enlarges the socket proximally. The lateral ligaments (*collateral ligaments*) originate at the lateral surfaces of the heads of the metacarpal bones, course dorsal to the axis of flexion towards the palm and distally, and are attached laterally at the articular margins of the proximal phalanges (Figs. **99** and **103**).

The **proximal metacarpophalangeal joint of the thumb** is a hinge joint. It corresponds to an interphalangeal joint with regard to the shape of its articular surfaces, the arrangement of the collateral ligaments and the execution of movement.

A radial and an ulnar *sesamoid bone* (Fig. **98 a**) are regularly contained in the capsule of the proximal metacarpophalangeal joint of the thumb on the palmar side – at the level of the head of the metacarpal. At the proximal metacarpophalangeal joint of the little finger, an ulnar sesamoid bone also develops frequently (over 80%). Likewise, radial or ulnar sesamoids can be present at the remaining proximal joints of the fingers.

The **middle** and **distal joints of the fingers** (interphalangeal joints, including the thumb articulations) are purely hinge joints (Fig. **99**).

A firm fibrous plate, the *palmar ligament*, which completes the socket proximally, is also woven into the *capsule* of the middle and terminal joints on the palmar side. The strong *collateral ligaments* ensure the direction of movement (Figs. **99** and **103**). In each joint position a part of its fibers is stretched.

The *innervation* of the metacarpophalangeal joints takes place on the palmar side via branches of the deep ramus of the ulnar nerve and the proper palmar digital nerves and on the dorsal side via branches of the deep ramus of the ulnar nerve and by the dorsal digital nerves. The ulnar branches arrive on the dorsal side between the two heads of origin of the dorsal interossei. The middle and terminal joints are supplied by the corresponding cutaneous nerves.

In joint effusions, the *relaxation position* of the joints of the fingers is a moderate flexion. In this position the joints are also immobilized (prevention of unfavorble contraction in the extended position) and, if necessary, stiffened (functionally the most favorable position for grasping).

Joint effusions are always visible on the dorsal side since the thin dorsal wall of the capsule protrudes outward.

Luxations of the finger segments appear almost exclusively on the dorsal side (from overextension, e.g. in basketball players). Frequently, a dislocation of the proximal phalanx of the thumb is dorsal after a fall on the free hand (close to 5% of all luxations).

Position relationships of finger folds. The flexion folds of the fingers (Fig. **98 a**) lie in the region of metacarpophalangeal joints 2 – 5 distal to the joint cavity; in the region of the distal interphalangeal joints they are proximal to the joint cavity. The proximal flexion folds at the metacarpophalangeal joint of the thumb and the flexion folds at the proximal interphalangeal joints correspond to the joint cavities. On the extensor side when the fingers are flexed, the heads of the metacarpal bones and phalanges jut out in all joints; the joint cavity always lies distal to the knuckles of the fingers.

There are **movement possibilities at the metacarpophalangeal joint of the thumb** for:
– *flexion* (about 70°) or *extension* (up to an extended position or – varying individually – up to a more or less distinct hyperextension) around a "*transverse*" axis.

There are **movement possibilities at the metacarophalangeal joints of fingers 3–5** for:
– *flexion* (about 90°) or *extension* (actively about 20° or more individually) around *transverse* axes, and
– *radial* or *ulnar abduction* (in the extended basal joint) around *dorso-palmar* axes.

The index finger can be abducted from the true axial position about 15° radially and can be carried toward the ulnar side about 45° over the flexed middle finger (in the normal position). The middle finger can be abducted toward the radial and ulnar sides about 20° respectively. Ring and little fingers can be abducted approximately 20° or 25° and adducted so far toward the neighboring finger that they cross somewhat over or under it.

With increasing palmar flexion, the capability to abduct the fingers is restricted more and more and finally ceases. The reason for the inhibition of abduction of the fingers is the tension of the collateral ligaments, for during palmar flexion the origin and insertion points for the ligaments are withdrawn. Moreover, they then pass over the broad palmar segment of the articular head.

At the metacarpophalangeal joint, the extended finger can be rotated passively around its longitudinal axis (up to 50°). A voluntary rotation is not possible since the central nervous system sends no suitable command to the musculature. An unavoidable rotation at this joint of the fingers takes place with mixed movements (combination of pure flexion and pure abduction).

Movement possibilities in the middle and distal joints of the fingers. The *middle phalanges* can be:

– *flexed* (up to about 110°) or *extended* (usually only up to the plane of the dorsum of the hand).

At the *intephalangeal joints of the thumb* and the *fingers*, it is possible to:

– *flex* (up to about 80°) or *extend* (frequently up to an insignificant hyperextension).

c) Organization and Innervation of the Short Muscles of the Hand

The powerful movements of the fingers are carried out by the long forearm muscles. The short muscles which originate in the region of the hand are available for the fine action of the fingers. They are all derivatives of the ventral muscles of the upper limb and thus in the genetic sense are flexors. For the particular tasks of the thumb and the little finger, special muscle groups have developed whose muscle mass forms two eminences on the palmar surface: the *ball of the thumb* (*thenar eminence*) and the *ball of the little finger* (*hypothenar eminence*). The tendons of the long flexors of the fingers and the lumbrical muscles arising at the tendons of the deep flexors are located in a middle compartment between these two groups of muscles. The spaces between the metacarpal bones (*metacarpal interosseous spaces*) are filled up by the interossei muscles.

The muscles of both thenar and hypothenar eminences are enclosed by fasciae which are fixed at metacarpals 1 and 5 respectively (Fig. **106**). The portions of these fasciae turned toward the palmar surface simultaneously form the marginal parts of the *superficial palmar fascia*, the middle part of which is strengthened into the *palmar aponeurosis*. The interosseous margins of the metacarpals are occluded by a *deep palmar fascia* on the palmar side and by a deep *dorsal fascia* on the dorsal side. Both fasciae are anchored at the metacarpal bones. In addition to the four metacarpal interosseous spaces, there are three *chambers* (compartments) in the palm which are bordered by fascia: *middle, thenar* and *hypothenar*. The middle compartment (chamber for the flexors of the fingers) communicates proximally with the connective tissue spaces of the forearm via the carpal canal (along the flexor tendons). Distally, there are connections to the palmar side of the fingers (routes for the spread of inflammation).

The thenar and hypothenar compartments are closed proximally. They communicate with the middle chamber via openings for nerves and vessels, which are so narrow that they permit no rapid spread of inflammation. As infections in the thenar and hypothenar compartments, therefore, cannot spreadout to the forearm, they rapidly cause painful turgor. Arterial and venous branches, which connect the vascular system of the dorsum with branches of the deep palmar arch and the accompanying veins (→ p. 287), pass through the occluded interosseous spaces of the metacarpals. Infections can be spread along these vessels from the palm to the dorsum of the hand. Edemas (=swelling by increased, diffuse water accumulation in tissue spaces) which result from infectious processes in the region of the palm of the hand always appears at the back of the hand since the palmar aponeurosis does not permit them to spread to the surface on the palmar side.

The **palmar aponeurosis**, the middle part of the superficial palmar fascia between the thenar and hypothenar eminences, forms a firm, tense, triangular connective tissue plate, which is attached proximally at the flexor retinaculum and which spreads out distally like a fan (Figs. **95 a** and **106**). It consists of longitudinal tracts and transverse fiber bundles (*transverse fasciculi*). The longitudinal fiber tracts end at the heads of the metacarpals, in the fibrous sheaths of the long flexor tendons, and at the subcutaneous connective tissue above the base of the proximal phalanges. The transverse tract located most distally, the *superficial transverse metacarpal ligament*, forms the ligamentous foundation of the interdigital folds of the skin ("web"). Numerous fibers (*retinacula cutis*) pass from the surface of the aponeurosis to the skin through the subcutaneous fat between the palmar aponeurosis and the dermis and demarcate small, almost immovable compression chambers.

The palmaris longus radiates proximally into the palmar aponeurosis, which it can stretch. The *palmaris brevis muscle* passes from the ulnar margin of the strengthened middle portion of the aponeurosis to the skin of the hypothenar eminence. Its contraction firms up the pad formed by adipose tissue and dermis; at the same time the muscle protects the ulnar vessels.

The palmar aponeurosis protects the muscles, tendons, vessels and nerves of the palm of the hand from local pressure damage. Together with the subcutaneous compression chambers and the particularly tough, strongly-cornified skin of the palm, it forms a solid abutment when an object is held by a strong closed fist.

A scarred shrinkage of the palmar aponeurosis (Dupuytren's contracture) forces the fingers into a flexed position at the proximal joints and leads to a restriction of mobility in the joints of the fingers.

Muscles of the Thenar Eminence

The arrangement and differentiation of the short muscles of the thumb correspond to the special movement possibilities at the 1st carpometacarpal joint. Their chief task is to oppose the thumb, to place it opposite to the remaining fingers and also to the palm of the hand, so that the hand can act as a prehensile pincer.

In addition to the short thumb muscles (opponens pollicis, flexor pollicis brevis, abductor pollicis brevis and abductor pollicis [oblique head]), the long flexors of the thumb cooperate in this opposition. On the other hand, reposition is only produced by the long extensor muscles: the extensor pollicis longus, extensor pollicis brevis and abductor pollicis longus.

Except for the abductor pollicis, all the muscles of the thenar eminence arise from the flexor retinaculum and from the radial margin of the sulcus carpi (tubercles of the scaphoid and the trapezium).

The **abductor pollicis brevis** (Figs. **102**, **104** and **106**) lies superficially and almost completely covers the opponens pollicis. It originates from the flexor retinaculum and the tubercle of the scaphoid and inserts at the radial sesamoid bone embedded in the capsule of the proximal joint of the thumb, at the lateral margin of the base of the proximal phalanx, and in the dorsal aponeurosis.

Innervation: median nerve.

The median nerve ramifies beneath the flexor retinaculum into the branches to the muscles of the thenar eminence and the common palmar digital nerves.

The **opponens pollicis** (Figs. **102**, **104** and **106**) crosses under the abductor pollicis brevis at an acute angle and passes from the flexor retinaculum and the trapezium to the radial side of the 1st metacarpal.

Innervation: median nerve.

The **flexor pollicis brevis** (Figs. **102**, **104** and **106**) lies medial to the abductor pollicis brevis. The portion at its origin is separated by the tendon of the flexor pollicis longus into a superficial head, which is attached at the flexor retinaculum, and a deep head, which arises from the radial distal carpal bones. (The two heads are genetically of different origin). The terminal tendon of the flexor pollicis brevis fuses with the tendon of the abductor pollicis brevis and inserts, like the latter, at the radial sesamoid bone, at the proximal phalanx of the thumb and at the dorsal aponeurosis.

Innervation: superficial head by the median nerve, deep head by the deep ramus of the ulnar nerve.

The **adductor pollicis** (Figs. **102**, **104** and **106**), covered by the palmar aponeurosis, the tendons of the long flexors of the fingers, and by lumbricals 1 and 2, has two heads of origin. Its *oblique head* arises from the capitate, the ligamentous tracts radiating from it and the base of metacarpal 2; its *transverse head* originates from the palmar surface of metacarpal 3 and passes transversely through the depth of the palm. The common terminal tendon of both heads inserts at the ulnar sesamoid bone of the proximal metacarpophalangeal joint and at the base of the proximal phalanx of the thumb.

During abduction of the thumb, the distal muscular margin is pushed into the "web" stretched out between the thumb and index finger; included within the "web" is the 1st dorsal interosseus muscle.

Innervation: deep ramus of the ulnar nerve.

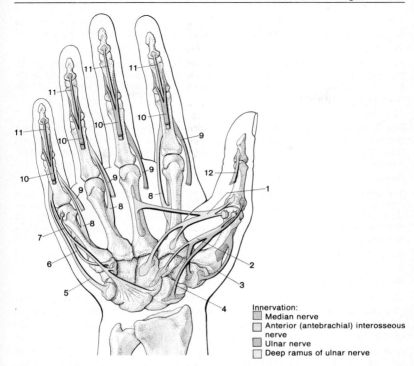

Innervation:
- Median nerve
- Anterior (antebrachial) interosseous nerve
- Ulnar nerve
- Deep ramus of ulnar nerve

Fig. 104. Short muscles of hand and tendons of long flexors of fingers, palmar view (Dorsal interossei muscles → Fig. 105)

1 Adductor pollicis
2 Flexor pollicis brevis
3 Opponens pollicis
4 Abductor pollicis brevis
5 Abductor digiti minimi
6 Opponens digiti minimi
7 Flexor digiti minimi brevis
8 Palmar interossei 1–3
9 Lumbricals 1–4
10 Tendons of flexor digitorum superficialis
11 Tendons of flexor digitorum profundus
12 Tendon of flexor pollicis longus

Muscles of the Hypothenar Eminence

The muscles of the hypothenar eminence are arranged in three tiers. The **palmar brevis** lies most superficially (1st layer), outside the hypothenar compartment (Fig. **106**). It passes from the ulnar margin of the palmar aponeurosis to the skin of the hypothenar eminence and is supplied by the superficial ramus of the ulnar nerve.

The muscles of the 2nd and 3rd layers, which are innervated by the deep ramus of the ulnar nerve, pass from the flexor retinaculum and from the ulnar margin of the carpal groove to the proximal phalanx of the 5th finger (2nd layer: abductor digiti minimi, flexor digiti minimi brevis) and to the 5th metacarpal (3rd layer: opponens digiti minimi).

The **abductor digiti minimi** (Figs. **102**, **104** and **106**) arises from the pisiform, from the pisohamate ligament and from the flexor retinaculum. It inserts at the ulnar margin of the base of the proximal phalanx of the little finger and radiates into the dorsal aponeurosis.

Innervation: deep ramus of the ulnar nerve.

The **flexor digiti minimi brevis** (Figs. **102**, **104** and **106**) attaches – usually without a sharp boundary – on the radial side and goes out from the flexor retinaculum and from the hook of the hamate. It fuses at the insertion with the abductor digiti minimi.

Innervation: deep ramus of the ulnar nerve.

The **opponens digiti minimi** (Figs. **102**, **104** and **106**) lies beneath the two previously mentioned muscles. It passes from the hook of the hamate and from the flexor retinaculum to the ulnar margin of the 5th metacarpal and can raise the 5th metacarpal somewhat toward the palmar side so that the curvature of the palm is deepened (water scoop).

Innervation: deep ramus of the ulnar nerve.

Muscles of the Middle Compartment

The **four lumbricals** (Figs. **103** – **106**) each arise at the radial side of the tendons of the flexor digitorum profundus and are therefore tensed during contraction of this muscle. They course distally on the palmar side of the deep transverse metacarpal ligament – and thus also palmar to the axis of flexion of the corresponding proximal joints of the fingers. Their tendons enter the dorsal aponeurosis from the radial side. The proximal fibers of the tendon of insertion pass in an almost transverse direction on the dorsal surface of the proximal phalanx, whereas the distal fibers pass obliquely to the dorsal surfaces of the middle and distal phalanges.

Innervation: both radial lumbricals (1, 2) are innervated by the median nerve, the ulnar lumbricals (3, 4) by the deep branch of the ulnar nerve. Frequently, the 3rd lumbrical receives a branch from the median nerve.

Muscles in the Metacarpal Interosseous Space

The *interossei* are derivatives of the deep, short digital flexor muscles of lower vertebrates (thus ventral limb muscles). Like the lumbricals, they cross the axis of flexion of the metacarpophalangeal joints on the palmar side.

Innervation of interossei: deep ramus of the ulnar nerve.

The three palmar interossei have retained their original position on the palmar side. The four dorsal interossei have shifted dorsally and they become visible on the dorsum of the hand in the depth between the extensor tendons after the deep dorsal fascia covering them is removed.

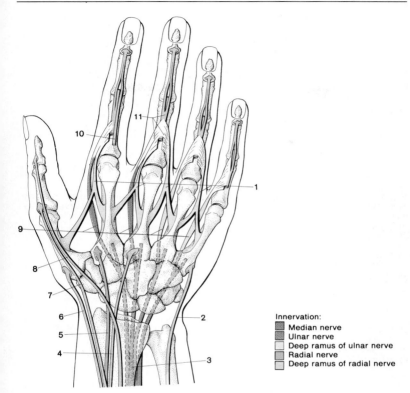

Fig. 105. **Muscles of forearm and hand, dorsal aponeurosis** dorsal view (palmar interossei → Fig. 104)

1 Dorsal interossei 1–4
2 Extensor carpi ulnaris
3 Flexor digitorum profundus (traced from palmar side, tendons severed distal to origin of lumbricals)
4 Extensor carpi radialis brevis
5 Extensor carpi radialis longus

6 Abductor pollicis longus
7 Extensor pollicis brevis
8 Extensor pollicis longus
9 Lumbricals 1–4
10 Tendon of extensor indicis
11 Dorsal aponeurosis of finger (cut open)

Innervation:
Median nerve
Ulnar nerve
Deep ramus of ulnar nerve
Radial nerve
Deep ramus of radial nerve

The **palmar interossei** (Figs. **104** and **106**) each arise at a metacarpal bone and insert at the dorsal aponeurosis of the corresponding finger. They are so arranged that they can adduct the 2nd, 4th and 5th fingers toward the middle finger, which lacks a palmar interosseus muscle.

The 1st palmar interosseus, therefore, lies on the ulnar side of the 2nd metacarpal, while the 2nd and 3rd palmar interossei originate from the radial side of meta-

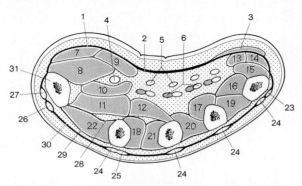

Fig. 106. **Cross-section in region of middle of hand**, arrangement of fasciae, muscles and tendons, distal view of section surface (Designation of vessels and nerves → Fig. 108)

1 Superficial palmar fascia
2 Palmar aponeurosis
3 Palmaris brevis
4 Tendon of flexor pollicis longus
5 Tendons of flexor digitorum superficialis
6 Tendons of flexor digitorum profundus and lumbricals
7 Abductor pollicis brevis
8 Opponens pollicis
9 Superficial head ⎫ of flexor pollicis brevis
10 Deep head ⎭
11 Oblique head ⎫ of adductor pollicis
12 Transverse head ⎭
13 Flexor digiti minimi brevis
14 Abductor digiti minimi

15 Opponens digiti minimi
16 Palmar interosseus 3
17 Palmar interosseus 2
18 Palmar interosseus 1
19 Dorsal interosseus 4
20 Dorsal interosseus 3
21 Dorsal interosseus 2
22 Dorsal interosseus 1
23 Tendon of extensor digiti minimi
24 Tendons of extensor digitorum
25 Tendon of extensor indicis
26 Tendon of extensor pollicis longus
27 Tendon of extensor pollicis brevis
28 Deep palmar fascia
29 Deep fascia of dorsum of hand
30 Dorsal fascia of hand
31 Metacarpal 1

carpals 4 and 5. The palmar interossei insert toward the longitudinal axis of the middle finger, and the dorsal interossei away from this axis. (The "palmar interosseus" of the thumb is incorporated in the adductor pollicis.)

The **dorsal interossei muscles** (Figs. **94**, **103**, **105** and **106**) each originate two-headed at the facing sides of two metacarpals and radiate into the dorsal aponeurosis of the 2nd, 3rd and 4th fingers. Two dorsal interossei muscles attach at the 3rd finger. At the 2nd finger the dorsal tendon approaches the dorsal aponeurosis from the radial side and at the 4th finger from the ulnar side.

d) Action of Muscles and Muscle Groups on Carpometacarpal Joint 1

At carpometacarpal joint 1 the thumb can be:
– *abducted* by the abductor pollicis longus and brevis with cooperation from the flexor pollicis brevis,

– *adducted* by the adductor pollicis and 1st dorsal interosseus with the collaboration of the opponens pollicis and extensor pollicis longus,
– *flexed* by the flexor pollicis longus and brevis with the help of the abductor pollicis brevis, adductor pollicis (oblique head) and opponens,
– *extended* by the extensor pollicis longus and brevis, as well as the abductor pollicis longus,
– *opposed* by the opponens and adductor pollicis, as well as the flexor pollicis longus and brevis, and
– *reposed* by the abductor pollicis longus and the extensor pollicis longus and brevis.

Paralyses. In the case of suitable injury to the radial nerve, the thumb is in opposition because of the paralysis of the reposing *extensors*; it can no longer be abducted with the same strength.

A paralysis of the *thenar muscles* innervated by the median nerve diminishes the expenditure of force in the opposition and abduction of the thumb and causes this muscle group to atrophy.

In the case of an interruption of excitatory conduction via the deep ramus of the ulnar nerve, an object can no longer be held fast between the thumb and index finger owing to the paralysis of the *adductor pollicis* and the *1st dorsal interosseus muscle*.

With a *combined paralysis* of the median and ulnar nerves, the abducted thumb can no longer be adducted to the index finger.

e) Action of Muscles and Muscle Groups on the Joints of the Fingers

The *thumb* at the *metacarpophalangeal joint* can be:
– *flexed* by the flexor pollicis longus and brevis,
whereby the abductor pollicis brevis and adductor pollicis can both assist; and
– *extended* by the extensor pollicis longus and brevis.

The *thumb* at the *interphalangeal joint* can be:
– *flexed* by the flexor pollicis longus, and
– *extended* by the extensor pollicis longus.

In contrast to the other fingers, a largely isolated flexion or extension of an individual thumb segment is possible.

Fingers 2–5 at the *metacarpophalangeal joint* can be:
– *flexed* by the flexor digitorum superficialis and profundus, the lumbricals, and the palmar and dorsal interossei,
the proximal phalanx of the 5th finger additionally by the flexor digiti minimi brevis and abductor digiti minimi;
– *extended* by the extensor digitorum,
the index finger additionally by the extensor indicis and the little finger additionally by the extensor digiti minimi;
– *abducted* by the dorsal interossei, the 5th finger by the abductor digiti minimi; and

– *adducted* (carried toward the middle finger) by the palmar interossei with the help of the extensor indicis (at the index finger) and the extensor digiti minimi (at the little finger).

From the extreme spreading position, all long muscles of the fingers also adduct until the fingers lie in the direction of the metacarpal bones. The palmar interossei then have the sole task of adducting the fingers from this slight spreading position (specific position of long extensors) toward the middle finger. They can therefore be considerably weaker than the dorsal interossei, which abduct fingers 2 – 4 from the axis of the middle finger and are supported by the long finger muscles only for the short distance to the characteristic position of the long extensors.

Fingers 2 – 5 at the *proximal interphalangeal joint* can be:
– *flexed* by the flexor digitorum superficialis and profundus, and
– *extended* by the extensor digitorum, lumbricals and interossei,
the index finger, in addition, by the extensor indicis, and the little finger also by the extensor digiti minimi and the tendon fibers of the abductor digiti minimi radiating into the dorsal aponeurosis.

Fingers 2 – 5 at the *distal interphalangeal joint* can be:
– *flexed* by the flexor digitorum profundus,
– *extended* – as in the proximal interphalangeal joint – by the extensor digitorum and the muscles radiating into the dorsal aponeurosis.

The *long flexors of the fingers* cannot be sufficiently contracted to flex maximally all joints over which they pass. The *flexor digitorum superficialis* flexes chiefly at the proximal joint, and the *deep flexor* at the proximal and distal interphalangeal joints.

Both muscles act to a noteworthy degree on the metacarpophalangeal joints only when the wrist joint is "dorsiflexed" or the middle and distal phalanges are extended. Fist closure is therefore much stronger in the dorsally-flexed hand than in the palmar flexed wrist joint. In powerful passive flexion at the wrist joint, an object can be wrested more easily from fingers closed into a fist.

The isolated flexion of the distal joint (flexor digitorum profundus) is not possible for most people without special training. For flexion of the middle and distal phalanges, the sliding collars formed by the perforating tendons of the superficial flexors of the fingers prevent the tendons of the flexor digitorum profundus from lifting off the bone.

A solitary flexion at the metacarpophalangeal joint can be effected by the *lumbricals* and *interossei* since their tendons enter into the lateral end of the dorsal aponeurosis on the palmar side of the axis of rotation of this joint. A palmar flexion of this joint is only possible when the extensor digitorum is not contracted.

The *extensor digitorum* extends primarily at the metacarpophalangeal joint. In the extended wrist and metacarpophalangeal joints, it is already largely insufficient, so that the middle and distal phalanges are extended by the *lumbricals* and *interossei*. Since the tendons of the long extensors of the fingers are connected with each other by the intertendinous connections, an isolated extension of individual fingers is possible only to the extent permitted by these "transverse ligaments." In this process, the index finger has the greatest freedom and the 4th finger the least. The tendons of the extensors of the fingers (like the extensor indicis proprius and extensor digiti minimi) try to bring the longitudinal axis of the trisegmented finger in line with that of the metacarpals. Depending on the starting position, they can slightly abduct or adduct the fingers at the metacarpophalangeal joint.

In the position of rest, the fingers are slightly flexed at all three joints (predominance of flexors), and the thumb lies in the mid-opposition position.

Paralysis of the nerves supplying the long and short flexors of the fingers produces characteristic forms.

In a paralysis of the *deep ramus of the radial nerve*, the fingers can no longer be extended at the metacarpophalangeal joint. The interossei and the lumbricals flex the proximal phalanges (since the extensor digitorum muscles do not respond). Both interphalangeal joints, on the other hand, are extended (incompletely, however, due to the resistance of the long flexors). The thumb stands in opposition. If the main trunk of the radial nerve is involved, the hand hangs downwards when the forearm is flexed and pronated: "wrist drop".

With a *paralysis of the median nerve*, the middle and distal phalanges of the index finger can no longer be flexed, and those of the middle finger weakly at best. The thumb lies close to the extended index finger (adductor pollicis). The attempt to make a fist results in the typical *"swearing hand" position*.

When the opponens pollicis and the two *flexors of the thumb* are paralyzed, contact between the thumb and little finger (thumb-little finger test) is no longer possible. Owing to the atrophy of the thenar muscles, a paralysis of the median nerve is also referred to as *"ape hand"*.

In a *paralysis of the deep ramus of the ulnar nerve*, the interossei and the ulnar lumbricals, among others, do not respond. At the metacarpophalangeal joint of the finger, the tonus of the long extensors leads to an extension (they have a more favorable active force here than the finger flexors), whereas the middle and terminal joints of the fingers are flexed (here the long flexors surpass the extensors): *"claw hand"*.

By the loss of the *adductor pollicis* and the *musculature of the hypothenar eminence*, the thumb-little finger test is no longer possible. When the main trunk of the ulnar nerve is injured, the little finger can no longer be actively flexed. The distal phalanx of the 4th finger and usually also the distal phalanx of the 3rd finger can still be flexed, but only weakly.

f) Neurovascular Routes in the Hand

Radial Artery in the Hand

On the palmar side of the wrist, the **radial artery** gives off the *superficial palmar ramus*, which courses above or through the thenar muscles as a variable, usually weak tributary of the superficial palmar arch. With its accompanying veins, it courses around the trapezium to the dorsum of the hand. Here it passes distally into the fossa designated as the "snuffbox," which is bordered by the tendons of the extensor pollicis longus (ulnar), the extensor pollicis brevis and the abductor pollicis longus (radial); at the proximal end of the 1st metacarpal interosseous space it passes between the two heads of the 1st dorsal interosseus to the palmar side of the palm (Fig. **94**).

In the "snuff-box", the radial artery lies close to the bone and deep, covered by compact connective tissue. As a rule, the arterial pulse can be palpated through the fascia.

At the dorsum of the hand the *radial artery* gives off (in addition to the *dorsal carpal ramus* to the dorsal carpal network) the *1st dorsal metacarpal artery* shortly before reaching the 1st interosseous space. The latter divides into the *dorsal digital arteries* for the dorsal side of the thumb and the radial margin of the index finger (Fig. **109**.)

The radial artery at the back of the hand and the dorsal metacarpal arteries (from the dorsal carpal network) pass together with the tendons (and tendon sheaths) of the extensors situated superficial to them in the "chamber of the extensors of the fingers", which is bordered by the superficial and the deep fascia of the dorsum of the hand. The *superficial fascia* is the distal continuation of the antebrachial fascia and communicates with the extensor retinaculum. A cutaneous venous network (dorsal venous network of the hand), superficial lymphatic vessels and branches of the superficial ramus of the radial nerve and the dorsal ramus of the ulnar nerve course on the fascia.

The **dorsal carpal network** lies on the dorsal side of the carpals (on the ligamentous collar of the wrist joint) and receives tributaries from the:
– anterior interosseous artery,
– posterior interosseous artery,
– dorsal carpal ramus of the radial artery, and
– dorsal carpal ramus of the ulnar artery.

From the dorsal carpal network the (weak) *dorsal metacarpal arteries* (Fig. **108**) arise, which course to the fingers in the 2nd – 4th interosseous space; each divides into two *dorsal digital arteries* to the margins of the two fingers facing each other (Fig. **109**). They supply the dorsal side of the proximal phalanges and the proximal half of the middle phalanges. The palmar metacarpal arteries open into the dorsal metacarpal arteries with their perforating branches and give rise to the dorsal metacarpal vessels when the dorsal carpal network is weakly developed.

Neurovascular Layers of the Palm

A superficial, *subfascial neurovascular layer* (between the palmar apo-neurosis and the flexor tendons) and a *deep neurovascular layer* (on the deep palmar fascia) can be distinguished in the palm of the hand.

Subfascial neurovascular layer. In the thin, subfascial fat and connective tissue layer there are (Fig. **107**):
– the *superficial palmar arch* – as terminal branch of the ulnar artery – with its branches and accompanying nerves;
– the *branches of the median nerve* to the thenar muscles, radial lumbricals and radial $3\frac{1}{2}$ fingers;
– the *superficial ramus of the ulnar nerve*, which gives off a branch to the palmaris brevis and divides into cutaneous nerves for the $1\frac{1}{2}$ ulnar fingers; and
– *one (or several) anastomoses* between the median and ulnar nerves.

Deep neurovascular layer. Beneath the tendons of the long flexors of the fingers and the lumbricals there are located on the deep fascia of the palm and the metacarpal bones (Fig. **107**):
– the *deep palmar arch* with its branches and accompanying veins fed chiefly by the radial artery, and
– the *deep ramus of the ulnar nerve* with muscular branches to the hypothenar muscles, adductor pollicis and the deep head of the short flexors of the thumb.

Lymphatic vessels. From the fine meshwork of the superficial lymphatic plexus and from the depth of the palm, the lymph – like venous blood – is conveyed to the back of the hand chiefly through the interosseous spaces of the middle of the hand, from which it is discharged via superficial lymphatic tracts. Delicate deep lymphatic pathways accompany the branches of the radial and ulnar arteries.

Subfascial Neurovascular Layers of the Palm

The terminal branch of the ulnar artery courses beneath the palmaris brevis and forms on the tendons of the long flexors of the fingers a distal convex vascular arch (**superficial palmar arch**, Fig. **107**), which can communicate with the superficial palmar ramus of the radial artery. The superficial palmar arch lies distal to the deep palmar arch. From the convexity of the superficial palmar arch the *proper palmar digital artery* for the ulnar side of the little finger and three (or four) *common palmar digital arteries* arise, each of which divides at about the level of the metacarpophalangeal joints into two (strong) *proper palmar digital arteries* to the margins of the 2nd to 5th fingers facing each other (Figs. **107–109**).

The ulnar artery supplies chiefly the $3\frac{1}{2}$ fingers on the ulnar side, whereas the $1\frac{1}{2}$ radial fingers receive their blood from branches of the radial artery (princeps pollicis and radialis indicis arteries).

The palmar vessels – just like the palmar cutaneous nerves – overlap at the distal half of the middle phalanx and at the distal phalanx on the dorsal side.

The **median nerve** (Fig. **107**) has already divided beneath the flexor retinaculum into the nerve branches to the muscles of the thenar eminence (except for the adductor pollicis and the deep head of the flexor pollicis brevis) and into three *common palmar digital nerves*, which diverge from one another distal to the carpal canal and pass underneath the

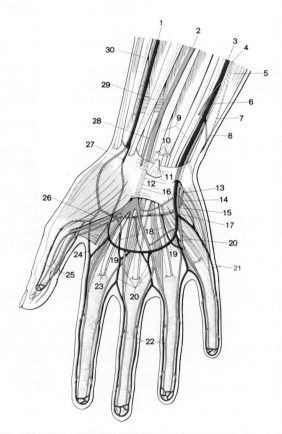

Fig. 107. **Arteries and nerves in forearm and hand**, palmar view (several forearm muscles, lumbricals, and muscles of thenar and hypothenar eminences shown but, for reasons of clarity, not labelled → Fig. 102)

superficial palmar arch. The common palmar digital nerves send branches to lumbricals I and II (occasionally also III) and ramify in the skin of the $3\frac{1}{2}$ radial fingers (Fig. **113 a**).

The common palmar digital nerve I divides into three cutaneous branches (proper palmar digital nerves), which course on the palmar side at both lateral margins of the thumb and on the radial side at the lateral edge of the index finger. The 2nd and 3rd common palmar digital nerves each bifurcate into two *proper palmar digital nerves*, which pass along the facing palmar margins of the 2nd and 3rd fingers and of the 3rd and 4th fingers.

The **ulnar nerve** (Fig. **107**) divides into its two terminal branches on the radial side of the pisiform. Whereas the *deep ramus* passes into the depth between the abductor digiti minimi and flexor digiti minimi brevis, the *superficial ramus of the ulnar nerve* courses on the ulnar side of the base of the superficial palmar arch, supplies the palmaris brevis, and ramifies in the skin of the $1\frac{1}{2}$ ulnar fingers. Between the superficial ramus of the ulnar nerve and the median nerve, a fibrous interchange normally exists by means of a *communicating ramus of the median nerve with the ulnar nerve* (*ramus communicans cum nervo ulnari*).

The *superficial ramus of the ulnar nerve* divides after the exit of the muscular branch for the palmar brevis into cutaneous branches, the *proper palmar digital nerve* to the ulnar margin of the little finger and the *common palmar digital nerve*, which bifurcates into two *proper palmar digital nerves*. They course to the palmar lateral margins of the 4th and 5th fingers facing one another (Fig. **113 a**).

Deep Neurovascular Layer of the Palm

The **radial artery** (Fig. **107**), which arrives at the palmar side of the hand through the 1st metacarpal interosseous space, gives off the *princeps*

◄ 1 Radial artery
2 Median nerve
3 Ulnar artery
4 Ulnar nerve
5 Flexor carpi ulnaris
6 Palmar branch of ulnar nerve
7 Dorsal branch of ulnar nerve
8 Dorsal carpal branch of ulnar artery
9 Flexor digitorum profundus
10 Tendons of flexor digitorum superficialis
11 Tendon of palmaris longus
12 Flexor retinaculum
13 Deep branch of ulnar nerve
14 Deep palmar branch of ulnar artery
15 Superficial branch of ulnar nerve
16 Communicating branch of median nerve with ulnar nerve
17 Deep palmar arch

18 Palmar metacarpal arteries
19 Superficial palmar arch
20 Common palmar digital arteries and nerves
21 Proper palmar digital artery and nerve to ulnar side of little finger
22 Proper palmar digital arteries and nerves
23 Tendons of superficial and deep flexors of fingers
24 Radialis indicis artery
25 Proper palmar digital arteries and nerves of thumb
26 Princeps pollicis artery
27 Superficial palmar branch of radial artery
28 Palmar branch of median nerve
29 Flexor carpi radialis
30 Brachioradialis

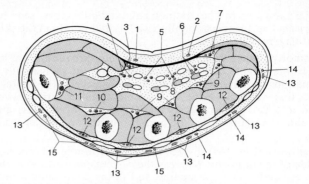

Fig. 108. **Cross section in region of middle of hand**, arrangement of nerves and
vessels, distal view of section surface (Designation of muscles and nerves → Fig. 106)

1 Palmar branch of median nerve
2 Palmar branch of ulnar nerve
3 Proper palmar digital artery and nerve
  to radial side of thumb (from median
  nerve)
4 Common palmar digital artery and nerve of
  thumb (from median nerve)
5 Common palmar digital arteries and
  nerves of fingers II, III (from median nerve)
6 Common palmar digital artery and nerve of
  finger IV (from superficial branch of ulnar
  nerve)

7 Proper palmar digital artery and nerve, to
  ulnar side of little finger (from superficial
  branch of ulnar nerve)
8 Communicating branch of median nerve
  with ulnar nerve
9 Palmar metacarpal arteries
10 Radialis indicis artery
11 Princeps pollicis artery
12 Dorsal metacarpal arteries
13 Subcutaneous dorsal metacarpal veins
14 Dorsal digital nerves (from dorsal branch
   of ulnar nerve)
15 Dorsal digital nerves (from superficial
   branch of radial nerve)

pollicis artery in the depth of the thenar eminence. Its terminal branch –
covered on the radial side by the adductor pollicis – forms the *deep palmar
arch* at the bases of the metacarpals and the palmar interossei.

The *princeps pollicis artery* (Fig. **108**) courses beneath the opponens
pollicis and branches into two *1st proper palmar digital arteries* to the
radial and ulnar margins of the thumb.

The *radialis indicis artery* to the radial margin of the index finger can arise from
the princeps pollicis artery or from the deep palmar arch (occasionally also from
the superficial palmar arch).

The **deep palmar arch** (Fig. **107**) lies proximal to the superficial palmar
arch. The usually delicate *deep palmar ramus*, which leaves the ulnar
artery radial to the pisiform, forms the ulnar crus of the deep vascular
arch and penetrates into the depth between the abductor digiti minimi
and flexor digiti minimi brevis. The deep palmar arch dispatches from its
convex side 3–4 *palmar metacarpal arteries* (Fig. **108**), each of which
unites with a common palmar digital artery from the superficial palmar
arch.

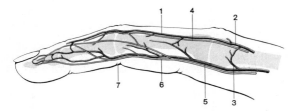

Fig. 109. **Arteries and nerves of fingers**, view of index finger from radial side.

1 Dorsal digital artery
2 Dorsal metacarpal artery
3 Perforating branch
4 Dorsal digital nerve (to index finger from superficial branch of radial nerve)
5 Proper palmar digital artery
6 Proper palmar digital nerve (to index finger from median nerve)
7 Flexure crease at middle joint (corresponds to position of articular cavity)

In each interosseous space, a *perforating ramus* passes through the interossei muscles and anastomoses with a dorsal metacarpal artery (Fig. **109**).

The *variability in the development of both palmar arches* is extraordinarily great. The pattern described occurs in less than 30% of the cases. Frequently, the superficial palmar arch is formed only by the ulnar artery; occasionally it is fed by the median artery (instead of by the superficial palmar ramus). Both arches can be incomplete. Often the blood supply of the thumb and index finger is completely taken over by the superficial palmar arch.

The **deep ramus of the ulnar nerve** (Fig. **108**) courses through the hypothenar eminence with the arterial *deep palmar branch*. It passes in the middle compartment of the palm proximally and below the deep vascular arch toward the thumb. It provides for the muscles of the hypothenar eminence (except for the palmaris brevis), the ulnar lumbricals, the adductor pollicis, and (usually) the deep head of the short thumb flexor and all interossei in the interosseous spaces. Sensory branches pass to the wrist and metacarpophalangeal joints.

g) Organization of the Vessels and Nerves in the Fingers

A respective total of *four digital arteries* and *nerves* course in the subcutaneous connective tissue at both lateral surfaces of each finger – each near the edge. Apart from the thumb, the dorsal arteries and nerves are weaker than the palmar vessels and nerves, which take over the blood and nerve supply at the three-segmented fingers in the regions of the distal phalanx and a part of the middle phalanx (also on the dorsal side of the fingers, i.e. fingernail bed, Fig. **109**).

The dorsal *digital arteries* arise from the dorsal metacarpal arteries, and the palmar vessels from the superficial palmar arch and from the princeps pollicis artery.

The *innervation* of the dorsum of the $2\frac{1}{2}$ radial fingers is provided by the superficial ramus of the radial nerve and of the ulnar fingers by the dorsal ramus of the ulnar nerve (Fig. **113 b**). Displacements of the border between the supply regions in favor of the radial nerve are not rare. The palmar digital nerves of the $3\frac{1}{2}$ radial fingers are branches of the median nerve; the proper palmar digital nerves of the $1\frac{1}{2}$ ulnar fingers are branches of the superficial ramus of the ulnar nerve (Figs. **107** and **113 a**).

Numerous anastomoses exist between the four arteries of a finger so that in the case of severance of a digital artery both the proximal and the distal vascular stumps must be cared for. In the hand region, the innervation areas of the digital nerves are partially overlapping. This is especially true for the thumb and ring finger, the nerve of which can lack an autonomous cutaneous field. In the case of a nerve block, one must therefore interrupt the conduction of excitation into all four proper digital nerves of a finger.

The *veins* in the finger do not accompany the arteries. Instead, they form a weak palmar and a more strongly-developed dorsal venous network. The venous blood is carried off chiefly by the dorsal venous network of the hand and the subcutanous veins of the forearm.

The *lymphatic vessels* of the fingers accompany the veins and form corresponding networks. The main drainage of lymph from the finger region takes place via the lymphatic tracts of the dorsum of the hand.

Pathways spreading inflammation. Since a typical superficial fascia is absent on the fingers and thus the subcutaneous connective tissue is not separated from the structures of the locomotor apparatus (dorsal aponeurosis, tendons, tendon sheaths, bone), inflammations can easily be spread from the subcutaneous connective tissue to the locomotor apparatus. On the flexor side of the fingers, the connective tissue septa, which demarcate the subcutaneous connective tissue and body fat into compression chambers, are anchored to the periosteum. Therefore, inflammatory processes are rapidly transported from the subcutaneous connective tissue into the deeper-lying tissues where they can destroy the bones or can spread to the tendon sheaths.

h) Cooperation of Arm, Hand and Fingers

By the combination of movement possibilities in the individual joints, an extraordinary variety and an extensive range of movements are possible for the upper limb, and these can be expanded still further by movements of the vertebral column and the lower limb. Thus, it is possible to reach (almost) any point on the surface of the body with the fingers. For a specific movement, the shoulder girdle assumes the most favorable position from which the free limb can work. In movements in front of the body (in the field of vision), the upper arm is rotated inward, the elbow joint more or less flexed. The hand, as a rule, is in the pronation position. Together with the other fingers, the thumb forms a grasping tool for everyday use. Decisive for the organized execution of a movement are temporal coordination and the accurately synchronized intensity of muscular activity, whereby the diminution of muscle tone of the antagonists is just as important as the contraction of the synergists.

D. Superficial Anatomy of the Upper Limb

1. Surface Morphology of the Upper Limb and Palpable Bony Points

Surface morphology is determined by the individually-different development of the musculature and the deposition of subcutaneous fatty tissue. As a consequence of heavy bodily work or specific sports training, a strongly developed deltoid muscle can accentuate the curvature of the shoulder. The upper arm is then flattened outside and inside by the powerful development of the flexors (biceps brachii) and the extensors, and the forearm can exhibit a very distinct conical constriction toward the wrist. An ample development of subcutaneous fat (especially in infants, small children and, as a rule, in women) can obscure the muscle contour. Upper arm and forearm appear rounded (instead of flattened or transversely oval). In flexion of the elbow, the three characteristic muscle bulges (biceps, radial extensors and forearm flexors) are more or less obliterated, and the subcutaneous veins are concealed.

The skeleton also plays a significant role in the formation of the surface morphology. On the extensor side of the elbow, the olecranon and both epicondyles of the humerus stand out through the skin. The part of the forearm near the wrist appears broad and plump or slender and graceful, depending upon the bone structure. When the upper arm is dislocated and the greater tubercle is no longer at its usual site, the characteristic shoulder curvature disappears.

The skin is moderately thick over the lateral shoulder region and in males occasionally exhibits adult hairiness. On the extensor side of the elbow, the skin is rough, folded, more strongly cornified and usually appears somewhat reddish. The heavily cornified skin of the palm and the palmar side of the fingers is especially thick and resistant, lacks hair (or sebaceous glands) and is rich in sweat glands.

On the palmar side of the terminal segment of the fingers, tracts and septa of collagenous connective tissue, which pass from the dermis to the subcutaneous layer, mark off the compression chambers filled with body fat (similar to those in the palm). The system of compression chambers at each finger forms a tactile elevation (*finger pad*), the skin of which is richly innervated and intensively vascularized. The fingernails serve as abutments for the finger pads.

In the remaining arm regions, the skin is relatively thin (especially on the flexor side), displaceable and can be lifted into folds. Hairs are often present in older men on the extensor side of the forearm and on the ulnar side of the dorsum of the hand. The transverse compression folds formed in the vicinity of joints are mentioned in the description of the joints. The subcutaneous layer of the dorsum of the hand is free of fat. Edema can spread into the connective tissue interstices here.

The *cleavage lines* (tension lines) of the skin, the directions of which are to be considered as far as possible in surgical operations, exhibit a complicated course – particularly in the forearm and hand. In the shoulder region, they converge toward the axilla. In the upper arm, they course steeply downward from the dorsal side toward the ulnar and radial sides (Fig. **71**).

Skin creases of the hand. The skin folds of the palm, which appear as the fist is closed, are bordered by *palm lines* which – since the skin is thinner here – are also distinctly visible when the fingers are extended (Fig. **98 a**). Of course, these lines, which remain recognizable even in the case of swelling, can offer the physician no noteworthy diagnostic assistance.

Instead of the two transverse creases, which do not cover the entire width of the palm, a line designated as the *four-finger crease* (simian crease) can appear (usually unilaterally) as a genetic variation; it runs proximal to the heads of the metacarpals from the radial to the ulnar margin of the palm. This crease is found more frequently in mongoloids or anencephalics than in healthy individuals.

Palpable bony points. With the exception of the lunate and trapezoid, there are individual segments or surfaces of the elements of the arm skeleton which can be palpated through the skin and soft parts so that a picture can be formed of the approximate form of nearly all bones.

The bony points whose contours can be recognized through the skin and are therefore especially accessible to the palpating fingers (Fig. **110**) are the following:

– at the *shoulder girdle*: clavicle, acromion and spine of scapula (the medial margin and superior angle of the scapula can also be palpated through the trapezius and latissimus dorsi; in the abducted arm, the coracoid process in the infraclavicular fossa);

– at the *upper arm*: both epicondyles (whereas in the adducted upper arm, the greater tubercle is usually not palpable from the axilla through the deltoid and the head of the humerus with equal precision);

– at the *forearm*: the olecranon, the dorsal edge of the ulna, and the styloid processes of the ulna and radius (the head of the radius in pronation and supination movements); and

– at the *hand*: tubercles of scaphoid and trapezium, pisiform, hook of hamate, dorsal surfaces of capitate and metacarpal bones, heads of

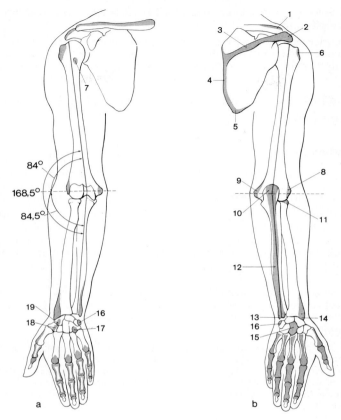

Fig. 110. **Palpable bony points on skeleton of upper limb** (after *von Lanz-Wachsmuth*)
a Ventral view
b Dorsal view

 1 Clavicle
 2 Acromion
 3 Spine of scapula
 4 Medial margin of scapula
 5 Inferior angle of scapula
 6 Greater tubercle of humerus
 7 Lesser tubercle of humerus
 8 Lateral epicondyle of humerus
 9 Medial epicondyle of humerus
10 Olecranaon
11 Head of radius
12 Posterior margin of ulna
13 Styloid process of radius
15 Capitate
16 Pisiform
17 Hook of hamulus
18 Tubercle of trapezium
19 Tubercle of scaphoid

metacarpals on the palmar side, as well as the lateral and dorsal surfaces of the phalanges.

In measuring the lengths of parts of the dangling arm (palmar surface in front), the acromion, lateral epicondyle of the humerus, styloid process of the radius, and tip of the third finger are used as *measuring points.*

2. Cutaneous Vessels and Nerves of the Upper Limb

a) Cutaneous Veins

The venous blood of the arm is carried off by (usually weak) *deep veins* (subfascial accompanying veins of arteries), as well as by superficial *cutaneous veins* (subcutaneous veins) lying on top of the fascia (Fig. **111**).

The cutaneous venous system consists of extensive, variable venous networks that are especially well-developed on the dorsum of the hand and fingers, as well as on the forearm. They are recognizable in part through the skin – especially in older people. The most important longitudinal trunks of the subcutaneous venous network of the arm are the *cephalic* and *basilic veins* (both from the cutaneous *dorsal venous network of the hand*) and the (often absent) *intermediate antebrachial vein* (from a venous plexus on the flexor side of the forearm). In the upper arm, the diameter of the cephalic and basilic veins exceeds that of the deep companion veins.

Numerous (partly variable) connections exist between the subfascial companion veins and the cutaneous veins. For example, a tight fist can cause the blood to flow from the deep veins of the palm through the valveless *intercapitular vein* (between the heads of the metacarpal bones) into the subcutaneous venous network on the dorsum of the hand. A second, regularly-formed (also valveless) anastomosis connects the intermediate veins in the bend of the elbow with the deep brachial veins.

Inflammatory processes can be spread from the subcutaneous into the deep tissues (or vice versa, e.g. palm → dorsum of the hand) along the "deep venous connections", which are accompanied also by lymphatic vessels passing from the superficial to the deep lymphatic tracts.

When a ring-shaped tourniquet is applied to moderately compress the upper arm, the cutaneous veins can be dammed up so that they become prominent (withdrawal of blood). Muscular activity (opening and closing the hand – "pumping") increases the flow of blood and, at the same time leads to a compression of the deep veins owing to the thickening of the contracting muscles and to a stronger filling of the superficial veins.

The subcutaneous venous network of the dorsum of the hand (*dorsal venous network of the hand*) consists of the *dorsal metacarpal veins* and their transverse

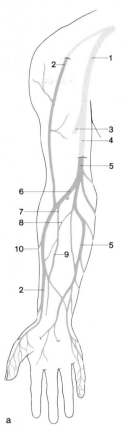
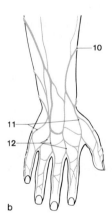

Fig. 111. **Cutaneous veins of upper limb**
a Palmar side
b Dorsum of hand

1 Axillary vein
2 Cephalic vein
3 Brachial vein (radial side)
4 Brachial vein (ulnar side)
5 Basilic vein
6 Intermediate (median) cubital vein

7 Intermediate (median) cephalic vein
8 Intermediate (median) basilic vein
9 Intermediate (median) antebrachial vein
10 Accessory cephalic vein
11 Dorsal venous network of hand
12 Subcutaneous dorsal metacarpal veins

anastomoses (Fig. **111 b**). It receives blood from the fingers and the palm of the hand. The drainage of blood takes place via longitudinal trunks that join the *cephalic vein* on the radial side of the venous network, which is a usually more strongly developed, and the *basilic vein* on the ulnar side. Occasionally, an *accessory cephalic vein* can arise from the middle of the venous network; it courses first across the dorsal side of the forearm before entering the cephalic vein.

The **cephalic vein** (Figs. **96** and **111 a**) forms the radial main trunk of the cutaneous venous network of the arm. It arrives proximal to the wrist joint on the flexor side of the forearm and passes on its radial margin to the bend of the elbow. In the upper arm, it usually courses at the lateral surface of the biceps brachii (Fig. **88**), arriving proximal to the clavipectoral triangle between the deltoid and pectoralis major; it then pierces the clavipectoral fascia to enter the axillary vein.

The **basilic vein** (Figs. **96** and **111 a**) arises from several longitudinal veins on the ulnar side of the forearm and becomes a single strong trunk when it reaches the proximal third of the forearm. At the bend of the elbow it anastomoses with the cephalic vein via the *intermediate cubital vein*, courses in the medial bicipital sulcus, and penetrates the brachial fascia (basilic hiatus) in the middle of the forearm. The basilic vein empties into the (ulnar) brachial vein.

The **intermediate antebrachial vein** (Figs. **96** and **111 a**) courses between the cephalic and the basilic veins on the flexor side of the forearm. In the bend of the elbow, it divides into two branches, the *intermediate cephalic* and *intermediate basilic veins*, which empty into the large cutaneous venous trunks, or it enters the intermediate cubital vein, more rarely the basilic vein.

The *organization of the cutaneous veins in the elbow* can vary considerably. In the typical case, the forearm segments of the cephalic and basilic veins form a letter "M" with the two opening branches of the intermediate antebrachial vein. If, however, the intermediate cubital vein receives the intermediate antebrachial vein, this venous connection, coursing obliquely toward the ulnar side and proximally, can be quite large, especially when the cephalic vein is only weakly formed in the upper arm.

A transverse connection of both longitudinal veins, however, can also be completely absent. In all variations, a connection to the brachial veins exist in the elbow (deep intermediate cubital vein from the intermediate basilic vein or, more rarely, from the intermediate cephalic vein, from the intermediate cubital vein, from the intermediate antebrachial vein or from an independent cephalic or basilic vein).

For a *venous puncture*, the superficial veins at the dorsum of the hand, the forearm and at the upper arm are preferred. The relatively large lumina of the cutaneous veins of the elbow and their easy accessibility make them likewise suitable for taking blood samples or for the injection of limited amounts of fluid, although possible variations of the brachial artery and the close proximity to the median nerve necessitate appropriate precautions. The veins of the elbow are less suited for infusions because the elbow joint must be placed at rest.

b) Superficial Lymphatic Tracts

The organization into cutaneous veins and accompanying veins corresponds to the differentiation between *superficial* (epifascial) and *deep lymphatic tracts* in the lymphatic vascular system of the upper limb. The *deep lymphatic vessels* course together with the arteries and the deep veins. The *superficial lymphatic vessels* come from the skin and subcutaneous tissues.

The lymph from the finely-meshed networks of the palm and the palmar side of the fingers drains via the lymphatic tracts of the fingers and dorsum of the hand, which also receives lymph from the deep tissues (bones, joints, tendon sheaths).

At the forearm, the longitudinal trunks of the superficial lymphatic tracts, which anastomose many times among each other, course mainly in the vicinity of the cephalic and basilic veins (Fig. **112**). Inflammations of the

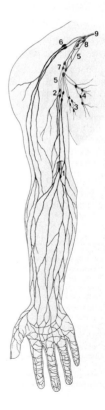

Fig. 112. **Superficial lymphatic tracts of arm and axillary lymph nodes**, ventral view
Superficial lymphatic vessels and nodes: (▬)
Deep vessels and nodes: (▬)
1 Cubital axillary lymph nodes
2–4 *Superficial axillary lymph nodes*
2 Lateral axillary lymph nodes
3 Subscapular axillary lymph nodes
4 Pectoral axillary lymph nodes
5 Axillary lymphatic plexus
6 Brachial axillary lymph nodes
7, 8 *Deep axillary lymph nodes*
7 Central axillary lymph nodes
8 Apical axillary lymph nodes
9 Subclavian trunk

lymphatic vessels are visible through the skin as red stripes. Connections existing between the deep and the superficial lymphatic vessels conduct lymph to the *superficial* lymphatic tracts. In the ulnar lymphatic vessels proximal to the medial epicondyle of the humerus, (one or several) *cubital axillary lymph nodes* can be deposited (in about 1/3 of the cases). Some of the lymphatic vessels accompanying the basilic vein pass with the vein through the fascia into the deep tissues. The ulnar lymphatic vessels, which continue in their superficial course, are joined by radial lymphatic vessels (from the vicinity of the cephalic vein) and pass on the surface of the fascia to the *lateral axillary lymph nodes* (Fig. **210 a**). A small number of radial lymphatic vessels accompany the cephalic vein to the infraclavicular fossa and conduct the lymph (via *brachial axillary lymphatic nodes*) to the *apical axillary lymph nodes*.

c) Cutaneous Nerves

Regions of innervation. The typical distribution areas of cutaneous nerves of the upper (and lower) limbs are not cutaneous bands which course transversely, as in the trunk wall, but irregularly-formed cutaneous fields.

Their extension can vary since the distribution of segmental nerve fibers differs somewhat individually in certain peripheral nerves and since anastomoses are formed between the branches of the cutaneous nerves in different dimensions. A clear border between neighboring cutaneous areas cannot be drawn because the areas occupied by the individual cutaneous nerves overlap (→ cutaneous innervation in the plexus region, p. 000); moreover, the nerve fibers for the various sensory perceptions (pain, touch, temperature) extend into the regions of adjacent nerves to varying degrees. In contrast to the nerves of the trunk wall, the "overlapping" of pain fibers is particularly pronounced.

The following description of the areas of innervation of cutaneous nerves of the upper limb reproduces the so-called anatomical cutaneous fields, i.e. the regions of ramification of cutaneous nerves in the subcutaneous

---

1 Lateral supraclavicular nerves
2 Medial brachial cutaneous nerve
3 Posterior ramus of medial antebrachial cutaneous nerve
4 Anterior branch of medial antebrachial cutaneous nerve
5 Palmar branch of ulnar nerve
6 Common and proper palmar digital nerves from superficial branch of ulnar nerve
7 Palmar branch of median nerve
8 Common and proper palmar digital nerves from median nerve
9 Lateral antebrachial cutaneous nerve from musculocutaneous nerve

10 Superior lateral brachial cutaneous nerve from axillary nerve
11 Inferior lateral brachial cutaneous nerve from radial nerve
12 Posterior brachial cutaneous nerve from radial nerve
13 Posterior antebrachial cutaneous nerve from radial nerve
14 Superficial branch of radial nerve
15 Dorsal digital nerves from superficial branch of radial nerve
16 Dorsal digital nerves from dorsal branch of ulnar nerve
17 Dorsal branch of ulnar nerve

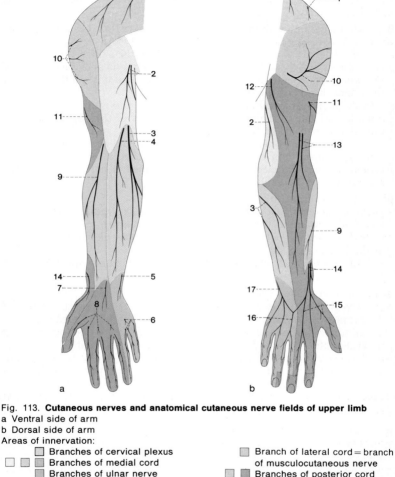

Fig. 113. **Cutaneous nerves and anatomical cutaneous nerve fields of upper limb**
a Ventral side of arm
b Dorsal side of arm
Areas of innervation:

☐ Branches of cervical plexus
☐ ☐ ☐ Branches of medial cord
☐ Branches of ulnar nerve
☐ Branches of medial and lateral cords = branches of median nerve

☐ Branch of lateral cord = branch of musculocutaneous nerve
☐ ☐ Branches of posterior cord
☐ Branches of radial nerve

connective tissue prepared from dissections. The clinically-ascertained autonomic regions are much smaller. For the radial nerve, for example, the autonomic cutaneous field is confined to the back of the thumb or is completely absent.

The skin of the upper limb receives sensory innervation (Fig. **113**) at the **upper arm** from the:

– *superior lateral brachial cutaneous nerve* (from the axillary nerve) in the lateral region of the shoulder (above the deltoid) and an adjacent area of the skin on the dorsolateral side (over the proximal third of the long and the lateral heads of the triceps brachii),
– *inferior lateral brachial cutaneous nerve* (from the radial nerve) at the dorsolateral side in the middle and distal third of the upper arm (over the lateral head of the triceps brachii).
– *posterior brachial cutaneous nerve* (from the radial nerve) at the dorsal side in the distal half of the upper arm, and the
– *medial brachial cutaneous nerve* (from the medial cord, T1, 2) at the medial side of the axilla up to the elbow;

at the **forearm** from the:

– *posterior antebrachial cutaneous nerve* (from the radial nerve) in the elbow region and at the dorsal side of the forearm,
– *lateral antebrachial cutaneous nerve* (from the musculocutaneous nerve) at the lateral side, and the
– *medial antebrachial cutaneous nerve* (from the medial cord, C8, T1) at the medial side;

at the **dorsum of the hand** from the:

– *superficial ramus of the radial nerve* at the lateral side and (via the dorsal digital nerves) at the $2\frac{1}{2}$ radial fingers (up to the middle segment),
– *dorsal ramus of the ulnar nerve* at the medial side and (via dorsal digital nerves) at the $2\frac{1}{2}$ ulnar fingers (up to the middle segment),
– *median nerve* (via the proper palmar digital nerves) at the distal segment of the thumb and at the middle and terminal segments of the 2nd and 3rd fingers, as well as the radial side of the 4th finger, and the
– *superficial ramus of the ulnar nerve* (via proper palmar digital nerves) at the middle and end segments of the $1\frac{1}{2}$ ulnar fingers;

at the **palm of the hand** from the:

– *median nerve* at the thenar eminence (palmaris branch), at the lateral side of the palm and the $3\frac{1}{2}$ radial fingers, and the
– *ulnar nerve* (palmaris and superficial rami) at the hypothenar eminence, at the medial side of the palm and the $1\frac{1}{2}$ ulnar fingers.

Segmental innervation of the skin of the upper limb (dermatomes, Fig. **114**) cannot be demonstrated by the dissection of multisegmental cutaneous nerves, but can only be revealed through clinical findings (e.g. by severance of the posterior roots of individual spinal nerves). The anlage of the arm arises as a derivative of the ventrolateral body wall at the level of the lower cervical somites. The skin of the upper limb is the area of distribution of (fibers of the ventral rami of) segmental spinal nerves (C5-T2(3)). With the elongation of the limb during ontogenesis, the cutaneous segments (to a varying degree) are stretched in length and

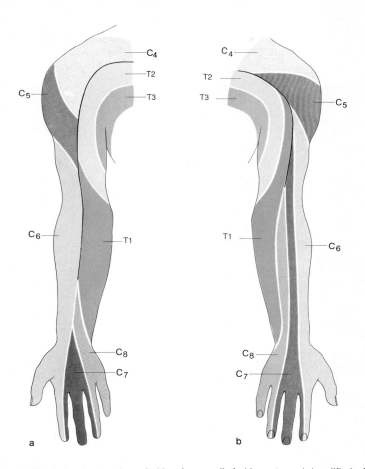

Fig. 114. **Segmental innervation of skin of upper limb** (dermatomes) (modified after *Hansen* and *Schliack*)
a Ventral side of arm
b Dorsal side of arm

drawn out into narrow bands. Thus, with the exception of T2 and T3, they are segmented off from the region of the body wall. Cutaneous segments C7 and C8 – corresponding to the middle of the limb anlage – reach the farthest distally (dividing line at about the 4th finger).

Segments C6 (thumb region, forearm and upper arm) and C5 (upper arm and shoulder) lie at the radial side of the arm, and segments T1 (forearm, upper arm), T2 (upper arm) and T3 (upper arm) at the ulnar side. The original metameric organization and the fundamental conformity with the belt-like arrangement of the cutaneous segments of the body wall become recognizable when the cutaneous segments are shown in color on a drawing of the abducted arm.

9. Lower Limb

The lower limb is the supporting column and the locomotor organ of the human body. The skeleton of the limb girdle, the *hipbone*, is inserted into the trunk wall and almost rigidly connected with the sacrum. Ventrally, both hipbones are fused at the *pubic symphysis* by fibrocartilage so that a closed osseous ring, the *bony pelvis*, is formed from the sacrum and both hipbones. It transfers the load of the trunk and the upper limbs on both sides to the free lower limbs, the legs.

Many textbook authors designate the "pelvic girdle" as the two hipbones – connected by a cartilaginous joint. In this interpretation our definition of pelvic girdle would correspond to half a girdle. Occasionally, both hipbones *and* the sacrum are defined as the "pelvic girdle", i.e. "pelvic girdle" and "bony pelvis" are synonymous. This definition is certainly not correct, for the sacrum is a segment of the axial skeleton and not a part of the lower limb.

Muscles of the pelvic girdle uniting the vertebral column and pelvic girdle are lacking; a movable sacro-iliac joint would be uneconomical to the highest degree. Movements of the pelvic girdle are possible only indirectly when the pertinent segment of the axial skeleton, the sacrum, is put into motion.

The place of movement between the trunk (+ pelvic girdle) and the free limb is the *hip joint*, which is a ball and socket joint like the shoulder joint.

The organization of the free lower limb corresponds to that of the free upper limb (→ p. 177). The leg skeleton consists of the *thigh bone* (femur), the two *leg bones* and the *skeletal elements of the foot*.

A. Pelvic Wall

1. Pelvic Girdle

a) Skeletal Elements of the Pelvic Girdle

The **skeleton of the pelvic girdle** is formed in the adult by a single large bone, the *hipbone*.

The **hipbone** (Figs. **115** and **117**) is formed by the synostosis of three individual bones, the cranially-situated *ilium*, the caudally-lying *ischium* and the ventrally-directed *pubis*. Up to about the 18th year of life, the three bones are still separated from one another by cartilaginous joints (Fig. **9**), which come together within the *socket of the hipbone (acetabulum)* to form the letter "Y".

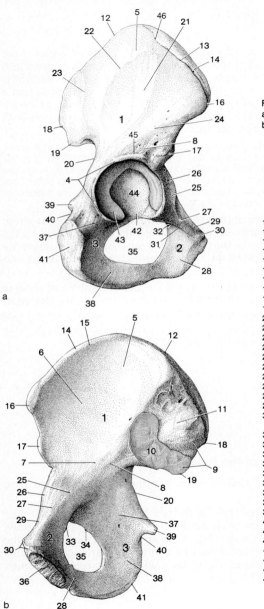

Fig. 115. **Hipbone**
a Lateral view (♀)
b Medial view (♂)

1 Ilium
2 Pubis
3 Ischium
4 Acetabulum
5 Ala (wing) of ilium
6 Iliac fossa
7 Arcuate line
8 Body of ilium
9 Sacropelvic surface
10 Auricular surface
11 Iliac tuberosity
12 Iliac crest
13 External lip of iliac crest
14 Intermediate line
15 Internal lip of iliac crest
16 Anterior superior iliac spine
17 Anterior inferior iliac spine
18 Posterior superior iliac spine
19 Posterior interior iliac spine
20 Greater sciatic notch
21 Gluteal surface
22 Anterior gluteal line
23 Posterior gluteal line
24 Inferior gluteal line
25 Body of pubis
26 Iliopubic eminence
27 Superior ramus of pubis
28 Inferior ramus of pubis
29 Pecten pubis (pectineal line)
30 Pubic tubercle and pubic crest
   (toward symphysis)
31 Obturator crest
32 Obturator sulcus
33 Anterior obturator tubercle
34 Posterior obturator tubercle
35 Obturator foramen
36 Symphysial surface
37 Body of ischium
38 Ramus of ischium
39 Ischial spine
40 Lesser sciatic notch
41 Ischial tuberosity
42 Acetabular notch
43 Lunate surface
44 Acetabular fossa
45 Supra-acetabular sulcus
46 Iliac tubercle

The **ilium** is distinguished by a large, flat bony plate directed cranially, the *ala (wing) of the ilium,* and a massive base, the *body,* whose caudal segment forms the upper sector of the acetabulum.

The slightly concave inner surface of the ala of the ilium, the *iliac fossa,* serves as the surface of origin of the iliacus muscle and contains the visceral centers dorsolaterally. Caudally, it is demarcated from the body of the ilium by a bony trabecula, the *arcuate line.* Dorsal to the iliac fossa the *sacropelvic surface* is situated. It bears the *auricular articular surface* for the sacro-iliac joint and dorsocranial to it the *iliac tuberosity* for the attachment of the sacro-iliac ligament. The field of origin of the gluteal muscles (Fig. **123**) is marked off on the external surface of the ala of the ilium (*gluteal surface*) by the *anterior* and *inferior gluteal lines,* both of which course more horizontally, and by the more vertically-directed *posterior gluteal line.*

The thickened cranial margin of the ala of the ilium is called the *iliac crest.* It ends ventrally at the *anterior superior iliac spine* (origin of the sartorius and tensor fasciae latae muscles, attachment of the inguinal ligament), which is palpable through the skin, and extends dorsally to the *posterior superior iliac spine.* The iliac crest has three bony lines: the *external lip* (outside, attachment of the external abdominal oblique muscle), the *intermediate line* (middle, origin of the internal abdominal oblique muscle) and the *internal lip* (inside, origin of the transversus abdominis muscle). At the external lip – about 5 cm posterior to the anterior superior iliac spine – a palpable bony prominence, the *iliac tubercle,* juts out where the anterior gluteal line reaches the iliac crest.

At the anterior margin of the ilium, a small notch marks off the *anterior inferior iliac spine* from the anterior superior iliac spine. The anterior inferior iliac spine serves as the place of origin of the rectus femoris muscle and the iliofemoral ligament. At the dorsal margin of the ala, the *posterior inferior iliac spine* lies caudal to the posterior superior iliac spine. The sacroiliac and sacrotuberous ligaments arise from both of these posterior spines. Caudal to the posterior inferior iliac spine, the posterior margin of the ilium and adjacent ischium is indented, producing the *greater sciatic notch,* the caudal margin of which is formed by the ischial spine.

The *body* of the **pubis** borders dorsocranially on the body of the ilium and dorsocaudally on the body of the ischium. It forms the ventral segment of the acetabulum. At the iliopubic border on the anterior margin of the hipbone, it forms the *iliopubic eminence* for the attachment of the iliopectineal arch.

The *superior ramus of the pubis* projects medially and somewhat ventrocaudally from the body of the pubis toward the region of the symphysis where it turns and becomes continuous with the *inferior ramus of the pubis*.

The superior margin of the superior ramus is drawn out into a sharp ventrocranially-directed pubic ridge, the *pecten pubis* (*pectineal line*), which ends at the *pubic tubercle* located lateral to the symphysis. From the pubic tubercle, the *pubic crest* passes as a narrow ridge medial to the symphysis. The inferior margin of the superior ramus sharpens into the *obturator crest*, which exhibits a sulcus, the *obturator groove* (bounded anteriorly and posteriorly by the *anterior* and *posterior obturator tubercles*).

The inferior ramus of the pubis passes laterocaudal to the *symphysial surface* and becomes continuous with the ramus of the ischium. The inferior pubic rami on both sides and the lower margin of the symphysis form the *pubic arch*. In females the enclosed arch is obtuse and rounded at the apex. In males the inferior rami of the pubes project more steeply downwards, the angle amounting to somewhat less than 90°. It is called, therefore, the *subpubic angle*.

The **ischium** participates in the structure of the acetabulum with its *body* and in the dorsocaudal boundary of the obturator foramen with its ramus. By means of a bony projection at the posterior margin of the ischial ramus, the *ischial spine*, the deeply-indented *greater sciatic notch* is separated from the shallow *lesser sciatic notch*, the caudal boundary of which represents the *ischial tuberosity*. This tuberosity lies at the apex of the arch formed by the ischial ramus and serves as the field of origin of the ischiocrural musculature. In a standing position, the ischial tuberosity is covered by caudal bundles of fibers of the gluteus maximus muscle. When the hip joint is flexed, these fiber tracts shift cranially so that in a sitting position the tuberosity is supported only by a subcutaneous fat pad.

The *obturator foramen* the "occluded hole", is framed by the bodies and rami of the pubis and ischium (Fig. **115**) and closed by the *obturator membrane* (Fig. **117**), the fibrous tracts of which course predominantly in a transverse direction. At its mediocranial circumference, it possesses a recess which, together with the obturator groove of the pubis, forms the *obturator canal* (place of passage of obturator vessels and nerves). The obturator externus muscle originates on the external surface of the membrane, and the obturator internus on the internal surface.

The **acetabulum** lies at the thickest part of the hipbone and exhibits a hemispherical cavity (Fig. **115 a**). The acetabulum receives the head of the femur and is formed by the bodies of all three bones which have combined into the hipbone. The well-developed bony, marginal elevation, the *acetabular rim*, is marked off from the body of the ilium by a sulcus, the *supra-acetabular groove*. At the caudal circumference, it is interrupted by the *acetabular notch* and replaced here by the *transverse acetabular* *ligament* (Figs. **9** and **123**), which closes the notch. Within the acetabular cavity there is only a marginally-situated, cartilage-covered, sickle-shaped band, the *lunate surface* of the acetabulum, with which the head of the femur articulates. The thin-walled central floor of the socket (*acetabular fossa*) is filled with adipose tissue and opens caudally into the acetabular notch.

Radiography. The acetabulum is markedly flat until the 5th year of life. Radiologists designate one or several radiologically-discernible, small bony shadows at the superior margin of the acetabulum as "acetabular bones", whereas anatomists use this term for one of three ossific centers in the synchondroses of the hipbone.

Ossification. The primary centers of ossification in the cartilaginous *hipbone* appear successively in the 3rd–7th fetal month in the ilium, ischium and pubis (Fig. **116**) and fuse at about the 6th–10th year of life – except for the Y-shaped synchondrosis in the acetabulum. Although bone formation has begun at the acetabulum at birth, it is only between the 10th and 13th year of life that three ossific centers, isolated at first, arise in the broad cartilaginous joint then synostose with one another and with the primary centers between ages 13 and 18. The epiphysial ossification of the iliac crest and the appearance of apophysial nuclei in the anterior inferior iliac spine and in the ischial tuberosity occur between the ages of 13 and 16. In the pubic tubercle and between the ischium and the inferior ramus of the pubis, apophysial ossific centers can be demonstrated between ages 16 and 20.

b) Connections of the Pelvic Girdle

In the *sacro-iliac joint* (Fig. **117**), the auricular surfaces of the sacrum and the ilium are in a rigid, virtually immovable union (amphiarthrosis).

The cartilaginous investment of the articular surfaces consists of fibrocartilage and, more deeply, hyaline cartilage; the surfaces are frequently interdigitated in a complicated way and are connected with each other by intra-articular fibers.

Ligaments. The *anterior sacro-iliac ligaments* cover the joint cavity on the ventral side. The powerful, short-fibered, *interosseous sacro-iliac ligaments* pass behind the joint from the sacral tuberosity to the iliac tuberosity. The *posterior sacro-iliac ligaments* follow dorsally with broad, short tracts coursing obliquely from the lateral part of the sacrum to the iliac tuberosity and to the posterior inferior iliac spine. Superficial, long bundles of fibers also pass steeply upward toward the posterior superior iliac spine.

Cranially, the *iliolumbar ligament* is attached at the sacro-iliac ligaments. It courses from the costal process of the 5th lumbar vertebra (i.e. from the rib rudiment homologous to the lateral part of the sacrum) to the iliac crest.

The shape of the articular surfaces and the powerful mass of fibers prevent any noteworthy movement at the sacro-iliac joint.

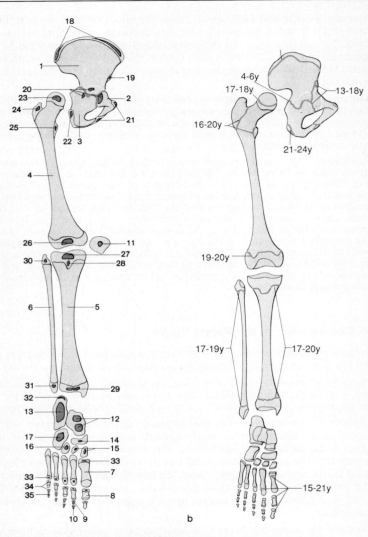

Fig. 116. Ossification of skeleton of lower limb (after *von Lanz-Wachsmuth*)
a Closure of epiphysial and apophysial synchondroses
b Time of appearance of centers of ossification
(EW . embryonic week, EM . embryonic month, M . postnatal month,
Y . postnatal year)

Only during pregnancy are the ligamentous bands loosened sufficiently to allow a slight tipping movement around a frontal axis, passively – not through active muscular effort. This movement can be stimulated by the so-called Walcher's position and effects a very slight expansion of the pelvic inlet.

Ligamentous connections between the sacrum and ischium (Fig. **117**). In the sacro-iliac union, the pressure exerted on the sacrum by the body weight is transferred to the hipbone. This occurs both directly across the articular surface of the sacro-iliac joint and indirectly across the sacro-iliac ligaments, by means of which the sacrum is suspended to some extent from the lateral parts of the pelvic girdle. Under the weight of the body, the sacrum has the tendency to be rotated around a frontal axis so that the promontory (anterior margin of the base of the sacrum) tips downward ventrocaudally, while the apex of the sacrum is moved outward from the pelvis dorsocranially. This movement is largely hindered by two strong ligamentous bands, the sacrospinous and sacrotuberous ligaments.

The *sacrospinous ligament* passes as a triangular fibrous plate from the lateral margin of the sacrum and the coccyx to the ischial spine and separates the greater sciatic foramen from the lesser.

The powerful *sacrotuberous ligament* possesses an extensive line of origin at the lateral margin of the sacrum and coccyx. Cranial bundles of fibers come from the posterior superior iliac spine. The ligament is attached to the ischial tuberosity and, together with the sacrospinous ligament,

◄ 1–10 *Onset of diaphysial ossification*
1 Ilium, 3 EM
2 Pubis, 6–7 EM
3 Ischium, 4–5 EM
4 Femur, 8 EW
5 Tibia, 7–8 EW
6 Fibula, 8 EW
7 Metatarsals I–V, 9 EW
8 Proximal phalanges, 5 EW
9 Middle phalanges, 8 EW
10 Distal phalanges, 9 EW
11–17 *Appearance of ossific centers in patella and tarsal bones*
11 Patella, 3–4 Y
12 Talus, 7 EM
13 Calcaneus, 5–6 EM
14 Navicular, 4 Y
15 Cuneiform I, II, 3–4 Y
16 Cuneiform III, 1 Y
17 Cuboid, 10 EM
18–35 *Appearance of epiphysial and apophysial ossific centers*

18 Iliac crest, 13–15 Y
19 Anterior inferior iliac spine, 16 Y
20 Acetabulum, 10–13 Y
21 Pubic tubercle, as well as between ischial ramus and inferior pubic ramus, 16–20 Y
22 Ischial tuberosity, 13–15 Y
23 Head of femur, 1 Y
24 Greater trochanter, 3–5 Y
25 Lesser trochanter, 9 Y
26 Distal epiphysis of femur, 10 EM
27 Proximal epiphysis of tibia, 10 EM
28 Tibial tuberosity, 1–13 Y
29 Distal epiphysis of tibia, 2 Y
30 Head of fibula, 4–6 Y
31 Lateral malleolus, 2 Y
32 Tuber calcanei, 9–11 Y
33 Epiphysis in metatarsal I (proximal), in metatarsals II–V (distal), 3–4 Y
34 Epiphyses in proximal and middle phalanges, 1–2 Y
35 Epiphyses in distal phalanges, 3–5 Y

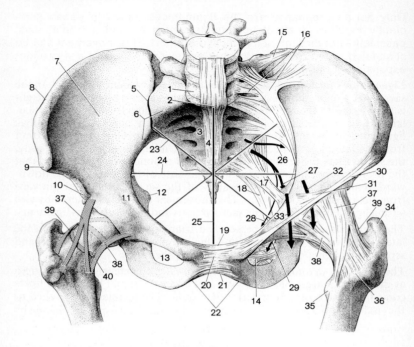

Fig. 117. **Bony female pelvis,** left side with ligaments, diameter of pelvic inlet, neurovascular passageways (arrows), **hip joint**

1 Fifth lumbar vertebra
2 Promontory
3 Pelvic surface of sacrum
4 Anterior longitudinal ligament
5 Sacroiliac joint
6 Linea terminalis
7 Iliac fossa
8 Iliac crest
9 Anterior superior iliac spine
10 Anterior inferior iliac spine
11 Iliopubic eminence
12 Ischial spine
13 Obturator foramen
14 Obturator membrane
15 Iliolumbar ligament
16 Anterior sacroiliac ligaments
17 Sacrospinous ligament
18 Sacrotuberous ligament
19 Superior pubic ligament
20 Interpubic disc
21 Arcuate pubic ligament
22 Pubic arch

23–25 Diameters of pelvic inlet
23 Oblique diameter
24 Transverse diameter
25 Conjugate diameter
26–29 *Neurovascular trunks* through
    suprapiriform division of greater sciatic
    foramen (26)
    infrapiriform division of greater sciatic
    foramen (27)
    lesser sciatic foramen (28)
    obturator canal (29)
30 Inguinal ligament
31 Iliopectineal arch
32 Arrow in muscular lacuna
33 Arrow in vascular lacuna
34 Greater trochanter
35 Lesser trochanter
36 Intertrochanter line
37 Iliofemoral ligament
38 Pubofemoral ligament
39 Ischiofemoral ligament
40 Zona orbicularis

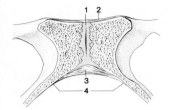

Fig. 118. **Frontal section through symphysis pubis of female pelvis**, ventral view
1 Interpubic disc
2 Superior pubic ligament
3 Arcuate pubic ligament
4 Pubic arch (>90°)

converts the greater sciatic notch into the *greater sciatic foramen* and the lesser sciatic notch into the *lesser sciatic foramen*.

The fiber tracts at the lower margin of the ligament continue medially into the *falciform process*, a marginal band of the fascia of the obturator internus muscle attached at the inner surface of the ischial ramus.

The piriformis muscle passes through the greater sciatic foramen from the pelvis and, in so doing, establishes slit-like openings (*suprapiriform* and *infrapiriform foramina*) for nerves and vessels. The obturator internus traverses the lesser sciatic foramen on the external side of the pelvis, while the pudendal nerve and internal pudendal vessels arrive again in the interior of the pelvis through this opening.

In the **pubic symphysis**, both pubic bones are united by the *interpubic disc* (Fig. **117** and **118**). In the adult, this disc consists almost exclusively of fibrocartilage; the hyaline cartilage which was originally present is preserved on each side only as a thin disc bordering directly on the bone.

An irregularly-formed cavity filled with synovial fluid appears in the disc after birth. At the upper and lower margins, the symphysial cartilage (broadened on the anterior surface) projects somewhat above the osseous boundary of the pubic symphysis.

The *superior pubic ligament* connects the upper margin of both pubic bones; the *arcuate pubic ligament* lines the pubic angle. Both strong ligaments are usually solidly fused with the periosteum of the bone and with the perichondrium of the symphysial cartilage.

In a standing position on both legs, the *symphysis* is stressed especially by traction and on one leg chiefly by shearing. In a sitting position, the stress on the symphysis varies according to the shape of the pelvis.

In the typical male pelvis, in which the distance between the ischial tuberosities is less than the distance between both sacroiliac joints, the symphysis is stressed in a sitting position especially by pressure. In the typical female pelvis, on the other hand, in which the interval between the ischial tuberosities is greater than the distance between the sacroiliac joints, it is stressed by traction.

The histological structure of the symphysis conforms to the diverse and alternating mechanical stresses. The cartilage absorbs compressive stresses, the transverse bundles of fibrils resist tension forces, and the oblique fiber bundles crossing the midline counter shearing forces.

2. Pelvis

The **skeleton of the pelvis** (Fig. 117) is a tripartite bony ring consisting of the two hipbones and the sacrum. The *greater pelvis* is formed by the two iliac alae, which enclose the visceral centers dorsally. The *lesser pelvis*, whose bony wall comprises all of the elements of the pelvic skeleton, circumscribes the *pelvic cavity*, in which the pelvic organs reside.

The boundary line (*linea terminalis*) separating the greater and lesser pelvis is composed of the promontory, the arcuate line and the pecten of the pubis. In the region of the hipbone, it corresponds to a strong osseous trabecula, the "main trabecula," which passes from the sacroiliac joint to the symphysis and in which the acetabulum is inserted on the external surface. It transfers to the head of the femur the pressure which the weight of the body exerts on the sacrum. The anterior part of the trabecula absorbs the tensions occurring in the symphysis. A bony frame is attached cranially and caudally at the main trabecula and is formed at the greater pelvis by a thickened margin of the ala of the ilium and at the lesser pelvis by the rami of the pubis and the ischium. The middle part of both framed constructions serves as an area of origin for muscles and is of slight importance for the stability of the pelvis.

In the center of the caudal part of the pelvis, the bone is completely reduced and replaced by the obturator membrane. The central part of the ala of the ilium consists of a thin bony plate, especially in the dorsal region. On its outer surface the abductors of the hip joint (gluteus medius and minimus) arise, which fix the pelvis during periods of single leg support and prevent it from tipping toward the side of the unsupporting leg. The enlargement and the position changes of its surface of origin, the ala of the ilium, represent a significant adaptation to man's erect gait.

Changes in the shape of the pelvic skeleton can also be caused in infants and children when they are not promptly treated for rickets, in which newly-formed osteoid is not sufficiently mineralized owing to a deficiency in vitamin D. Under the pressure of body weight on the sacrum and the counterpressure of the head of the femur on the acetabulum, the pelvis is flattened (flat, rachitic pelvis) or heart-shaped (e.g. in severe rickets, a condition seldom existing today). Since the deformations remain even after the disease is completely healed they can impede childbearing.

Pelvic canal (Fig. 119). At birth, the child's head must pass through the lesser pelvis of the mother. The pelvic canal (birth canal) forms a tube curved ventrally around the pubic symphysis and is broadest (pelvic width) at the level of the 3rd sacral vertebra. The *axis of the lesser pelvis* courses through the midpoint of the median diameter (*conjugate diameter*) of the pelvic inlet, the middle of the pelvis and the pelvic outlet

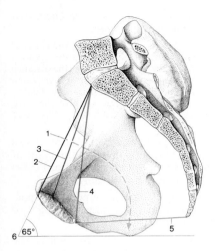

Fig. 119. **Axis and diameter of pelvis**, median section
1 Pelvic axis
2 Conjugate diameter of pelvic inlet ≈ 11.7 cm
3 True conjugate diameter ≈ 11 cm
4 Diagonal conjugate diameter ≈ 13 cm
5 Conjugate diameter of pelvic outlet ≈ 9 cm
6 Inclination of pelvis ≈ 55–75°

respectively. The *pelvic inlet* (*superior pelvic aperture*) is bordered by the linea terminalis. The plane of the pelvic inlet is inclined about 65° toward the horizontal plane when the body posture is in the "normal," erect position (*the inclination of the pelvis*). The pelvis, however, can be positioned considerably steeper or flatter without a change in body posture because the altered position of the pelvis can be compensated for by a corresponding increase or decrease in the lumbosacral angle. In a sitting position, the plane of the pelvic inlet is approximately horizontal. The *pelvic outlet* (*inferior pelvic aperture*) is bordered by the tip of the coccyx, the ischial tuberosity and the inferior ramus of the pubis.

Dimensions of the female pelvis (Fig. **119**). The birth canal exhibits the smallest sagittal diameter at the pelvic outlet between the tip of the coccyx and the posterior surface of the symphysis (conjugate diameter of the pelvic outlet, about 9 cm); however, the head of the child can push back the tip of the coccyx about 2.5 cm. Effectively, the narrowest point in the birth canal lies between the promontory and the posterior surface of the symphysis and is designated as the *true conjugate diameter*. Measured directly, of course, only in anatomical preparations, it amounts to an average of 11 cm in females (somewhat less in males). According to experience, it is about 1.5–2 cm less than the *diagonal conjugate diameter* (distance between the promontory and the lower margin of the symphysis) measurable in the living woman, which amounts to about 13 cm. The *transverse pelvic diameter* (Fig. **117**) is the greatest (about 13.5 cm); the *oblique diameter*, which connects the sacroiliac joint with the iliopubic eminence of the opposite side, measures about 12 to 12.5 cm. These two measurements cannot be determined in the living woman.

In obstetrics, a series of *external pelvic measurements* are known, e.g. the *external conjugate* (distance from the anterior surface of the symphysis to the spinous process of the 5th lumbar vertebra, about 20 cm), the *spinous distance* (the distance between the anterior superior iliac spines of both sides), the *distance of iliac crests*, etc. All of these distances can be measured in the living woman without difficulty. However, they do not provide any absolute certainty on the width of the birth canal since the measurements mentioned are not always sufficiently correlated with the dimensions of the lesser pelvis.

Sexual differences of the pelvis. In the typical adult, the bony pelvis exhibits characteristic sexual differences. The development of the shape of the female pelvis (as a prerequisite for uncomplicated parturition) takes place at the time of puberty under the influence of sex hormones.

The *pelvic inlet* in the sexually-mature female is more rounded or transversely oval. In the male, the promontory projects stronger ventrally so that the pelvic inlet exhibits a heart-shaped outline.

The *subpubic angle* in males amounts to maximally 90°. In females, the symphysis is lower, the pubic arch rounded like a bow, and the angle is greater than 90° (Figs. **117** and **118**).

At the *obturator foramen*, the greatest diameter in males is in the vertical direction; in females, the foramen is extended further in a transverse direction.

The *alae of the ilia* in females project farther laterally than in males, and the entire pelvis is relatively lower and wider.

The *interval between ischial tuberosities* is relatively less in males than in females.

In females, the *sacrum* is often absolutely, but always relatively, wider than in males. The transverse diameter of *Michaelis's rhomboid* (→ p. 498), i.e. the distance between the articular cavities of the sacroiliac joints, is therefore, in females not much smaller than the vertical diameter.

B. Hip

1. Hip Joint

a) Skeletal Elements of the Thigh

In the hip joint, the *hipbone* articulates with the *femur*.

The **femur** (Figs. **120 a** and **b**), the longest bone of the body, consists of a spherical *head*, a slender *neck*, a strong *shaft* and a distal extremity which bears two articular cartilages, the *medial* and *lateral condyles*.

The femur is a typical tubular bone, which plays an essential role in determining the height of the body. The *head* articulates in the acetabulum (Fig. **9**). On its cartilage-covered surface, somewhat distal to the middle of the axis of the shaft, there is a small pit (*fovea*), to which the ligament of the head of the femur is anchored. The neck of the femur forms an obtuse angle with the axis of the shaft called the *angle of inclination* (Fig. **121**). This term is not quite correct insofar as the neck also belongs to the diaphysis and the epiphysial joint lies between the head and the neck. In the newborn, the angle of inclination amounts to about 150°; in the infant, it still has an average value of over 140°, which diminishes from the age of 3 onward to approximately 125°.

When the angle of inclination exceeds the norm (138° and more), the condition is known as *coxa valga*; when the angle is below average (less than 120°), it is known as *coxa vara*.

The *femoral neck* – especially when supported by one leg – is strained on bending. The tensile pressures and stresses appearing during this phase of movement are taken up by the spongy trabeculae, which course in the direction of the tensile trajectories, as demonstrated in model experiments on homogeneous comparison bodies (Figs. **7a** and **b**).

In suitable sectioned preparations and radiograms of the proximal end of the femur, at least two spongy systems can be recognized (with the normal angle of inclination). One system ascends steeply from the medial cortex of the neck to the upper segment of the head of the femur (pressure absorption); the other courses in a bow from the lateral cortex of the shaft to the lower head region and, in so doing, crosses the spongy trabeculae of the first system almost at a right angle (traction bundles of the spongiosa). The rarified area of spongiosa enclosed in the pointed arch formed by the two trabecular systems appears in the radiogram (less shadow density) as Ward's triangle.

The tubular *shaft of the femur* consists of compact osseous tissue. It has a slightly convex curve anteriorly and on its posterior surface a longitudinal ridge, the *linea aspera*, which is divided into *lateral* and *medial lips*. It serves as a surface for the origin and insertion of muscles and, at the same time, increases the bearing strength of the femoral shaft since its transverse diameter broadens at the place where the greatest tensions caused by the curvature appear. Both lips of the linea aspera withdraw from one another at the upper and lower ends of the shaft. Distally, the *popliteal surface* situated above the femoral condyle lies between them. Proximally, the medial lip is turned onto the anterior side of the shaft and merges into the *intertrochanteric line* distal to the lesser trochanter. The lateral lip passes to the base of the greater trochanter and is raised to the *gluteal tuberosity* (occasionally also to a *third trochanter*), a roughness, at which a portion of the gluteus maximus inserts.

The *greater trochanter* sits laterocranially on the proximal end of the shaft (Fig. **117**). It provides a process at which several hip muscles attach. The *lesser trochanter*, at which the iliopsoas inserts, projects medially from the posterior surface of the shaft at the border of the body and neck. Both protuberances are connected on the posterior surface by the strong *intertrochanteric crest* and on the anterior surface by the intertrochanteric line. The *trochanteric fossa* (insertion of the obturators and gemelli muscles) is a depression in the medial surface of the greater trochanter. A short, narrow ridge, the *pectineal line*, at which the pectineus muscle attaches, passes distally from the lesser trochanter.

At the *distal extremity* of the femur, the more slender *medial condyle* is separated on the posterior surface from the broader *lateral condyle* by the deep *intercondylar fossa*, which is marked off from the popliteal surface by the *intercondylar line*. On the anterior surface, a cartilage-covered recession, the *patellar surface*, unites the cartilaginous articular surfaces of both condyles. The patella glides on it. The lateral guidance area of the patellar surface formed by the lateral condyle projects a bit more than the medial guidance region built by the medial condyle and counteracts the lateral traction component of the vastus lateralis muscle. The femoral condyles are more strongly curved in the posterior region than in their anterior segment. The lateral view of the outline of the condyle, which is nearly identical for both, therefore resembles a spiral line.

Proximal to the articular surface, a prominence projects outward from each condyle to form processes, the *lateral* and *medial epicondyles*, for the attachment of muscles and ligaments. A small protuberance above the medial epicondyle, the *adductor tubercle*, serves for the attachment of the "epicondylar" portion of the adductor magnus muscle.

If the femoral shaft is held perpendicularly, the medial condyle extends further distally. In the upright position, however, both articular condyles lie at the same height since the axis of the shaft is oblique and forms an obtuse angle with the axis of the tibia that opens laterally (frontal knee angle, Fig. **133 a**).

In the adult, the projection of the axis of the femoral neck on a horizontal plane forms an angle of about 12° with the transverse axis of the condyles, indicating the anteversion of the neck (Fig. **122**). Frequently referred to as

1 Head of femur	15 Medial lip of linea aspera
2 Fovea in head of femur	16 Popliteal surface
3 Neck of femur	17 Intercondylar line
4 Greater trochanter	18 Medial condyle
5 Trochanteric fossa	19 Adductor tubercle (attachment of adductor
6 Intertrochanteric line	magnus)
7 Intertrochanteric crest	20 Medial epicondyle
8 Lesser trochanter	21 Patellar surface
9 Body of femur	22 Intercondylar fossa
10 Gluteal tuberosity	23 Lateral condyle
11 Pectineal line	24 Lateral epicondyle
12 Nutrient foramen	25 Base of patella
13 Linea aspera	26 Apex of patella
14 Lateral lip of linea aspera	27 Articular surface of patella

▶

femoral torsion, which is not completely correct, the *anteversion* of the neck becomes more and more pronounced from the 4th fetal month onward. It attains its highest value after birth (34° on the average) and then retrogresses.

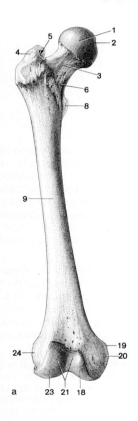

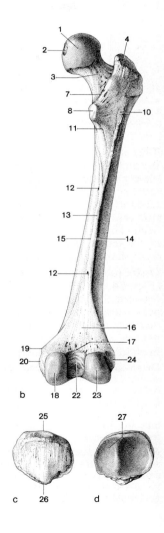

Fig. 120. **Skeletal elements of thigh**
a Femur, view from in front
b Femur, view from behind
c Patella, view from in front
d Patella, view from behind

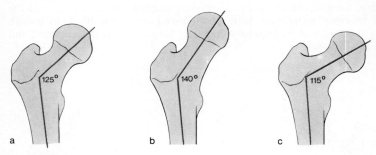

Fig. 121. **Angle of inclination in adults**
a Average value
b Coxa valga
c Coxa vara

The *knee cap* (*patella*, Figs. **120 c, d** and **139**) is embedded in the tendon of the quadriceps femoris muscle as a sesamoid bone. The triangular bony plate possesses a broad rounded *base* proximally and a blunt-edged, tapered *apex* distally, from which the distal extremity of the quadriceps tendon (*ligamentum patellae*) originates. On its cartilage-covered posterior *articular surface*, a guiding ridge marks off two slightly grooved fields. The larger area lies laterally and articulates with the lateral condyle of the femur. The patella prevents the tendon fibers of the quadriceps from sliding on the articular cartilage of the femur.

Ossification. The center of ossification of the distal epiphysis of the *femur* (Figs. **6 b** and **116**), from which the condyles and epicondyles ossify, arises between the 9th fetal month and the 2nd postnatal month. Since it is demonstrable in 95% of all newborn children, it is one of the *signs of maturity* and has forensic significance. The radiogram of this ossific nucleus is frequently used to clarify the diagnosis of growth disturbances in childhood or to evaluate the course of the disease, rickets.

Diaphysial ossification begins at the end of the 2nd embryonic month. It is not confined to the body of the femur, but also continues into the neck of the femur. The ossific center in the proximal epiphysis (femoral head) appears in the 2nd half of the 1st postnatal year; the epiphysial joint closes by the 18th year (somewhat earlier in girls, in boys somewhat later). The centers for the processes appear very late: 3rd–5th postnatal year in the greater trochanter, at about the 9th year in the lesser trochanter.

Epiphysial fractures at the proximal end of the femur can be observed in newborn children as a result of birth trauma. They can also appear in adolescence, however, in the form of a loosening of the synchondrosis, whereby the neck of the femur is slowly displaced toward the femoral head in the acetabulum.

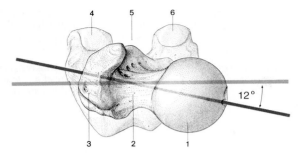

Fig. 122. **Anteversion of femoral neck**
(angle between axis of neck of femur and
horizontal axis of condyles, viewed from
above)
Axis of neck of femur ▬▬
Axis of frontally-placed condyles ▬▬

1 Head of femur	4 Lateral condyle
2 Neck of femur	5 Intercondylar fossa
3 Greater trochanter	6 Medial condyle

b) Capsule and Ligaments of the Hip Joint

The **hip joint** is a ball and socket joint with three degrees of freedom. Since, however, the articular head projects so deeply into the socket that the latter surrounds it beyond the equator, the hip joint is also referred to as a *spheroidal articulation*.

The *joint socket* (Figs. **9** and **123**) is formed by the acetabulum and the transverse ligament of the acetabulum and is completed by a ring-shaped, fibrocartilaginous *acetabular lip*. The lip is fastened to the margin of the socket, surrounds the spherical head of the femur beyond its equator, and forms an airtight seal for the articular cavity with its free margin. The head of the femur articulates only with the crescent-shaped, cartilage-covered lunate surface. It curves around the fat-lined acetabular fossa, in which the *ligament of the head of the femur* is embedded. This ligament arises at the margin of the base of the socket in the acetabular notch and at the transverse ligament. It is attached at the pit of the femoral head and carries branches from the acetabular ramus of the obturator artery or the medial circumflex femoral artery to the head of the femur. These small branches are often obliterated in old age.

The *joint capsule* is fixed at the osseous margin of the acetabulum and at the transverse ligament. In contrast to the shoulder joint, however, it is generally not attached at the lip. At the femur, the capsule attaches on the anterior side at the intertrochanteric line so that the anterior surface of the femoral neck lies completely within the capsule. On the posterior side, it remains about 1.5 cm from the intertrochanteric crest (the neck of the femur·is longer posteriorly than anteriorly). The epiphysial joint of the femoral head lies completely within the capsule.

In a fracture of the neck of the femur, the fracture line can course outside of the capsule posteriorly, whereas it must always lie within the capsule on the anterior side – as long as the fracture line does not pass into the shaft of the femur from the posterior side of the neck.

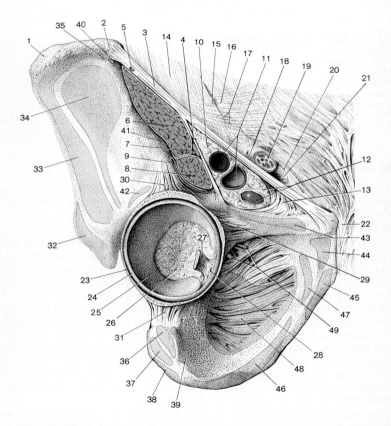

Fig. 123. **Muscular and vascular compartments between inguinal ligament and upper margin of pelvis**
External surface of hipbone and acetabulum, view from in front

Ligaments (Figs. **117** and **123**). In the fibrous layer of the wall of the joint capsule, powerful strengthening ligaments are inserted, which decisively influence the movement potential of the hip joint.

The *iliofemoral ligament*, one of the strongest ligaments of the human body, passes fan-shaped on the anterior side of the hip joint from the anterior inferior iliac spine to the intertrochanteric line. A lateral "transverse" band and a medial "longitudinal" band are especially pronounced and give the ligament the shape of an inverted "V". The iliofemoral ligament stretches during extension of the bone and permits only an insignificant retroversion of the femur. (Elevation of the back of the unsupporting leg is produced by a flexion in the hip joint of the supporting leg). In a standing position, the ligament prevents the pelvis from dropping backwards. The lateral band of the iliofemoral ligament hinders excessive external rotation and adduction; the medial band prevents internal rotation to a lesser degree.

The weaker *pubofemoral ligament* arises from the superior ramus of the pubis. Its fibers radiate into the medial band of the iliofemoral ligament, one portion reaching the intertrochanteric line. The ligament hinders the

◀ 1 Iliac crest
2 Anterior superior iliac spine
3 Inguinal ligament
4 Iliopectineal arch
5 Lateral femoral cutaneous nerve, can also pass underneath inguinal ligament via the muscular compartment
6–8 Contents of *muscular compartment*
6 Iliacus
7 Femoral nerve
8 Psoas major
9 Iliopectineal bursa
10–12 Contents of *vascular compartment*
10 Femoral branch of genitofemoral nerve
11 Femoral artery and vein
12 Femoral septum (closes femoral ring) and Rosenmüller's lymph node
13 Lacunar ligament, continues as pectineal ligament to pecten pubis
14 Aponeurosis of external oblique
15 Lateral crus ⎱ of external oblique
16 Medial crus ⎰
17 Intercrural fibers
18 Ilio-inguinal nerve
19 Spermatic cord (with ductus deferens, testicular artery, pampiniform plexus, cremaster muscle, among others)
20 Superficial inguinal ring
21 Reflected ligament
22 Fundiform ligament of penis

23 Articular capsule of hip joint, cut surface
24 Lip of acetabulum
25 Lunate surface
26 Adipose tissue in acetabular fossa
27 Ligament of head of femur
28 Transverse ligament of acetabulum
29 Pubofemoral ligament
30 Iliofemoral ligament
31 Ischiofemoral ligament
32–48 *Fields of muscle origin* for:
32 Gluteus maximus
33 Gluteus medius
34 Gluteus minimus
35 Tensor fasciae latae
36 Semimembranosus
37 Biceps femoris
38 Semitendinosus
39 Quadratus femoris
40 Sartorius
41 Rectus femoris, straight head
42 Rectus femoris, reflected head
43 Pectineus
44 Adductor longus
45 Gracilis
46 Adductor magnus
47 Adductor brevis
48 Obturator externus on obturator membrane and its bony margin
49 Obturator artery and vein, anterior and posterior branches of obturator nerve

excessive abduction of the thigh. The part of the femoral head which projects downward from the acetabulum during extreme abduction is braced against the pubofemoral ligament. In the abduction position, the pubofemoral ligament is also stretched during external rotation.

The *ischiofemoral ligament* is stronger than the pubofemoral ligament. It lies on the posterior surface of the joint capsule, arises from the ischium and courses spirally above the neck of the femur to the zona orbicularis and to the trochanteric fossa. Proximal fibers reach the "transverse" band of the iliofemoral ligament. The ligament hinders internal rotation and, together with the iliofemoral ligament, prevents a noteworthy retroversion at the hip joint.

The *zona orbicularis* (Figs. **9** and **117**) forms a fibrous ring which closely surrounds the neck of the femur at its thinnest site. Situated adjacent to the inner membrane of the joint, it is fused on its external surface with the spiral fibrous tracts of the three ligaments mentioned above. The head of the femur cannot leave the acetabulum so long as the zona orbicularis is intact and the joint capsule is not torn proximal to this circular elevation.

On the whole, the joint capsule exhibits four *weak spots* between the wall segments strengthened by the external ligaments and between the zona orbicularis and the base of the two trochanters, where it possesses an outpocketing comparable to the recessus sacciformis of the elbow joint.

Arterial supply of the hip joint. The blood supply of the joint capsule is provided by branches of the medial and lateral circumflex femoral arteries (Fig. **128**), as well as by delicate branches of the inferior gluteal artery in the dorsal region of the wall. The contribution of the obturator artery (via the acetabular branch) is variable and slight.

Innervation of the joint capsule. Branches of the femoral and obturator nerves run to the ventral side of the joint capsule, whereas branches of the sciatic nerve innervate the dorsal side.

When there is fluid accumulation in the articular cavity, the *relaxation position* of the hip joint is in slight flexion, abduction and external rotation of the femur (mid-position of the hip joint). In this position, the strengthening ligaments of the joint are uniformly relaxed.

Traumatic dislocations of the hip joint are relatively rare (5% of all luxations), since the strong ligaments secure the joint and the strong muscle covering furnishes active protection. Dislocations of the hip joint are due to heavy, traumatic forces on the femur, which cause the head to extrude from the socket. The luxation results from a force striking one of the weak areas of the capsule, depending on the direction – more often posteriorly than inferiorly or anteriorly. The capsule tears between the pubofemoral and ischiofemoral ligaments. The iliofemoral ligament is preserved and determines decisively the position of the femoral head and the leg after luxation. The pubofemoral ligament usually suffers an incomplete tear, and the ligament of the head of the femur a complete one.

When a child with a so-called *cogenital dislocation of the hip* first attempts to walk, the head of the femur moves from the incongruent and too flat acetabulum to the ala of the ilium without rupturing the capsule. In a walking posture, the pelvis can no longer be securely fixed by the abductors of the hip joint on the side of the supporting leg and drops down toward the side of the unsupported leg. With bilateral luxation, the so-called *waddling gait* is evident (Trendelenburg's sign).

Movement possibilities at the hip joint. In the utilization of all movement possibilities at the hip joint, the femur describes a cone, the base of which forms an oval which is only slightly asymmetrical. The long axis of this ellipse lies perpendicular when the body is erect, i.e. the extent of the flexion and extension movement is greater than the range of movement by abduction and adduction.

From the normal position (upright body posture, legs placed next to one another, feet at an angle of 45°, center of gravity of upper body and points of rotation of hip joints lie in a frontal plane), the movements possible at the hip joint in the principal planes are:
– *flexion* (anteversion, about 120°) or *extension* (retroversion, at most 15°) around a *frontal* axis:
– *abduction* (up to 45°) or *adduction* (up to 10°) around a sagittal axis; and
– *internal rotation* (about 35°) or *external rotation* (15°) around a "*longitudinal*" axis which passes through the midpoint of the hip and knee joints.

The *flexion potential* becomes less in the case of adduction and abduction of more than 20°. Extension movement increases in an abduction of up to about 40° and then amounts to 45°. In the untrained, the ischiocrural musculature (when the knee joint is extended) becomes prematurely passively insufficient; the possibility of active flexion at the hip joint is therefore essentially restricted when the knee is extended. Even when the knee joint is flexed, the thigh can be brought up to the trunk only passively or by utilization of momentum (active insufficiency of the flexor muscles of the hip joint).

The possibility of *abduction* is greatest when the hip joint is flexed to 60° and amounts then to almost 90°. The true transverse splits of course, is not possible. It is simulated by a compensatory lumbar lordosis when both legs are maximally abducted and the hip joint flexed. The maximal *adduction* can reach about 55° when the thigh is flexed.

When the hip joint is flexed, the extent of movement for *internal rotation* can be increased to 40°, and for *external rotation*, to 60°.

Movements of the pelvis can be carried out in the corresponding way when the leg is fixed. In a person standing on both legs, the pelvis can be inclined anteriorly or (to a slight degree) posteriorly. In a person standing on one leg, the pelvis can be tipped additionally inward or outward, as well as turned anteriorly or posteriorly.

In a person standing on both legs, the hips can be swung anteriorly or posteriorly, if the lower ankle joints work together with the hip joints.

Mucous bursae. In the vicinity of the hip joint there are several mucous bursae which underlie the tendons before their osseous insertions at the greater or lesser trochanter. Yet of these, only the *iliopectineal bursa* (Fig. **123**) occasionally communicates with the joint cavity. It lies on the joint capsule beneath the iliopubic eminence, between the medial band of the iliofemoral ligament and the pubofemoral ligament, and prevents friction between the capsule and the iliopsoas muscle passing over it.

c) Arrangement and Innervation of the Hip Musculature

The muscles of the hip surround the joint as a narrow, circularly-closed muscular mantle. They originate almost exclusively at the pelvis and attach chiefly at the proximal end of the femur. When the pelvis is fixed, they move the femur. When the femur is fixed, they act on the pelvis, which they either bring into a certain position or – a feature of special significance for the upright gait – hold in a certain position (phase of support by one leg).

The hip musculature is genetically autochthonous limb musculature. Transition muscles, as they have so strongly evolved in the border region of the trunk and upper limb, are absent; the firm anchorage of the vertebral column in the closed pelvic ring permits no movement of the pelvic girdle against the axial skeleton. While the genetic arrangement into extensor and flexor groups at the thigh and leg can be realized relatively simply, however, a corresponding division of the hip muscles is difficult. Since only the iliopsoas muscle arises from a primary blastema situated within the pelvis and since the adductors innervated by the obturator nerve occupy a special position because of their innervation and their location between the extensors and flexors in the thigh, it appears most appropriate to organize the muscles of the hip joint according to a topographical point of view. The following groups are thus distinguishable: *inner hip muscles, outer hip muscles* and *muscles of the adductor group.*

Depending upon the course of the muscles (or their active terminal extensions) with respect to the three main axes, we can distinguish flexors and extensors, abductors and adductors, and internal and external rotators. This character- ization is valid, however, only for an exactly marked position of the joint; for during the course of a movement, more and more fiber bundles of a muscle can wander across a fixed axis of movement and, in so doing, reverse its action on the joint. In addition, such a classification does not take into account that parts of the same muscle can have an antagonistic effect on each other. It also neglects the fact that the muscles, for example, designated as abductors can simultaneously take part in movements around the other two main axes of the joint.

Inner Hip Muscles

The **iliopsoas** (Figs. **124** and **126**) consists of two parts. The medial part (*psoas major*: long fibers, great lift) arises with a deep layer from the lateral surfaces of the 12th thoracic and first four lumbar vertebrae and with a superficial portion of origin from the costal processes of all lumbar vertebrae. (Between the two portions a large part of the lumbar plexus is located). The lateral part of the iliopsoas (*iliacus*: large number of fibers, therefore, large power component) fills up the iliac fossa. An extrapelvic head arises from the capsule of the hip joint (capsule tensor). The undivided terminal tendon of the iliopsoas inserts at the lesser trochanter.

The psoas major and the iliacus leave the pelvis together through the *muscular lacuna* (with the femoral nerve, Fig. **123**). They curve around the neck of the femur medially and are separated from the joint capsule by the *iliopectineal bursa*, which occasionally communicates with the joint cavity. Frequently, another mucous bursa, the *subtendinous iliac bursa*, is found between the tendon of insertion and the lesser trochanter. The thin psoas fascia in the cranial region becomes stronger caudally and, together with the firm iliac fascia (Fig. **205**), which is strongly fused with the lateral portion of the inguinal ligament, forms a rigid connective tissue covering for the muscle up to its insertion.

Innervation: branches of the lumbar plexus and femoral nerve.

A third inner muscle, the *psoas minor* (Fig. **124**), is inconstant in humans. It arises from the 12th thoracic and 1st lumbar vertebrae. Its long tendon passes caudally on the psoas major and radiates into the iliopsoas fascia, specifically into the iliopectineal arch.

Innervation: branches of the lumbar plexus.

The *pectineus* arises from the same blastema as the iliopsoas. On account of its close functional affiliation with the adductor group, this muscle is discussed with them.

Outer Hip Muscles

The external muscles of the hip form a stratified muscular compartment which covers over the hip joint from the side, from in front and from behind. From an extensive field of origin, the muscle tracts converge at the outer and inner surfaces of the pelvis to a relatively limited area of insertion at the femur, especially in the region of the greater trochanter.

During ontogenesis, the piriformis and obturator internus have pushed their origin forward to the anterior side of the sacrum and to the inner surface of the obturator membrane and its osseous perimeter.

Like the gluteus medius and minimus (small muscles of the buttocks), the **gluteus maximus**, the large muscle of the buttocks (Figs. **123** and **125**), belongs genetically to the extensor group. It originates at the sacrococcygeal margin, from the iliac crest posterior to the posterior gluteal line, from the thoracolumbar fascia and especially from the sacrotuberous ligament. The thick bundles of fibers coursing obliquely downward merge

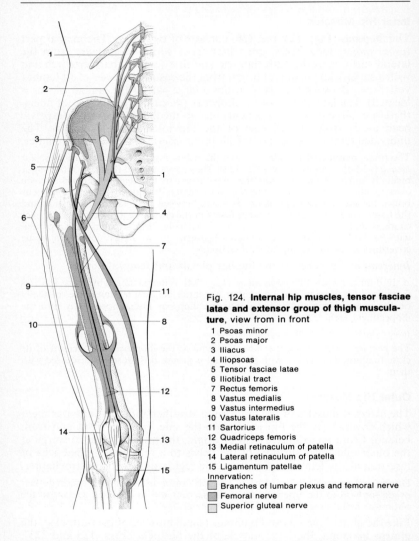

Fig. 124. **Internal hip muscles, tensor fasciae latae and extensor group of thigh musculature**, view from in front
1 Psoas minor
2 Psoas major
3 Iliacus
4 Iliopsoas
5 Tensor fasciae latae
6 Iliotibial tract
7 Rectus femoris
8 Vastus medialis
9 Vastus intermedius
10 Vastus lateralis
11 Sartorius
12 Quadriceps femoris
13 Medial retinaculum of patella
14 Lateral retinaculum of patella
15 Ligamentum patellae
Innervation:
☐ Branches of lumbar plexus and femoral nerve
▨ Femoral nerve
☐ Superior gluteal nerve

into a broad terminal tendon, which radiates proximally into the fascia lata and the iliotibial tract and inserts at the lateral lip of the linea aspera distal to the gluteal tuberosity and above the lateral intermuscular septum.

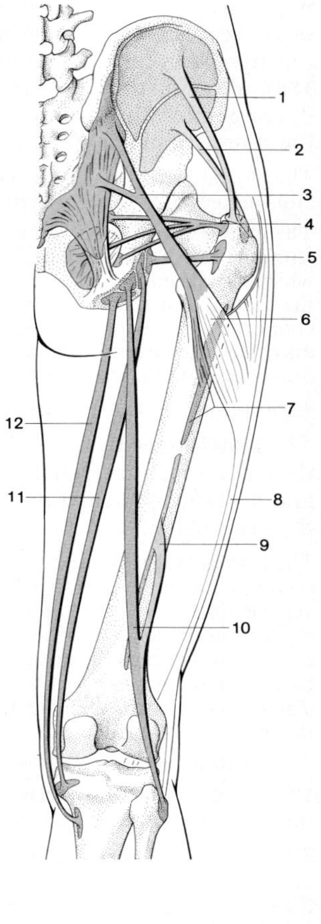

Fig. 125. **External hip muscles and flexor group of thigh musculature**, view from behind (Tensor fasciae latae → Fig. 124, Piriformis → Fig. 127)

1 Gluteus medius
2 Gluteus minimus
3 Gluteus maximus
4 Obturator internus + gemelli
5 Quadratus femoris
6 Tendon of attachment of gluteus maximus to iliotibial tract
7 Tendon of attachment of gluteus maximus to gluteal tuberosity
8 Iliotibial tract
9 Short head ⎫
10 Long head ⎬ of biceps femoris
11 Semimembranosus
12 Semitendinosus

Innervation:
▢ Superior gluteal nerve
▨ Inferior gluteal nerve
▩ Tibial portion of sciatic nerve
▢ Peroneal portion of sciatic nerve

The *ischial bursa* (Fig. **130**) lies between the ischial tuberosities and the fascia at the inferior surface of the gluteus maximus. As a result of chronic irritation (weaver's knot, miner's knot), it can become inflamed in people, who must sit on unpadded surfaces at work. The inflamed bursa then presses on the posterior femoral cutaneous nerve.

The terminal tendon of the gluteus maximus is separated from the greater trochanter by the *trochanteric bursa*. At the gluteal tuberosity, it usually glides over several *intermuscular bursae* between the other gluteal muscles (Fig. **130**).

In a standing position, the muscle covers the ischial tuberosity with its caudal portion. When the thigh is flexed, the lower margin of the gluteus maximus is pushed cranialwards so that in a sitting position the tuberosity lies directly on the subcutaneous fat pad and can be palpated through the skin. The *gluteal furrow* coursing almost horizontally (Fig. **188**), which distinctly indents during contraction of the gluteus maximus, does not mark the lower margin of the muscle, but crosses the direction of the muscle bundles at an acute angle.

The gluteal furrow forms the boundary line between the *gluteal region* (proximal) and the *posterior femoral region* (distal).

The gluteal furrow corresponds to the fibers coursing bow-like in the fascia lata from the region of the ischial tuberosities to the greater trochanter. These fibers, which have been formed as a result of muscular and fascial tension at the border of the gluteal and thigh regions, are designated as a *seat halter*. From them short connective tissue fibers pass to the skin. During contraction of the gluteus maximus, they transfer the fascial tension to the skin so that the gluteal furrow is drawn in. The buttocks protrude cranial to them.

Innervation: inferior gluteal nerve.

The **gluteus medius** (Figs. **123** and **125**) arises on the external surface of the ala of the ilium from a field bordered by the iliac crest and the anterior and posterior gluteal lines. It inserts at the external surface of the apex of the greater trochanter.

The fiber bundles of the muscle, which appears triangular when viewed laterally, converge to the greater trochanter. In the process, the tracts coming from the ventral side cross over the posterior muscle bundle before they merge into the short terminal tendon. Mucous bursae (*trochanteric bursae of the gluteus medius*) are present between the muscle and bone (Fig. **130**). The gluteus medius is covered by the fascia lata, from whose undersurface the fiber bundles of the muscle arise. The posterior portion of the muscle lies underneath the anterior marginal part of the gluteus maximus.

The **gluteus minimus** (Figs. **123**, **125** and **130**) arises from the external surface of the ilium between the anterior and inferior gluteal lines. It inserts at the lateral edge of the anterior surface of the greater trochanter.

The gluteus minimus is almost completely covered by the gluteus medius. Both muscles are fused at their anterior margin and form a pouch which is open toward the back. The *trochanteric bursa of the gluteus minimus lies* between the tendon of insertion and the apex of the trochanter.

Innervation of both muscles: superior gluteal nerve.

The nerve leaves the suprapiriform division of the greater sciatic foramen on the surface of the gluteus minimus and ramifies at both muscles.

The gluteus medius and minimus originate from the same blastema, from which the tensor fasciae latae muscle also arises. They are contrasted with the gluteus maximus as the *small gluteal muscles* and form the "abductor group" of the hip musculature since they – except in the case of a strongly flexed thigh – abduct at the hip joint. Far more significant than the movement of the thigh, however, is their action on the pelvis with regard to the supporting leg when walking or in one-legged standing. They prevent the pelvis on the side of the unsupported leg from sinking down (and incline it slightly toward the supporting leg side).

The **tensor fasciae latae**, a flat, parallel-fibered muscle, arises lateral to the anterior superior iliac spine and inserts at the fascia lata (Figs. **123**, **124** and **129**).

At its origin, it still preserves the original connection with the gluteus medius. In the fascia lata, its tendon fibers form a part of the iliotibial tract. In it, they can be followed to the lateral condyle of the tibia and to the head of the fibula. They reach the femur via the lateral intermuscular septum and radiate into the lateral patellar retinaculum.

Innervation: superior gluteal nerve.

The nerve branch proceeds from a muscular branch to (or in) the gluteus minimus and passes downward to the lower surface of the tensor fasciae latae.

The **iliotibial tract** (Figs. **124**, **125**, **129** and **132**), as a broad strengthening layer of the fascia of the thigh (fascia lata), passes along the lateral circumference of the fascia from the iliac crest across the hip and knee joint to the lateral condyle of the tibia. It arises from tendinous fibers of the tensor fasciae latae, the gluteus maximus and the aponeurotic fascia of the gluteus medius and attaches – aside from at the tibia – at the femur via the lateral intermuscular septum; it dispatches fibers to the head of the fibula and to the lateral patellar retinaculum. The iliotibial tract represents a traction belt of the femur. In the supported leg period, the body weight tries to bend the femur into a medially concave curve. The tension of the iliotibial tract produces a tendency to bend in the opposite direction so that the resulting compressive stresses (medial) and especially the tensile stresses (lateral) are decisively reduced. The contraction of the gluteus medius, which prevents the dropping of the pelvis, simultaneously tenses the tract so that the releasing action of the traction belt sets in synchronously with the increased burden on the supporting leg.

The **piriformis** (Fig. **126** and **127**) arises at the pelvic fascia of the sacrum (lateral to the anterior sacral foramina and between their openings) and at the capsule of the sacro-iliac joint, with several fiber bundles also derived from the upper margin of the greater sciatic notch. It passes through the greater sciatic foramen, which it divides into suprapiriform and infrapiriform portions (Fig. **130**), to the external surface of the pelvis and courses – covered by the gluteus maximus – to the inner side of the apex of the greater trochanter.

From its extensive surface of origin, the muscle tapers down continuously, and the narrow terminal tendon is usually separated from the capsule of the hip joint by a *bursa*.

Innervation: nerve to the piriformis from the sacral plexus.

The **obturator internus** and the two **gemelli muscles** form a genetic unit.

The *obturator internus* (Figs. **125**, **126** and **130**) has pushed its origin forward into the intrapelvic space on the obturator membrane and the osseous frame bordering it. It passes externally at an acute angle around the margin (cartilage-covered at this site) of the lesser sciatic foramen, which serves as a fulcrum and is protected by the *bursa of the obturator internus*. With its extrapelvic part, it covers the two deep heads of the tripartite muscle, the gemelli, more or less extensively. The *superior gemellus* comes from the ischial spine, the *inferior gemellus* from the ischial tuberosity (Figs. **125** and **130**). The terminal tendon of the obturator internus, at whose upper and lower margins both gemelli attach, is inserted into the trochanteric fossa.

The endopelvic part of the obturator internus is covered by the firm *obturator fascia* (Fig. **126**), which gives rise to the tendon fibers of the levator ani muscle.

The fascia can be strengthened at the origin of these fibers by a tendon-like fascial band (*tendinous arch of the levator ani*), which follows a curved course. The portion of the obturator internus situated above this muscle origin forms the muscular wall of the lesser pelvis, its fascia being a part of the parietal pelvic fascia. Caudal to this, muscle and obturator fascia delimit laterally the connective tissue space beneath the pelvic floor, the *ischio-anal fossa* (→ vol. 2).

Innervation: internal obturator nerve, occasionally (though rarely exclusively) also pudendal or sciatic nerves.

The inferior gluteal nerve ramifies directly after exiting from the infrapiriform division of the greater sciatic foramen.

The **quadratus femoris** (Figs. **123**, **125** and **130**) is a predominantly fleshy muscle, which is rectangular in shape when the femur is in its normal

1 Iliacus
2 Psoas major
3 Piriformis
4 Obturator internus
5 Levator ani (severed)
6 Coccygeus
7 Tendinous arch of levator ani
8 Tendinous fiber tracts of obturator fascia which radiate into tendon of origin of levator ani
9 Arcuate line (sheath of rectus abdominis)
10 Linea alba
11 Rectus abdominis
12 Transversus abdominis
13 Abdominal aorta
14 Median sacral artery
15 Common iliac artery
16 External iliac artery
17 Internal iliac artery
18 Iliolumbar artery

19 Superior gluteal artery
20 Lateral sacral artery
21 Obturator artery and nerve
22 Pubic branch of obturator artery (unites with pubic branch of inferior epigastric artery)
23 Inferior gluteal artery
24 Internal pudendal artery and pudendal nerve in pudendal canal
25 Pubic branch of inferior epigastric artery
26 Inferior epigastric artery
27 Deep circumflex iliac artery
28 Inguinal ligament and iliopectineal arch
29 Lateral femoral cutaneous nerve
30 Genitofemoral nerve
31 Sacral plexus
32 Sympathetic trunk
33 Ureter
34 Ductus deferens and artery of ductus deferens

position; it passes in a transverse direction from the ischial tuberosity to the intertrochanteric crest. In spite of its moderate size, the muscle is an effective external rotator of the hip joint since almost all of its muscular power is available for rotation because of the favorable course direction of its fibers.

Innervation: nerve to quadratus femoris, occasionally additionally, or exclusively, via the tibialis portion of the sciatic nerve.

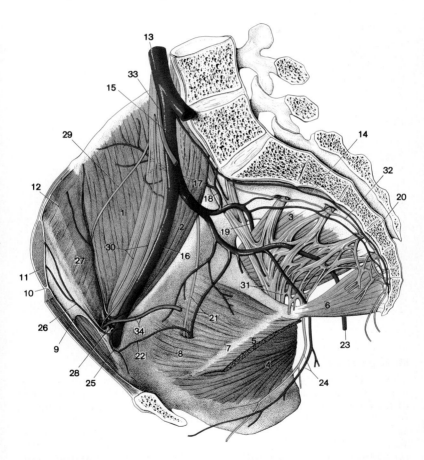

Fig. 126. **Muscles, arteries and nerves in wall and floor of male pelvis**, medial view of sagittal section

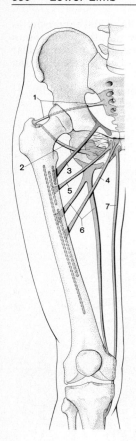

Fig. 127. **Adductor group**, view from in front
1 Piriformis
2 Obturator externus
3 Pectineus
4 Adductor longus
5 Adductor brevis
6 Adductor magnus
7 Gracilis
Innervation:
☐ Obturator nerve
■ Femoral nerve and anterior ramus of obturator nerve
☐ Nerve to the piriformis from the sacral plexus

Muscles of the Adductor Group and the Pectineus

The muscles of the adductor group fill the space contoured in the shape of a triangle when viewed anteriorly. This space is bordered by the inner side of the femur, the anterior surface of the lesser pelvis and a line running from the ischial tuberosity to the medial epicondyle of the femur. All of these muscles are capable of adducting the thigh. Of more practical significance, however, is their action on the position of the pelvis. Since the adductors are arranged with a part of their muscle mass in front of the axis of flexion and the greater portion behind it, they can balance the pelvis on the supporting leg or, in the bipedal position, on both femoral heads — together with the small gluteal muscles.

The obturator externus attaches at the obturator membrane, while all the remaining muscles of the adductor group derive in the form of a semicircle from the osseous margin of the obturator foramen (Fig. 123). With the exception of the gracilis, they are all single-jointed and insert at the femur.

The **obturator externus** (Fig. 123 and 127) arises at the external surface of the obturator membrane and the mediocaudal circumference of its bony margin. Coming ventrally and medially, it turns around the femoral neck and head on the dorsal surface of the hip joint before its conically-shaped terminal tendon finally passes ventrolaterally to the trochanteric fossa.

The muscle lies very hidden: it is covered anteriorly by the adductor longus, adductor brevis and iliopsoas, and posteriorly by the obturator internus, gemellus inferior and quadratus femoris.

Innervation: obturator nerve.

The muscular branch separates from the trunk of the obturator nerve in front of the entrance into the obturator canal and courses through the canal with it (or with the anterior and posterior rami of this nerve).

The **adductor longus** (Figs. 123, 127, 129 and 132) originates with a long tendon from a small area of the pubis below the pubic crest and from the fibrocartilage of the pubic symphysis. It widens distally and inserts with a thin, broad tendon at the middle third of the linea aspera (medial lip).

Distal marginal bundles of the tendon of insertion participate to a varying degree in the structure of the vasto-adductor membrane and border the entrance to the adductor canal.

Innervation: anterior ramus of the obturator nerve.

The **adductor brevis** (Figs. 123, 127 and 130), which arises from the anterior surface of the inferior ramus of the pubis between the obturator externus and gracilis, is almost completely covered by the pectineus and adductor longus and attaches at the medial lip of the linea aspera proximal to the insertion of the adductor longus.

Innervation: anterior ramus of the obturator nerve.

The **adductor magnus** (Figs. 123, 127, 129 and 132) is the strongest muscle of the adductor group and one of the largest muscles of the human body. It arises – dorsal to the other adductors – from the inferior ramus of the pubis and the adjacent portion of the ischial ramus up to the ischial tuberosity. The muscular portion emanating from the ischial tuberosity attaches with a strong tendon at the adductor tubercle in the vicinity of the medial epicondyle of the femur, while the remaining bundles of fibers have predominantly fleshy insertions at the medial lip of the linea aspera.

Innervation: posterior ramus of the obturator nerve; the muscular portion attaching at the adductor tubercle is additionally supplied by the sciatic nerve (tibialis portion).

Adductor canal. The two insertions of the adductor magnus and the femur border an elongated opening, the *hiatus tendineus* (*adductor hiatus*). Together with the vastus medialis and the vasto-adductor membrane, it forms the *adductor canal* through which the femoral vessels arrive at the popliteal space (Fig. **129**). The vasto-adductor membrane represents an aponeurotic intermediate tendon between the adductor magnus and the adductor longus on one side, and the vastus medialis on the other. It is formed from tendinous fibers which are derived both from the muscular portion inserting at the linea aspera and from the part of the adductor magnus attaching at the adductor tubercle and is completed in the proximal segment by distal marginal fibers of the adductor longus.

The **gracilis** (Figs. **123**, **127**, **129** and **132**) is the only two jointed muscle of the adductor group. It arises with a thin, flat tendon from the medial edge of the inferior ramus of the pubis, directly distal to the symphysis, courses with parallel bundles of fibers at the medial surface of the thigh and ends in a long terminal tendon in the distal third of the femur. It passes behind the medial condyle of the femur distally and attaches via the pes anserinus (Fig. **142**) at the medial surface of the tibia, posterior to the tibial tuberosity, and at the deep fascia of the leg.

Innervation: anterior ramus of the obturator nerve.

The **pectineus** (Figs. **123**, **127** and **129**) originates from the superior ramus of the pubis between the iliopubic eminence and the pubic tubercle and inserts at the pectineal line of the femur.

The muscle is derived primarily from the blastema of the iliopsoas group. The contribution of the adductor group to the construction of the muscle varies individually.

The pectineus is covered by the pectineal fascia, a caudal continuation of the iliac fascia, and, together with the iliopsoas, delimits a depression, the iliopectineal fossa, in which the femoral vessels course.

Innervation: regularly by the femoral nerve, additionally by a variable branch from the anterior ramus of the obturator nerve.

d) Action of Muscles and Muscle Groups on the Hip Joint

As at the shoulder joint, parts of several muscles always cooperate at the hip joint as synergists, whereby effective movement is decisively influenced by the antagonists. In addition, the hip joint is especially susceptible to the effects of centrifugal force and the force of gravity since this joint has a fairly large dead muscular space; this means that the range of joint movement in large part (up to 30% in the case of flexion) cannot be utilized during active muscular contraction (Fig. **17 c**). Decisive for the function of a muscle in a certain phase of movement or from a certain position, as in any ball-and-socket joint, is the position of the joint in each case, since not only the torque, but, in the case of many muscles or parts of muscles, also the direction of the pull depends upon it. The piriformis, for example, is an external rotator in its normal position; it rotates internally, however, when the femur is flexed above the horizontal plane.

The extensor muscles carry out the most important task at the hip joint. They must raise the total body mass in climbing stairs, whereas in walking the weaker flexors (considered absolutely) must swing forward only the much lighter mass of the leg which bears no weight. The torque of the abductors and especially of the adductors is also quite great (fixation of the pelvis in the supporting leg period). The torque of the rotators is distinctly less, with that of the external rotators of the hip joint exceeding that of the internal rotators.

At the hip joint the thigh is:

–*flexed* by the iliopsoas, rectus femoris and tensor fasciae latae,

whereby the sartorius and pectineus, as well as the ventral parts of the small gluteal muscles collaborate (and the abductors can join in the flexion of the **femur** from the extended position to the standard position);

– *extended* by the gluteus maximus, the ischiocrural muscles (especially by the semimembranosus) and the posterior fiber bundles of the small gluteal muscles,

whereas the action of extension by the piriformis and obturator internus is slight, and the obturator externus, quadratus femoris and (especially powerful) the dorsal part of the adductor magnus can bring the flexed **femur** to the standard position;

– *abducted* particularly by the small gluteal muscles, the tensor fasciae latae (when the knee is extended), the cranial fiber bundles of the gluteus maximus (attached at the iliotibial tract) and (when the knee is flexed) by the rectus femoris,

whereby the piriformis and sartorius cooperate to a slight degree;

– *adducted* by the muscles of the adductor group (most effectively by the adductor magnus) and the pectineus, the caudal fiber tracts of the gluteus maximus (attached at the femur), the iliopsoas and semimembranosus,

whereas the obturator internus (when the hip joint is extended), quadratus femoris, semitendinosus and long head of the biceps have only an auxiliary function;

– *rotated internally* by the ventral portions of the small gluteal muscles, the tensor fasciae latae, the adductor magnus and the adductor longus (via the fiber tracts of the vasto-adductor membrane),

the iliopsoas also assisting as a weak internal rotator from the normal position (when the femoral neck is anteverted by $12°$); and

– *rotated externally* by the gluteus maximus and the dorsal parts of the small gluteal muscles, the adductor magnus, obturator internus, piriformis (when the hip is extended) and quadratus femoris,

whereby the remaining muscles of the adductor group and the pectineus can act as auxiliary muscles – from extreme internal rotation also the iliopsoas, from the standard position the sartorius, rectus femoris and the long head of the biceps.

In walking, the *iliopsoas* throws the **femur** of the unsupporting leg forward and thus influences the length of the step. When the leg is fixed and contraction is bilateral, it inclines the pelvis and lumbar vertebral column anteriorly (flexion of the lumbar vertebral column and the hip joint against resistance, raising of the trunk from the horizontal dorsal position). When the contraction is one-sided, it draws the lumbar vertebral column laterally.

The *gluteus maximus* prevents the pelvis and, thus, also the trunk from tipping anteriorly when the center of gravity lies in front of the axis of rotation of the hip joint. In a relaxed standing position, the muscle is also relaxed. It contracts immediately, as soon as the center of gravity moves ventrally above the axis of flexion of the hip joint.

Through bilateral contraction, the gluteus maximus is able to move the pelvis forward immediately. When the hip joints are fixed, the large, stretched gluteal muscles press toward the anal furrow and complement the closing mechanism of the anus.

In a standing position on one leg, the *small gluteal muscles* hold the pelvis firmly and prevent it from sinking down on the side of the unsupported leg. Together with the muscles of the adductor group, they carry out the fine balancing of the pelvis on the heads of both femora.

The *tensor fasciae latae* is often especially strongly developed in sprinters ("sprinter's muscle"). When the leg is fixed, it inclines the pelvis anteriorly, whereas the *piriformis* turns the pelvis so that the hip is carried posteriorly on the side of the unsupported leg.

Capsule tensor. From the innermost layer of the muscular mantle that surrounds the hip joint, tendinous fibers radiate into the joint capsule and act as a capsule tensor (cranial: gluteus minimus; dorsal: obturator internus and quadratus femoris). On the ventral side, fibers of the iliacus and rectus femoris arise at the joint capsule.

Paralyses. In the case of *failure* of the *iliopsoas*, the thigh cannot be lifted above the horizontal plane from a sitting position. Walking is extraordinarily difficult, and a long stride is no longer possible.

With a *paralysis of the gluteus maximus*, all powerful movements of extension (walking on an uneven floor, jumping, standing up from a sitting or squatting position, climbing stairs, climbing, etc.) can no longer be executed. External rotation is possible only to a limited degree. If the *small gluteal muscles* are paralyzed or if the head of the femur and, with it, the great trochanter are displaced proximally in a "congenital" luxation of the hip joint so that the muscular contraction remains ineffective, the pelvis sags toward the side of the unsupported leg (Trendelenburg's sign). When both sides lack "abductors", the typical waddle occurs. If the *tensor fasciae latae* is also paralyzed owing to the severance of the superior gluteal nerve, the thigh is distinctly rotated toward the outside in walking.

Even with a complete severance of the obturator nerve, the *adductors* are not always completely paralyzed (innervation of the pectineus from the femoral nerve and of the adductor magnus from the sciatic nerve). Usually, however, the abductors predominate to such an extent that an abduction contracture occurs.

2. Vascular and Nerve Routes to the Lower Limb

From the pelvis, vascular and nerve routes lead:
– to the *ventral region of the hip* between the inguinal ligament and the superior margin of the pelvis,
– to the *medial region of the hip* through the obturator canal, and
– to the *deep gluteal region* through the greater sciatic foramen.

a) Vascular and Nerve Routes in the Ventral Hip Region

Inguinal ligament. In the border region between the trunk and the free lower limb, the *inguinal ligament* forms the boundary line between the ventral abdominal wall and the thigh (Figs. **117** and **123**). The connective tissue band, which has a slightly convex curvature on the caudal side, stretches from the anterior superior iliac spine to the pubic tubercle and is not a uniformly-shaped, typical ligament. The lateral third is basically nothing but a rigid, transverse bundle of fibers in the iliac fascia, which covers the iliopsoas. The medial two-thirds of the ligament are formed from the caudal margin of the aponeurosis of the external abdominal oblique muscle. Part of the fibers of the lateral portion continue into the medial portion, and another part separates from the inguinal ligament as the *iliopectineal arch* and passes to the iliopubic eminence.

In very lean persons, the flexion crease between the trunk and the leg (*inguinal furrow*, Figs. **207** and **210 a**) corresponds to the course of the inguinal ligament at the cutaneous surface. With increasing deposits of fat in the abdominal wall, the inguinal furrow is displaced distally onto the leg and is organized into secondary folds.

Muscular and **vascular compartments**. The place of passage for muscles, vessels and nerves circumscribed by the inguinal ligament and the superior margin of the pelvis (between the pubic tubercle and the anterior superior iliac spine) is subdivided by the *iliopectineal arch* into the lateral *muscular compartment* (*lacuna musculorum*) and the medial *vascular compartment* (*lacuna vasorum*) (Figs. **117** and **123**).

The following pass through the *muscular compartment* (Fig. **129**):
- the *lateral femoral cutaneous nerve* (close beside the anterior superior iliac spine, occasionally also through the inguinal ligament) to the skin on the external side of the thigh;
- the *iliopsoas muscle* to the lesser trochanter; and
- the *femoral nerve* (in the medial region of the compartment, embedded in the groove bordered by the psoas and iliacus muscles) to the extensors at the thigh, as well as to the skin at the anterior and inner side of the thigh and leg.

The following pass through the *vascular compartment* (Figs. **123** and **129**):
- the *femoral ramus of the genitofemoral nerve* (lateral to the femoral vessels) to the skin beneath the inguinal ligament, especially in the region of the saphenous hiatus;
- the *femoral artery*, which lies lateral to the femoral vein and sends branches to the ventral side of the hip, to the thigh and into the deep layers of the gluteal region before it reaches, via the hiatus tendineus, the popliteal fossa as the popliteal artery;
- the *femoral vein*, which lies medial to the artery of the same name and is enclosed with it in a connective tissue vascular sheath, passes toward the pelvis and continues into the external iliac vein; and
- the efferent *lymphatic vessels* of the deep inguinal lymph nodes (furthest medially), which conduct lymph to the external iliac lymph nodes from the entire lower limb, from the abdominal wall beneath the umbilicus, from the caudal part of the back, form the gluteal region, from the perineum and from the genital region.

Femoral ring (Fig. **123**). The vascular compartment has the form of an obtuse-angled triangle standing on its apex. The base is formed by the medial two thirds of the inguinal ligament (i.e. by the lower margin of the aponeurosis of the external abdominal oblique), whereas the iliopectineal arch and the superior ramus of the pubis form the obtuse angle of the triangle. The medial angle of the vascular compartment is covered by a fibrous plate, the *lacunar ligament*. This ligament extends between the inguinal ligament and the superior ramus of the pubis and continues to the pecten pubis (pectineal line) as the *pectineal ligament*. The sharp crescent-shaped margin of this fibrous plate forms the medial boundary of the *femoral ring*. The ring is bordered laterally by the vascular sheath of the femoral vessels, ventrocranially by the fibers of the lacunar ligament radiating into the inguinal ligament, and dorsocaudally by the pectineal ligament.

The femoral ring is closed by the delicate *femoral septum*, which is formed from fibers of the transversalis and iliac fasciae. Lymphatic vessels pass through the ring in a cranial direction (lacuna lymphatica). Usually a lymph node, Rosenmüller's lymph node, lies in the ring.

A *femoral hernia* (about 10% of all herniae) protrudes from the femoral ring, which represents a point of least resistance. Viscera evaginate the peritoneum and the femoral septum as a hernial sac; they can penetrate below the fascia lata up to the saphenous hiatus and cause the cribriform fascia to bulge. The canal created by the hernial sac is called the *femoral canal*. Femoral herniae always lie *below* the inguinal ligament and lateral to the lacunar ligament, which can strangulate the herniae with its sharp margins. In women, with their relatively broader pelvis and relatively wider vascular opening than males, femoral herniae are 3 to 4 times as frequent as in males. The inguinal canal passes through the abdominal wall cranial to the inguinal ligament. *Inguinal herniae*, therefore, always protrude *above* the inguinal ligament.

Gravitational abscesses. Abscesses (pus accumulations) as the result of an inflammation (usually tuberculous) of the lumbar vertebral column can penetrate the psoas muscle and migrate downwards in its fascial investment. They pass through the muscular compartment and can be palpated beneath the inguinal furrow. The contracture resulting from the irritation of the psoas leads to a constrained position of the hip joint (slight flexion, abduction and external rotation, → relaxation position of the hip joint, p. 000).

Vessels and Nerves in the Femoral Triangle

The **femoral triangle** is a triangular area bordered cranially by the inguinal ligament, laterally by the sartorius and medially by the gracilis (Fig. **129**). The muscular floor of this region is formed laterally by the iliopsoas, rectus femoris and vastus medialis and medially by the pectineus, adductor longus and adductor magnus.

The term *groin* (subinguinal region) is essentially used as a synonym for femoral triangle. Many authors, however, define it as being only the proximal segment of the femoral triangle and regard the extrapelvic section of the iliopsoas as the lateral border and the pectineus as the medial boundary.

The **subinguinal** or **iliopectineal fossa** is designated as the connective tissue *space* situated beneath the inguinal ligament and bordered laterally by the fascia of the iliopsoas and medially by the pectineus and the adductors. It is traversed by the femoral vessels and closed off from the subcutaneous tissue by the fascia of the thigh (fascia lata).

In the subinguinal fossa, there are proximal branches of the *femoral vessels* near their origins or openings (including the profunda femoris vessels) and branches of the *femoral nerve*, which enter the fossa through the iliopsoas fascia. In the distally-directed apex of the triangular fossa, the *saphenous nerve* adheres to femoral vessels laterally so that a united neurovascular cord exists for a limited distance.

The *femoral artery* (Figs. **123**, **128** and **129**), the distal continuation of the external iliac artery, lies rather superficially in the subinguinal fossa as it

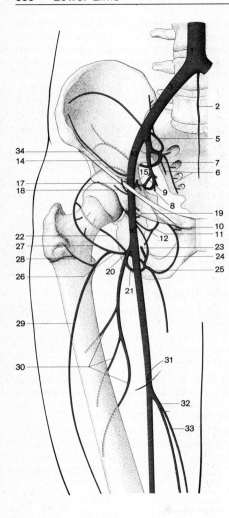

Fig. 128. **Arteries in region of hip and thigh**, view from in front

 1 Abdominal aorta
 2 Median sacral artery
 3 Common iliac artery
 4 Internal iliac artery
 5 Iliolumbar artery
 6 Lateral sacral arteries
 7 Superior gluteal artery
 8 Inferior gluteal artery
 9 Obturator artery
10 Anterior branch ⎫ of
11 Posterior branch ⎬ obturator
12 Acetabular branch ⎭ artery
13 External iliac artery
14 Deep circumflex iliac artery
15 Inferior epigastric artery
16 Femoral artery
17 Superficial epigastric artery
18 Superficial circumflex iliac artery
19 External pudendal arteries
20 Profunda femoris artery
21 Medial circumflex femoral artery
22 Ascending branch ⎫ of medial
23 Deep branch ⎪ circumflex
24 Acetabular branch ⎬ femoral
25 Transverse branch ⎭ artery
26 Lateral circumflex femoral artery
27 Ascending branch ⎫ of lateral
28 Transverse branch ⎬ circumflex
29 Descending branch ⎭ femoral artery
30 Perforating arteries
31 Entrance of femoral artery into
   adductor canal
32 Descending genicular artery
33 Exit of saphenous branch of
   descending genicular artery from
   adductor canal
34 Inguinal ligament

exits from the vascular compartment, in the middle of a line connecting the pubic symphysis with the anterior superior iliac spine. It is covered only by the fascia lata and skin. Behind the sartorius the femoral artery passes distally into the groove (Fig. **132**) formed by the vastus medialis and adductor longus, enters the adductor canal and, after passing through the hiatus tendineus, arrives at the popliteal fossa where it is called the *popliteal artery*.

The *femoral vein* (Fig. **123**) lies in the vascular compartment. In the subinguinal fossa, it passes medial to the femoral artery, in the middle of the thigh behind the femoral artery and in the adductor aperture dorsolateral to it. The *femoral nerve* is separated from the artery by the iliopectineal arch. The *saphenous nerve* (Fig. **129**) lies in the subinguinal fossa at the lateral side of the artery, further distally in front of it, and passes with it into the adductor canal. It then leaves the artery, penetrates the vasto-adductor membrane and passes to the knee joint and to the medial side of the tibia with the saphenous branch of the descending genicular artery.

The **femoral artery** (Fig. **128**) sends "cutaneous" arteries (*superficial epigastric, superficial circumflex iliac* and the *external pudendal arteries*) into the subinguinal fossa, which enter via the cribriform fascia. As a deep vessel it gives off the main artery of the thigh, the *profunda femoris artery*. The *descending genicular artery* arises in the adductor canal.

In the hip region, the femoral artery communicates with branches of the internal iliac artery via numerous anastomoses so that in ligatures of the external iliac artery or the femoral artery (proximal to the exit of the profunda femoris), an extensive collateral circulation can form. Bleeding from the femoral artery can be stopped by pressing the vessel firmly against the iliopubic eminence.

The *superficial epigastric artery* passes above the inguinal ligament to the abdominal skin (up to the umbilicus) and anastomoses with branches of the internal thoracic artery. The *superficial circumflex iliac artery* courses laterally, parallel to the inguinal ligament. The *external pudendal arteries* (usually two vessels) turn medially, give off *inguinal branches* to the skin of the inguinal region and to the inguinal lymph nodes, and end in males with *anterior scrotal branches* in the scrotum, in females *anterior labial branches* in the labium majus.

The **profunda femoris** originates 2–3 transverse finger lengths beneath the inguinal ligament at the lateral side of the femoral artery, crosses under this artery medially and passes distally between the vastus medialis and the muscles of the adductor group.

Still in the region of the subinguinal fossa, the *profunda femoris* gives off two large lateral branches, the *circumflex femoral arteries*, the branches of which curve around the femur and hip joint and supply the muscles of the adductor group and parts of the gluteal musculature, as well as the extensors and flexors at the thigh. They anastomose with one another and with branches of neighboring arteries.

The *medial circumflex femoral artery* arrives at the medial side of the femoral neck between the iliopsoas and pectineus. The *ascending ramus* encircles the neck of the femur on the posterior surface, anastomoses with the ascending ramus of the lateral circumflex femoral artery, and thus closes the arterial ring around the femoral neck. The *deep ramus* supplies the quadratus femoris, adductor magnus and the flexors at the thigh; the *transverse ramus* ramifies in the muscles of the adductor group; and the variable *acetabular ramus* passes through the acetabular notch into the acetabular fossa and can supply blood to the femoral head via the ligament of the head of the femur.

The *lateral circumflex femoral artery* courses laterally, dorsal to the sartorius and rectus femoris, and divides into the *ascending branch* passing upward above the neck of the femur, the *transverse branch* encircling the femur just below the greater trochanter, and the *descending branch* coursing downward in the quadriceps femoris.

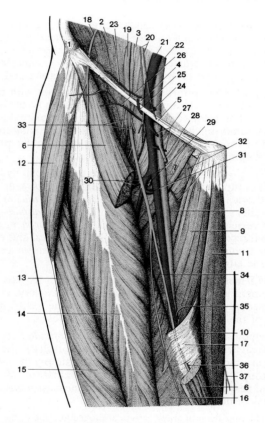

Fig. 129. **Vessels and nerves in femoral triangle**, view from in front
(Cutaneous branches shown for only a short distance, muscular branches and veins either absent of incompletely shown)

The *circumflex femoral arteries* can also arise directly from the femoral artery (close to 20% of the cases).

As the terminal branches of the profunda femoris artery, 3 (−5) *perforating arteries* near the linea aspera pass through the adductors, ramify in them and in the ischiocrural muscles, and communicate with one another and with adjacent arterial rami.

The 1st and 3rd (or last) perforating artery usually gives off a *nutrient artery* to the femur.

Femoral vein. At the leg, as at the arm, a cutaneous venous network is formed in addition to the system of accompanying veins. This network anastomoses many times with the deep veins and possesses well developed longitudinal veins in the venous saphenous system.

The *femoral vein* (Fig. **129**), the companion vein of the femoral artery, enters the adductor groove from the popliteal vein. It turns from the dorsolateral side of the femoral artery to its medial side and receives the great saphenous vein in the saphenous hiatus. The femoral vein passes medial to the artery into the vascular compartment and continues as the external iliac vein proximal to the inguinal ligament.

The femoral vein and the proximal part of the popliteal vein are single, whereas their lateral branches and the distal portion of the popliteal vein are double. The tributaries of the femoral vein and the popliteal vein accompany the branches of the same-named arteries.

Although the femoral vein possesses, via the superficial epigastric vein, an anastomosis with the drainage area of the superior vena cava (via thoraco-

1 Anterior superior iliac spine
2 Iliacus } Iliopsoas
3 Psoas major
4 iliopectineal arch
5 Inguinal ligament
6 Sartorius
7 Pectineus
8 Adductor brevis
9 Adductor longus
10 Adductor magnus
11 Gracilis
12 Tensor fasciae latae
13 Iliotibial tract, cut edge
14 Rectus femoris
15 Vastus lateralis
16 Vastus medialis
17 Vasto-adductor membrane
18 Lateral femoral cutaneous nerve
19 Femoral nerve
20 Femoral and genital branches of genitofemoral nerve
21 External iliac artery, at other side of vascular compartment: femoral artery
22 External iliac vein, at other side of vascular compartment: femoral vein
23 Deep circumflex iliac artery
24 Inferior epigastric artery
25 Superficial epigastric artery
26 Superficial circumflex iliac artery
27 External pudendal arteries
28 Great saphenous vein
29 Profunda femoris artery and vein
30 Ascending and descending branches of lateral circumflex femoral artery
31 Medial circumflex femoral artery and muscle branch
32 Anterior branches of obturator artery and obturator nerve
33 Anterior cutaneous branches of femoral nerve
34 Saphenous nerve
35 Adductor canal
36 Saphenous branch of descending genicular artery
37 Cutaneous branch of obturator nerve

epigastric veins – axillary vein), a high degree of venous obstruction still appears when the femoral vein is ligated in the vicinity of the inguinal ligament. Extensive anastomoses are present distally. Since the femoral vein is free of valves proximal to the junction of the great saphenous vein, considerable bleeding occurs when the vessel is opened near the inguinal ligament. The connective tissue struts supporting the veins in the vascular sheath promotes the reflux of blood and holds the vascular lumen somewhat open even during extreme flexion or extension of the hip joint. An aspiration of air during an injury to the venous wall is prevented (under the influence of gravity) by the venous pressure prevailing in this vascular region.

Deep *lymphatic vessels* accompany the femoral vessels and their branches. In the subinguinal fossa small lymphatic trunks (8–12 coursing predominantly on the medial side of the femoral vein) enter the *deep inguinal lymph nodes* (Fig. **204**). The 3–4 deep inguinal lymph nodes lie at the medial side of the femoral vein near the junction of the great saphenous vein. They receive lymph from the skeleton and the musculature of the lower limb, as well as (the greatest part of the lymph) from the superficial inguinal lymph nodes, and conduct it further to the external iliac lymph nodes.

Considerable clinical significance is attributed to Rosenmüller's lymph node located in the femoral ring since it intervenes between the groups of lymph nodes situated in the subinguinal fossa and along the external iliac vessels. It can be infiltrated by pus-forming organisms from the drainage area of the deep inguinal lymph nodes or be the site of tumor metastases (from bone, rectum, uterus, etc.). When Rosenmüller's lymph node is swollen, symptoms similar to a femoral hernia can appear.

The **femoral nerve** (Figs. **123** and **128**) passes through the muscular compartment with the iliopsoas and divides immediately into its branches, which enter the iliopsoas fascia.

While still inside the greater pelvis, the femoral nerve gives off *muscular rami* to the psoas and iliacus muscles and, cranial to the inguinal ligament, dispatches a thin muscular branch to the pectineus, which courses through the fibrous layers of the iliopectineal arch dorsal to the femoral vessels.

At the thigh, the femoral nerve gives off *muscular branches* to the extensor muscles (sartorius and quadriceps femoris) and *anterior cutaneous branches*, which pass through the fascia lata to the skin at the medial and anterior surfaces of the thigh and which can anastomose with branches of the femoral ramus of the genitofemoral nerve and the lateral femoral cutaneous nerve.

The *saphenous nerve* is the terminal branch of the femoral nerve. It ramifies in the skin at the medial side of the leg and at the medial margin of the foot.

b) Neurovascular Routes in the Medial Hip Region

The **obturator canal** (Fig. **117**) which is bordered by the obturator groove and the obturator membrane, is about 2–3 cm long. It connects the subperitoneal connective tissue space at the wall of the lesser pelvis with the fascial chamber of the adductor group in the medial region of the hip and harbors the conduction pathways embedded in adipose tissue, occasionally also a small fat body.

The following course in this neruovascular route (Figs. **123** and **126**):

– the *obturator artery*, which supplies blood especially to the adductors and the deep layer of external hip muscles and whose branches anastomose with branches of the medial circumflex femoral artery and the inferior gluteal artery;

– the *obturator veins*, which drain blood from the medial region of the hip into the internal iliac vein, but which also possess extensive anastomoses with branches of the femoral vein and the external iliac vein;

– *lymphatic vessels* accompanying the obturator vessels, which convey the lymph from the medial hip region to the iliac lymph nodes; and

– the *obturator nerve*, which innervates the adductors and provides sensory innervation for a small area of skin at the medial side of the thigh (autonomic region: above the knee joint).

In the case of an *obturator hernia* (not infrequent in older women), the hernial sac can press medially on the obturator nerve, which courses in the obturator canal cranial to the vessels, and cause paresthesia (tingling, numbness) or pain at the inner surface of the thigh. The rarer motor disturbance produces a forced position characterized by adduction and external rotation of the flexed thigh.

The obturator nerve can be easily damaged in fractures of the hip because of its relatively long course along the bony wall of the lesser pelvis and in the obturator canal.

Before entering the obturator canal, the **obturator artery** gives off branches to the iliopsoas and obturator internus, as well as the *pubic branch*, which passes to the symphysis at the posterior surface of the superior ramus of the pubis (Fig. **126**). A lateral branch of the pubic branch anastomoses with the pubic ramus of the inferior epigastric artery.

Not infrequently, the obturator artery arises from this connection or obtains an additional origin in this way, the *accessory obturator artery*. This strong vessel courses at the medial margin of the vascular compartment. Since it was frequently incised in the early days of surgical operations for femoral herniae, resulting in fatal bleeding, this accessory origin of the obturator artery received the name *corona mortis* (crown of death).

In the obturator canal, the *obturator artery* (Fig. **128**) – like the nerve of the same name – gives off an *anterior branch* (to the muscles of the adductor group and to the skin of the external genitalia) and a *posterior branch*. The latter passes above the ischial tuberosity to the deep layers of the external muscles of the hip and dispatches the *acetabular branch*, which reaches the head of the femur in the ligament to the head of the femur.

The anterior branch anastomoses with branches of the medial circumflex femoral artery, and the posterior branch with branches of the inferior gluteal artery.

Before entering into the obturator canal, the **obturator nerve** gives off a muscle branch for the obturator externus which passes through the canal with the nerve (Fig. **126**). Either before or at the exit from the obturator canal, the obturator nerve divides into *anterior* and *posterior rami* (Fig. **123**).

The *anterior ramus* courses between the adductors brevis and longus, both of which it innervates. It supplies the gracilis, usually – in addition to the femoral nerve – also the pectineus, and gives off the *cutaneous branch* to the skin at the inner side of the thigh (autonomic region) and the knee joint (maximal region). The *posterior branch* innervates the adductor magnus, on which it passes distally.

c) Neurovascular Routes in the Deep Gluteal Region

The vascular and nerve routes which travel dorsally from the lesser pelvis into the deep gluteal region pass through the greater sciatic foramen (Figs. **117** and **130**) and lead into the *subgluteal connective tissue layer*. This connective tissue space, which contains abundant adipose tissue, lies between the gluteus maximus and the deep muscle layer consisting of the piriformis and obturator internus, together with the gemelli and quadratus femoris. It is bordered on one side by the fascia at the inferior surface of the large gluteal muscle and the other side by a deep fascial layer, which provides the digital continuation of the fascia of the gluteus medius, covers the deep muscles, and goes over into the fascial covering of the ischiocrural muscles. The subgluteal connective tissue layer is both a movable layer and a broad neurovascular route for vessels and nerves of the gluteal region, which ramify here, and for conduction paths, which course to the ischio-anal (ischiorectal) fossa or to the thigh.

In the connective tissue which encloses the vessels and nerves passing through the greater sciatic foramen, inflammation can be spread from the subperitoneal connective tissue space of the lesser pelvis into the gluteal region, as well as along the sciatic nerve into the movable layers between the muscles at the posterior side of the thigh.

Sciatic hernia. Hernial formations in the region of the greater sciatic foramen are extremely rare. In the case of such a hernia, specific symptoms usually appear only if there is a strangulation of the hernia. If the hernial sac is evaginated beneath the piriformis, it can press on the sciatic nerve and in so doing can cause pain in the leg.

The following course through the *suprapiriformis division of the greater sciatic foramen* (Figs. **126**, **130** and **131**):
– the *superior gluteal artery* (with accompanying veins) to the cranial part of the gluteus maximus, to the small gluteal muscles and to the piriformis, and

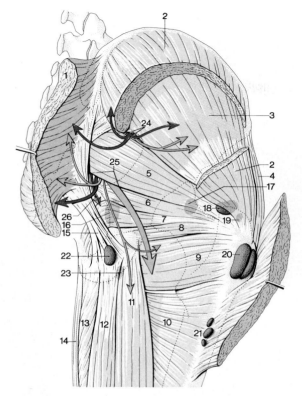

Fig. 130. Muscles, bursae and neurovascular routes in gluteal region (Gluteus maximus severed and retracted on both sides, middle third of gluteus medius removed)

1 Gluteus maximus
2 Gluteus medius
3 Gluteus minimus
4 Tensor fasciae latae
5 Piriformis
6 Superior gemellus
7 Obturator internus
8 Inferior gemellus
9 Quadratus femoris
10 Adductor magnus
11 Biceps femoris, long head
12 Semitendinosus
13 Adductor longus
14 Gracilis
15 Sacrotuberous ligament
16 Bursa of obturator internus
17 Bursa of piriformis
18 Trochanteric bursa (of gluteus medius)

19 Trochanteric bursa (of gluteus minimus)
20 Trochanteric bursa (of gluteus maximus)
21 Intermuscular gluteal bursae
22 Ischial bursa (between ischial tuberosity and gluteus maximus)
23 Bursa of biceps femoris (between tendon of long head and ischial tuberosity)
24–26 *Neurovascular routes* through:
suprapiriform division of greater sciatic foramen (24):
superior gluteal vessels and nerve
infrapiriform division of greater sciatic foramen (25):
sciatic nerve, posterior femoral cutaneous nerve, inferior gluteal vessels and nerve, internal pudendal vessel, pudendal nerve
lesser sciatic foramen (26):
internal pudendal vessels, pudendal nerve

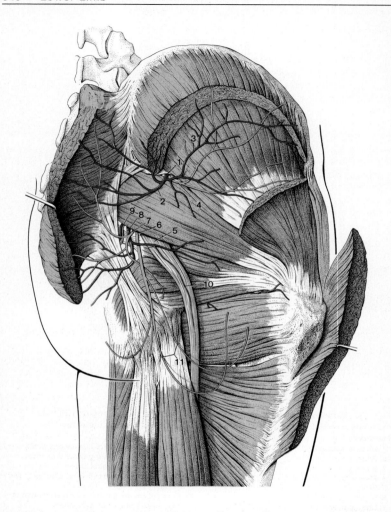

Fig. 131. **Arteries and nerves in subgluteal fascial layer** (muscle depiction → Fig. 130)

1 Superior gluteal artery
2 Superficial branch of superior gluteal artery
3 Deep branch of superior gluteal artery
4 Superior gluteal nerve
5 Sciatic nerve
6 Posterior femoral cutaneous nerve
7 Inferior gluteal nerve
8 Inferior gluteal artery
9 Pudendal nerve and internal pudendal artery
10 Companion artery of sciatic nerve
11 Inferior clunial nerves

– the *superior gluteal nerve* to the small muscles of the gluteal region and to the tensor fasciae latae.

The following pass through the *infrapiriformis division of the greater sciatic foramen* (Figs. **126, 130**, and **131**):

– at the *lateral angle*, the *sciatic nerve*, which courses distally on the obturator internus, gemelli, quadratus femoris and adductor magnus and is covered in the gluteal region by the gluteus maximus, and the *posterior femoral cutaneous nerve* to the skin of the buttocks, thigh and the popliteal fossa (occasionally also to the calf of the leg);

– in the *middle*, the *inferior gluteal artery* (with companion veins) to the caudal two-thirds of the gluteus maximus, and the *inferior gluteal nerve*, which innervates mainly the large gluteal muscle; and

– in the *medial angle*, the *internal pudendal artery* (with accompanying veins) and the *pudendal nerve*, both of which wind around the ischial spine, pass into the ischio-anal fossa through the lesser sciatic foramen, and supply the muscles and skin of the genito-anal region.

During intramuscular injections, for which the voluminous gluteal musculature is well-suited, the sciatic nerve is vulnerable to improper techniques.

As a rule, injections are made in the superior, external quadrant of the gluteal region. They should not be placed distal to a line connecting the posterior and anterior superior iliac spines.

Vessels and Nerves in the Subgluteal Connective Tissue Layer

The **superior gluteal artery** (Figs. **128** and **131**) gives off a nutrient artery to the ilium in its passage through the greater sciatic foramen; it divides at the upper margin of the greater sciatic notch into a *superficial branch* (to the cranial part of the gluteus maximum and to the gluteus medius) and a *deep branch*. From these two branches, the *superior branch* ramifies in the small gluteal muscles and in the tensor fasciae latae, and the *inferior branch* in the gluteus medius and piriformis, as well as at the capsule of the hip joint.

The superior gluteal artery possesses numerous anastomoses with other branches of the internal iliac artery and with twigs from the lateral circumflex femoral artery.

The **inferior gluteal artery** (Figs. **128** and **131**) supplies the caudal two-thirds of the gluteus maximus.

It sends fine branches to the small rotator muscles and to the capsule of the hip joint, anastomoses with numerous twigs of adjacent arteries, and can give off the *companion artery to the sciatic nerve* (Figs. **131** and **132**), which accompanies this nerve to the thigh.

The **superior gluteal nerve** (Fig. **131**) passes between the gluteus medius and gluteus minimus and gives off short muscular branches to both. Its terminal branch courses (frequently through the gluteus minimus) to the tensor fasciae latae.

The **inferior gluteal nerve** (Fig. **131**) courses lateral to the inferior gluteal vessels and branches off like a fan at the lower surface of the gluteus maximus.

The cranial rami of the nerve interweave with branches of the superficial branch of the superior gluteal artery, and the caudal bundles of nerve fibers accompany the twigs of the inferior gluteal artery. As a rule, small muscular branches pass into the obturator internus, gemelli and quadratus femoris.

At the lower margin of the gluteus maximus, the **posterior femoral cutaneous nerve** (Fig. **131**) gives off 2–3 *inferior clunial nerves*, which turn back to the skin of the buttocks and dispatch weak individual *perineal branches* to the skin of the perineum and to the scrotum (labium majus in females). Its main branch courses distally beneath the fascia between the semitendinosus and the biceps femoris and ramifies in the skin of the back of the thigh, of the popliteal space and (occasionally also) of the calf of the leg.

The **sciatic nerve** (Fig. **131**) lies in the gluteal region somewhat medial to the midpoint of a line connecting the greater trochanter and the ischial tuberosity. It passes distally on the fascia of the adductor magnus, first between adductors and flexors, then above the popliteal fossa between the medial and the lateral flexors, and divides into the tibial and common peroneal nerves at the latest at the entrance into the popliteal fossa.

The sciatic nerve innervates, in exceptional cases, the obturator internus, gemelli and quadratus femoris and, as a rule, the ischiocrural musculature and all the muscles at the leg and foot. It supplies sensory innervation to the entire skin of the leg and foot, except for a band-shaped field over the medial surface of the tibia (close to the medial malleolus) which is innervated exclusively by the saphenous nerve.

d) Vessels and Nerves in the Ischio-Anal Fossa

The **internal pudendal vessels** and the **pudendal nerve** wind around the ischial spine and the inferior margin of the sacrospinous ligament and pass through the lesser sciatic foramen into the *pudendal canal* (*Alcock's canal*, Figs. **117**, **126** and **130**). This canal lies in the lateral wall of the ischio-anal fossa and is formed by a duplication of the obturator fascia. It conveys vessels and nerves along the medial side of the ischial tuberosity and ramus – caudal to the pelvic diaphragm – up to the posterior margin of the urogenital diaphragm.

The *internal pudendal artery* – still dorsal to the ischial tuberosity – gives off the *inferior rectal artery* at the entrance into the pudendal canal. Occasionally it has several branches of origin. It penetrates the medial layer of the duplicated fascia and passes through the fat body into the anal canal where it anastomoses with the artery of the opposite side and the middle rectal artery.

The *internal pudendal vein* is usually formed doubled. Its branches accompany the branches of the internal pudendal artery.

The *pudendal nerve* – usually organized into bundles – courses in the pudendal canal somewhat more superficially than the internal pudendal vessels.

Sequence of branches of the internal pudendal vessels and pudendal nerve → vol. 2.

C. Thigh and Knee Region

1. Thigh

a) Arrangement and Innervation of the Thigh Musculature

As in the upper arm, *extensor* (*dorsal* muscles) and *flexor* (*ventral* muscles) *groups* are also distinguished in the **thigh** (*femur*). The muscle mass of the extensors considerably surpasses those of the flexor group. The *extensors* lie on the *anterior*(!) side of the thigh and almost completely enclose the femur except for the narrow ridge of the linea aspera on its posterior surface. Laterally, the extensors and flexors are separated by the femoral intermuscular septum; medially, the adductor group lies between them. The extensor group consists of the sartorius and of the four individual muscles of the quadriceps femoris, all of which are innervated by the femoral nerve. Of the flexors, the long head of the biceps, as well as the semitendinosus and semimembranosus are supplied by the tibialis portion of the sciatic nerve, whereas the short head of the biceps femoris is innervated by the peroneal component of the sciatic nerve.

The **fascia lata** (Figs. **132** and **204**) encloses the muscle groups at the thigh like a stocking. It is attached proximally to the inguinal ligament and iliac crest and continues distally into the fascia of the leg. The fascia is relatively firm on the lateral and ventral sides of the thigh, consisting of connective tissue fibers arranged primarily in roughly circular fashion. At the lateral circumference of this fascia, strong longitudinally-coursing tracts of fibers are woven in to form the *iliotibial tract*. In a standing position, the thin fascia on the medial side of the thigh is protruded by the uncontracted medial head of the quadriceps femoris (vastus medialis): *suprapatellar swelling*.

In the gluteal region, the fascia lata is also called the gluteal fascia. It covers the gluteus medius and gluteus maximus and attaches along the line of origin of the large gluteal muscle, as well as at the sacrum and coccyx.

Thin connective tissue membranes go into the depth from the fascia lata, enclose the muscle groups and individual muscles, and form a movable separation for the muscles from one another (Fig. **132**). Special compartments are formed for the sartorius, tensor fasciae latae and gracilis which give these muscles a strong guidance. The strong, partly aponeurotic *lateral femoral intermuscular septum* unites the fascia lata with the lateral lip of the linea aspera and separates the extensors from the flexors. The *medial femoral intermuscular septum*, which passes to the medial lip

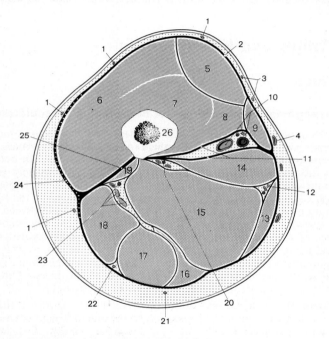

Fig. 132. **Cross section in middle third of thigh**, distal view of section surface

1 Branches of lateral femoral cutaneous nerve
2 Fascia lata
3 Anterior cutaneous branches of femoral nerve
4 Great saphenous vein
5–8 *Quadriceps femoris*
5 Rectus femoris
6 Vastus lateralis
7 Vastus intermedius
8 Vastus medialis
9 Sartorius
10 Saphenous nerve, femoral artery and vein
11 Medial femoral intermuscular septum
12 Anterior branch of obturator nerve
13 Gracilis
14 Adductor longus
15 Adductor magnus
16 Semimembranosus
17 Semitendinosus
18 Long head of biceps femoris
19 Short head of biceps femoris
20 Terminal branch of profunda femoris artery: tertiary perforating artery
21 Branch of posterior femoral cutaneous nerve
22 Posterior femoral cutaneous nerve
23 Sciatic nerve and companion artery of sciatic nerve
24 Iliotibial tract
25 Lateral femoral intermuscular septum
26 Femur

between the extensor and adductor groups, is in part an extensive connective tissue layer, in which the femoral vessels and the saphenous nerve course. A relatively delicate connective tissue layer, which is more strongly developed only in the region of the sciatic nerve, extends between the flexor and adductor groups dorsal to the fascia lata.

The fascia lata and the connective tissue partitions, in which a large part of the "annular" fibers of the fascia of the thigh join, mark off three muscle chambers. The extensive *chamber of extensors* lies at the anterior surface and on both sides of the femur. It is bordered by the fascia lata and the two intermuscular septa and is largely closed, apart from the places of entry of the femoral vessels and their branches, as well as the branches of the femoral nerve. The *chamber of flexors* occupies the dorsolateral sector (in a cross section of the thigh) behind the lateral intermuscular septum. It communicates proximally with the connective tissue space of the lesser pelvis through the infrapiriform division of the greater sciatic foramen and continues distally into the connective tissue layer of the popliteal fossa. In the *chamber of adductors* (behind the medial femoral intermuscular septum, at the dorsomedial circumference of the thigh), a connective tissue route leads through the obturator canal from the lesser pelvis.

Saphenous hiatus. The great saphenous vein passes through the fascia lata directly below the inguinal ligament and enters the femoral vein. The place of entry, the *saphenous hiatus* (Fig. **204**), is bordered laterally, distally and (somewhat less pronounced) proximally by a strong C-shaped fascial band, the *falciform margin,* and closed by a sieve-like, perforated membrane, the *cribriform fascia.* This fascia covers the femoral vessels as part of the fascia lata and in this region closes the subinguinal fossa ventrally.

In addition to the great saphenous vein, the "cutaneous" branches of the femoral artery and their companion veins, the femoral ramus of the genitofemoral nerve and an anterior cutaneous branch of the femoral nerve which accompanies the great saphenous vein, pass through the perforations of the **cribriform fascia**, together with numerous lymphatic vessels.

On the anterior side of the knee joint, the fascia lata is fixed at the patella, the patellar retinacula and the ligamentum patellae. Over the patella it is separated from the skin by the extensive *prepatellar subcutaneous bursa* (Fig. **139**). On the posterior side of the knee joint, a thin popliteal fascia, a distal portion of the fascia lata strengthened by circular fiber tracts, separates the structural contents of the popliteal fossa.

Extensor Group (Dorsal Muscles)

The **quadriceps femoris** (Fig. **124** and **132**) arises with four heads: the *rectus femoris,* which passes over the hip and knee joints, and the three one-jointed *vasti muscles,* which largely surround the femur. The four muscles unite in a broad common terminal tendon, in which the patella is embedded as a sesamoid bone. From the apex of the patella, the *ligamentum patellae* – as a continuation of the terminal tendon – proceeds to the tibial tuberosity (Figs. **124** and **140**). Owing to the patella, the distance of the quadriceps tendon from the axis of flexion of the knee joint is increased, thus increasing the torque of the muscle. The *patellar retinaculum* denotes the lateral tendinous tracts of the muscle, which flank the patella on each side as longitudinal bands and which course to the upper margin of the tibia. They prevent the patella from slipping off the gliding tract formed by the patellar surface of the femur and transfer a limited part of the extension action of the quadriceps femoris to the tibia.

The bipennate **rectus femoris** (Figs. **124**, **129** and **140**) originates with the *straight head* at the anterior inferior iliac spine, with the *reflected head* at the upper margin of the acetabulum and at the joint capsule. The fibers from the central region of the tendon of attachment insert at the upper margin of the patella or pass across its anterior surface into the ligamentum patellae. The lateral fiber tracts radiate into the retinaculum on both sides of the patella.

The **vastus medialis** (Figs. **124**, **129** and **132**) arises at the proximal two-thirds of the medial lip of the linea aspera and from the terminal tendons of the adductor longus and adductor magnus. The proximal fibers of the muscle course obliquely downwards, and the distal fibers almost transversely. In addition to the common terminal tendon of the quadriceps femoris, fibers of the vastus medialis pass to the medial margin of the patella and to the medial patellar retinaculum.

The **vastus lateralis** (Figs. **124**, **129** and **132**), the largest head of the quadriceps, takes its origin from the base of the greater trochanter, from the lateral lip of the linea aspera and from the superficial aponeurosis of the muscle arising from the greater trochanter. The terminal tendon merges into the common tendon field of the quadriceps situated proximal to the patella, and a portion of the tendinous fibers radiates into the patellar retinaculum.

The **vastus intermedius** (Figs. **124** and **132**) passes from the anterior and the lateral surfaces of the femur to the common terminal tendon. Its field of origin reaches from the intertrochanteric line to the border between the middle and distal thirds of the shaft of the femur.

Medially and laterally, the vastus intermedius is arched over by the vastus medialis and vastus lateralis muscles. The rectus femoris glides on its aponeurotic tendon of attachment, which extends far proximally at the anterior surface of the muscle. The muscle bundles of the vastus intermedius originating most distally insert at the capsule of the knee joint as the *articularis genus muscle* (Fig. **139**) and prevent the joint capsule from being pinched during extension at the joint.

Innervation: femoral nerve.

The femoral nerve fans out directly beneath the inguinal ligament into cutaneous branches and branches to the sartorius and to the four heads of the quadriceps femoris. The branch to the vastus medialis is united with the saphenous nerve for a short distance and gives off short twigs to the distal portion of the sartorius.

The **sartorius** (Fig. **123**, **124**, **129** and **132**) passes spirally from the anterior superior iliac spine over the anterior and medial surfaces of the thigh in a fascial sheath formed by the fascia lata. Owing to its arched course, the muscle crosses the axis of flexion of the knee joint on the dorsal side. The terminal tendon, which is obliquely directed distally and ventrally, inserts via the pes anserinus (Fig. **142**) at the medial surface of the tibia (behind the tibial tuberosity) and at the fascia of the leg.

The pes anserinus originates through the common location of the widened terminal tendons of the sartorius (superficial layer) and the gracilis and semitendinosus (deep layer); it resembles the folded web membranes of the foot of a goose. From the pes anserinus, which is separated from the tibial collateral ligament by the *bursa anserina*, the tendon fibers radiate into the medial surface of the tibia, and superficial fiber tracts continue into the fascia of the leg.

Innervation: femoral nerve.

Flexor Group (Ventral Muscles)

With the exception of the short head of the biceps femoris, the muscles of the flexor group pass over the hip and knee joints. They originate at the ischial tuberosity and attach at both leg bones. Thus, they represent the *ischiocrural musculature*. The biceps femoris is the only muscle to insert at the fibula, and it forms the lateral boundary of the popliteal fossa. The semitendinosus and semimembranosus attach at the tibia and delimit the popliteal fossa on the medial side. The ischiocrural muscles can flex at the knee joint and extend at the hip joint or assist in fixing the pelvis in a definite position. Their contractility does not suffice to flex the leg maximally when the hip joint is extended: *active insufficiency*. On the other hand, the muscles cannot be extended enough to permit a maximal flexion at the hip joint when the knee joint is extended: *passive insufficiency* (Fig. **17 b, c**).

The **biceps femoris** (Figs. **123**, **125** and **132**) arises with its *long head*, together with the semitendinosus, from the posterior surface of the ischial tuberosity. The *short head* comes from the middle third of the lateral lip of the linea aspera. It continues the fiber direction of the adductor longus, which inserts at the medial lip at the level of the muscle origin. The common terminal tendon of both heads of the biceps attaches at the head of the fibula. A portion of the tendon fibers passes to the lateral condyle of the tibia and into the fascia of the leg.

The biceps tendon is separated from the fibular collateral ligament by a *subtendinous bursa*.

Innervation: long head from the tibialis component of the sciatic nerve, short head from the peroneal division of the sciatic nerve.

The muscular branches from the tibialis component of the sciatic nerve, which pass to the ischiocrural musculature, frequently leave the sciatic nerve as a uniform trunk after it has divided beneath the long head of the biceps. After a short course, the muscular branches separate from one another distally and divide so that, as a rule, two nerve twigs enter into a muscle.

The **semitendinosus** (Figs. **123**, **125** and **132**) arises from the ischial tuberosity in close vicinity to the long head of the biceps and attaches via the pes anserinus at the medial surface of the proximal end of the tibia and at the fascia of the leg.

The muscle courses distally in a groove formed by the semimembranosus. The long terminal tendon, beginning already at the thigh (hence the name "semi-tendinosus"), radiates into the deep layer of the pes anserinus.

Innervation: tibialis component of the sciatic nerve.

The **semimembranosus** (Figs. **123**, **125** and **132**) arises from the ischial tuberosity between the long head of the biceps and the quadratus femoris. It inserts at the medial condyle of the tibia, at the posterior wall of the capsule of the knee joint and at the fascia of the popliteus muscle.

The muscle is muscular only in the two middle quarters. The long tendon of origin broadens to an extensive tendinous plate, and the terminal tendon is likewise flat. It ends in three tendinous cords. The tibial cord bends back ventrally and attaches at the medial condyle of the tibia under the tibial collateral ligament, whereas the middle cord continues the direction of the muscle and inserts partly at the posterior surface of the proximal end of the tibia, partly in the fascia of the popliteus muscle (Fig. **142**). The fibular terminal tendon strengthens the posterior wall of the articular capsule of the knee joint. It passes obliquely and laterally toward the lateral condyle of the femur as the *oblique popliteal ligament*. A *mucous bursa* regularly lies between the tendon of insertion (at its division) and the medial condyle of the tibia.

Innervation: tibialis component of the sciatic nerve.

b) Neurovascular Routes in the Thigh

Vessels and Nerves on the Extensor Side of the Thigh

A true neurovascular cord exists on the extensor side of the femur only in the distal region of the subinguinal fossa and in the proximal segment of the adductor canal (Fig. **129**). The saphenous nerve approaches the femoral artery in the subinguinal fossa from the lateral side and accompanies the vascular bundle in this space. Formed by the femoral vessels and several deep lymphatic trunks, this bundle is enveloped in a tough connective tissue sheath.

The **saphenous nerve** lies more superficially in the region of the adductor canal than the femoral vessels. Before the femoral vessels leave the canal through the hiatus tendineus and enter the popliteal fossa, the nerve penetrates the vasto-adductor membrane, passes below the sartorius between the vastus medialis and adductor magnus to the medial side of the knee, and accompanies the great saphenous vein up to the medial margin of the foot.

The sartorius is the conducting muscle for the femoral vessels, which pass in a nearly straight line from the subinguinal fossa to the popliteal fossa in the groove bordered by the vastus medialis and the adductors. The sartorius winds in a long-drawn helical line from the lateral to the medial side across the ventral surface of the vascular bundle.

In the adductor canal, the **femoral artery** (Figs. **128** and **129**) gives off only the *descending genicular artery* as a strong derivative. This artery, which passes downward in the vastus medialis to the knee joint, provides small branches to this muscle, as well as to the adductor magnus, and gives off *articular branches* to the articular network of the knee. While still in the adductor canal, the descending genicular artery dispatches the *saphenous branch*, which – together with the saphenous nerve or near its exit – penetrates the vasto-adductor membrane and ramifies in the skin of the leg at the medial side of the tibia.

The femoral artery should be ligated distal to the exit of the profunda femoris artery only in an emergency since the development of an extensive collateral circulation between the branches of the profunda femoris and descending genicular arteries is possible, but not absolutely certain.

The **femoral vein** (Fig. **129**), which arises from the popliteal vein, lies in the hiatus tendineus dorsal to the artery. Further proximally, it moves increasingly to the medial side so that it courses beneath the inguinal ligament medial to the femoral artery.

Vessels and Nerves on the Flexor Side of the Thigh

Vessels. On the flexor side of the thigh, there are no large vessels passing through the limb segment in a longitudinal direction. The blood vessels to muscles, skin and bones are branches of the profunda femoris artery, which arrive at the back of the thigh distal to the quadratus femoris (deep ramus of the medial circumflex femoral artery) and through the adductors (perforating arteries). They are accompanied by root branches of the profunda femoris vein and deep lymphatic vessels.

The **posterior femoral cutaneous nerve** (Fig. **131**) courses beneath the fascia up to the popliteal fossa and gives off branches through the fascia lata to the skin on the dorsal side of the thigh on both sides.

The **sciatic nerve** (Figs. **131** and **132**) passes distally in the connective tissue layer which separates the adductor and flexor groups.

Directly at the lower margin of the gluteus maximus and at the entrance into the popliteal fossa, the nerve lies relatively superficial and close to the fascia lata. For the entire remainder of its course, it is covered by the long head of the biceps, which passes obliquely over it distally and laterally. The sciatic nerve is not accompanied by a continuous artery in its entire extent. It is accompanied in sequence by its companion artery and by branches of the deep ramus of the medial circumflex femoral artery and the perforating arteries.

Whereas the sciatic artery forms the chief artery of the leg in nonmammals, in humans only the proximal segment of it is preserved during ontogenesis as the (usually) thin *companion artery to the sciatic nerve* (Figs. **131** and **132**). In a gradual closure of the femoral artery, a collateral circulation can be established under certain conditions between the pelvic artery and the popliteal artery, the distal segment of the embryonic sciatic artery. The anastomotic formation is facilitated if the sciatic artery is only partially degenerated.

Within its connective tissue sheath, the sciatic nerve is already organized into its tibial and common peroneal components at its emergence from the greater sciatic foramen. This division into tibial and common peroneal nerves becomes outwardly visible shortly before their entry into the popliteal fossa. The tibial component dispatches muscles branches successively to the portion of the adductor magnus inserting at the adductor tubercle, to the long head of the biceps and to the semitendinosus and semimembranosus. The muscular branch for the short head of the biceps leaves the peroneal component or (when the division is higher) the common peroneal nerve at the distal end of the sciatic nerve's extension in the thigh.

2. Knee Joint

a) Skeletal elements of the Leg

In the knee joint the femur articulates with the *tibia*, but not the *fibula*. The fibula is substantially thinner than the tibia, lies at the lateral (fibular) side of the tibia, and is connected with it by the *interosseous membrane of the leg* (Fig. **134**). With the distal end of the tibia, the distal end of the fibula forms the bifurcated joint for the superior ankle joint. For this reason, the distal segment of the fibula is always developed, even in those mammals (e.g. hoofed animals, bats) in which the shaft of the fibula is reduced.

In the adult, the axis of the shaft of the femur forms a laterally open angle (frontal knee angle, tibiofemoral angle) with the longitudinal axis of the tibia of about 175° (Fig. **133**). Thereby, the axis of the femoral shaft is inclined around 82° toward a horizontal plane through the articular cavity, whereas the axis of the tibia forms an angle of 93° with the horizontal. Under these normal conditions, the *weight-bearing line of the leg*, which at any given time runs through the middle of the hip joint and the superior ankle joint, lies in the middle of the knee joint.

If the frontal knee angle is distinctly smaller than 175° so that the knees scrape one another when walking, then a knock-knee (*genu valgum*) exists, and the weight-bearing line has moved laterally. In the opposite condition, bowlegs (*genu varum*), the weight-bearing line has moved medially.

In genu valgum, the inner collateral ligament is overstretched, and the cartilage in the lateral half of the joint is damaged by excessive compression

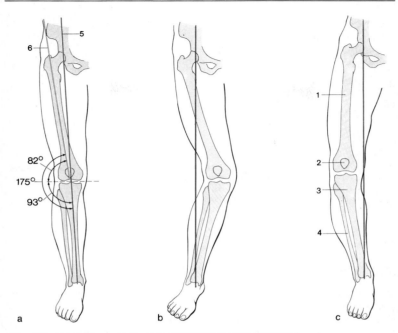

Fig. 133. **Frontal knee angle and weight-bearing line of bones (━━━)**
a Normal condition
b Genu valgum
c Genu varum

1 Femur	4 Fibula
2 Patella	5 Weight-bearing line
3 Tibia	6 Axis of shaft of femur

stress. In genu varum, the reverse is true: the external collateral ligament and the cartilage of the medial portion of the joint are involved.

A slight bowleggedness is completely physiological in newborn children and infants. Owing to the different linear growth at the epiphysial joints, this physiological genu varum is transformed in the pre-school child into a mild genu valgum (the frontal knee angle in the 5-year-old child amounts to 170°). At the beginning of puberty, the weight-bearing line of the leg once more returns to the middle of the knee joint.

The **tibia** (Fig. **134**) consists of a strong shaft, or *body*, which is triangular in cross section, a broadened proximal end, which bears two cartilaginous protuberances, the *medial* and *lateral condyles*, and a distal terminal piece, which forms the *medial malleolus* and a part of the bifurcated joint.

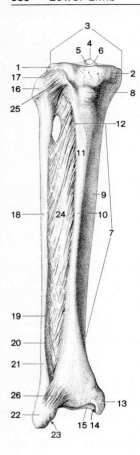

Fig. 134. **Skeletal elements of leg and interosseous membrane**, view from in front
1 Lateral condyle of tibia
2 Medial condyle of tibia
3 Superior articular surface of tibia
4 Intercondylar eminence
5 Lateral intercondylar tubercle
6 Medial intercondylar tubercle
7 Body of tibia
8 Tuberosity of tibia
9 Medial surface of tibia
10 Anterior margin of tibia
11 Lateral surface of tibia
12 Interosseous margin of tibia
13 Medial malleolus
14 Articular surface of medial malleolus
15 Inferior articular surface of tibia
16 Head of fibula
17 Apex of head of fibula
18 Body of fibula
19 Interosseous margin of fibula
20 Anterior margin of fibula
21 Lateral surface of fibula
22 Lateral malleolus
23 Articular surface of lateral malleolus
24 Interosseous membrane of leg
25 Anterior ligament of head of fibula
26 Anterior tibiofibular ligament

At the *body of the tibia* a distinction is made between the sharp-edged *anterior margin* located directly beneath the skin, the laterally-directed *interosseous margin*, to which the interosseous membrane is attached, and the rounded *medial margin*. The anterior margin (tibial crest) is broader proximally and ends in a bony projection, the *tibial tuberosity*, to which the ligamentum patellae is attached. (In a kneeling position, the tibial tuberosity transfers a large part of the pressure exerted by the weight of the body to the ground. The tuberosity is protected by a *subcutaneous mucous bursa*.)

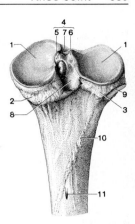

Fig. 135. **Proximal end of tibia**, view from behind
and above
 1 Superior articular surface
 2 Medial condyle
 3 Lateral condyle
 4 Intercondylar eminence
 5 Medial intercondylar tubercle
 6 Lateral intercondylar tubercle
 7 Anterior intercondylar area
 8 Posterior intercondylar area
 9 Articular surface of fibula
10 Soleal line
11 Nutrient foramen

The three tibial margins delimit three surfaces: the *medial surface*, which is not covered by muscles and lies directly beneath the skin, the *lateral surface*, and the *posterior surface*. Passing obliquely across the proximal segment of the posterior surface is a rough bony ridge, the *soleal line* (Fig. **135**), which gives rise to tendon fibers of the soleus muscle.

The triangular cross-sectional shape of the tibia is suited for the special flexion stresses of the bone. The main mass of the bone lies in the posterior part of the cross section, where the greater compressive stresses also occur. The tensile stresses at the apex of the triangular cross section are slighter.

The *proximal surface* of both tibial condyles, the *superior articular surface* (Figs. **135** and **138**), does not lie centrally over the middle axis of the tibial shaft, but is shifted posteriorly (Fig. **136**). It consists of two cartilage-covered articular surfaces, the medial surface of which is somewhat more extensive in the sagittal direction than the lateral surface. The cartilage-free intermediate zone is divided by the *intercondylar eminence* into an anterior and a posterior field (*anterior* and *posterior intercondylar areas*). The intercondylar eminence ends in two peaks, the *medial* and *lateral intercondylar tubercles*. The anterior cruciate ligament attaches at the anterior intercondylar area, and the posterior cruciate ligament at the posterior intercondylar area. At the lateral surface of the lateral tibial condyle there is the *articular fibular surface*, which is turned somewhat dorsally and adjoins the corresponding joint surface of the head of the fibula.

The proximal surface of the tibia in the newborn child inclines somewhat more than 25° posteriorly (*retroversion of the tibia*). Young infants, therefore, cannot completely extend the knee joint. During postnatal development, the retroversion

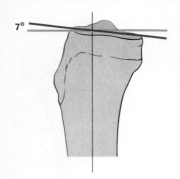

7°

Fig. 136. **Retroversion of proximal tibial surface**, view from medial side
Horizontal plane ——
Plane of superior articular surface ——
Central axis of shaft of tibia ——

is largely eliminated. In the adult, the posterior inclination of the proximal surface of the tibia amounts to only 3–7° (Fig. **136**).

Together with the fibula, the distal end of the tibia forms the bifurcated joint of the superior ankle joint, the *malleolar fork*, which encloses the trochlea of the talus from above and from the sides. The fibula rests in a shallow excavation of the tibia (the *fibular notch of the tibia*). The *medial malleolus* forms the medial prong of the fork (Fig. **134**). It distinctly projects medially and possesses on its laterally-directed surface a cartilage-covered *malleolar articular surface*, which merges into the transversely-situated, sagittally-concave *inferior articular surface* of the tibia. Dorsally, the medial malleolus is indented by the *malleolar groove* for the tendons of the tibialis posterior and the flexor digitorum longus.

The distal end of the tibia in the adult is turned outward against the proximal end so that the greatest transverse diameter of both ends of the tibia form a variable angle (on the average, about 23°) with one another (*torsion of the tibia*, Fig. **137**). The tip of the foot is directed somewhat outward when the transverse axis of the upper end of the tibia is frontal. Owing to the angular position of both feet (normally about 45°), the stability of the standing position is increased.

The torsion of the tibia – in contrast to the anteversion of the femur – is first developed postnatally during the first year of life. In anthropoid apes (and in human fetuses), the tibia is twisted inwardly.

The **fibula** (Fig. **134**), a narrow, slightly pliable bony rod, is covered by the muscles of the lower leg over almost its entire length. The shaft is quadrangular in cross section. The interosseous membrane attaches at its dorsomedially-directed *interosseous margin*.

On the *posterior surface*, the *medial crest* separates the areas of origin of the tibialis posterior and flexor hallucis longus muscles.

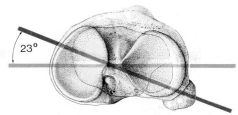

Fig. 137. **Torsion of tibia in the adult** (proximal end of tibia projected on malleolar fork)
Transverse axis of knee joint ━━━
Transverse axis of the upper ankle joint ━━━

The *head of the fibula* ends in a short *apex* and possesses medially a small, cartilage-covered *articular surface*, which lies adjacent to the corresponding articular surface on the lateral condyle of the tibia.

The distal end of the fibula forms the external *lateral malleolus*, which represents the lateral prong of the malleolar fork. It extends somewhat further distally than the medial malleolus. Its medial surface contains the *malleolar articular surface*, which articulates with the lateral surface of the trochlea of the talus and dorsal to it exhibits a cavity, the *malleolar fossa*, in which the posterior talofibular ligament is anchored. On the external surface of the lateral malleolus there is a groove, the *malleolar groove*, for the tendons of the peroneus longus and peroneus brevis.

Ossification. The center of ossification in the proximal epiphysis of the *tibia* (Fig. **116**), which appears just before birth in about 80% of the cases, is valued as another maturity indicator like the ossific center in the distal epiphysis of the femur.

The distal epiphysial nucleus appears in the tibia in the 2nd postnatal year. The ossification of the tibial shaft begins in the 7th–8th embryonic week. Proximal and distal epiphysial joints usually close by the 17th (females) or 18th year (males), although individual variants of $\pm 2 - 3$ years are common. The tibial tuberosity ossifies (at ages $11 - 13$) from the proximal tibial epiphysis in the form of a tongue-shaped osseous cone or possesses its own ossific center.

The ossification of the attachment site of the ligamentum patellae can be disturbed – especially in male adolescents (Osgood-Schlatter disease).

The shaft of the *fibula* ossifies in the 8th embryonic week, only slightly later than the tibial diaphysis. Ossific centers appear in the head of the fibula in the 4th – 6th postnatal year and in the lateral malleolus at the beginning of the 2nd year. The closure of the epiphysial joint takes place at about the same time as in the tibia. An additional bony nucleus can appear in the apex of both the medial and the lateral malleolus in the 6th–12th year, which soon fuses with the distal epiphysis.

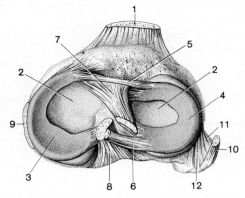

Fig. 138. **Menisci and ligaments of knee joint**, view of superior articular surface of tibia (articular capsule not shown)

1 Ligamentum patellae
2 Superior articular surface of tibia
3 Medial meniscus
4 Lateral meniscus
5 Transverse ligament of knee
6 Posterior meniscofemoral ligament
7 Anterior cruciate ligament

8 Posterior cruciate ligament
9 Tibial collateral ligament (fuses with medial meniscus by means of joint capsule)
10 Fibular collateral ligament
11 Anterior ligament of head of fibula
12 Posterior ligament of head of fibula

b) Menisci, Capsule and Ligaments of the Knee Joint

In the *knee joint* (Figs. **138 – 141**), the largest joint of the human body, flexion and extension movements are possible, as well as rotation when the knee is flexed. With regard to form, the knee joint is thus a combination of hinge and pivot joints and is, therefore, also designated as a *trochoginglymus* joint.

The cartilage-covered surfaces of both femoral condyles articulate with the superior articular surface of the tibia. The fibula does not participate at the knee joint. Since the curvature of the joint surfaces of the femoral condyles increases from anterior to posterior, the bearing surface of the femur is all the more extensive, the more the knee joint is extended.

The *menisci* are deformable, C-shaped discs, whose structural materials resemble fibrocartilage. In cross section they are wedge-shaped: their outer margin is thickened and grown together with the joint capsule. The *lateral meniscus* forms an almost closed ring. The *medial meniscus*, on the other hand, is more crescent-shaped. Both menisci are fixed with their anterior horns at the anterior intercondylar area and with their posterior horns at the posterior intercondylar area. The fields of attachment of both ends of the medial meniscus enclose the narrower attachment places of the lateral meniscus.

At the anterior margin, both menisci can be connected by a *transverse ligament*. From the posterior horn of the lateral meniscus a strong bundle of fibers, the *posterior meniscofemoral ligament*, passes behind the posterior cruciate ligament medial and cranial to the lateral surface of the medial femoral trochlea. A weak *anterior meniscofemoral ligament* can connect the posterior end of the lateral meniscus with the medial condyle of the femur in front of the posterior cruciate ligment.

During movements in the knee joint, the menisci with their flat, free undersurfaces are displaced on the superior articular surface of the tibia. They form transportable joint sockets for the femoral condyles and distribute the circumscribed pressure to the larger joint surfaces of the tibial condyles. The menisci subdivide the knee joint incompletely into the (upper) meniscofemoral articulation and the (lower) meniscotibial articulation.

Excursion possibilities of the medial articular disc are limited more strongly than those of the lateral meniscus; for the medial collateral ligament is inserted in the joint capsule and thus is also connected with the medial meniscus, whereas the lateral collateral ligament has not grown together with the articular capsule.

For these reasons, meniscus injuries affect the medial articular disc much more frequently. Tears or detachments occur in the weaker anterior crescentic margin of the less mobile medial meniscus (sport injuries) particularly during maximal flexion with simultaneous external rotation of the leg.

After operative removal of a meniscus, the load capacity of the knee joint is initially reduced. Suitable therapy, however, promotes the formation of a replacement tissue and usually results in an extensive restoration of functional capacity.

The *joint capsule* is attached at the tibia along the cartilage-bone border. At the femur the attachment line of the inner membrane does not correspond, for the most part, to the attachment of the external fibrous layer. The inner membrane of the joint lies on the anterior surface of the femur, usually a finger's width proximal to the patellar surface (suprapatellar recess) and is connected with the bone by displaceable fatty tissue. The replication fold lies at individually varying levels in the region of the distal fourth of the femoral shaft. Laterally, the attachment line does not involve the epicondyle and follows on the dorsal side of the cartilage-bone border. The inner membrane of the joint capsule invaginates here (on the dorsal side) into the intercondylar fossa and surrounds the front and sides of the cruciate ligaments. At the ventral side, the patella borders directly on the joint cavity with its cartilage-covered articulate surface.

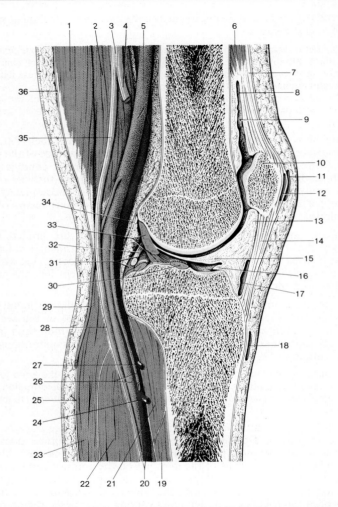

Fig. 139. Sagittal section through knee joint in region of lateral femoral condyle,
lateral view of section surface
Preparation of muscles, vessels and nerves in popliteal space

1 Semitendinosus
2 Semimembranosus
3 Sciatic nerve
4 Common peroneal nerve, severed
5 Popliteal artery and vein
6 Articularis genus
7 Tendon of quadriceps femoris
8 Suprapatellar bursa
9 Suprapatellar recess
10 Patella

Distal to the patella, the synovial membrane of the joint is displaced from the fibrous layer formed here by the ligamentum patellae and the patellar retinaculum by the wedge-shaped *infrapatellar fat body* and pushed into the interior of the joint. The fat body curves around the lower margin of the patella and pushes forward with two fatty folds (*alar folds*) into the two fossae bordered by the inner surfaces of the femoral condyles, by the menisci and by the patella and separated from one another by the cruciate ligaments. As the vestige of an embryonic, distinctly developed anterior partition, there is a slender fatty fold (the *infrapatellar synovial fold*) covered by the synovia, which passes from the fat body to the cruciate ligaments. The fat body forms a deformable padding material which fills up a space that shifts according to the position of the joint and is caused by positional changes in the ends of the joint and the menisci. Since the front of the articular cavity opens wide during flexion, atmospheric pressure presses the fat body deeply into the interior of the joint, and the skin caves in slightly on both sides of the patella. During extension of the leg the fat body causes the skin to bulge on both sides of the ligamentum patellae.

The knee joint is particularly vulnerable to infection owing to the dimensions of the articular cavity and its abundant fossae. Because of the large surface of the synovial membrane, pathogens and bacteriotoxins can be taken up very rapidly into the blood stream.

The *anterior capsular wall* is strengthened by tendinous bands that are connected directly or indirectly with the tendon sheath of the quadriceps femoris: ligamentum patellae and retinacula patellae. The *ligamentum patellae* is the terminal tendon of the quadriceps femoris and connects the patella, which is embedded in it as a sesamoid bone, with the tibial tuberosity.

Superficial fibers from the shiny tendon pass over the patella and radiate into the ligament. The *retinacula patellae* are broad, ligamentous tracts,

11 Subcutaneous prepatellar bursa
12 Subfascial prepatellar bursa
13 Infrapatellar fat pad
14 Ligamentum patellae
15 Infrapatellar synovial fold
16 Alar fold
17 Deep infrapatellar bursa
18 Subcutaneous bursa of tibial tuberosity
19 Tibialis posterior (section surface)
20 Posterior tibial artery and tibial nerve
21 Popliteus (section surface)
22 Soleus (section surface)
23 Medial head of gastrocnemius (section surface)
24 Peroneal artery, severed
25 Crural fascia (section edge)

26 Posterior tibial veins
27 Anterior tibial artery, severed
28 Deep layer of crural fascia (section edge)
29 Small saphenous vein
30 Lateral meniscus, severed near attachment
31 Posterior cruciate ligament
32 Posterior meniscofemoral ligament
33 Anterior cruciate ligament (partly section surface, partly view from above, synovial membrane removed)
34 Fibrous membrane of posterior wall of capsule (connective tissue which pushes ventrally against cruciate ligaments is mostly removed)
35 Tibial nerve
36 Fascia lata (section edge)

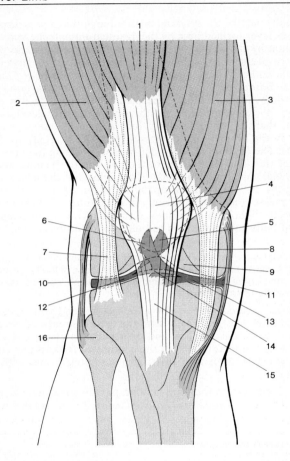

Fig. 140. **Knee joint**, view from in front
(Articular capsule not shown, structural elements made partly transparent)

1 Rectus femoris
2 Vastus lateralis
3 Vastus medialis
4 Patella
5 Posterior cruciate ligament
6 Anterior cruciate ligament
7 Lateral retinaculum of patella
8 Medial retinaculum of patella
9 Patellar surface of femur
10 Fibular collateral ligament
11 Tibial collateral ligament
12 Lateral meniscus
13 Medial meniscus
14 Transverse ligament of knee
15 Ligamentum patellae
16 Head of fibula

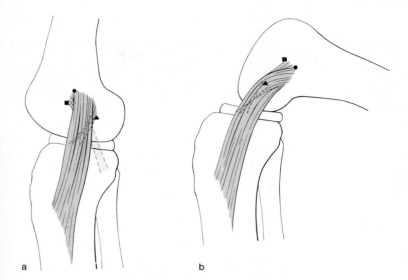

Fig. 141. **Internal collateral ligament of knee joint**
a In extended position, external collateral ligament transparent
b Involution of tibial collateral ligament in flexed position (identical points of
  attachment of internal collateral ligament marked with same symbols in both
  illustrations)

which can be clearly defined only artificially; they pass along both sides of
the patella from the shiny tendon of the quadriceps tendon to the tibia.
To a limited extent, they can transmit the traction of the contracted
quadriceps femoris to the tibia even when the true terminal tendon of the
muscle is interrupted by a transverse fracture of the patella: reverse
extension apparatus of the tibia.

The *lateral retinaculum patellae* is strengthened by radiating fibers of the iliotibial
tract. The superficial longitudinal fibers of the retinacula counteract a luxation of
the patella only when the quadriceps femoris is contracted. Deep fibers passing
from the epicondyles of the femur at the lateral margins of the patella guide the
patella like two reins. A luxation is only possible when a rein tears. In transverse
fractures of the patella, the traction transmitted through the retinacula makes it
possible to walk on level ground. For walking uphill or climbing stairs, however,
the traction transmitted is insufficient since it is not capable of carrying the body
weight.

The *posterior wall of the capsule* of the knee joint (Fig. **142**) is strengthened and protected against impaction by tendinous bundles from the

semimembranosus, popliteus and gastrocnemius and by ligamentous tracts of the tibiofibular joint, which radiate laterally into the capsule of the knee joint. The *oblique popliteal ligament*, a bundle from the terminal tendon of the semimembranosus, passes into the posterior wall of the capsule obliquely upward toward the lateral femoral condyle; the *arcuate popliteal ligament*, which courses at right angles to it, gives off fibrous tracts to the tendon of origin of the popliteus and can be continued up to the head of the fibula.

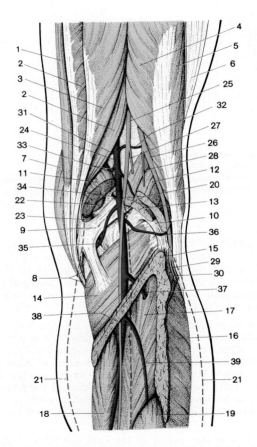

Fig. 142. **Arteries and nerves in popliteal fossa** (muscular branches not shown)

Ligaments (Figs. **138–141**). *External* and *internal ligaments* are distinguished at the knee joint. Traction of these ligaments plays a more important role in the management of movements at the knee joint than at any other joint of the human body since the guidance of muscles and bones is largely absent. Thanks to the strong ligamentous apparatus, dislocations of the knee joint are extremely rare, yet injuries resulting from unphysiological strain on the ligaments occur not infrequently.

The *external ligaments* of the knee joint are the *collateral ligaments* on the lateral and medial sides of the joint, the *ligamentum patellae* and the *patellar retinacula* on the anterior side, as well as the *oblique* and *arcuate popliteal ligaments*, which are crossed in the posterior wall of the capsule as strengthening bands.

The lateral (external) ligament, the *fibular collateral ligament*, passes – at some distance from the articular capsule – as a rounded cord from the lateral epicondyle of the femur to the head of the fibula.

The tendon of the popliteus and a fibrous cord segmented off from the tendon of the biceps femoris, which inserts at the lateral condyle of the tibia, pass through the fissure between the joint capsule and the ligamentous tract.

The medial (internal) collateral ligament, the *tibial collateral ligament*, is firmly attached to the joint capsule and thus also with the medial meniscus. This broad ligament arises with an anterior portion from the medial epicondyle of the femur and with a short, posterior part from the medial side of the internal femoral trochlea. The short, dorsal fibrous tracts course to the medial meniscus (meniscus tracts). The main part of the internal collateral ligament passes to the medial surface of the

1 Gracilis
2 Semimembranosus
3 Semitendinosus
4 Long head ⎱ of biceps femoris
5 Short head ⎰
6 Iliotibial tract
7 Sartorius
8 Pes anserinus
9 Oblique popliteal ligament
10 Arcuate popliteal ligament
11 Medial head ⎱ of gastrocnemius
12 Lateral head ⎰ (severed)
13 Plantaris
14 Popliteus
15 Soleus (severed near its origin)
16 Peroneus longus
17 Tibialis posterior
18 Flexor digitorum longus
19 Flexor hallucis longus
20 Distal boundary of popliteal fossa

21 External contour line of triceps surae
22 Subtendinous bursa of medial head of gastrocnemius
23 Bursa of semimembranosus
24 Popliteal artery
25 Tibial nerve
26 Common peroneal nerve
27 Medial sural cutaneous nerve
28 Lateral sural cutaneous nerve
29 Deep peroneal nerve
30 Superficial peroneal nerve
31 Medial superior genicular artery
32 Lateral superior genicular artery
33 Sural arteries
34 Middle genicular artery
35 Medial inferior genicular artery
36 Lateral inferior genicular artery
37 Anterior tibial artery
38 Posterior tibial artery
39 Peroneal artery

proximal end of the tibia (tibial tracts) and, in so doing, covers the tendon bundles of the semimembranosus radiating toward the tibia.

Since the anterior fibrous tracts are attached to the femur further proximally than the posterior portion, the internal collateral ligament, which spreads broadly in the extended position, is pushed together during flexion at the knee joint and twisted into itself (Fig. 141). When the knee is extended, the medial collateral ligament passes somewhat obliquely from posterosuperior to antero-inferior, whereas the lateral collateral ligament follows an opposite course from antero-superior to postero-inferior.

The collateral ligaments fix the knee in the extended position and prevent abduction and adduction. In the flexed knee joint, only the posterior portion of the medial collateral ligament is stretched, and voluntary rotation is therefore possible. Since the medial collateral ligament is not completely relaxed, however, and the medial meniscus is fused with it, the mobility of the medial condyle is restricted more strongly than that of the lateral femoral trochlea. The axis of rotation is moved, therefore, somewhat medially.

In the case of *tearing* of a collateral ligament (most often the internal collateral ligament), merely the attempt to abduct the leg toward the opposite side is extremely painful, whereas when a *detachment* occurs, the leg can be abducted toward the healthy side. In the radiogram, the articular cavity gapes on the damaged side. "Overstretched" collateral ligaments (e.g. as the result of a persistent effusion or a traction bandage of more than one week) also permit abnormal movements of the knee joint: loose or flail knee joint.

The *internal ligaments* are represented by the *cruciate ligaments*, which thrust into the articular cavity from the posterior wall of the capsule. They lie extracapsularly, but are separated anteriorly and laterally from the joint cavity only by the synovial membrane covering them.

The *anterior cruciate ligament* ascends from the anterior intercondylar area of the tibia to the medial surface of the lateral femoral condyle. The *posterior cruciate ligament* passes from the posterior intercondylar area to the lateral surface of the medial femoral trochlea. The anterior cruciate ligament thus courses obliquely from anterior, inferior and medial to posterior, superior and lateral, while the posterior cruciate ligament runs in the opposite direction from posterior, inferior and lateral to anterior, superior and medial.

Both cruciate ligaments arise at the tibia in the frontal plane. The anterior ligament twists in such a way that in the extended position the fibers arising laterally attach most dorsally at the medial surface of the lateral condyle, whereas the fibers of the posterior ligament are attached most ventrally at the lateral surface of the medial femoral trochlea.

The cruciate ligaments secure the articular contact of the femur and tibia and prevent the femoral condyles from sliding off the articular surface of the head of the tibia. When the knee joint is flexed, they prevent abduction and adduction; when it is extended, they collaborate with the collateral ligaments to counteract hyperextension. In each position of the knee joint, portions of the cruciate ligaments are stretched (the medial partial tracts of both ligaments during extension; the lateral part of the anterior and the medial fiber bundles of the posterior ligament during flexion). They twist around each other during internal rotation and unwind during external rotation. A parallel position of the cruciate ligaments, however, is normally not reached because the medial collateral ligament does not permit such an extensive external rotation.

When the cruciate ligaments are detached – their anchorage is generally torn away from the tibia together with the intercondylar eminence, the tibia can be pushed back and forth against the femur when the knee is flexed: drawer phenomenon.

The *arterial supply of the knee joint* is effected by a finely-meshed network (*articular network of the knee*) which surrounds the capsule of the knee joint. It is fed by branches of the femoral, popliteal, anterior tibial and posterior tibial arteries.

Innervation of the articular capsule. The nerve branches to the knee joint arise from the tibial nerve (and course with the middle, medial superior, and medial inferior arteries of the knee), common peroneal nerve (together with the lateral superior and lateral inferior arteries of the knee) and saphenous nerve (together with the descending genicular artery), or from the obturator nerve.

The *relaxation position of the knee joint* consists of a slight flexion (about 25°), as is attained when the knee is supported by a knee roll. In this position, all parts of the capsule, the rectus femoris (owing to the slight flexion at the hip joint) and the flexors (owing to flexion at the knee joint) are relieved of tension. The *normal position* of the knee joint, however, is the extended position. In the case of joint effusion, the knee is held slightly flexed (relaxation position); the joint capsule bulges above and on both sides of the patella. The patella is raised off the underlying tissues by the accumulation of fluid in the articular cavity. If the patella is pressed intermittently and then freed, the patella then "dances". On the other hand, when an effusion occurs in a prepatellar bursa, its position is not altered.

The following **movement possibilities exist at the knee joint:**
- *from the normal* (= *extension*) *position, flexion* around approximately *frontal* axes, and
- *with increasing flexion* at the knee joint, the voluntary *internal* or *external rotation* of the tibia (or in the case of firmly placed feet, the external or internal rotation of the femur) around a *longitudinal* axis of the leg, which courses through the medial condyle of the tibia.

Flexion is actively possible by about 130°, and then the flexors of the knee joint are actively insufficient (Fig. **17 c**). The knee can be flexed passively on the average by about 155° before a soft part inhibition ends the movement. During flexion, especially the cruciate ligaments are stretched.

During the first phase of the flexion movement (up to 20°), the femoral condyles are rotated downward, the axis thereby moving posteriorly. The main part of the movement then takes place as a stationary rotary gliding of the femoral trochlea, since the cruciate ligaments prevent a further unrolling of the condyles. The medial and particularly the lateral meniscus are displaced backward during flexion and slide forward during extension.

Extension of the knee joint is retarded by the stretching of the collateral ligaments and by parts of the cruciate ligaments. A noteworthy hyperextension is possible under physiological conditions only in small children (round shape of the condyles). If the knee joint is extended up to about 170°, an external rotation of the tibia of about 5° automatically takes place (or an internal rotation of the femur when the foot is firmly placed in position) before the extension movement can be completed (further extension of 10° to 180°). In this so-called *terminal rotation*, the cruciate ligaments are slightly unwound from one another to permit further extension. If the knee joint is flexed from the extended position, the rotation is reversed.

When the knee is strongly flexed, the patella lies on the patellar surface of the femur; when the knee is extended, the patella is shifted proximally by several centimeters and adjoins the suprapatellar bursa.

Voluntary *internal* or *external rotation* of the tibia takes place essentially in the articular cavity between the menisci and the superior articular surface of the tibia. The circumference of movement is the greater, the stronger the knee joint is flexed. With a flexion of 90°, the inner rotation of the leg is possible up to about 10° and is stopped by the cruciate ligaments. The circumference of outer rotation can amount to somewhat more than 40° and is limited by the tension of both collateral ligaments (especially the medial).

During external rotation, the lateral condyle of the tibia is carried backwards, and during internal rotation, the medial condyle is shifted. The menisci are displaced in opposing directions whereby the more movable lateral intra-articular disc travels the greater distance and is simultaneously deformed. Through the possibility of voluntary rotation of the leg, the transport space of the foot in walking (e.g. on uneven stony ground) is expanded.

Mucous bursae (Figs. **139** and **142**). Numerous mucous bursae lie in the vicinity of the knee joint. They prevent the tendons passing over the joint from rubbing against the underlying bones and protect the projecting bony parts from circumscribed pressure and friction. The *suprapatellar bursa* is developed proximal to the patella as a movable space for the quadriceps tendon and is almost always in more or less extensive communication with the proximal segment of the articular cavity (suprapatellar recess). The *deep infrapatellar bursa* situated distal to the patella above the tibial tuberosity ensures a frictionless gliding of the ligamentum patellae. This bursa rarely communicates with the joint cavity.

At the posterior wall of the capsule, the *subpopliteal recess*, which is located below the tendon of origin of the popliteal muscle, always communicates with the articular cavity, frequently also with the joint cavity of the tibiofibular joint. Likewise, the *semimembranosus bursa* and the *subtendinous bursa of the medial gastrocnemius* communicate frequently with the joint. The remaining mucous bursae (below the tendons of the lateral gastrocnemius, biceps femoris, sartorius and below the pes anserinus), on the other hand, like the subcutaneous, subfascial or subtendinous *prepatellar bursa*, have no connection with the articular cavity.

c) Action of Muscles and Muscle Groups on the Knee Joint

The torque of the extensors of the knee joint is about three times greater than that of the flexors. The quadriceps femoris not only must move almost the total body weight in climbing stairs, it must also punctually inhibit movement during flexion of the knee joint and fix the desired position (flexed knee). In standing up from a sitting position, in raising the body from a supine or a squatting position, no other muscle can replace the quadriceps femoris.

In the knee joint:
- *flexion* is accomplished by the ischiocrural muscles (semimembranosus, semintendinosus and biceps femoris),
  whereby they are supported by the gracilis, sartorius, popliteus, and gastrocnemius;
- *extension* is produced by the quadriceps femoris,
  whereby support by the tendon fibers of the tensor fasciae latae radiating into the lateral patellar retinaculum is negligible;
- *rotation* (with the leg flexed) of the tibia *inwards* is provided by the semimembranosus, semitendinosus and popliteus,
  whereby the gracilis and sartorius, as well as the lateral head of the gastrocnemius, can assist: and
- *rotation* (with the leg flexed) of the tibia *outwards* is produced especially by the biceps femoris,
  whereas the action of the tensor fasciae latae and the medial head of the gastrocnemius is limited.

The torque of the ischiocrural musculature, aside from the short head of the biceps, is increased by simultaneous flexion at the hip joint. In the extended hip joint, it increases up to the right-angled flexion of the knee joint, then rapidly decreases, and is exhausted at a flexion of over 130°. The *semimembranosus* is the strongest flexor of the knee joint and also the most effective internal rotator. The *biceps femoris* acts as an external rotator of the leg when the knee joint is flexed. Its torque is almost as great as that of the numerous internal rotators.

The action potential of the two-jointed *rectus femoris* on the knee joint is greatest when the hip is extended, but is far surpassed by the torque of the *vasti muscles*. The lateral traction produced by the contraction of the vastus lateralis is equalized by the transverse traction of the vastus medialis and the tension of the vasto-adductor membrane system. Moreover, the elevation of the external femoral condyle counteracts a luxation of the patella laterally. When the knee is flexed, the holding function is carried out primarily by the vasti muscles. At the same time, they form a tension belt for the femur which decisively diminishes the bending stress on this bone caused by body weight.

Paralyses. When the *ischiocrural musculature* is paralyzed, the knee joint can no longer be flexed with power. The tip of the foot of the free leg cannot be sufficiently lifted from the ground on the paralyzed side and drags. At the same time, there is a failure of the stretching action of these muscles on the hip joint. The patient therefore attempts to walk as erect as possible, that is, to shift the body's line of gravity backward, in order not to fall forward.

When the *quadriceps femoris* is paralyzed, an active extension at the knee joint is not possible. The patient usually cannot rise from the sitting position without help when there is a unilateral paralysis, and certainly not when it is bilateral. However, the patient can stand on the paralyzed leg as long as the center of gravity of the body falls in front of the transverse flexion-extension axis. As soon as the center of gravity moves backwards across this axis, the leg gives way at the knee joint. In walking, the leg of the paralyzed, unsupported leg is extended with the help of gravity and centrifugal force and is moved forward only a limited distance so that only short steps are possible. With bilateral paralysis, a patient cannot sit down slowly or maintain a standing position with flexed knees.

3. Popliteal Fossa

The *popliteal fossa* (Fig. **142**) is the area on the dorsal side of the knee joint which is deepened into a diamond-shaped fossa bordered by muscular elevations when the knee is flexed. Proximally, the muscular rhombus is bordered at the lateral side by the biceps femoris, on the medial side by the semimembranosus and the semitendinosus lying dorsal to it. Distally, the fossa is closed by the two origins of the gastrocnemius (as well as the plantaris at the lateral edge).

The popliteal fossa extends in a longitudinal direction from the femur up to the tibia, proximal to the origin of the soleus muscle. In the superior and the middle portions, the base of the popliteal fossa is formed by the popliteal surface of the femur and the posterior wall of the capsule of the knee joint with its strengthening tracts. The lower part of the popliteal fossa is only accessible when both heads of the gastrocnemius are artificially pushed apart. At the base (at the anterior wall in an erect posture) of this distal portion the popliteus and the fascia covering it are situated.

The space of the popliteal fossa bordered by the muscular rhombus is filled with a deformable fat body. The superficial closure of this connective tissue space is effected by the distal portion of the fascia lata designated as the popliteal fascia. This tough, predominantly transversely-fibered portion of the fascia lata, which stretches tautly and is bulged out by the fat body when the knee is extended, separates the skin and the subcutaneous tissue of the popliteal fossa from the deep connective tissue space; it continues ventrally into the fascial covering of the knee joint and distally into the fascia of the leg.

The short transverse axis of the rhomboidal popliteal fossa lies somewhat proximal to the intercondylar line; the apex of the distal portion of the rhombus (triangle of the calf muscles) marked off by the transverse axis lies at the level of the articular cavity of the knee joint when the leg is extended and when the heads of the gastrocnemius are not spread artificially.

The large conducting pathways connecting the thigh and leg (common peroneal nerve and tibial nerve, which are loosely connected with the vascular cord formed from the popliteal vessels and deep lymphatic vessels) and smaller subfascial vessels and nerves to the skin of the leg and foot (small saphenous vein, superficial lymphatic vessels, medial and lateral sural cutaneous nerves) course within the connective tissue space of the popliteal fossa.

The connective tissue in the popliteal fossa communicates proximally with the connective tissue stroma at the flexor side of the thigh via the hiatus tendineus (adductor hiatus) and continues distally below the tendinous arch of the soleus into the connective tissue layer between the peroneal muscles and the deep flexors at the leg. Inflammatory processes can spread rapidly in this connective tissue route. Abscesses can settle unhindered without necessarily being discernible externally through the rigid popliteal fascia.

Vessels and Nerves in the Popliteal Fossa

The large conducting pathways pass through the fat body of the popliteal fossa (Fig. **142**). The *tibial nerve* (in the middle) and the *common peroneal nerve* (at the lateral margin) lie superficially, whereby the common peroneal nerve increasingly approaches the popliteal fascia distally. The tibial nerve, which courses in the longitudinal axis of the popliteal rhombus, gradually crosses over the *popliteal vessels*, which are enclosed in a connective tissue vascular sheath, so that it arrives on the dorsomedial side of the vessels at the exit from the popliteal fossa. The nerve is united with the tough vascular sheath of the popliteal vessels by loose connective tissue to form a neurovascular cord. The *popliteal artery* lies deepest (Fig. **139**). It is separated from the popliteal fascia of the femur by a spongy fat pad, although it comes quite close to the posterior wall of the capsule of the knee joint. Two accompanying veins – as proximal continuations of the anterior and posterior tibial veins – flank the popliteal artery in the distal third of the popliteal fossa on both sides and are united at various levels into a single *popliteal vein*. It courses – first between artery and nerve, then further proximally at the dorsolateral side of the popliteal artery – into the lower opening of the adductor canal.

By extreme flexion of the knee joint, the blood flow in the popliteal artery can be slowed down, but not completely interrupted. Since the fat body cannot protect the vessel very much, the popliteal artery is vulnerable to supracondylar fractures of the femoral shaft.

The *common peroneal nerve* (Figs. **142** and **143**) has separated from the tibial nerve, at the latest, at the entrance into the popliteal fossa. Covered at first by the biceps femoris, it then passes along the tibial side of the tendon of insertion of this muscle and over the lateral head of the gastrocnemius distally. The nerve courses more and more superficially, covered only by the popliteal fascia, and leaves the popliteal fossa in its lower portion. It winds itself around the fibula directly beneath its head, where it is fixed in the periosteum by connective tissue tracts. It then enters the peroneal compartment, where it divides into the *superficial peroneal nerve* (for the peroneal muscles and the skin at the dorsum of the foot and toes) and the *deep peroneal nerve*, which passes distally into the extensor compartment and innervates all extensors and the skin at the facing margins of the 1st and 2nd toes.

Because of its superficial course, the common peroneal nerve is very endangered dorsal and distal to the head of the fibula. Covered only by skin and fascia and, at the same time, fixed at the bone, it can be crushed by pressure and blows against the proximal end of the fibula, damaged by sharp bone fragments in the case of a fracture of the fibular head and affected by excessive callus formation during fracture healing.

In addition to a branch to the capsule of the knee joint in the upper or in the middle third of the popliteal fossa, the *common peroneal nerve* gives off the *lateral sural cutaneous nerve*, which penetrates the fascia at the lateral head of the gastrocnemius and innervates the lateral side of the leg with several twigs.

A medial branch of the lateral sural cutaneous nerve (rarely a direct branch of the common peroneal nerve) anastomoses, usually as a *peroneal [fibular] communicating branch,* with the medial sural cutaneous nerve (from the tibial nerve) and forms the *sural nerve.*

The **popliteal artery** (Fig. **139**, **142** and **143**) retains its deep location near bones and joints during its course through the superior and middle portions of the popliteal fossa, passes distally over the popliteus, and divides at the upper margin of the soleus into the anterior and posterior

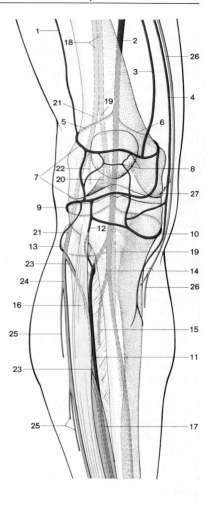

Fig. 143. **Arteries and nerves in region of knee joint**, view from in front (Cutaneous nerves and peroneal artery severed, middle genicular artery and muscular branches of arteries not shown)

1 Descending branch of lateral circumflex femoral artery
2 Popliteal artery
3 Articular branch ⎫ of descending
4 Saphenous branch ⎬ genicular artery
5 Lateral superior genicular artery
6 Medial superior genicular artery
7 Articular network of knee
8 Patellar network
9 Lateral inferior genicular artery
10 Medial inferior genicular artery
11 Anterior tibial artery
12 Anterior tibial recurrent artery
13 Circumflex fibular branch
14 Posterior tibial artery
15 Peroneal artery
16 Extensor digitorum longus
17 Extensor hallucis longus
18 Sciatic nerve
19 Tibial nerve
20 Medial sural cutaneous nerve
21 Common peroneal nerve
22 Lateral sural cutaneous nerve
23 Deep peroneal nerve
24 Superficial peroneal nerve
25 Muscular branches of superficial peroneal nerve to peroneal muscles
26 Saphenous nerve
27 Infrapatellar branch of saphenous nerve

tibial arteries. The popliteal artery gives off branches to the portions of the thigh muscles near the knee joint (particularly the flexors), dispatches the *sural arteries* distally to both heads of the gastrocnemius (each with a branch to the skin and fascia of the leg), and supplies the knee joint with five *genicular arteries*.

The *middle genicular artery* arises in the middle third of the popliteal fossa, penetrates the wall of the capsule of the knee joint posteriorly, and supplies the cruciate ligaments. Four *articular branches* of the popliteal artery pass to the *articular network of the knee*, which is developed as a fine meshwork, particularly in the region of the patella (*patellar network*) and below the retinacula and the ligamentum patellae.

The *superior medial genicular artery* courses proximal to the medial condyle of the femur below the tendons of the adductor magnus and vastus medialis. The *superior lateral genicular artery* passes anterior to the patella below the biceps tendon and proximal to the lateral femoral trochlea. The *inferior medial genicular artery* arises at the proximal margin of the popliteus and, covered by the tendon of the semimembranosus and by the medial collateral ligament, curves around the medial condyle of the tibia. The *inferior lateral genicular artery* passes over the origin of the popliteus laterally, crosses under the lateral head of the gastrocnemius, the biceps tendon and the fibular collateral ligament before it reaches the vascular network on the anterior side of the knee joint above the head of the fibula.

The *articular network of the knee* receives the following

branches of the *femoral artery*:
– descending ramus of the lateral circumflex femoral artery, and
– descending genicular artery;

branches of the *popliteal artery*
– twigs of the muscular branches to the flexors at the thigh and to the vasti muscles,
– superior medial genicular artery,
– superior lateral genicular artery,
– inferior medial genicular artery, and
– inferior lateral genicular artery;

branches of the *anterior tibial artery*:
– anterior tibial recurrent artery, and
– posterior tibial recurrent artery (inconstant);

branch of the *posterior tibial artery*:
– circumflex fibular branch.

The articular network of the knee is thus fed by branches of the femoral, popliteal, anterior tibial and posterior tibial arteries. The anastomoses between the vessels entering the arterial network proximally and distally, however, are not able to provide sufficient blood to the leg in the case of a sudden interruption of the popliteal artery. The popliteal artery, therefore, may not be ligated.

The companion veins (*veins of the knee*) coursing with the branches of the popliteal artery pass to the **popliteal vein** (doubled in the distal portion of the popliteal fossa). In the upper third of the popliteal fossa, the popliteal vein receives the *small saphenous vein* (Fig. **139**), which conveys blood from the venous network of the dorsum of the foot, passing behind the lateral malleolus to the fibula and then coursing to the popliteal fossa beneath the fascia in the groove between the two heads of the gastrocnemius.

Lymphatic vessels. Superficial lymphatic pathways accompany the small saphenous vein and carry off lymph from the lateral margin of the foot, from the region of the lateral malleolus and from the fibular region. They course subfascially in the popliteal fossa and enter (1–2) *superficial popliteal lymph nodes,* which lie adjacent to the small saphenous vein.

Epifascial lymphatic pathways can convey a portion of the lymph, however, to the lymphatic tracts accompanying the great saphenous vein and, thus, directly into the superficial inguinal nodes.

Lymph from the skeleton and the musculature of the leg, as well as from the region of the knee joint flows via deep lymphatic paths coursing in the vascular cord of the popliteal fossa to the *deep popliteal lymph nodes* (3–4) situated along the popliteal vein.

The lymph from the superficial and deep lymph nodes of the popliteal fossa arrives at the deep lymphatic vessels, which course with the femoral vein, through the lower opening of the adductor canal.

The **tibial nerve** (Figs. **139**, **142** and **143**), located superficially in the neurovascular cord, leaves the popliteal fossa together with the blood vessels and passes below the tendinous arch of the soleus in the connective tissue layer between the peroneal muscles and the deep flexors. It innervates all flexors at the leg and foot, as well as the skin in a band of varying width at the dorsomedial side of the leg and at the sole of the foot.

In the popliteal fossa, the *tibial nerve* gives off – besides branches to the joint capsule and *muscular branches* (to both heads of the gastrocnemius, plantaris, soleus and popliteus) – the *medial sural cutaneous nerve,* which courses with the small saphenous vein in the groove between the two heads of the gastrocnemius, penetrates the deep fascia of the leg in the middle of the fibula and, as a rule, anastomoses with the peroneal [fibular] anastomotic branch. It supplies – now designated as the *sural nerve* – the skin over the tendo calcaneus, at the lateral malleolus and (as the *lateral dorsal cutaneous nerve*) at the lateral margin of the foot.

D. Leg and Foot

1. Leg

a) Connections of the Two Leg Bones

The two skeletal elements of the leg articulate with one another at their proximal ends in the tibiofibular joint and communicate syndesmotically in the diaphysial region by an *interosseous membrane* and at the distal end by the *tibiofibular syndesmosis* (Figs. **134** and **150**).

At the **tibiofibular joint**, the fibular articular surface of the tibia articulates with the articular surface of the head of the fibula.

The joint capsule, which stretches beyond the cartilage-bone border ventrally at the tibia and dorsally at the fibula, is strengthened at the anterior side by the *anterior ligament of the head of the fibula* consisting of transverse and oblique fibrous tracts and at the posterior side by the weaker *posterior ligament of the head of the fibula* formed predominantly of transverse tracts (Fig. **138**). The proximal epiphysial joint of the tibia borders on the articular cavity.

The tibiofibular joint permits, at most, insignificant sliding movements between the almost flat articular surfaces. Since the articular cavity communicates indirectly with the joint cavity of the knee in about 20% of the cases (by the subpopliteal recess), inflammatory processes can transmigrate.

The **interosseous membrane of the leg** is a firm fibrous plate which connects the two leg bones with one another (Figs. **134** and **148**). The majority of fibers pass from the interosseous margin of the tibia obliquely downward to the interosseous margin of the fibula. Oppositely-coursing bundles of fibers accumulate in this layer both dorsally and ventrally. The interosseous membrane serves as an extensive field for muscular origins. The arrangement of its fibers does not permit the leg bones to move appreciably from one another and counteracts distally-directed muscle traction.

At the **tibiofibular syndesmosis**, the strong *anterior* and *posterior tibiofibular ligaments* coursing from the tibia distally to the fibula in an oblique manner (Figs. **150** and **151c**) connect the distal ends of both leg bones into a firm, resistant, but not completely inflexible, *malleolar fork*. Both ends of the bones can slide somewhat against each another and withdraw slightly from one another. With strong dorsiflexion of the foot, the broader anterior segment of the trochlear surface of the talus presses the two prongs of the malleolar fork somewhat apart.

Between the distal ends of the tibia and fibula, the articular cavity of the talocrural (superior ankle) joint continues proximally as a fissure (Fig. **153**) about 1 cm long. The bony surfaces here are (usually) not covered by cartilage, but by an inner-articular membrane. A fold of synovial membrane underlaid by adipose tissue pushes into the fissure.

Injuries of the malleolar fork are relatively frequent. It almost always involves damage to the malleolus, whereby one or both of the bones are cracked or torn off. A laceration of the tibiofibular ligaments is very rare.

b) Arrangement and Innervation of the Musculature of the Leg

The leg musculature can be arranged in two genetic groups. The *extensor group* lies at the anterior (and lateral) surfaces of the leg, and the *flexor group* at the posterior surface. Among the extensors, a further distinction is made between the *anterior muscle group* (often also designated by itself as extensor group), which is innervated by the deep peroneal nerve, and the *lateral* or *peroneal group*, which is supplied by the superficial peroneal nerve. The flexor group, innervated by the tibial nerve, is divided by a connective tissue layer (occasionally designated as the deep layer of the fascia of the leg) into the superficially-situated *peroneal muscles* and into the group of *deep flexors*.

The genetic classification of the peroneal group among the extensors does not correspond to their function since the peroneal muscles plantar flex at the superior ankle joint just as the superficial and deep flexors do.

The **fascia cruris** (deep fascia of the leg) (Fig. **148**) is the continuation of the fascia lata distal to the knee joint. It fuses with the medial surface of the tibia, encloses the leg muscles superficially, and communicates with the fibula (anterior and posterior margins) via the *anterior* and *posterior crural intermuscular septa*. Three osteofibrous chambers for the leg musculature are delimited by the fascia cruris and the two intermuscular septa, as well as the tibia, fibula and interosseous membrane.

The *chamber for the peroneal group* is bordered by the fascia cruris, the two intermuscular septa and the lateral surface of the fibula. The *extensor* and *flexor compartments* are separated by the tibia, interosseous membranes, fibula and peroneal group.

The large flexor chamber is divided by a connective tissue layer which is aponeurotic in the proximal region. It conducts the posterior tibial vessels and the tibial nerve between the peroneal muscles and deep flexors behind the medial malleolus.

Inflammations spread chiefly within the muscle chambers in the direction of the malleolar region and the dorsum of the foot. From the chamber of the peroneal muscles, suppurations (pus formations) can ascend into the connective tissue space of the popliteal fossa.

In the distal region of the leg and at the level of the malleoli, the part of the fascia cruris and fascia of the dorsum of the foot covering the extensors is strengthened by transverse and oblique fibrous tracts. The *superior extensor retinaculum* can be dissected out as a transverse band, and the *inferior extensor retinaculum* as a cross-shaped or ypsiliform (located at the dorsum of the foot) fascial reinforcement (Fig. **145**, **147** and **159**). Both retinacula prevent the muscles from being lifted off their substrate during contraction.

Between the medial malleolus and the calcaneus, the fascia cruris is strengthened by taut connective tissue fibers into a *flexor retinaculum* (Fig. **146 b** and **147**), the superficial layer of which encloses the neurovascular bundle. The deep layer covers the tendons of the deep flexors, which are enclosed in separate tendon sheaths, and forms the lateral wall of the three tendon compartments. The tendons of the deep flexors are carried to the dorsum of the foot behind the *medial* malleolus. They cross the axis of the talocrural joint on the posterior side and that of the inferior ankle (subtalar) joint posteriorly and medially.

Behind the *lateral* malleolus, the peroneal tendons are likewise directed behind the transverse axis of the talocrural joint by the fascial reinforcement designated as the *superior peroneal retinaculum* (Fig. **145** and **159**).

At the dorsum of the foot, the fascia cruris is continued as the dorsal fascia of the foot.

Anterior Muscle Group (Extensor Group)

The **tibialis anterior** (Figs. **144** and **148**) arises from the lateral condyle of the tibia, from the lateral surface of the tibia (proximal two-thirds), from the fascia cruris and from the interosseous membrane. It inserts at the plantar surface of the 1st metatarsal and 1st cuneiform bones.

During contraction, the muscle belly projects over the edge of the proximal third of the tibia. Its tendon, which is formed at the boundary to the distal third of the tibia, passes under the extensor retinaculum to the medial margin of the foot. Its *tendon sheath* (Fig. **145**) begins proximal to the extensor retinaculum and extends distally up to the level of the articular cavity of the talocrural joint. It covers the proximal and distal portions of the tendon superficially and envelops the middle part.

The proximal muscular branches for the tibialis anterior and extensor digitorum longus already separate from the deep peroneal nerve in the peroneal compartment. After it has penetrated the extensor digitorum longus, distal branches pass to each of the two muscles named and muscular branches (usually two) to the extensors of the big toe.

The **extensor digitorum longus** (Figs. **144** and **148**) arises from the lateral condyle of the tibia, the anterior margin of the fibula and a narrow area of the interosseous membrane. It passes to the *dorsal aponeuroses* of the 2nd – 5th toes, which are similar in their basic form to the dorsal aponeuroses of the fingers (both marginal bundles of each tendon end at the distal phalanx, the middle part at the middle phalanx).

The *dorsal aponeuroses* (Fig. **156**) are not always completely delineated at the toes. Since the tendons of the interossei usually insert only at the proximal phalanges and the tendinous tracts of the lumbricals frequently do not reach the middle and distal phalanges of the 2nd–5th toes, the active extension of these toe segments is often not completely possible. Only the distal phalanx of the big toe can be truly dorsiflexed by the extensor hallucis longus.

The extensor digitorum longus fills the lateral recess of the extensor compartment of the leg. Superficial fibers come from the aponeurotic fascia cruris. The fiber bundles of the muscle approach the tendons of insertion obliquely, which – enclosed in a single *tendon sheath* (Fig. **145**) – pass the lateral division of the extensor retinaculum as an enclosed cord before separating from one another distal to it.

The **peroneus tertius**, as a distal portion of the extensor digitorum longus which is more or less segmented off, can send a 5th tendon to the base of the 5th (and 4th) metatarsal (Fig. **145**).

Innervation: deep peroneal nerve.

The **extensor hallucis longus** (Fig. **144**) is covered completely by the two adjacent muscles in the region of its origin at the medial surface of the

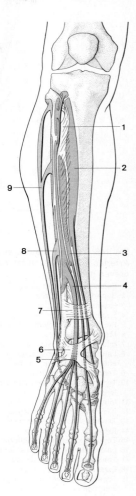

Fig. 144. **Extensor and peroneal muscle groups of leg**, view from in front
1 Interosseous membrane of leg
2 Tibialis anterior
3 Extensor hallucis longus
4 Extensor digitorum longus
5 Inferior peroneal retinaculum
6 Inferior extensor retinaculum
7 Superior extensor retinaculum
8 Peroneus brevis
9 Peroneus longus
Innervation:
☐ Superficial peroneal nerve
▨ Deep peroneal nerve

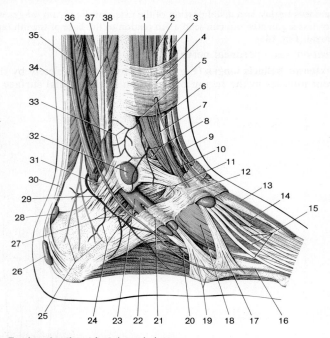

Fig. 145. **Tendon sheaths at foot**, lateral view
Arteries and nerves in lateral region of ankle (terminal branching of arteries and nerves not shown)

1 Extensor digitorum longus
2 Superficial peroneus
3 Extensor hallucis longus
4 Superior extensor retinaculum
5 Perforating branch of peroneal artery
6 Medial dorsal cutaneous nerve
7 Intermediate dorsal cutaneous nerve
8 Lateral anterior malleolar artery and anterior tibiofibular ligament
9 Tendon sheath of tibialis anterior
10 Tendon sheath of extensor digitorum longus
11 Interosseous talocalcanean ligament
12 Inferior extensor retinaculum
13 Tendon sheath of extensor hallucis longus
14 Extensor hallucis brevis
15 Tendons of extensor digitorum longus
16 Lateral dorsal cutaneous nerve
17 Tendon of peroneus tertius
18 Extensor digitorum brevis
19 Tuberosity of metatarsal V with tendinous insertion of peroneus brevis

20 Plantar tendon sheath of peroneus longus
21 Inferior peroneal retinaculum
22 Abductor digiti minimi
23 Common synovial sheath of peroneal muscles
24 Calcanean branches of peroneal artery
25 Lateral calcanean branches of sural nerve
26 Subcutaneous bursa of calcaneus
27 Lateral talocalcanean ligament and calcaneofibular ligament
28 Bursa of tendo calcaneus
29 Superior peroneal retinaculum
30 Tendo calcaneus
31 Synovial tendon sheath of flexor hallucis longus
32 Subcutaneous bursa of lateral malleolus
33 Arterial network of lateral malleolus
34 Small saphenous vein
35 Sural nerve
36 Soleus
37 Peroneus longus
38 Peroneus brevis

fibula and at the interosseous membrane (2nd and 3rd quarters). Its tendon passes to the surface only above the superior extensor retinaculum and attaches at the distal phalanx, partly also at the proximal segment of the big toe, which possesses no dorsal aponeurosis.

The *tendon sheath* begins only at the level of the malleolus, but extends far distally up to the base or head of the 1st metatarsal (Fig. **145**).

Innervation: deep peroneal nerve.

Lateral Muscle Group (Peroneal Group)

The **peroneus longus** (Figs. **144** and **148**), a bipennate muscle, arises from the proximal portion of the wall of the peroneal compartment (fibula, intermuscular septum, fascia cruris) and inserts at the tuberosity of the 1st metatarsal and at the 2nd cuneiform.

Its tendon courses distally on the muscle belly and the tendon of the peroneus brevis. Posterior to the lateral malleolus, the tendons of both peroneal muscles are enclosed in a common *tendon sheath* (Fig. **145**), which is fixed at the lateral malleolus by the superior peroneal retinaculum. At the lateral surface of the calcaneus, the tendon sheath separates, the tendon of the peroneus brevis coursing above the peroneal trochlea to the 5th metatarsal and the tendon of the peroneus longus passing behind this bony prominence to its turning point at the lateral margin of the foot. Both peroneal tendons are held securely by the inferior peroneal retinaculum.

The tendon of the peroneus longus glides on the tuberosity of the cuboid with a fibrocartilaginous covering and – enclosed by a tendon sheath (Fig. **145**) – passes to the 1st (2nd) metatarsal and to the 2nd cuneiform (Fig. **155**) across the plantar surface of the foot in a groove covered over by the long plantar ligament.

The **peroneus brevis** (Figs. **144** and **148**) originates from the distal half of the fibula and from both intermuscular septa, passes behind the lateral malleolus together with the peroneus longus, and attaches at the tuberosity of the 5th metatarsal.

As a phylogenetic vestige of a long deep, extensor group which is well-developed in lower mammals, a weak terminal tendon passes to the dorsal aponeurosis of the 5th toe.

Innervation of both peroneal muscles: superficial peroneal nerve.

The superficial peroneal nerve gives off branches (2–3) to the peroneus longus directly distal to the head of the fibula. The muscular branch to the peroneus brevis leaves the main trunk of the nerve, as a rule, only after the latter has left the peroneus longus and courses between the two peroneal muscles.

Superficial Layer of Flexors: Muscles of the Calf

The *calf muscles* are represented by the gastrocnemius, arising with two heads and the soleus, which insert at the posterior surface of the calcaneus with a common tendon, the Achilles' tendon. They form the **triceps surae**

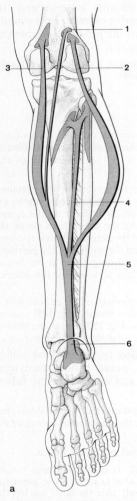

Fig. 146. **Flexor group of leg**, view from behind
a Superficial layer (calf muscles)
b Deep layer

1 Plantaris
2 Lateral head ⎫ of gastrocnemius
3 Medial head ⎬
4 Soleus
5 Triceps surae
6 Tendo calcaneus
7 Popliteus
8 Tibialis posterior

9 Flexor digitorum longus
10 Flexor hallucis longus
11 Crossing of flexor tendons of leg
12 Flexor retinaculum
13 Crossing of flexor tendons in sole of foot
Innervation:
▨ Tibial nerve

(Fig. **146 a**), an extremely strong muscle which bulges the posterior surface of the leg as the "calf".

The **gastrocnemius** (Figs. **142**, **146** and **148**) arises with both heads at the popliteal surface, above the femoral condyle, the stronger medial head somewhat more proximal than the lateral head. The terminal tendon of the muscle unites with the tendon of the soleus into the *Achilles' tendon* (*tendo calcaneus*), which inserts at the tuber calcanei (Fig. **145**).

The *bursa of the tendo calcaneus* (Figs. **145** and **147**) cushions the tendon against the upper margin of the tuber calcanei and permits it to be lifted off its base during plantar flexion of the foot.

Innervation: tibial nerve.

The muscular branches to the three heads of the triceps surae already leave the tibial nerve in the upper third of the popliteal fossa.

The **soleus** (Figs. **146 a** and **148**), which is largely covered by the gastrocnemius, takes its origin from the head and the adjacent posterior surface of the fibula, from a tendinous arcade (*tendinous arch of the soleus*), which passes from the fibula to the tibia and bridges over the neurovascular cord, and from the tibia (soleal line and medial margin). It inserts at the tuber calcanei via the Achilles' tendon (Fig. **145**).

The belly of the soleus extends further distally than the muscular belly of the gastrocnemius and is covered by a fine tendinous layer on which the gastrocnemius glides. The soleus is a complex pennate muscle and is organized into a superficial and a deep muscular layer by a frontally-situated tendinous sheet.

Innervation: tibial nerve.

The **plantaris** (Figs. **142** and **146 a**) arises medial to the lateral head of the gastrocnemius and proximal to the lateral condyle of the femur. From its short muscle belly, a long, narrow terminal tendon passes between the gastrocnemius and soleus to the tuber calcanei (via the Achilles' tendon); it occasionally extends to the crural fascia or, more rarely, to the plantar aponeurosis.

The muscle, a phylogenetic vestige of a muscular tract passing directly to the plantar aponeurosis still found in lower primates, can occasionally be absent in humans or fused with the lateral head of the gastrocnemius.

Innervation: tibial nerve.

Situated between the gastrocnemius and soleus, the plantaris is enveloped in a connective tissue which communicates with the vascular sheath of the posterior tibial artery and vein. The muscle forms a protective bow over the vessels above the tendinous arcade. During flexion of the knee joint, its task is to raise the neurovascular bundle, bring it into an arched course and help to protect the vessels from kinking.

Deep Layer of Flexors

The **tibialis posterior** (Figs. **146** and **148**) possesses a broad field of origin at the interosseous membrane. Narrow marginal parts come from the

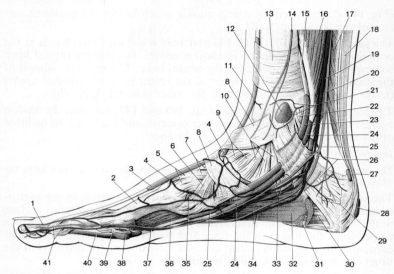

Fig. 147. **Tendon sheaths in foot**, medial view, arteries and nerves in medial region of ankle

1 Medial dorsal digital artery of toe
2 Metatarsal I
3 Tendon sheath of extensor hallucis longus
4 Medial tarsal arteries
5 Dorsal tarsometatarsal ligaments
6 Tendon of tibialis anterior
7 Dorsal cuneonavicular ligaments
8 Inferior extensor retinaculum
9 Talonavicular ligament
10 Medial ligament (tibionavicular, anterior tibiotalar, tibiocalcanean parts)
11 Tendon sheath of tibialis anterior
12 Subcutaneous bursa of medial malleolus
13 Superior extensor retinaculum
14 Saphenous nerve
15 Tendon of tibialis posterior
16 Flexor digitorum longus
17 Soleus
18 Tendo calcaneus
19 Posterior tibial artery
20 Tibial nerve
21 Medial malleolar arterial network
22 Posterior tibiotalar part of medial ligament

23 Synovial tendinous sheath of tibialis posterior
24 Tendon sheath of flexor digitorum longus
25 Synovial tendinous sheath of flexor hallucis longus
26 Flexor retinaculum, superficial and deep layers
27 Bursa of tendo calcaneus
28 Subcutaneous bursa of calcaneus
29 Calcanean branches of posterior tibial artery and medial calcanean branches of tibial nerve
30 Abductor hallucis, severed
31 Flexor digitorum brevis, severed
32 Quadratus plantae
33 Medial plantar artery and nerve
34 Lateral plantar artery and nerve
35 Subtendinous bursa of tibialis anterior
36 Flexor hallucis brevis
37 Superficial branch of medial plantar artery
38 Subcutaneous bursa of head of metatarsal I
39 Sesamoid bone
40 Synovia tendon sheath of digits of feet
41 Medial plantar artery and nerve of toe

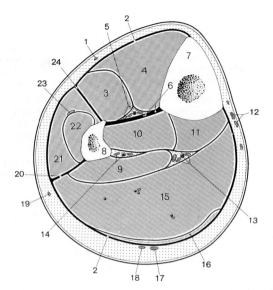

Fig. 148. **Cross section in middle third of right leg,** distal view of section surface

1 Branch of lateral sural cutaneous nerve
2 Fascia cruris
3 Extensor digitorum longus
4 Tibialis anterior
5 Anterior tibial artery and vein, deep peroneal nerve in extensor compartment
6 Interosseous membrane and interosseous nerve of leg
7 Tibia
8 Fibula
9 Flexor hallucis longus
10 Tibialis posterior
11 Flexor digitorum longus
12 Great saphenous vein, saphenous nerve

13 Posterior tibial artery and vein, tibial nerve in deep flexor compartment
14 Peroneal artery and vein
15 Soleus
16 Gastrocnemius
17 Small saphenous vein
18 Sural nerve
19 Lateral sural cutaneous nerve
20 Posterior intermuscular septum of leg
21 Peroneus longus
22 Peroneus brevis
23 Superficial peroneal nerve in peroneal compartment
24 Anterior intermuscular septum of leg

proximal portion of the tibia and fibula, and superficial fiber tracts also arise from the connective tissue sheet between the superficial and deep flexors. Its tendon, which crosses under the tendon of the flexor digitorum longus above the medial malleolus (crural chiasma, Fig. **146 b**), attaches with its main bundle at the tuberosity of the navicular bone (Fig. **147**), with its lateral tracts at the plantar surface (often) of all distal tarsal bones and the bases of metatarsals 2–4 (Fig. **155**).

In the malleolar groove, the tendon is enclosed by a *tendon sheath* and covered below the medial malleolus by the flexor retinaculum.

Innervation: tibial nerve.

Of the muscular branches to the deep flexors, the branch to the tibialis posterior originates farthest proximally, at about the level of the tendinous arch of the soleus. The proximal branches to the long flexors of the big toe and the toes leave the tibial nerve at the transition to the middle third of the leg. Muscular branches are usually also given off by the tibial nerve in the distal half of the leg.

The **flexor hallucis longus** (Figs. **146** and **148**), the flexor muscle which inserts farthest medially (main tendon to the base of distal phalanx I), arises farthest laterally at the leg: at the distal two-thirds of the posterior surface of the fibula, at a narrow band of the interosseous membrane and at the posterior intermuscular septum. Its tendon crosses under the tendon of the flexor digitorum longus (plantar chiasma) on the plantar surface of the foot where it gives off tendinous endings to the distal phalanx of the 2nd and 3rd (more rarely the 4th) toes.

At the posterior surface of the talus and at the undersurface of the sustentaculum tali, the tendon of the long flexor of the big toe courses in its own groove. It is enclosed by a *tendon sheath* (Fig. **150**) which begins at the level of the apex of the medial malleolus and extends distally up to the base of the 1st metatarsal. The tendon of insertion is covered in a tendon sheath from the head of the 1st metatarsal to the distal phalanx. The sheath is anchored to the segments of the big toe by a fibrous covering.

Innervation: tibial nerve.

The **flexor digitorum longus** (Figs. **146** and **148**) arises from the posterior surface of the tibia distal to the soleal line and from a tendinous arcade, which passes to the fibula proximal to the point at which the tibialis posterior in its fascia crosses under it. The terminal tendons of the muscle perforate the tendons of the flexor digitorum brevis in the region of the proximal phalanges (Fig. **160**) and insert at the distal phalanges of the 2nd–5th toes.

Enclosed by its own *tendon sheath*, the tendon of the flexor digitorum longus courses through the malleolar groove dorsolateral to the tendon of the tibialis posterior and, covered over by the flexor retinaculum, passes to the sole of the foot along the medial margin of the sustentaculum tali (Fig. **147**). At the level of the navicular tuberosity, it crosses under the tendon of the flexor hallucis longus, which contributes tendinous bundles to it. Distal to the crossing, the quadratus plantae attaches to the tendon of the flexor digitorum longus. This accessory flexor muscle correlates the direction of traction of the terminal tendons of the long flexors of the toes with the longitudinal direction of the toe radiations.

The terminal tendons of the flexor digitorum longus ("perforating muscle") and the flexor digitorum brevis ("perforated muscle") coursing to the same toes are enclosed in *tendon sheaths* (synovial sheaths, Fig. **147**), which begin above the head of the 1st metatarsal and extend up to the distal phalanx. These *synovial sheaths* are covered by *fibrous sheaths*, which – as in the fingers – exhibit transverse and crisscrossing fibrous tracts (*anular* and *cruciform parts*).

Innervation: tibial nerve.

The **popliteus** (Fig. **146 b**) belongs genetically to the deep flexors of the leg. In non-mammals it connects the tibia and fibula. In mammals – and thus also in humans – it has developed a close connection to the knee joint and helps to rotate the flexed leg inward.

The popliteus arises below the lateral collateral ligament of the knee joint at the external surface of the lateral condyle of the femur. Its attachment surface lies at the posterior surface of the tibia, proximal to the soleal line.

The muscle courses in the depth of the popliteal fossa (Fig. **139**) and is covered by the heads of the gastrocnemius, as well as by vessels and nerves. Its tendon of origin, over which the arcuate popliteal ligament passes, lies above the sub-popliteal recess, which in the adult always communicates with the cavity of the knee joint. A portion of the tendon of the semimembranosus radiates into the fascia of the popliteus.

Innervation: tibial nerve.

c) Vascular and Nerve Routes in the Leg

Typical *neurovascular routes* course in the *extensor compartment* (anterior tibial, deep lymphatic tracts + deep peroneal nerve) to the dorsum of the foot and in the posterior wall of the *deep flexor compartment* (posterior tibial vessels, deep lymphatic vessels + tibial nerve) to the sole of the foot. In the latter muscle compartment – closely adjacent to the fibula and interosseous membrane – the peroneal vessels (accompanied by several deep lymphatic tracts) pass distally for a variable distance. Only the superficial peroneal nerve passes through the *peroneal compartment* in a longitudinal direction. The vascular supply for the peroneal muscles is provided by short branches from the anterior tibial (proximal) and peroneal (distal) arteries.

Neurovascular Routes in the Extensor Compartment

The **anterior tibial artery** arrives at the extensor compartment via the superior margin of the interosseous membrane (Figs. **142** and **147**). It continues on the dorsum of the foot as the dorsalis pedis artery.

The *anterior tibial artery* gives off two recurrent branches to the articular network of the knee.

The inconstant *posterior recurrent tibial artery* arises behind the interosseous membrane and passes below the popliteus and around the head of the fibula obliquely upward to the knee joint. The *anterior recurrent tibial artery* passes proximally through the origin of the tibialis anterior.

Aside from numerous muscular branches to the extensors at the leg, the anterior tibial artery dispatches two arteries into the malleolar region. The *anterior medial malleolar artery* courses below the tendon of the tibialis anterior to an *arterial network* on the medial malleolus. The *anterior lateral malleolar artery* passes below the tendons of the long extensor of the toes to the *similar network* on the lateral malleolus.

The anterior lateral malleolar artery anastomoses with the perforating branch of the peroneal artery from the posterior tibial artery. The arterial networks on both malleoli communicate with one another on the anterior and posterior sides so that a collateral circulation can be formed in the case of occlusion of a tibial artery.

The **anterior tibial veins** and deep *lymphatic vessels* accompany the artery on the anterior surface of the interosseous membrane (Fig. **148**).

In the lymphatic tracts, an *anterior tibial node* can be present, which lies on the anterior surface of the interosseous membrane in the proximal third of the leg and directs lymph toward the popliteal lymph nodes.

The **deep peroneal nerve** (Figs. **143** and **148**), which innervates the extensors at the leg and foot, passes laterally through the anterior intermuscular septum to the lateral side of the vascular bundle. The neurovascular cord passes distally between the tibialis anterior and extensor digitorum longus, from the middle third of the leg the extensor hallucis longus (Fig. **159**). At the level of the superior ankle joint, the extensor hallucis longus crosses over the neurovascular bundle, and the deep peroneal nerve passes over the artery at its medial side.

Nerves in the Peroneal Compartment

The **common peroneal nerve** (Figs. **142** and **143**) enters the peroneal compartment from the dorsal side directly distal to the head of the fibula and divides immediately. The deep peroneal nerve and its branches to the tibialis anterior and the extensor digitorum longus leave the compartment through the anterior intermuscular septum.

The **superficial peroneal nerve** (Figs. **143**, **148** and **159**) gives off muscular branches to the peroneus longus; it first passes between the two peronei, then distalward on the peroneus brevis, to which it sends a twig. Before or after entering the distal third of the leg through the fascia cruris, it divides into the *medial dorsal cutaneous* and the *intermedial dorsal cutaneous nerves* for the skin at the dorsum of the foot and toes.

Neurovascular Routes in the Deep Flexor Compartment

The *posterior tibial artery* (Figs. **139**, **142** and **148**), a continuation of the popliteal artery on the flexor side of the leg, passes into the deep flexor compartment below the tendinous arch of the soleus. It courses distalward with the *posterior tibial veins*, deep lymphatic vessels and the *tibial nerve* (at the lateral side of the vascular bundle) directly under the connective tissue sheet covering the deep flexor. In the proximal region of the leg, the neurovascular bundle courses distally between the flexor digitorum longus and tibialis posterior and posterior to the medial malleolus, which is covered by the flexor retinaculum (Fig. **147**), between the tendons of the muscles mentioned and the tendon of the flexor hallucis longus. Below the medial malleolus, the posterior tibial artery divides into the medial and lateral plantar arteries, which course under the origin of the abductor hallucis to the sole of the foot. The tibial nerve divides behind the medial malleolus into the medial and lateral plantar nerves.

The **posterior tibial artery** supplies the superficial and the deep flexors at the leg with *muscular branches* and the tibia with the *nutrient artery* and dispatches the *circumflex fibular branch* around the head of the fibula to the articular network of the knee. The *peroneal artery* branches off distal to the tendinous arch of the soleus and – covered by the flexor hallucis – passes along the fibula to the *network of the lateral malleolus*. Weaker branches pass from the posterior tibial artery as *medial malleolar branches* to the *network of the medial malleolus* and as *calcanean branches* to the medial side of the tuber calcanei and to the *calcanean network* situated at its dorsal side.

The **peroneal [fibular] artery** (Figs. **142**, **143** and **148**), which is webbed by a multireticulated network of companion veins and accompanied by several deep lymphatic tracts from the region of the lateral malleolus, can be larger than the posterior tibial artery, which it can supply with blood via the communicating ramus. With short branches, it supplies the peroneal muscles (through the posterior intermuscular septum), the soleus and the deep flexors. It sends out a *nutrient artery to the fibula*, the *perforating ramus* which perforates the interosseous membrane above the lateral malleolus and passes to the network of the lateral malleolus, and the *communicating ramus* which connects the peroneal and posterior tibial arteries and courses medially on the interosseous membrane proximal to the two malleoli.

Lateral malleolar branches pass to the network on the lateral malleolus, and *calcanean branches* to the lateral surface of the calcaneus and to the *calcanean network*.

The **posterior tibial veins** are enclosed with the artery in a firm vascular sheath. They receive tributaries from the companion veins of the branches of the posterior tibial artery and communicate with the great and small saphenous veins via the venous networks at the medial and lateral malleoli.

The **tibial nerve** sends *muscular branches* at the leg to the deep flexors (the branches for the peroneal muscles already separate in the popliteal fossa), branches to the capsule of the talocrural joint, and *medial calcanean branches* to the skin covering the calcaneus and to a portion of the skin of the sole of the foot near it.

The *interosseus cruris nerve* proceeds usually from the "popliteal ramus", which already separates from the tibial nerve in the popliteal fossa and not only supplies the muscle of the same name, but also gives off a branch to the marrow cavity of the tibia. This interosseous nerve of the leg innervates the capsule of the tibiofibular joint with a proximal branch, courses distally on the interosseous membrane or between its fibrous layers (Fig. 148) to the tibiofibular syndesmosis, and sends branches to the periosteum of the distal end of the tibia.

2. Joints of the Foot

a) Skeletal Elements of the Tarsus and Metatarsus

At the *foot* – as at the hand – three successively organized segments are distinguished: *tarsus*, *metatarsus* and *digits* (toes). Their corresponding skeletal elements (Fig. 149) are: *tarsal bones*, *metatarsal bones* and *phalanges*. The big toe has only *two phalanges*, the remaining toes possess a *proximal*, *middle* and *distal phalanx*. The *sole of the foot* is designated as the *plantar (inferior) surface*, the *back* or upper surface as the *dorsum of the foot*.

Topographically, the foot is delimited from the leg by a horizontal plane which courses just above the two malleoli (i.e. corresponds to the projection of the articular cavity of the talocrural joint onto the skin).The dorsum of the foot goes over into the sole of the foot at the medial (tibial) and at the lateral (fibular) margins of the foot. The free margin of the interdigital folds (webs) is considered as the distal border of the dorsum of the foot, the inclined surface of which tapers down toward the toes to the plantar side. According to this definition, the metatarsophalangeal joints lie in the region of the dorsum of the foot.

Better suited for clinical needs is a classification of the foot into:

- the *back of the foot*, comprising the talus, calcaneus and soft covering parts;
- the *middle of the foot*, including all of the remaining tarsals together with the soft parts; and
- the *front of the foot*, consisting of the metatarsals, phalanges and their soft tissue coverings.

Tarsal bones (Fig. 149). The specialization of the hand and foot, the hand for grasping, the foot for standing, which resulted from the acquisition of erect posture, has also led to divergent development of the carpal and tarsal bones. Although they can be traced back to the same basic structural plan, they differ in their organization and composition.

The *proximal row of tarsal bones* consists of only two bones, the *talus* and the *calcaneus*. They are not beside one another in the same plane, but rather the talus has pushed above the calcaneus. The talus rests on the subtalar footplate, with which it articulates in the lower ankle joint (talocalcaneonavicular joint), and is solely responsible for the articulation with the two leg bones at the upper ankle joint (talocrural joint).

The *distal row of tarsal bones* consists of four elements: *medial, intermediate* and *lateral cuneiforms* and the *cuboid*. The *navicular*, which corresponds to the os centrale of the vertebrate structural plan, lies between the talus and cuneiforms. This element has disappeared in the skeleton of the human hand.

The *body* of the **talus** bears the *trochlea* and projects toward the toes with a constricted *neck*, upon which a spherical *head* rests. The trochlea is broader in front than behind. Its cartilage-covered *superior articular surface* and the *medial* and *lateral malleolar articular surfaces* form the undivided articular head of the talocrural joint, which is embraced by the malleolar fork (joint socket).

A small process, the *posterior process of the talus*, projects from the posterior surface of the body of the talus; its two eminences, the *lateral* and *medial tubercles*, border a *groove for the tendon of the flexor hallucis longus*. The lateral tubercle is larger and has its own ossific center. It can be separated from the talus by a joint cavity and can appear as an independent ossicle *os trigonum* (about 13%).

The lower surface of the body of the talus is hollowed out by the extensive *posterior calcanean surface*. It forms the joint socket for the posterior compartment of the lower ankle joint. The *middle articular surface for the calcaneus* (at the lower surface of the neck of the talus) and the *anterior articular surface for the calcaneus* (at the head of the talus) are separated from it by a groove, the *sulcus tali*. This groove, together with a corresponding groove on the calcaneus, the sulcus calcanei, forms a canal which widens laterally into the *sinus tarsi*. As an extensive articular facet, the head of the talus bears the *navicular articular surface* for the articulation with the navicular bone and the fibrocartilaginous coating of the plantar calcaneonavicular ligament.

The **calcaneus** is the largest tarsal bone. Its *tuberosity (tuber calcanei)* projects posteriorly and forms the short strong lever of the foot skeleton (Fig. **154 b**).

On the lower surface of the tuber are two raised prominences, with which the calcaneus rests on the supporting surface: the larger *medial process of the tuber* gives origin to the abductor hallucis and the flexor digitorum brevis, and the *lateral process* to the abductor digiti minimi.

The calcaneus possesses three joint surfaces for articulation with the talus (Fig. **154 a**). The *posterior talar articular surface*, which forms the joint head of the posterior compartment of the lower ankle joint, lies behind the *sulcus calcanei*. The *middle* and *anterior talar articular surfaces*, together with the articular surface of the navicular and the plantar calcaneonavicular ligament, form the socket for the anterior compartment of the lower ankle joint. The middle articular facet lies, for the most part, on a laterally-projecting process of the calcaneus, the *sustentaculum tali*, which hooks under and supports the talus as far as its medial border.

The tendon of the flexor hallucis longus glides in its *sulcus* on the undersurface of the sustentaculum (Figs. **149** and **154 b**). On the lateral surface of the calcaneus there are two, usually shallow grooves for the tendons of the peroneal muscles, between which a more or less distinct, blunt process, the *peroneal trochlea*, rises. The anterior aspect of the calcaneus contains the *cuboid articular surface*.

The **navicular** possesses proximally a concave articular surface for the head of the talus (Fig. **154 a**) and distally three cartilage-covered facets for articulation with the cuneiforms. The medial margin of the navicular projects as its *tuberosity* and can be palpated through the skin.

An accessory ossicle, the *os tibiale externum*, lies behind this blunt bony projection in about 10% of the cases, usually enclosed in the plantar calcaneonavicular ligament.

The three **cuneiforms** articulate proximally with the navicular, distally with metatarsals 1–3. They articulate with one another at their adjoining

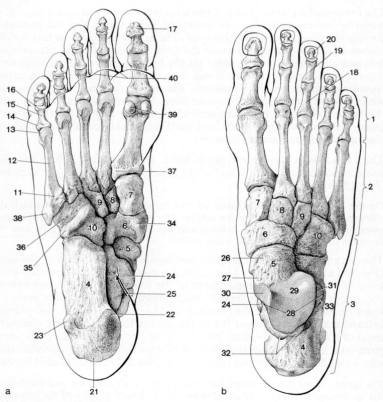

Fig. 149. **Skeleton of foot**
a Plantar view, relative position of transverse skin creases of toes
b Dorsal view

surfaces. The lateral cuneiform possesses a small articular surface for the cuboid.

The medial cuneiform is the strongest of the three and broader on its plantar aspect than on its dorsal. In contrast to this, the edges of the 2nd and 3rd cuneiform are directed toward the plantar side so that the plantar surface of the foot skeleton is curved here into a transverse concavity (Fig. 155). The apex of the transverse curvature of the foot lies in the region of the intermediate cuneiform since its dorsoplantar diameter is less than that of its two neighbors. The 2nd cuneiform, moreover, is shorter than the 1st and 3rd so that the base of the 2nd metatarsal is displaced partly between these two bones.

The **cuboid** fits in the skeleton of the foot between the calcaneus, lateral cuneiform and metatarsals IV and V. It occasionally articulates with the navicular.

On its inferior surface the *groove for the tendon of the peroneus longus* is evident laterally. Behind it there is the elevated *cuboid tuberosity*, which is covered by fibrocartilage. The tendon of the peroneus longus glides over this tuberosity on a fibrocartilaginous pad and passes medially into the groove. The proximomedial angle of the cuboid on the plantar aspect is drawn out into the *calcanean process*. The osseous apex hooks under the plantar part of the cuboid articular surface of the calcaneus with its portion of the joint surface passing obliquely dorsad.

Each of the five **metatarsal bones** (Fig. 149 and 153) – like the metacarpals – features a *base*, *body* and *head*. The *bases* articulate proximally with the cuneiforms (metatarsals I – III) and the cuboid (metatarsals IV and V). They possess articular surfaces on one or both sides for the adjacent metatarsals.

1 Bones of the digits of the foot (phalanges)
2 Metatarsals
3 Tarsals
4 Calcaneus
5 Talus
6 Navicular
7 Medial cuneiform
8 Intermediate cuneiform
9 Lateral cuneiform
10 Cuboid
11 Base of metatarsal V
12 Body of metatarsal V
13 Head of metatarsal V
14 Base of phalanx
15 Body of phalanx
16 Head of phalanx
17 Tuberosity of distal phalanx
18 Proximal phalanx
19 Middle phalanx
20 Distal phalanx
21 Tuberosity of calcaneus
22 Medial process of calcanean tuberosity
23 Lateral process of calcanean tuberosity
24 Sustentaculum tali
25 Groove for tendon of flexor hallucis longus
26 Head of talus
27 Neck of talus
28 Trochlea of talus
29 Superior surface of talus
30 Facet for medial malleolus
31 Facet for lateral malleolus
32 Posterior process of talus with medial and lateral tubercles, between which is groove for tendon of flexor hallucis longus
33 Lateral process of talus
34 Tuberosity of navicular
35 Tuberosity of cuboid
36 Groove for tendon of peroneus longus
37 Tuberosity of metatarsal I
38 Tuberosity of metatarsal V
39 Sesamoid bones
40 Transverse skin crease

The base of the 2nd metatarsal, which is inserted between the medial and lateral cuneiforms, articulates medially only with the 1st cuneiform, laterally with the 3rd cuneiform and the 3rd metatarsal.

On the plantar side, the first metatarsal exhibits a strong process, the *tuberosity of the 1st metatarsal*, which projects laterally and serves for the insertion of the tendon of the peroneus longus. The base of the 5th metatarsal is drawn out laterally and proximally to form the *tuberosity* of this bone, which gives attachment to the tendon of the peroneus brevis and causes a distinct bulge in the skin of the fibular margin of the foot (Figs. **145**, **149** and **154 a**).

The *shaft* of the metatarsals is weaker than their respective proximal and distal ends. The lateral surfaces of metatarsals 2–5 are sloped dorsally.

The articular surface of the *head* of each metatarsal bone is extended further proximally on the plantar aspect than on the dorsal side and ends in two bilateral grooves on the plantar side. Two sesamoid bones regularly glide on these at the 1st metatarsal (Figs. **147** and **149**).

Occasionally, an unpaired sesamoid bone is present at the 5th metatarsal, usually on the fibular side. The heads of metatarsals II – V are relatively narrow. The flattened surface on each side possess small prominences and indentations to which the collateral ligaments of the metatarsophalangeal joints are attached.

Of the five metatarsals, the tibial marginal ray (metatarsal I) is the strongest. Metatarsal V is stronger than IV (often also III), and metatarsal II is the longest.

Luxations of the talus are generally combined with malleolar fractures. *Fractures* of the talus often involve the neck, whereas those of the calcaneus affect the tuber calcanei. Extreme fatigue fractures (march fractures) can appear at the metatarsal bones (usually II or III) as a result of excessive strain even without direct traumatic force.

Ossification of the *calcaneus* begins in the 5th–6th fetal month and of the *talus* about 2 months later (Fig. **116**). The *cuboid* frequently has an ossific center at the time of birth, whereas ossification of the *lateral cuneiform* begins in the 1st postnatal year and of the remaining *tarsal elements*, as a rule, in the 3rd to 4th year.

Within the *metatarsals*, the diaphysial centers of ossification appear in the 9th embryonic week, the epiphysial nuclei in the 3rd year (females) or toward the beginning of the 4th year (males). Like the metacarpals, the metatarsals possess only one epiphysial center, which is developed at the proximal end of the 1st metatarsal and at the distal ends of metatarsals II – V (Fig. **154 a**). The epiphysial joints ossify between the 15th to 20th year in girls and two or three years later in boys.

Construction of the foot skeleton (Fig. **150**). The skeleton of the foot can be regarded as a two-armed lever with an axis of rotation which courses transversely through the trochlea of the talus. The short posterior part of the lever is joined together from the body of the talus and the posterior

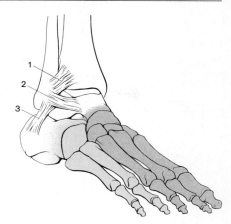

Fig. 150. Construction of
foot skeleton
▨ Main brace for tibia
▨ Accessory brace for
    fibula
1 Anterior tibiofibular ligament
2 Anterior talofibular ligament
3 Calcaneofibular ligament

segment of the calcaneus. The longer anterior portion consists of a larger
number of skeletal elements which form an open concave margin on the
plantar side.

A *tibial main strut* and a *fibular accessory strut* are distinguished at the
anterior part. The tibial main strut is formed by metatarsals I–III, the
cuneiforms and the navicular, which articulates with the head of the talus.
It bears the principle weight of the body in a normal standing posture.
The fibular accessory brace, which is especially-stressed by a standing
posture with the feet placed parallel, runs from metatarsals IV and across
the cuboid to the anterior portion of the calcaneus.

The foot skeleton is arched both longitudinally and transversely. (Longitudinal and transverse arches of the foot are distinguished even though
the construction of the arch does not completely meet an engineer's
standards.) The longitudinal curvature of the tibial arch is more strongly
pronounced than that of the fibular accessory arch. The longitudinal
curvature of the foot is secured by ligaments (plantar calcaneonavicular,
long plantar ligaments) and to a special degree by muscular traction
(short plantar muscles of the foot, flexor hallucis longus, flexor digitorum
longus, plantar aponeurosis). The transverse curvature is maintained
particularly by the transverse tension provided by the tendons of the
peroneus longus and tibialis posterior.

In the newborn child, the foot still retains a position adjusted to the intrauterine
spatial conditions. The calcaneus is angled inward; the tuber calcanei faces
medially on the plantar aspect (Fig. **151**). During postnatal development, the
calcaneus is lifted almost completely from this supination position. The directional axis (longitudinal diameter) of the calcanean tuberosity is approximately
vertical in the adult.

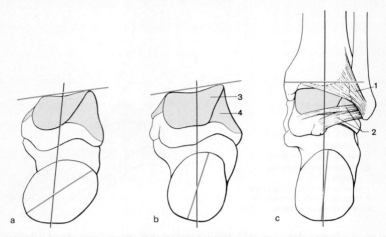

Fig. 151. **Change in orientation of axis of calcanian tuberosity during postnatal development**, dorsal view (a and b after *von Lanz-Wachsmuth*)
Direction of axis (longitudinal diameter) of tuber calcanei and inclination of superior surface of trochlea of talus in frontal plane ——
Weight-bearing line of bone ——
a Talus and calcaneus in newborn child
b Talus and calcaneus in two-year-old child
c Tibiofibular syndesmosis, talus and calcaneus in adult
(skeletal elements in a–c shown approximately the same size by differential enlargement)

1 Posterior tibiofibular ligament   3 Superior surface of trochlea of talus
2 Posterior talofibular ligament   4 Lateral malleolar surface

If the plantar bracing of the arch of the foot is not provided by muscles, tendons and ligaments when a load is applied, a reshaping of the foot is forcefully induced by a progressive pronation of the calcaneus. The talus sinks deeper and threatens to slide off the sustentaculum tali. The tibial main strut gives way, and the subtalar basal plate flexes toward the fibular side. The longitudinal and transverse curvature of the foot is lost: *flatfoot*.

In flat-footedness, the arch of the medial contour typical for the normal footprint has largely or completely disappeared (Fig. **152**). A similar form of soleprint is produced in the small child by the extensive deposition of subcutaneous fat in the region of this arch. A particularly strong development of the muscles of the sole of the foot can likewise reduce the contour and falsely indicate a flattening of the arch.

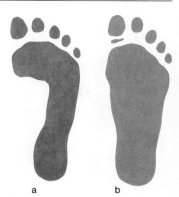

Fig. 152. **Footprints**
a Normal
b Flatfoot   a   b

In *splayfoot*, the transverse curvature of the foot in the region of the meta-tarsals is leveled off or abolished. The heads of metatarsals II–IV are subjected to stronger loads. The front of the foot is broadened.

In *clubfoot*, the foot is in the extreme supinated position with the lateral margin of the foot directed toward the plantar side and the sole of the foot facing medially.

b) Capsules and Ligamentous Apparatus of the Joints of the Foot

The **joints of the foot** (in the broader sense) here include all articulations in the tarsometatarsal region; the joints of the toes will be discussed separately.

The following are regarded as joints of the foot:
– *superior ankle joint* (*talocrural joint*);
– *inferior ankle joint*, comprising the posterior *subtalar joint*, and the anterior inferior *talocalcaneonavicular joint*;
– *calcaneocuboid joint*;
– *cuneonavicular joint*;
– *intercuneiform joints*;
– *cuneocuboid joint*;
– articular connections between the navicular and cuboid (inconstant);
– *tarsometatarsal joints*; and
– *intermetatarsal joints*, between the bases of the metatarsals.

Superior Ankle Joint

In the *talocrural articulation* (Fig. **153**), a single-axis joint, the two leg bones communicate with only one tarsal bone, the talus. The malleolar

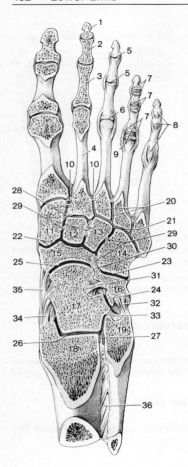

Fig. 153. Flat section through foot: joints of foot and toes, dorsal view
(Collateral ligaments shown for toes 3–5, articular capsule for toe 5. Articular capsule at toe 4 cut open and retracted)

◼ Articular cavity of talocrural (ankle) joint
◼ Articular cavity of intertarsal joint
◻ Articular cavity of tarsometatarsal joint and intermetatarsal joints

1 Distal phalanx
2 Middle phalanx
3 Proximal phalanx
4 Metatarsal II
5 Interphalangeal III joints
6 Metatarsophalangeal III joint
7 Collateral ligaments of interphalangeal joints
8 Articular capsules of interphalangeal joints
9 Articular capsule, cut open and retracted
10 Metatarsal interosseous ligaments
11 Medial cuneiform
12 Intermediate cuneiform
13 Lateral cuneiform
14 Cuboid
15 Navicular
16 Calcaneus
17 Talus
18 Tibia
19 Fibula
20 Intermetatarsal joints
21 Tarsometatarsal joints
22 Cuneonavicular joint
23 Calcaneocuboid joint
24 Subtalar joint
25 Talocalcaneonavicular joint
26 Talocrural joint
27 Fold of synovial membrane between distal end of tibia and fibula
28 Tarsometatarsal interosseous ligaments
29 Tarsal interosseous ligaments, named after tarsal bones to which they are attached
30 Calcaneonavicular ligament, part of bifurcate ligament
31 Talcalcanean interosseous ligament
32 Calcaneofibular ligament
33 Posterior talofibular ligament
34 Anterior tibiotalar part } of medial (deltoid)
35 Tibionavicular part   } ligament
36 Interosseous membrane of leg

fork formed by the tibia and fibula embrace the trochlea of the talus on three sides. The ligaments of the fork, the anterior and posterior tibiofibular ligaments, connect the tibia and fibula with each other on their anterior and posterior sides and supplement the joint socket with the fibrocartilaginous portion of their inner surfaces.

The *joint capsule* is attached at the cartilage-bone border of the articulating skeletal elements, except at the neck of the talus where it has advanced forward a bit onto the bone. On both sides, the otherwise thin-walled capsule is strengthened by fan-shaped collateral ligaments radiating out from the medial or from the lateral malleolus to the proximal tarsal bones.

Ligaments. The medial collateral ligament (*medial [deltoid] ligament*, Figs. **147**, **153** and **154 b**) unites the medial malleolus with the talus (*anterior* and *posterior talar parts*), the navicular (*tibionavicular part*) and the sustentaculum tali (*tibiocalcanean part*). The lateral collateral ligament (lateral ligament) can be grouped into the *anterior* and *posterior talofibular ligaments* and into the *calcaneofibular ligament* located between these two ligamentous tracts (Figs. **150**, **151 c** and **153**). The collateral ligaments, especially the medial ligament, are extraordinarily strong and prevent an angling of the foot at the superior ankle joint. Owing to their fan-shaped organization, portions of the collateral ligaments are stretched in each position of the joint.

If the leg is twisted against the foot fixed at the ground (e.g. in a wheel track or in tree roots, it results more frequently in a fractured malleolus than in a transverse tear of a collateral ligament.

Effusions in the superior ankle joint cause the skin at the dorsum of the foot to bulge more or less on the both sides of the extensor tendons and in front of the two malleoli.

Possibilities of movement of the superior ankle joint. The superior ankle joint is a hinge joint with a transverse axis of rotation that runs through the middle of the trochlea of the talus, meets the apex of the lateral malleolus on the fibular side and passes distal to the tibial malleolus on the tibial side. It permits:

– *flexion* (plantar flexion) of the foot (= lowering of the tip of the foot) by about 30° or
– *extension* (dorsiflexion) of the foot (= elevation of the tip of the foot) by around 25°.

With the foot firmly set, the leg can be inclined posteriorly or anteriorly. During plantar flexion the narrower posterior portion of the talar trochlea articulates so that the bony guidance is less fixed and lateral oscillating movements are possible (feeling one's way with the tip of the foot in the dark or in turbid water). When the foot is dorsiflexed, the broader anterior part of the trochlea presses apart the springy connection of the two prongs of the malleolar fork by about 2–3 mm. The extension movement ends when the trochlea is flexibly fixed in the malleolar fork (=maximal dorsiflexion of the foot.)

Inferior Ankle Joint

The *inferior ankle joint* (Figs. 153 and 154 a), which has no official designation in the Nomina Anatomica, but which could be called the

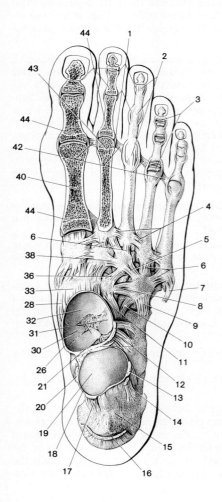

Fig. 154. Ligaments of joints of foot and toes
a Dorsal view
(Anterior and posterior compartments of lower ankle joint opened, bones removed. Skeletal elements of toe rays 1 and 2 sawed open, articular capsules shown closed at third toe, retracted at fourth toe)
b Medial view

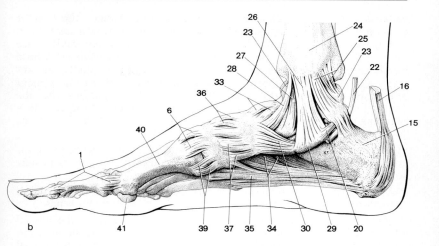

b

1 Collateral ligaments of joints of the toes
2 Articular capsules of joints of the toes, closed
3 Articular capsules of joints of the toes,
   retracted
4 Dorsal metatarsal ligaments
5 Dorsal cuneocuboid ligament
6 Dorsal tarsometarsal ligaments
7 Tendon of peroneus brevis
8 Dorsal cuboideonavicular ligment
9 Dorsal calcaneocuboid ligment
10, 11 *Bifurcated ligament*
10 Calcaneocuboid ligament
11 Calcaneonavicular ligament
12 Talocalcanean interosseous ligament
13 Lateral talocalcanean ligament
14 Calcaneofibular ligament
15 Calcaneus
16 Tendon of triceps surae = tendo calcaneus
17 Posterior talocalcanean ligament
18 Capsule of subtalar joint, cut margin
19 Posterior articular facet of calcaneus for talus
20 Medial talocalcanean ligament
21 Capsule of talcalocaneonavicular joint, cut
    edge
22 Tendon of flexor hallucis longus
23 Talus

24 Tibia
25–28 *Medial ligament*
25 Posterior tibiotalar part
26 Tibiocalcanean part
27 Anterior tibiotalar part
28 Tibionavicular part
29 Sustentaculum tali
30 Plantar calcaneonavicular ligament
31 Anterior and middle articular facets of
    calcaneus for talus
32 Articular facet of navicular for talus
33 Talonavicular ligament
34 Plantar calcaneocuboid ligament
35 Long plantar ligament
36 Dorsal cuneonavicular ligaments
37 Plantar cuneonavicular ligaments
38 Dorsal intercuneiform ligaments
39 Plantar tarsometatarsal ligaments
40 Metatarsal I
41 Sesamoid bone
42 Deep transverse metatarsal ligament (plantar
    connection of heads of metatarsals)
43 Distal epiphysial discs at metatarsals II–V
44 Proximal epiphysial disc at metatarsal I and
    phalanges

talotarsal articulation, consists of a posterior compartment, the *subtalar joint*, and an anterior compartment, the *talocalcaneonavicular joint*. Each articulation possesses an individual capsule. The articular cavities are completely separated by the *interosseous talocalcanean ligament*, whose partly cruciform fibers largely fill the sinus tarsi. Functionally, the anterior and posterior compartments form a uniform, single-axis movement site, in which the subtalar footplate moves toward the talus or – when the foot is firmly fixed – the talus moves toward the subtalar footplate. In a standing position on one leg, the body is balanced against the foot at this joint.

At the **subtalar joint** (Figs. **153** and **154 a**), the slightly concave posterior calcanean articular surface of the talus articulates with the convex posterior articular surface of the calcaneus.

The thin *joint capsule* is always fixed at the cartilage-bone border and is strengthened on all sides – more or less extensively – by ligamentous bands.

Ligaments. The *medial talocalcanean ligament* passes from the medial tubercle of the posterior process of the talus to the sustentaculum tali at the calcaneus. The *interosseous talocalcanean ligament* at the anterior wall of the joint capsule separates the two compartments of the inferior ankle joint and, at the same time, unites the capsules of both joints. The *lateral talocalcanean ligament* attaches at the interosseous ligament toward the lateral and calcanean sides as a reinforcement of the capsule. Dorsal fibrous tracts can be delimited as the posterior talocalcanean ligament. In addition, the *calcaneofibular ligament* passes over the subtalar joint.

In the **talocalcaneonavicular joint** (Fig. **154 a**), the spherical articular head is formed by the head and neck of the talus. The three articular facets of the talus articulate with the corresponding joint surfaces of the calcaneus (anterior and middle talar articular facets) and the navicular. The cartilage-covered surfaces of the sockets of both tarsal bones are supported by ligamentous tracts.

The *articular capsule* is fastened, for the most part, along the cartilage-bone border, but pushes forward proximally onto the bone at the neck of the talus. The portion of its wall directed toward the calcaneus is included in the interosseous talocalcanean ligament. The dorsal portion of the capsule is strengthened by the *talonavicular ligament,* which passes from the head of the talus across the talonavicular joint cavity to the navicular. The capsule is covered by the *tibionavicular part* of the *medial ligament* at its dorsomedial circumference and by the *tibiocalcanean part* at its medial side.

Ligaments. The *plantar calcaneonavicular ligament* (Fig. **154b**) passes from the sustentaculum tali to the plantar and medial surfaces of the navicular. It serves as a ligamentous clamp connecting the navicular with the calcaneus, secures the head of the talus in its position and, at the same time, permits it to have a limited mobility. The partially fibrocartilaginous plantar portion of the ligament completes the socket of the joint on the plantar side. The substantially stronger medial portion of the tract consists primarily of fibrocartilage. It is braced by fibrous tracts, which pass obliquely from its upper margin to the mediodorsal surface of the navicular, and forms a compression plate for the weighted head of the talus, which prevents the talus from sliding off the sustentaculum tali.

The *calcaneonavicular ligament*, which forms the medial portion of the tract of the bifurcated ligament, passes in the dorsolateral circumference of the anterior inferior ankle joint with short tense fibers from the dorsal surface of the distal end of the calcaneus to the lateral margin of the dorsum of the navicular and completes the joint socket in its dorsolateral segment.

Possibilities of movement in the inferior ankle joint. The axis of the inferior ankle joint courses – oblique to the orientation plane of the foot and of the whole body – from the dorsomedial circumference of the neck of the talus posteriorly, inferiorly and laterally to the lateral surface of the tuber calcanei. It crosses the talocalcanean interosseous ligament, whose surface is approximately at a right angle to the axis of the joint. The oblique course of the axis limits the movements in the inferior ankle to mixed movements.

The inferior ankle joint facilitates the following movements:
- *supination* of the foot, i.e. the lifting of the medial margin of the foot (= tilt inward) with simultaneous adduction and plantar flexion of the subtalar footplate, or
- *pronation* of the foot, i.e. the depression of the medial margin of the foor (= tilt outward), coupled with abduction and dorsiflexion of the subtalar footplate.

Supination and pronation of the foot are thus fundamentally different from hand movements of the same name which take place at the radio-ulnar joint. The circumference of movement in the inferior ankle joint is to a great extent dependent on age and also on training. The existing numerical data, therefore, vary considerably. The extent of possible abduction and adduction, as well as pronation and supination, hardly exceeds 30° in adults and is considerably less in the elderly.

Supination at the inferior ankle joint is passively inhibited mainly by the talocalcanean ligament. During strong supination, the calcaneofibular and lateral talocalcanean ligaments are also stretched (on the lateral side). During pronation, the tibiocalcanean part of the medial ligament and the medial talocalcanean ligament act (on the medial side) as inhibitory ligaments.

An active suppression of supination is possible at the leg by the contraction of the peronei muscles, whereas a suppression of pronation is achieved by the contraction of the deep flexors.

Remaining Joints of the Foot

No isolated movements occur at the remaining joints of the foot. With the exception of the calcaneus-cuboid joint, they act more in the manner of a spring joint and permit only minor displacements of the skeletal elements upon corresponding stress of the foot.

The **calcaneocuboid joint** (Fig. **153**), an independent joint with its own capsule and saddle-shaped articular surfaces, permits in the adult only insignificant sliding movements between the cuboid and the calcaneus, by means of which, however, the extensive angling of the subtalar footplate becomes possible.

Ligaments (Fig. **154**). The calcaneus and cuboid are united dorsally with one another by capsular reinforcements, the *calcaneocuboid ligaments*, and on the plantar side by the strong *plantar calcaneocuboid ligament*.

The *long plantar ligament* braces the tarsals on the fibular side of the sole of the foot. The long, superficial ligamentous tracts arise from the plantar surface of the calcaneus, pass over the sulcus tendineus of the peroneal longus, and attach at the bases of metatarsals II–V. The short, deep fibrous tracts of the long plantar ligament correspond to the above-mentioned plantar calcaneocuboid ligament.

Lying deeply below the superficial, *dorsal* ligamentous tracts, the *bifurcated ligament* fixes the navicular at the calcaneus with its medial bundle (*calcaneonavicular ligament*), whereas its lateral bundle of fibers (*calcaneocuboid ligament*) passes from the calcaneus to the cuboid.

The **transverse tarsal joint** comprises the anterior compartment of the inferior ankle joint (talocalcaneonavicular articulation) and the calcaneocuboid articulation. The slightly S-shaped, curved articular cavity coursing transversely through the tarsals (transverse tarsal or Chopart's joint line) lies between the talus and calcaneus (proximally) and the navicular and cuboid (distally). It is interrupted by the joint capsule and the bifurcated ligament.

In earlier times when amputation techniques and prosthesis structuring had not yet reached the high standards of today, an amputation of the foot was frequently carried out at Chopart's joint line. At this posterior amputation site, the articular cavity gapes only after the superficial ligamentous tracts, as well as the hidden bifurcated ligament (= retaining ligament of Chopart's joint) are severed. Modern operative techniques strive for a functionally sound stump that can be prosthetically equipped as soon as possible. The amputation of the foot is performed as far distally as possible.

The *cuneonavicular joint* (the articular unions of the lateral surfaces of the distal tarsals), the *tarsometatarsal joints*, and the *intermetatarsal joints* (between the bases of the metatarsals) are rigid amphiarthroses (Fig. **153**). Under the influence of external forces (e.g. the load of the body weight when standing), only insignificant displacements of the bones are possible; only in both marginal rays are the skeletal elements somewhat more movable.

Lisfranc's joint line (former anterior site of amputation) connects the tarsometatarsal articulations. It begins at the external margin of the foot behind the tuberosity of the 5th metatarsal, which is palpable through the skin. Owing to the proximally projecting base of the 2nd metatarsal, the line formed by these joints is angled off sharply in the region of the 2nd ray. Today, amputations along Lisfranc's joint are carried out only in an emergency situation (risk of foot drop because of a muscular imbalance).

Ligaments (Figs. **153** and **154**). The articular cavities between the distal tarsal bones are also bridged over by short, strong plantar and weaker dorsal tendinous tracts, which are named after the tarsal bones to which they are attached. In the region of the tarsus, all plantar ligaments are grouped as *plantar tarsal ligaments*, the dorsal tendinous tracts as *dorsal tarsal ligaments*, and the ligaments between the talus and calcaneus, as well as those spreading out between the distal tarsal bones, as *interosseous tarsal ligaments*.

The *interosseous intercuneiform ligaments* connect the cuneiform bones with one another; the *interosseous cuneocuboid ligament* passes from the 3rd cuneiform to the cuboid.

The *plantar, dorsal* and *interosseous tarsometatarsal ligaments* course from the distal tarsals to the bases of the metatarsals, which are held together by *plantar, dorsal* and *interosseous metatarsal ligaments*. The *interosseous tarsometatarsal ligaments* subdivide the joint line between the tarsals and metatarsals (Lisfranc's joint line) into three articular cavities. The 1st tarsometatarsal joint possesses an individual joint capsule. The undivided articular cavity between the 2nd and 3rd metatarsals and the 2nd and 3rd cuneiforms usually continues into the cuneonavicular joint. Tarsometatarsal joints IV and V are likewise enclosed in a common joint capsule.

Arterial supply of the joint capsules of the foot. Branches of all adjacent arteries pass to the joint capsules of the ankle joints (branches of the anterior and posterior tibial arteries, as well as the peroneal artery, form the arterial networks on the medial and lateral malleoli and on the calcaneus). Branches of the medial and lateral plantar arteries (on the plantar side) and the dorsalis pedis artery (on the dorsal side) ramify at the joint capsules of the distal tarsal and tarsometatarsal joints.

Innervation of the joint capsules of the foot joints. The capsule of the superior ankle joint is supplied by branches of the tibial nerve (medial side), deep peroneal nerve (dorsal side) and probably the sural nerve (lateral side). Branches of the deep peroneal nerve and the medial and lateral plantar nerves ramify at the other foot joints.

Movement possibilities at the foot joints. By the combination of movements at the superior and inferior ankle joints and at the transverse tarsal joints, the foot can be moved voluntarily around three primary axes. The cooperation of these joints provides the movement possibilities of a ball-and-socket joint, whereby the compulsory coupling of movements, as is the case in pronation and supination at the inferior ankle joint, is (largely) abolished.

From the normal position, in which the longitudinal axis of the foot (through the calcaneus and the 2nd metatarsal) is perpendicular to the weight-bearing line of the bone and to a line connecting the two malleoli, the foot in the adult can be:

- *plantar flexed* (over 60°) or *dorsiflexed* (about 45°);
- *abducted* and *adducted*, each by approx. 30°;
- *tilted*, so that the medial margin of the foot stands almost perpendicular above the lateral margin of the foot, whereas the lateral margin cannot be lifted to the same extent.

The range of movement in the foot joints is greatest in the newborn child and in the infant and decreases gradually with advancing age. It can be increased by training.

c) Action of Muscles and Muscle Groups on the Joints of the Foot

All muscles which pass over the foot joints cooperate in the movements of the foot by initiating, expediting, modifying or retarding these movements. Unlike true ball-and-socket joints, here the tendons cannot transmigrate the joint axes since they are fixed in their relationship to the bones (and thus to the axes) by retinacula.

In the normal position of the foot, the following course is taken by the effective terminal extensions of the tendons of:

- all flexors: *behind* the transverse axis of the superior ankle joint and *medial* to the oblique axis of the inferior ankle joint;
- the peroneal muscles: *behind* the transverse axis of the superior ankle joint and *lateral* to the oblique axis of the inferior ankle joint;
- the tibialis anterior: *in front of* the transverse axis of the superior ankle joint and *partly medial, partly lateral* to the oblique axis of the inferior ankle joint;
- the extensor digitorum longus (including the peroneal tertius) and the extensor hallucis longus: *in front of* of the transverse axis of the superior ankle joint and *lateral* to the oblique axis of the inferior ankle joint.

All muscles which dorsally cross the transverse axis of the superior ankle joint depress the tip of the foot or, when the foot is fixed, carry the leg backward. All muscles which course in front of the transverse axis raise the subtalar footplate or draw the leg toward the dorsum of the foot. The muscles which pass along the medial side of the oblique axis of the inferior ankle joint carry the foot toward the tibia and lift the medial margin of the foot. When the foot is on the ground, they rotate the leg externally and incline it internally. All muscles which laterally cross the oblique axis abduct the foot toward the fibula and lift the lateral margin of the foot. Conversely, they can rotate the leg somewhat inward and incline it externally.

By appropriate counter movements at the transverse tarsal joint, the supinator or pronator component in the inferior ankle joint can be suppressed during adduction or abduction of the foot or the foot can be turned around the longitudinal axis.

Since the tendons of the extensor hallucis longus and the lateral part of the tendon of the tibialis anterior cross the axis of the inferior ankle joint laterally and the longitudinal axis of the foot medially, they act on the inferior ankle joint as pronators and on the transverse tarsal joint as supinators when the foot is positioned normally.

Since no muscle is attached to it, the talus can neither be directly moved nor directly fixed by muscle traction.

The foot is:

– *plantar fixed* by the triceps surae, which produces almost 90% of the torque of all plantar flexors, and by the flexor hallucis longus (5%),

 while the remaining deep flexors and the two peroneal muscles do relatively little work and the peroneal muscles equalize the supinator action of the flexors;

– *dorsiflexed* by the extensors (particularly by the tibialis anterior, to a lesser degree by the extensor digitorum longus and the extensor hallucis longus;

– *supinated*, especially by the triceps surae (over 50% of the torque of all supinators) and the tibialis posterior,

 whereby the flexor hallucis longus, the flexor digitorum longus, the tibialis anterior (in the transverse ankle joint and – from a supination position – also in the inferior ankle joint), and the extensor hallucis longus (very little and only in the transverse ankle joint) assist;

– *pronated* by both peroneal muscles, which produce almost two-thirds of the torque of all pronators, by the extensor digitorum longus and – when present – by the peroneus tertius,

 whereby they are supported to a slight degree by the tibialis anterior and the extensor hallucis longis, both of which can pronate only at the inferior ankle joint.

The torque of the *triceps surae* is four times as great as that of all the dorsiflexors. It carries out the major work during locomotion, levers the calcaneus from the ground, and lifts the body weight from the tips of the feet (which the deep flexors cannot do alone).

Owing to the functional predominance of the plantar flexors, there is a risk of footdrop (extreme plantar flexion of the foot) in bedridden patients. The foot must always be encased in plaster in the flexed position at a right angle to the leg.

Although the triceps surae inserts at the short lever of the foot, its torque is much more favorable than that of the remaining plantar flexors, whose tendons course at a shorter distance to the frontal axis of the superior ankle joint (and whose virtual lever arm is therefore shorter). Only the tendon of the flexor hallucis longus courses at the posterior process of the talus at some distance from the axis of rotation. At the same time, the triceps surae is the strongest supinator (and adductor) of the foot: its torque is equal to that of all the pronators. (The torque of *all* supinators is about twice as great as that of the pronators.)

The *soleus* secures the extension of the knee joint in a standing position by pulling the upper portion of tibia and fibula posteriorly and thus locking the knee in place. The two-jointed *gastrocnemius* plays no essential role in the flexion of the knee joint. Through maximal flexion of the knee, however, the muscle can be so relaxed that its plantar flexing action on the ankle joint declines strongly (active insufficiency). Only in the extended knee joint does the full tendon power of the gastrocnemius come into play in plantar flexion of the foot.

The *extensors* are concerned in locomotion insofar as they shorten the free leg in its forward swing by dorsally flexing the foot and thus make possible a long stride. The *deep flexors* and the *peroneal muscles* adjust the foot on uneven ground to the actual shape and condition of the ground.

The *flexor hallucis longus* plays an essential role in rolling the foot off the big toe; at the same time, the *flexor digitorum longus* presses the toes against the ground. In a standing position, both muscles cooperate to brace effectively the longitudinal curvature of the foot. The flexor hallucis longus prevents the depression of the sustentaculum tali toward the plantar and medial sides. The *tibialis posterior* regulates the length and tension of the plantar calcaneonavicular ligament, which it covers on the plantar aspect with its tendinous fan.

The *transverse curvature of the foot* is secured by the transverse traction which the *tibialis posterior* and the *peroneus longus* each exert in opposing directions (Fig. **155**). If the balance between the supinators of the foot (particularly the triceps surae and the tibialis posterior) and the pronators

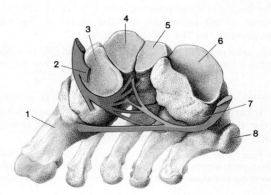

Fig. 155. **Muscular protection of transverse curvature of foot**, topview of distal series of tarsals from behind and from plantar aspect
Tendons of attachment of tibialis posterior ——
Tendons of attachment of peroneus longus ——

1 Metatarsal I
2 Tendon tract of tibialis posterior to navicular tuberosity
3 Medial cuneiform
4 Intermediate cuneiform
5 Lateral cuneiform
6 Cuboid
7 Tuberosity of cuboid
8 Tuberosity of metatarsal V

is disturbed in favor of the pronators, the peroneal muscles force the calcaneus into a position of increasing pronation, an important factor in the development of flatfeet.

Both peroneal muscles try to lift the lateral margin of the foot. With the failure of its antagonists, the peroneus longus attempts to depress the medial margin of the foot so that the arch of the sole of the foot is leveled off.

Paralyses. With a paralysis of the *extensors*, the tip of the foot can no longer be lifted. The patient must flex the thigh at the hip joint and the leg at the knee joint more strongly in the free leg phase of walking (tap-dancer's shuffle) in order to prevent the foot from sliding on the ground. Owing to the shortening of the flexors (as a result of the paralysis of the extensors), a footdrop (plantar flexion) is gradually produced. If the *peroneal muscles* are paralyzed, pronation is impossible. The foot remains plantar flexed and supinated (clubfoot).

In damage to the tibial nerve below the popliteal fossa which leads only to a paralysis of the *deep flexors* (and the *muscles of the sole of the foot*), plantar flexion and supination at the ankle joint are not significantly restricted. This paralysis is obvious in walking only insofar as the foot can no longer be correctly rolled off the big toe (in the heel to toe fashion of walking). The curved construction of the foot is decisively affected since, on the one hand, active longitudinal tension is impossible and, on the other hand, the transverse arch has broken down.

The *peroneal muscles* become predominant and flatten the middle and front of the foot. If the *triceps surae* is also paralyzed, powerful plantar flexion of the foot and standing on tiptoe are no longer possible. The foot can no longer be rolled off during walking. Since all supinators are unresponsive, the foot remains in the pronation position. Secondarily, a permanent shortening of the extensors can set in, which leads to a talipes calcaneus (dorsal flexion of the foot combined with pronation).

3. Foot and Toes

a) Skeletal Elements of the Toes

The **bones of the toes** (digits, phalanges) correspond in number, arrangement and basic shape to the bones of the fingers, but are substantially shorter. At the 2nd to 5th toes, *proximal, middle* and *distal phalanges* are distinguished and at the 1st toe (great toe, hallux) proximal and distal (Fig. **149** and **153**).

The proximal portion of each phalanx is designated as the *base of the phalanx*, the shaft as the *body*, and the distal end as the *head*. The distal phalanx is flattened and widened on the plantar side into the *tuberosity of the distal phalanx*. The phalanges of the great toe are extraordinarily strong. The great toe (in about 65%) or the 2nd toe (in about 21%) is the longest, and in about 13% of the cases they are of the same length. The middle and distal phalanges of the 5th toe are fused synostotically in over one third of the cases.

It is not uncommon for the distal phalanges to be underdeveloped. The number of phalanges can (in rare cases) increase to four, the number of toes to six.

The **ossification** of the *phalanges* (Fig. **116**) begins in the diaphysis of the distal phalanx in the 9th embryonic week, whereas the diaphyses of the proximal phalanges ossify around the 5th fetal month and those of the middle phalanges around the 8th fetal month. Proximal epiphysial centers (Fig. **154a**) appear in the proximal and middle phalanges usually between the 1st and 2nd postnatal year, in the distal phalanx after the 2nd year. Occasionally, the proximal ends of the phalanges ossify from the diaphysis. The epiphysial joints close between the ages of 13 and 20.

Deviations of the toes. Whereas in the newborn child and infant the toes continue the direction of the metatarsal bones, in the adult – due to the confining effect of stockings and footwear – the big and little toes are angled off toward the longitudinal axis of the foot coursing through the 2nd metatarsal and the 2nd toe. A lateral deviation of the big toe of 10–15° is still considered to be physiological, and this figure is frequently exceeded (in middle Europe by over two-thirds of the population).

This deviation of the big toe, which appears especially in women and increases with age, is designated as *hallux valgus*. It is accompanied by a decrease in the longitudinal curvature of the foot. With this condition the big toe can be subluxated at the metatarsophalangeal joint. In a similar manner the 5th toe can also be deviated (medially) whereby the 5th metatarsal is abducted laterally.

A *hammer toe* occurs when the toe (usually the 2nd) is superextended at the metatarsophalangeal joint and extremely flexed at the interphalangeal joints. It is generally accompanied by other foot deformities (e.g. splayfoot).

b) Capsules and Ligaments of the Joints of the Toes

The **metatarsophalangeal joints of the toes** (Figs. **153** and **154**), according to the shape of their articular surfaces, are ball-and-socket joints in which the spherical head of the metatarsal bone possesses a more extensive joint surface than the relatively small, flat socket at the base of the proximal phalanges.

The *articular capsules*, thin on the dorsal side, are strengthened on their plantar aspect by compact fibrous connective tissue plates, the *plantar ligaments*. In the plantar ligament of the big toe, two sesamoid bones are embedded (Fig. **147**); at the 5th toe one (fibular) sesamoid bone is frequently developed.

Ligaments (Figs. **153** and **154**). The *collateral ligaments* course somewhat obliquely from proximal and dorsal to distal and plantar. The heads of all metatarsals are united with one another on the plantar side by the *deep transverse metatarsal ligament.*

Movement possibilities. The *metatarsophalangeal joints* permit an active *plantar flexion* of up to 40° and a *dorsal flexion* of about 55° (passive almost 90°). Voluntary *splaying* of the toes, however, is possible to a varying individual extent only in the extended or superextended position. With increasing plantar flexion, spreading and (passive) rotation of the toes are limited more and more by the tension of the eccentrically organized collateral ligaments.

Active rotation movements cannot be carried out at the metatarsophalangeal joints (as is also true at the basal joints of the fingers).

Small *mucous bursae* are often present between the adjacent metatarsophalangeal joints.

Interphalangeal joints of the toes (Figs. **153** and **154**) – like the corresponding joints in the fingers – are pure hinge joints with a guidance groove at the proximally situated articular head and a guidance ridge at the distal joint socket. Flexion or extension movements are guided by *collateral ligaments.*

Movement possibilities. The *middle phalanges* can *flex* from the extended position by about 90°; the *distal phalanges* can be *plantar flexed* or *dorsiflexed* by 45° respectively.

Toe position. In the foot bearing no weight, the toes are slightly dorsiflexed at the metatarsophalangeal joint and somewhat plantar flexed at the interphalangeal joints. When pressure is exerted at the front of the foot, the middle and distal phalanges of toes II–IV are pressed against the ground and slightly flexed by the flexors of the toes. The hallux lies flat on the ground. In a tiptoe posture, which is mainly a standing position on the heads of the metatarsals, the proximal phalanges are (passively) strongly dorsiflexed, while the middle and distal phalanges of toes II–IV are plantar flexed. The heads of the metatarsals withdraw slightly from one another so that the standing surface is widened. The hallux, fixed by its flexor, forms a strong tibial supporting pillar.

At the joints of the toes, the *innervation* of the joint capsules corresponds to the nerve supply of the skin. Branches of the medial plantar nerve pass on the plantar side to $3\frac{1}{2}$ medial toes; the lateral plantar nerve supplies the remaining $1\frac{1}{2}$ lateral toes. Its deep ramus also provides branches to the metatarsophalangeal joints of toes II–V. On the dorsal side, branches of the superficial peroneal nerve supply the joints of the toes. Only at the sides of the 1st and 2nd toes facing one another are the joint capsules innervated dorsally by the cutaneous branch of the deep peroneal nerve, while the metatarsophalangeal joints of the 4th and 5th toes are supplied by the lateral dorsal cutaneous nerve (the terminal branch of the sural nerve).

Toe creases. At the soles of the feet, the balls of the big toe and the common balls for toes 2–5 are set off from the individual tips of the toes by the transverse toe crease (Figs. **149** and **157 a**). At the big toe, this crease is shallow, and a proximal and distal flexion fold can usually be distinguished, both of which lie in the region of the proximal phalanx. At the remaining toes, the toe crease is deeper. It is depressed toward the middle phalanx during plantar flexion of the toes. The proximal phalanges of the 2nd to 5th toes lie predominantly in the common toe ball. For the exact determination of the position of the joint cavity, the transverse toe crease cannot be used.

c) Organization and Innervation of the Short Muscles of the Foot

The musculature of the foot consists of the *muscles at the dorsum of the foot* (extensors), which are supplied by the deep peroneal nerve, and of the *muscles at the sole of the foot* (flexors), which are innervated by the tibial nerve. A dorsal musculature corresponding to that present on the dorsum of the hand is not developed in humans.

Muscles at the Dorsum of the Foot

The **dorsalis pedis fascia** (Fig. **158**), as the distal continuation of the fascia lata, covers the tendons of the long extensor muscles arising at the leg and the short extensors at the dorsum of the foot. The fascia is fixed at both malleoli, as well as by connective tissue tracts at the skeletal elements of the foot. Proximally, the dorsalis pedis fascia is strengthened by oblique and transverse bundles of fibers, which can be artificially isolated as the *inferior extensor reticulum*. Distally, it radiates into the dorsal aponeurosis of the toes.

In the depth of the dorsum of the foot, a layer of loose conective tissue, which is interwoven with the dorsal ligaments of the joints of the foot, is spread out on the foot skeleton. The connective tissue layer, occasionally also referred to as the deep layer of the dorsalis pedis fascia, delimits (incompletely) the dorsum of the foot in the region of the metatarsals from the *metatarsal interosseous space*. The dorsalis pedis artery, with its companion veins and deep lymphatic vessels, and the deep peroneal nerve course from the extensor compartment of the leg in the connective tissue layer as a continuation of the neurovascular trunk.

The tendons of the long extensors are protected against pressure and friction in the region of the extensor retinaculum by gliding *tendon sheaths* (Figs. **145** and **147**), which were described with the individual muscles. the synovial sheath of the extensor hallucis longus extends most distally up to the base of the 1st metatarsal.

The **extensor hallucis brevis** (Fig. **156**) arises on the dorsal surface of the calcaneus and from the interosseous talocalcanean ligament. It inserts at the proximal phalanx of the big toe.

Innervation: deep peroneal nerve.

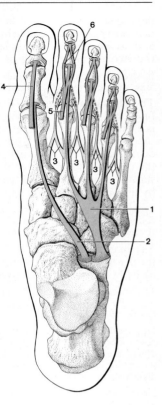

Fig. 156. **Muscles at dorsum of foot and dorsal interossei**
1 Extensor digitorum brevis
2 Extensor hallucis brevis
3 Dorsal interossei
4 Tendon of extensor hallucis longus
5 Tendon of extensor digitorum longus to 2nd toe
6 Dorsal aponeurosis of 2nd toe
Innervation:
☐ Deep peroneal nerve
☐ Lateral plantar nerve

The branches from the deep peroneal nerve to the extensor hallucis brevis and extensor digitorum brevis course beneath the inferior extensor retinaculum.

The **extensor digitorum brevis** (Fig. **156**) passes from the dorsolateral surface of the calcaneus to the dorsal aponeurosis of toes 2–4, sometimes also to toe 5.

Innervation: deep peroneal nerve.

Both muscles form an incompletely-organized unit. A corresponding tendinous tract usually also passes to the 5th toe from the peroneus brevis and occasionally also from the peroneus tertius.

Muscles at the Sole of the Foot

The muscles at the sole of the foot are formed much more strongly than one might expect from the movement possibilities of the joints which they pass over. They are first and foremost *holding muscles*, whose primary task is to provide an active brace for the longitudinal curvature of the foot and to increase its tonus as stress on the foot increases so that no (noteworthy) leveling off of the arch of the foot occurs.

In strongly-muscled individuals, the muscles at the sole of the foot largely fill the arch so that a reduced plantar recess does not indicate flatfoot in these cases.

The **plantar aponeurosis** (Fig. **158**) is the reinforced middle part of the fascia of the sole of the foot, which is relatively thin along the margins. It is a firm connective tissue plate. At the heel it is attached broadly at the tuber calcanei; at the front of the foot it is fixed with tongue-shaped extractions at the plantar ligaments of the metatarsophalangeal joints of the toes (including that of the big toe) and at the digital sheaths (fibrous sheaths of the toes). The tendinous ends are connected with one another by fibrous bundles coursing transversely (*transverse fasciculi*).

Transverse fiber tracts, which are situated further distally and which no longer communicate with the plantar aponeurosis, project into the interdigital skin folds In their totality, they are referred to as the *superficial transverse metatarsal ligament.*

The plantar aponeurosis forms an important passive bracing especially for the longitudinal curvature of the foot, while transverse fibrous tracts assist in securing the transverse curvature.

The aponeurosis protects the underlying muscles, tendons and conduction pathways. Its portion near the calcaneus also serves as a field of origin for the short flexors of the toes.

Numerous superficial connective tissue lamellae, which contain an abundance of elastic fibers, pass from the plantar aponeurosis to the dermis of the foot. They divide the subcutaneous fat tissue into well-filled, deformable compartments, which are immovable against the skin and the skeleton and which absorb and distribute the pressure.

From the plantar aponeurosis, a connective tissue septum is deeply submerged toward the foot skeleton at both the medial and lateral margins (medially toward the 1st metatarsal, medial cuneiform and navicular; laterally toward the 5th metatarsal and long plantar ligament). The two septa delimit (incompletely) three *muscular chambers* for the plantar muscles of the foot: the *big toe compartment* for the muscles of the hallux, the *middle compartment* for the muscles of the middle of the sole and the *little toe compartment* for the musculature of this digit.

The middle chamber carries the deep flexors from the leg. Distally, the connective tissue of this compartment continues into the subcutaneous tissue of the toes. At both margins of the compartment numerous connections to the adjacent compartments exist along the vessels and nerves passing through the septa.

In the depth of the sole of the foot, the middle muscular compartment is separated from the metatarsal interosseous space by a connective tissue layer. This layer, also designated as the deep fascia of the sole of the foot (Fig. **158**), lies on the foot skeleton at the plantar side and communicates proximally with the long plantar ligament, distally with the deep transverse metatarsal ligament. The (arterial) plantar arch, the venous plantar arch, lymphatic vessels and the deep ramus of the lateral plantar nerve course in this deep fascial layer.

Muscles of the Big Toe

The **abductor hallucis** (Figs. **157 a**, **158** and **161**) originates from the medial process of the tuber calcanei, from the flexor retinaculum and from the plantar aponeurosis. It attaches via the medial sesamoid bone at the capsule of the metatarsophalangeal joint of the hallux and at the 1st proximal phalanx.

Innervation: medial plantar nerve.

In the tarsal region, the medial plantar nerve gives off the branches for the abductor hallucis and flexor digitorum brevis. From its medial terminal branch, which enters the compartment of the big toe, a muscular branch is given off for the medial head of the short flexor of the hallux. The lateral terminal twig sends branches into the muscular compartment for the lumbricals I, II (III).

The **flexor hallucis brevis** (Fig. **157 a, b**) has its origin at the cuneiform bones, the plantar calcaneocuboid ligament and the tendon of the tibialis posterior. Together with the tendon of the abductor hallucis, it inserts with its medial head at the metatarsophalangeal joint via the medial sesamoid bone; together with the tendon of the adductor hallucis, it inserts with its lateral head at the proximal phalanx via the lateral sesamoid bone.

Innervation: medial head by the medial plantar nerve, lateral head by the lateral plantar nerve.

The **adductor hallucis** (Figs. **158** and **161**) arises with its *oblique head* from the cuboid, the lateral cuneiform, the deep ligaments, and the bases of metatarsals II–IV. Its *transverse head* comes from the metatarsophalangeal joints III–V and the deep transverse metatarsal ligament. The common terminal tendon of the two heads attaches via the lateral sesamoid bone to the capsule of the metatarsophalangeal joint and to the proximal phalanx of the big toe.

The muscle is covered almost completely by the tendons of the flexor digitorum longus and by the flexor digitorum brevis. Only the insertion and the medial marginal part of the oblique head lie in the big toe compartment.

Innervation: lateral plantar nerve.

Muscles of the Little Toe

The **abductor digiti minimi** (Figs. **157 a** and **158**) originates at the plantar surface of the calcaneus, especially from the lateral process of the tuber, from the plantar aponeurosis and from the tuberosity of the 5th metatarsal. It inserts at the proximal phalanx of the 5th toe.

Innervation: lateral plantar nerve.

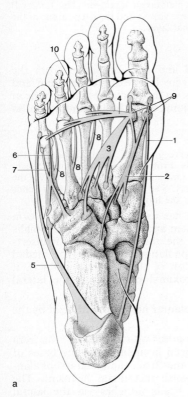

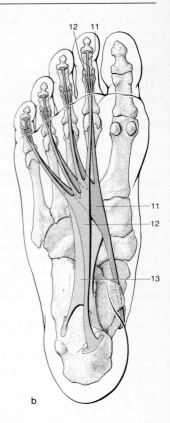

a

b

Fig. 157. Muscles at sole of foot
(Dorsal interossei →Fig. 156, lumbricals →Fig. 158)
Innervation:
☐ Tibial nerve
☐ Medial plantar nerve
☐ Lateral plantar nerve
a Mucles of big and little toe, plantar interossei
b Short and long flexors of toes

1 Abductor hallucis
2 Flexor hallucis brevis
3 Oblique head ⎫ of adductor
4 Transverse head ⎭ hallucis
5 Abductor digiti minimi
6 Flexor digiti minimi brevis
7 Opponens digiti minimi

8 Plantar interossei
9 Sesamoids
10 Transverse skin crease of toes
11 Flexor digitorum longus ("perforating flexor")
12 Flexor digitorum brevis ("perforated flexor")
13 Quadratus plantae (flexor accessorius)

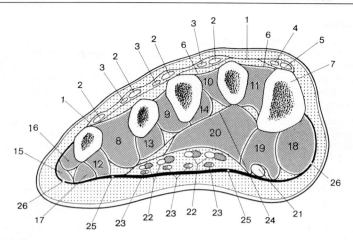

Fig. 158. **Transverse section in region of middle of foot, arrangement of fascia, muscles and tendons**, distal view of section surface (Designation of vessels and nerves → Fig. 160).

 1 Dorsal fascia of foot
 2 Tendons of extensor digitorum longus
 3 Tendons of extensor digitorum brevis
 4 Tendon of extensor hallucis brevis
 5 Tendon of extensor hallucis longus
 6 Deep fascia of dorsum of foot
 7 Metatarsal I
 8 Dorsal interosseus IV
 9 Dorsal interosseus III
10 Dorsal interosseus II
11 Dorsal interosseus I
12 Plantar interosseus III
13 Plantar interosseus II
14 Plantar interosseus I

15 Abductor digiti minimi
16 Opponens digiti minimi
17 Flexor digiti minimi brevis
18 Abductor hallucis
19 Flexor hallucis brevis
20 Adductor hallucis, oblique head
21 Tendon of flexor hallucis longus
22 Tendons of flexor digitorum longus and lumbricals
23 Flexor digitorum brevis
24 Deep fascia of sole of foot
25 Plantar aponeurosis
26 Superficial fascia of sole of foot

The lateral plantar nerve gives off branches to the abductor digiti minimi and the quadratus plantae in the region of the calcaneus, dispatches the muscular branch to the short flexor of the little toe via the superficial ramus, and supplies the lateral head of the flexor hallucis brevis, the adductor hallucis (II), III and IV, all interossei and the opponens digiti minimi via the deep ramus.

The **flexor digiti minimi brevis** and **opponens digiti minimi** (Figs. **157 a** and **158**) arise with a common tendon of origin from the base of the 5th metatarsal, from the long plantar ligament and from the tendon sheath of the peroneus longus. The short flexor of the little toe inserts at the base of the proximal phalanx of the 5th toe, and the opponens at the lateral surface of the 5th metatarsal.

In humans, the opponens often appears only as a weakly-defined muscle tract of the flexor digiti minimi brevis and is identifiable only on the basis of its insertion.

Innervation of both muscles: lateral plantar nerve.

Muscles of the Middle of the Sole

The **flexor digitorum brevis** (Figs. **157 b** and **158**) arises from the under-surface of the calcanean tuberosity and the portion of the plantar aponeurosis near the calcaneus. Its tendons split above the proximal phalanges of the 2nd–5th toes ("perforated flexor"), enclose the deeper-lying tendons of the flexor digitorum longus ("perforating flexor") between themselves, and insert at the middle phalanges of toes 2–5.

The tendons of the long and short flexors of the toes are enclosed in the region of the toes by *tendon sheaths* (*synovial sheaths*), which begin, however, only at the distal fourth of the metatarsals. The tendon of the flexor digitorum brevis can be absent at the 5th toe.

Innervation: medial plantar nerve.

The **quadratus plantae** (Fig. **157 b**) originates from the plantar surface of the calcaneus and inserts at the tendon(s) of the flexor digitorum longus. It is also designated as the *accessory flexor muscle* because it corrects the direction of traction of the terminal tendons of the long flexors of the toes (in the sense of a plantar flexion of the toes).

The tendons to the lateral toes pass mainly obliquely over the metatarsal bones before being fixed in the longitudinal direction of the toes by the fibrous tendon sheath. The oblique direction of traction of these tendons is diverted by the contraction of the quadratus plantae in the longitudinal direction of the metatarsals.

Innervation: lateral plantar nerve.

The four **lumbricals** (Fig. **158**) pass from the tendons of the flexor digitorum longus to the medial margin of the proximal phalanges of toes 2–5.

The 1st lumbrical arises with one head at the medial margin of the tendon for the 2nd toe; the bipennate lumbricals II–IV come from the surfaces of the tendons of the long flexor of the toes which face one another. The lumbricals course plantar to the deep transverse metatarsal ligament, from which they are separated by small mucous bursae.

Innervation: the 1st lumbrical (occasionally also the 2nd) is supplied by the medial plantar nerve; the lateral lumbricals are innervated by the lateral plantar nerve.

Muscles in the Metatarsal Interosseous Space

In the interosseous spaces of the metatarsus, the interossei muscles are separated from the muscles of the middle of the sole and the short extensors of the toes by deep connective tissue layers at the sole and dorsum of the foot. Genetically, both the plantar interossei and the dorsal interossei, which are situated more dorsally in the interosseous spaces, are ventral muscles.

The three **plantar interossei** (Figs. **157 a** and **158**) pass from the plantar surface of metatarsals III–V and from the long plantar ligament to the medial side of the bases of the proximal phalanges of toes 3–5, usually without reaching the dorsal aponeurosis of the toes.

Innervation: lateral plantar nerve.

The four **dorsal interossei** arise with two heads at the facing surfaces of all metatarsals and at the long plantar ligament. They also attach at the bases of the proximal phalanges, whereby the 2nd ray forms the axis of symmetry around which they are grouped. Rarely do tendon fibers radiate into the dorsal aponeurosis of the toes.

Innervation: lateral plantar nerve.

d) Action of Muscles and Muscle Groups on the Joints of the Toes

At the *metatarsophalangeal joint*, the *big toe* can be:
- *flexed* (plantar flexed) by the flexor hallucis longus and flexor hallucis brevis,
  whereby the abductor hallucis and adductor hallucis can work together in support;
- *extended* (dorsiflexed) by the extensor hallucis longus and extensor hallucis brevis;
- *abducted* (spread from the 2nd toe) by the abductor hallucis; and
- *adducted* (moved toward the 2nd toe) by the adductor hallucis.

At the *distal interphalangeal joint*, the *big toe* can be:
- *flexed* only by the flexor hallucis longus, and
- *extended* only by the extensor hallucis longus.

At the *metatarsophalangeal joint*, toes *II–V* can be:
- *flexed* by the flexor digitorum longus and flexor digitorum brevis, the interossei and the lumbricals; the 5th toe can be flexed additionally by the flexor digiti minimi brevis and abductor digiti minimi,
  whereby the simultaneous contraction of the 3rd plantar interosseus hinders the abduction of the little toe;
- *extended* by the extensor digitorum longus and extensor digitorum brevis;
- *carried laterally* by dorsal interossei II–IV and the abductor digiti minimi; and
- *carried medially* by dorsal interosseus I (2nd toe) and the plantar interossei.

In general, children are able to spread their toes strongly (dorsal interossei and abductor digiti minimi) or adduct again toward the 2nd toe (plantar interossei). In the adult this ability is more or less stunted.

At the *proximal interphalangeal joints, toes II–V* can be:
- *flexed* by the flexor digitorum longus and flexor digitorum brevis, and
- *extended* by the extensor digitorum longus and extensor digitorum brevis,

At the *distal interphalangeal joints, toes II–V* can be:
- *flexed* only by the flexor digitorum longus, and
- *extended* only by the extensor digitorum longus.

The lumbricals can assist in extending a toe at the proximal and distal interphalangeal joints if their tendon is continued into the dorsal aponeurosis up to the proximal or distal phalanx of the toe affected.

If the dorsal aponeurosis of a toe is not adequately formed, the active extension of the distal phalanx (possibly also the middle phalanx) of this toe is not possible.

Bracing of the Foot Skeleton by Muscles at the Sole of the Foot

The plantar muscles of the foot can only move the segments of the toes when the foot is not stressed. If, however, the weight of the body is supported by the foot, the short flexors at best are able to press the toes on the ground. The action of these muscles, together with the plantar ligaments, is primarily to ensure the curved construction of the foot in standing and walking and to prevent a flattening of the arch as much as possible. In common with the long flexors of the toes, the short muscles – especially the flexor digitorum brevis and the muscles of the hallux – try to brace the longitudinal curvature of the foot effectively and to "shorten" the foot. The plantar longitudinal strut is safeguarded additionally by the tibialis anterior, which exerts an upward (dorsal) traction near the apex of the longitudinal curvature. The transverse head of the adductor hallucis is the only source of transverse muscular traction in the front of the foot to counteract a spreading of the heads of the metatarsals, thus bracing the front of the foot in the transverse direction.

The importance of the opponens digiti minimi for the maintenance of this transverse bracing is probably slight.

Paralyses. A failure of the *extensors of the toes* does not lead to conspicuous motor disturbances. When the *plantar muscles of the foot* are paralyzed, the effective bracing of the longitudinal arch of the foot no longer suffices, and the recess of the sole of the foot sinks. The transverse curvature in the region of the front of the foot disappears, whereas it is preserved (at first) in the tarsal region.

In a paralysis of the *interossei*, the toes can no longer be spread and brought together. Like the clawhand resulting from a paralysis of the ulnar nerve, a clawfoot arises when the interossei fail to function (because of an injury to the lateral plantar nerve). The toes are dorsiflexed at the metatarsophalangeal joint since the tonus of the extensors predominates here, while the middle and distal phalanges are plantar flexed.

e) Neurovascular Routes in the Foot

Neurovascular Routes at the Dorsum of the Foot

The conduction pathways in the extensor compartment of the leg continue into the dorsum of the foot. In the deep connective tissue layer lying directly on the foot skeleton – lateral to the tendon of the flexor hallucis longus – the *dorsalis pedis artery* (a continuation of the anterior tibial artery) passes into the 1st interosseous space. It is entwined by *companion veins* and their transverse anastomoses and accompanied by *deep lymphatic tracts*. The *deep peroneal nerve* courses (usually) at the medial side of the vascular cord.

The *pulse* of the dorsalis pedis artery can be felt at the proximal end of the 1st interosseous space lateral to the tendon of the extensor hallucis longus.

In crossing over to the dorsum of the foot, the **dorsalis pedis artery** (Fig. **159**) crosses underneath the tendon of the extensor hallucis longus and, below the inferior extensor retinaculum, gives off the *lateral tarsal artery* to the lateral margin of the foot. At the distal tarsals, it sends several small *medial tarsal arteries* to the median margin of the foot and, in the tarsometatarsal region, the *arcuate artery*, which courses laterally on the bases of the metatarsal bones below the tendons of the long and short extensors of the toes. The arcuate artery gives off weak *dorsal metatarsal arteries* and anastomoses with the lateral tarsal artery. The terminal branch of the dorsalis pedis artery is the *1st dorsal metatarsal artery*, over which the tendon of the extensor hallucis brevis crosses. The artery passes distally on the 1st dorsal interosseus and, via the first interosseous space, gives off the deep plantar artery to the plantar side of the foot.

The *lateral tarsal artery* is covered by the extensor digitorum brevis muscle, ramifies on the distal tarsals, and dispatches a *dorsal digital artery* to the lateral side of the little toe.

The *dorsal metatarsal arteries II–IV* arise at the convex side of the vascular arch formed by the arcuate and lateral tarsal arteries, pass to the 2nd–4th interosseous spaces (Fig. **160**), and each divides into two *dorsal digital arteries* to the facing margins of toes 2–5.

The *1st dorsal metatarsal artery* supplies the dorsomedial margin of the 2nd toe with a *dorsal digital artery* and the dorsolateral margin of the big toe with the *dorsal lateral hallucis artery*. The *medial dorsal hallucis artery*, as a rule, comes from the medial plantar hallucis artery.

The *deep plantar artery* (Fig. **160**) arrives at the 1st interosseous space between the two heads of the 1st dorsal interosseus muscle at the plantar side of the foot and is united with the deep plantar arch from the lateral plantar artery.

The arterial network at the dorsum of the foot can be formed with considerable variation. Usually, two perforating rami (Fig. **159**) from the plantar metatarsal

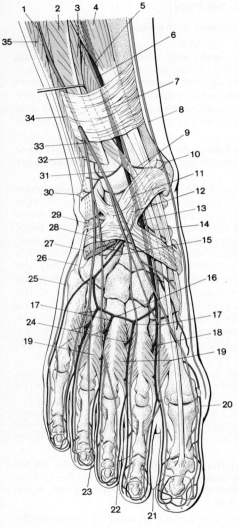

Fig. 159. **Arteries and nerves in leg and dorsum of foot**

 1 Superficial peroneus
 2 Extensor digitorum longus, severed distal to superior extensor retinaculum
 3 Extensor hallucis longus
 4 Tibialis anterior
 5 Anterior tibial artery
 6 Deep peroneal nerve
 7 Superior extensor retinaculum
 8 Saphenous nerve
 9 Medial anterior malleolar artery
10 Arterial network of medial malleolus
11 Inferior extensor retinaculum
12 Muscular branch of deep peroneal nerve to extensor digitorum and extensor hallucis brevis
13 Dorsalis pedis artery
14 Medial tarsal artery
15 Lateral tarsal artery
16 Arcuate artery
17 Dorsal metatarsal arteries
18 Deep plantar artery
19 Dorsal interossei
20 Medial dorsal hallucis artery, usually from medial plantar hallucis artery
21 Dorsal digital nerves (hallucis lateralis and digiti secundi medialis)
22 Dorsal digital nerves
23 Dorsal digital arteries
24 Perforating branches
25 Lateral dorsal cutaneous nerve
26 Tendon of peroneus brevis
27 Extensor digitorum brevis
28 Extensor hallucis brevis
29 Inferior peroneal retinaculum
30 Arterial network on lateral malleolus
31 Lateral anterior malleolar artery
32 Intermediate dorsal cutaneous nerve
33 Medial dorsal cutaneous nerve
34 Peroneus brevis
35 Peroneus longus

arteries enter each dorsal metatarsal artery. In case of a degeneration of the arcuate artery, the blood for the dorsal digital arteries comes entirely or partly from the plantar vessels. The anastomosis of the lateral tarsal artery with the arcuate artery can be absent; the lateral tarsal artery can also be developed in duplicate (proximal and distal).

The **deep veins at the dorsum of the foot** communicate with the plantar veins of the foot and with the *dorsal venous network of the foot* situated on the surface of the fascia. Blood from this network is carried off primarily by the subcutaneous great saphenous and small saphenous veins.

Inflammations on the plantar side of the foot and the toes are conducted to the dorsal side of the foot by means of numerous lymphatic pathways and veins, which course to this region in the interosseous spaces. They can cause extensive swelling in the loose subcutaneous connective tissue of the dorsum of the foot (collateral edema of the dorsum of the foot), while an inflammation on the plantar side remains largely hidden beneath the rigid skin of the sole of the foot (with the subcutaneous compression chambers).

The **deep peroneal nerve** (Figs. **159** and **160**) at the dorsum of the foot gives off branches to the short extensors of the toes and to the capsules of the tarsal and the tarsometatarsal joints, as well as to the metatarsophalangeal joints of the toes. It accompanies the 1st dorsal metatarsal artery and ramifies on the 1st dorsal interosseus muscle into the *dorsal digital nerves* to the adjacent margins of the big toe (*lateral dorsal digital nerve of the hallux*) and the 2nd toe (*medial dorsal digital nerve of the 2nd toe*).

Neurovascular Routes at the Sole of the Foot

From the compartment of the deep flexors at the leg, a *medial* (tibial) and a *lateral* (fibular) *neurovascular cord* pass dorsal and distal to the medial malleolus – superficial to the tendons of the deep flexors – into the middle compartment of the sole of the foot (Fig. **147**). The medial conduction paths consist of the *medial plantar artery*, *accompanying veins*, *deep lymphatic tracts* and the *medial plantar nerve*.

The *lateral plantar artery*, *accompanying veins*, *deep lymphatic vessels* and the *lateral plantar nerve* course in the lateral cord.

The deep veins, which weave around the branches of the plantar arteries, and their accompanying lymphatic vessels discharge mainly via the venous and lymphatic networks on the dorsum of the foot.

The lateral plantar nerve always lies at the medial side of the corresponding artery, whereas the medial plantar nerve does so in about 80% of the cases. The lateral plantar artery is larger than the medial plantar artery in two-thirds of the cases.

The **medial neurovascular cord** of the sole of the foot courses first near the skeleton in the connective tissue septum which separates the big toe and middle compartments. Toward the middle of the foot, the conduction pathways separate, and the **medial plantar nerve,** which has already

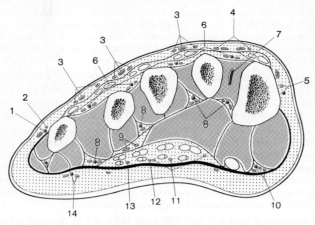

Fig. 160. **Transverse section in region of middle of foot, arrangement of nerves and vessels,** dorsal view of section surface
(Designation of muscles and tendons → Fig. 158)

1 Lateral dorsal digital artery V
2 Lateral dorsal digital nerve V (from lateral dorsal cutaneous nerve)
3 Dorsal digital nerves of toes (from superficial peroneal nerve) and subcutaneous dorsal metatarsal veins
4 Dorsal digital nerves (lateral hallucis and medial digiti secundi from deep peroneal nerve)
5 Medial dorsal hallucis artery and nerve
6 Dorsal metatarsal arteries
7 Deep plantar artery
8 Plantar metatarsal arteries

9 Branches of deep branch of lateral plantar nerve
10 Superficial branch of medial plantar artery and medial plantar hallucis nerve (from medial plantar nerve)
11 Common plantar digital nerves of first three toes from medial plantar nerve
12 Anastomosis between superificial branch of lateral plantar nerve and common plantar digital nerve of 3rd toe
13 Common plantar digital nerve of 4th toe from lateral plantar nerve
14 Lateral plantar digital artery and nerve of 5th toe

provided branches to the abductor hallucis and the flexor digitorum brevis, gives off several branches (Fig. **161**). Its area of sensory innervation corresponds to that of the median nerve in the hand.

The big toe compartment contains branches of the medial plantar nerve to the flexor hallucis brevis, to the capsule of the metatarsophalangeal joint, and a cutaneous branch to the medial side of the big toe (*medial plantar nerve to the hallux*), as well as the **medial plantar artery** (Fig. **161**). After a short course, the medial plantar artery divides between the abductor hallucis and flexor hallucis brevis into the *superficial ramus* (along the abductor hallucis to the big toe) and the *deep ramus*, which passes in the deep neurovascular layer of the sole of the foot and unites (as a rule) with the deep plantar arch.

In the middle compartment, the main trunk of the medial plantar nerve gives off the *common plantar digital nerves* coursing beneath the plantar aponeurosis (Figs. **160** and **161**). They supply the 1st lumbrical (occasionally also the 2nd), and each divides into two *proper plantar digital nerves* for the skin of the adjacent margins of two toes. Altogether, the medial plantar nerve innervates the skin on the plantar side of $3\frac{1}{2}$ medial toes.

The **lateral neurovascular cord** of the sole of the foot is covered by the flexor digitorum brevis and passes obliquely over the quadratus plantae toward the fibular side (Fig. **147**). It courses for only a short distance in the connective tissue septum separating the middle and little toe compartments at the level of the cuboid before it gives off the lateral plantar nerve. With respect to the supply of the skin and joints, the lateral plantar nerve corresponds to the ulnar nerve in the hand.

The **lateral plantar artery** (Fig. **161**) goes over into the *deep plantar arch* at the level of the base of the 5th metatarsal.

A *superficial plantar arch*, which is fed by a superficial branch of the medial and lateral plantar arteries and which corresponds to the superficial palmar arch, occurs as a well-developed arterial arch only in 2% of the cases. In 25% of the cases, it is formed as an extraordinarily thin, transverse anastomosis.

In a convex course which runs laterally and distally between the oblique head of the adductor hallucis and the interossei, the (deep) arch of the sole of the foot turns to the medial side and anastomoses in the 1st metatarsal interosseous space with the deep plantar artery from the dorsalis pedis artery. The *plantar metatarsal arteries*, which course in the interosseous spaces of the metatarsal bones and which are referred to as the *common plantar digital arteries* after they have given off the perforating branches, leave from the convex side of the vascular arch. Each splits into two *proper plantar digital arteries* for the margins of two toes facing each other.

The 1st plantar metatarsal artery generally also dispatches the medial *plantar hallucis artery*, which is occasionally connected with the superficial ramus of the medial plantar artery or which can proceed from it. The proper plantar digital artery to the lateral margin of the 5th toe comes from the base of the plantar arch.

Perforating branches of the plantar metatarsal arteries pass through the interosseous spaces and are united with the dorsal metatarsal arteries.

If the lateral plantar artery is weakly developed, the deep plantar arch is mainly fed by the deep plantar artery from the dorsalis pedis artery (43%). In rare cases, the arch of the sole of the foot is not closed.

In the region of the calcaneus, the **lateral plantar nerve** (Fig. **161**) gives off branches to the abductor digiti minimi and quadratus plantae. Then it divides into its superficial and deep rami.

The *superficial ramus* sends the *4th common plantar digital nerve* to the middle muscular compartment, with branches to the facing margins of the 4th and 5th toes and an anastomotic branch to the 3rd common plantar digital nerve. The lateral branch of the superficial ramus passes through the lateral compartment of the sole of the foot, innervates the flexor digiti minimi brevis, and proceeds to the skin at the lateral side of the 5th toe as the *5th proper plantar digital nerve*.

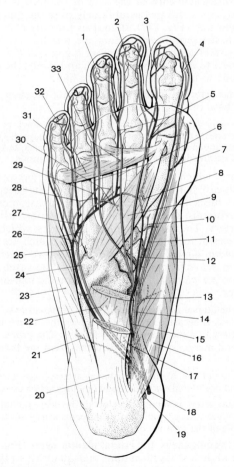

Fig. 161. **Arteries and nerves of sole of foot**

The *deep ramus* of the lateral plantar nerve courses with the plantar arch into the deep connective tissue layer of the sole of the foot. It innervates the lateral head of the flexor hallucis brevis, the adductor hallucis, (as a rule) lumbricals (II), III and IV, all interossei and the opponens digiti minimi.

Lumbricals III, IV and V, the interosseus in the 4th interosseous space, the flexor digiti minimi brevis, and the opponens digiti minimi can also be innervated by branches of the superficial ramus.

f) Arrangement of Vessels and Nerves in the Toes

As in each finger, a total of *four arteries* and *four nerves* also course in each toe in the subcutaneous connective tissue at both plantar and both dorsal margins. The plantar arteries and nerves are larger than the dorsal digital arteries and nerves. As in the fingers, the dorsal arteries of the toes terminate at the middle phalanges, while the dorsal nerves to the toes pass to the distal phalanges.

The *dorsal digital arteries* (Fig. **159**) originate (as a rule) from dorsal metatarsal artery I (adjacent margins of the 1st and 2nd toes), from dorsal metatarsal arteries II–IV arising from the arcuate artery (margins of toes 2–5 facing each other), and also from the medial plantar hallucis artery (medial margin of big toe) and the lateral tarsal artery (lateral margin of little toe). The *plantar arteries of the toes* obtain their blood from the plantar arch.

◀ 1 Proper plantar digital arteries
2 Proper plantar digital nerves
3 Lateral plantar hallucis artery and nerve
4 Medial plantar hallucis artery and nerve
5 Common plantar digital arteries and nerves
6 Plantar metatarsal arteries
7 Branch to medial dorsal hallucis artery
8 Deep plantar artery
9 Adductor hallucis, oblique head
10 Branch of medial plantar nerve to flexor hallucis brevis
11 Superficial branch of medial plantar artery
12 Deep branch of medial plantar artery
13 Branch of medial plantar nerve to abductor hallucis
14 Medial plantar nerve
15 Medial plantar artery
16 Abductor hallucis
17 Branch of medial plantar nerve to flexor digitorum brevis
18 Posterior tibial artery

19 Tibial nerve
20 Flexor digitorum brevis, severed
21 Branch of lateral plantar nerve to abductor digiti minimi
22 Quadratus plantae (severed) and muscular branch from lateral plantar nerve
23 Abductor digiti minimi
24 Lateral plantar nerve
25 Lateral plantar artery
26 Superficial branch (lateral) and deep branch (medial) of lateral plantar nerve
27 Deep plantar arch
28 Proximal perforating branches
29 Anastomosis between superficial branch of lateral plantar nerve and common plantar digital nerve of 3rd toe
30 Muscular branches of deep branch of lateral plantar nerve
31 Lateral plantar digital artery of 5th toe
32 Adductor hallucis, transverse head
33 Distal perforating branches

Regular connections between the dorsal and plantar arteries exist in the region of the metatarsals and phalanges. Likewise, both plantar arteries of a toe anastomose with each other.

Veins and *lymphatic vessels of the toes* form networks on the plantar and dorsal sides, which discharge at the dorsum of the foot via deep veins and lymphatic vessels, but mainly via subcutaneous vessels.

The *dorsal digital nerves of the foot* (Figs. **159** and **160**) are the terminal branches of the superficial peroneal nerve. Only the facing dorsal margins of the 1st and 2nd toes are (also) supplied by the deep peroneal nerve.

The *lateral dorsal cutaneous nerve*, the terminal branch of the sural nerve, passes to the dorsolateral margin of the 5th toe.

Anastomoses exist between the medial dorsal cutaneous nerve and the terminal branch of the deep peroneal nerve, as well as between the intermediate dorsal cutaneous nerve and the lateral dorsal cutaneous nerve.

The *proper plantar digital nerves* of the $3\frac{1}{2}$ medial toes are branches of the medial plantar nerve (Fig. **161**). To the $1\frac{1}{2}$ lateral toes there are branches of the lateral plantar nerve as plantar nerves to the toes.

Nerve fibers from the lateral plantar nerve to the medial side of the 4th toe are joined to the 3rd common plantar digital nerve by means of an anastomosis.

4. Lower Limb: Standing and Walking

In a standing posture, the tuber calcanei forms the skeletal foundation for the posterior part of the standing surface. The anterior part of the foot rests on the heads of the metatarsals. The most important points of support of the foot skeleton, the tuber calcanei and the heads of the 1st and 5th metatarsal bones, are frequently underlaid by subcutaneous mucous bursae (Fig. **147**). The distribution of pressure on the individual metatarsals depends on the type of standing posture and the position of the feet. For example, the 1st metatarsal is subjected to the most pressure when the apex of the foot is directed slightly outward and the knee joint is extended.

In an erect standing posture with the body positioned symmetrically, the weight of the body is borne equally by both feet, and the line of gravity courses in the median plane of the body. In order to prevent the body from losing its balance forward or backward, this line must strike within the supporting surface (Fig. **162**), which is bordered by tangents drawn along the convex sides of the standing surface.

In the so-called *normal posture* (Fig. **163 a**), which in reality is an artificial position and is seldom maintained for a long period, a plumb line passing through the center of gravity of the body bisects the line connecting the rotation points (pivots) of both hip joints. The *center of*

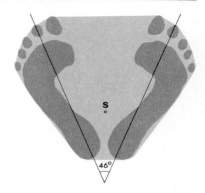

Fig. 162. **Supporting surface of body in relaxed standing position** (▢)
Standing surface.shaded
S = projection of center of gravity on the supporting surface (point of impact of line of gravity)

gravity of the body lies in the median plane somewhat in front of and below the promontory, at the level of the 2nd sacral vertebra. In this position, the pivots of both hip, knee and superior ankle joints lie in the same frontal plane, and the body is in *labile equilibrium*.

This labile equilibrium can be disturbed by even the smallest movement, e.g. a minimal depression of the head. The musculature of the trunk and the lower limb must, therefore, always be prepared to balance the body weight. Since the line of gravity in this position strikes the supporting surface close to its dorsal boundary, a slight push from the front already suffices to bring the body out of equilibrium.

When the body is held in a taut erect posture (also incorrectly called military bearing, Fig. **163 b**), the body is extended at the hip and knee joints, and the legs are inclined somewhat anteriorly at the superior ankle joints. The line of gravity hits at the middle of the supporting surface. However, in this position – as in any erect body posture – not only must the erector spinae muscle ensure the lordosis in the cervical and lumbar regions, but also the large gluteal muscle and the ischiocrural muscles must prevent a flexion at the hip joint and the flexors at the leg (especially the triceps surae) must prevent the body from falling forwards.

The so-called comfortable or *relaxed posture* (Fig. **163 c**) furnishes a high stability with economical muscular activity. The pelvis can be inclined so far backwards that the line of gravity passes behind the frontal axis of both hip joints and in front of the frontal axis of both knee joints. In this position, the iliofemoral ligaments are stretched at both hip joints, the collateral and cruciate ligaments at the knee joints.

The line of gravity passes to a point roughly within the posterior third of the sagittal diameter of the supporting surface and lies ventral to the axis of rotation through the superior ankle joints. In addition to the erector spinae muscle, only the plantar-flexing muscles at the leg must be stretched for the maintenance of equilibrium.

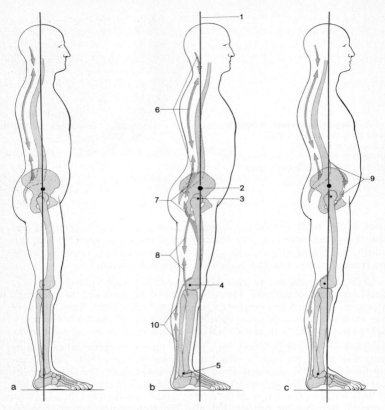

Fig. 163. **Standing in upright and symmetrical posture** (modified after *Kummer*)
a So-called normal posture
b Taut erect posture
c Relaxed posture

1 Line of gravity
2 Weight center of body (center of gravity)
3 Projection of frontal axis of hip joint
4 Projection of frontal axis of knee joint
5 Projection of axis of upper ankle joint
6 Erector spinae
7 Gluteal musculature
8 Ischiocrural musculature
9 Ilipsoas
10 Flexors of leg

An injurious maximal stretching of the above-mentioned ligaments, which could result from the action of the force of gravity at the hip and knee joints, is prevented by the retarding effect of the iliopsoas and gastrocnemius. Observations have shown, moreover, that any given pelvic position and the erect body posture coupled with it are always maintained for only a short time (usually less than a minute) and are then varied slightly.

In walking (Fig. **164**), the same leg alternates as the *supporting leg* and *free (swinging) leg*. As the supporting leg, it carries the body weight in the direction of the movement; as the free, unsupporting leg, it swings freely over the ground and reaches a new standing surface. In a walking stride (medium-sized step at an average tempo), the *standing phase* (supporting phase) and *swinging phase* of a leg are not equally long; for in the alternation of both phases, the body weight is distributed for a brief moment on both legs, on the "old" supporting leg, whose foot is being lifted from the ground to end its supporting phase, and on the "new" supporting leg, whose standing phase already began as the heel was set on the ground.

In a walking stride, the standing phase amounts to 61%, and the swinging phase to 39% of a stride cycle (= double stride, beginning with the heel contact of a leg and ending with the renewed heel contact of the same leg). The time interval in which both legs carry the body weight becomes shorter with increasing velocity of locomotion. In a running stride, there is a period in which both legs have no contact with ground, namely, between the lifting of the "old" and the putting down of the "new" supporting leg.

In walking, the feet are put down alternately (somewhat) to the right and the left of the walking line. Correspondingly, the center of gravity of the body swings with each individual step from one side to the other since otherwise the line of gravity cannot fall on the standing surface. With the shifting of the center of gravity to each new standing surface, critical importance belongs to the small gluteal muscles because they prevent the lowering of the body's center of gravity and hold it approximately in the horizontal plane.

In walking forward, the *standing phase* of a leg begins when the heel is set down. The foot is slightly flexed dorsally, and the knee joint is slightly bent; the vasti muscles prevent a stronger flexion. The hip joint is likewise flexed and, during normal walking, the trunk is inclined somewhat obliquely toward the ventral side. Then, the heel, the lateral margin of the foot and the heads of the metatarsals take over one by one the body weight. The knee and hip joint are extended (quadriceps femoris and gluteus maximus). The body is carried anteriorly over the supporting surface by the supporting leg. In about the middle of this phase, the foot is at a right angle to the extended leg. At the same time, the hip joint reaches the highest point in its undulating movement, and the center of gravity lies perpendicularly over the supporting surface. The small gluteal muscles prevent the pelvis from descending toward the side of the free leg and incline it slightly toward the side of

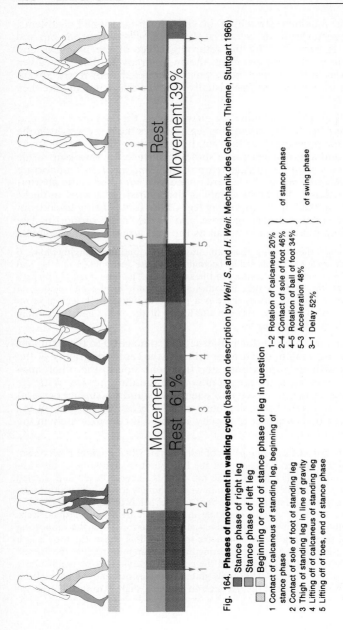

Fig. 164. **Phases of movement in walking cycle** (based on description by *Weil, S.,* and *H. Weil:* Mechanik des Gehens. Thieme, Stuttgart 1966)

■ Stance phase of right leg
■ Stance phase of left leg
□ Beginning or end of stance phase of leg in question

1 Contact of calcaneus of standing leg, beginning of stance phase
2 Contact of sole of foot of standing leg
3 Thigh of standing leg in line of gravity
4 Lifting off of calcaneus of standing leg
5 Lifting off of toes, end of stance phase

1–2 Rotation of calcaneus 20% ⎫
2–4 Contact of sole of foot 46% ⎬ of stance phase
4–5 Rotation of ball of foot 34% ⎭
5–3 Acceleration 48% ⎫ of swing phase
3–1 Delay 52% ⎭

the supporting leg. The upper body is also inclined somewhat toward the side and thus facilitates the balance of the body, which rests on the small supporting surface of the foot placed beside the median line.

The heel-to-toe movement of the foot on the ground takes place via the 1st metatarsal and the big toe. (In contrast to the movable connection of the 1st metacarpal with the trapezium, the 1st metatarsal is relatively firmly fixed in the tarsometatarsal skeleton.) The foot is plantar flexed more and more strongly (especially by the triceps surae), and the heel thereby lifted from the ground. The toes are dorsiflexed passively at the metatarsophalangeal joint. The plantar flexion at the superior ankle joint causes the supporting leg, which is extended at the knee joint and stands obliquely, to be "lengthened". The body is shoved forward, and this forward movement produced by the muscular contraction is complemented by the action of gravity. Toward the end of the standing phase, the knee joint is already slightly flexed again. Before the swinging phase begins, the previous supporting leg is relieved of its load, and the body weight is shifted to the future supporting leg.

In the *swinging phase*, the thigh of the free leg flexes at the hip joint, the toe of the foot is lifted off the ground, the free leg is carried forward past the supporting leg and its heel is placed on the ground. The forward swinging of the free leg occurs as a pendular movement under the influence of the force of gravity; it is controlled by muscle action and modified as the situation dictates. So that the foot does not slide on the ground, the leg must be held flexed long enough against the action of gravity when the thigh swings forward (ischiocrural muscles) until it can also swing through unhindered. The foot (during almost the entire swinging phase) is at an approximate right angle to the leg. The extensors at the leg prevent a plantar flexion of the foot and, therefore, a sliding of the toe of the foot on the ground. When the heel is set down, the knee joint is already slightly flexed again, and the foot slightly dorsiflexed at the superior ankle joint.

From the structural characteristics of the limb skeleton (e.g. femoral length, tibial torsion) and the slight differences in the control of muscular action, a *typical individual gait* results. With an increase in the velocity of locomotion, the basic elements of the motion described here are correspondingly modified. By alternating collateral movements of the arms (free leg and arm of the opposite side), the balancing of the body and the displacement of the body's center of gravity to the alternate side (especially during fast walking and running) are facilitated.

E. Surface Anatomy of the Lower Limb

1. Surface Relief of Lower Limb and Palpable Bony Points

Surface relief. On the ventral side of the hip, the inguinal fossa marks the boundary between trunk and thigh. It lies at the level of the inguinal ligament only in very lean people. With increasing deposits of fat in the subcutaneous tissue, it clearly shifts more and more distally toward the thigh. In lean, well-built men, the tensor fasciae latae and the sartorius, as well as the adductor group, stand out through the skin. Over the iliac crest, the inguinal bulging is arched. The shape of the buttocks varies greatly according to the development of the large gluteal muscle and the thickness of the subcutaneous fat tissue. The thigh is conically-shaped and tapers toward the knee.

A strong development of the thigh musculature causes a slight bulging of the anterior, lateral and posterior surfaces of the thigh. The medial contour line of the thigh is approximately straight and slightly concave above the knee (sartorius). Pathological curvatures of the shaft of the femur can strikingly alter its typical conical shape. The course of the sartorius, the muscle bellies of the vastus medialis and vastus lateralis, and the biceps femoris are visible in muscular individuals. At the border between the extensors and flexors (attachment of the lateral femoral intermuscular septum at the fascia lata), the lateral surface of the thigh can be depressed in the form of a longitudinal groove. On the rounded dorsal side of the thigh, the tendons of insertion of the ischiocrural muscles appear against the popliteal fossa on both sides and border the proximal part of this fossa.

In the popliteal fossa, the skin is depressed into a rhomboidal fossa only when the knee is flexed, the muscular marginal swellings of this fossa being especially apparent during active flexion. When the knee is extended, the fat body in the connective tissue space of the fossa causes the skin to bulge and, in so doing, sets off the marginal swellings formed by the ischiocrural muscles by longitudinal furrows.

The flexion creases in the popliteal fossa are not reliable indicators for the location of the articular cavity. The main bow-shaped crease, which is also recognizable in the extended knee, generally lies proximal to the joint cavity.

The patella, the infrapatellar fat body and the tendons of the quadriceps femoris, among others, can be recognized through the skin. In women, the contours are smoother owing to the more abundant fatty deposits in the subcutaneous tissue. With a well-developed bone structure and a weaker musculature, the normal knee joint appears relatively thick. With fatty thighs and legs, on the other hand, it appears thin since not very much fat is deposited between the skin and joint capsule. In the leg, the medial surface of the tibia lies directly beneath the skin. The shape of the calf is determined by the muscle bellies of the triceps surae. If the muscle tissue of the gastrocnemius reaches far distally or is layered on both sides of the tendo calcaneus with abundant, subcutaneous fat, the calf appears ungainly.

When the skin in front of and behind both malleoli is depressed, the Achilles' tendon projects distinctly. The external form of the foot is determined essentially by the skeleton of the foot. The dorsum of the foot is curved in a transverse and longitudinal direction. The height of the instep is determined by the tibial main strut. The dorsum of the foot is broader toward the toes. At the sole of the foot, the heel prominence, lateral margin of the foot, ball of the big toe and the common ball of the toes form the supporting surfaces. The medial margin of the foot is highly arched to form the recess of the sole. A transverse groove (Fig. **157 a**) separates the two toe balls from the bulgings of the toes, the toe pads.

In a standing position with the feet close together, the malleoli, calves and knee touch if the legs are "straight" (the bearing line courses through the middle of the knee joint on each side). Diamond-shaped intervals exist proximal to the malleolar region and distal to the knee; in males, there is another midway up the thigh, whereas in females the thighs lie close together.

The skin of the lower limb is firm at the dorsolateral side of the thigh and in the region of the knee joint. It is thick and heavily cornified at the heel, at the lateral margin of the foot, at the common ball of the toes and at the ball of the big toe. The skin is strikingly thin at both malleoli. Hairs and sebaceous glands are absent in the plantar region. In the adult male, the thighs (anteriorly, posteriorly and at the sides) and the legs (especially anteriorly) can be heavily covered with hair. Adult hairiness is also often pronounced on the legs of women.

The ridged skin of the sole of the foot and the pads of the toes shows – as in the palm of the hand and the finger pads – an individualistic dermal ridge system. In the gluteal region and at the supporting surfaces of the sole of the foot, the subcutaneous fat tissue is compartmentalized. Here, the skin cannot be lifted off into folds. At the thigh and leg, the skin is easily moved. The looser texture of the subcutaneous tissue permits extensive fluid accumulations in the malleolar region and on the dorsum of the foot.

With circulatory disturbances, edemas occur particularly in the malleolar region and at the dorsum of the foot. In standing for a long period, the "feet" swell.

The *cleavage lines* of the skin course longitudinally on the thigh and leg, transversely in the popliteal fossa (Fig. **71**).

Palpable bony points. Of all the skeletal elements of the lower limb, at least the bony prominences, marginal contours or partial surfaces can be palpated through the skin and through soft tissues that are only moderately thick. The dorsal and the dorsolateral walls of the pelvis can be felt from the rectum (also from the vagina in females). In contrast to these areas, the margins of the acetabulum of the hip joint and of the femoral neck and shaft, as well as the greater part of the fibular diaphysis are completely covered by muscles.

Structures lying close to the skin and therefore easy to palpate are the following (Fig. **165**):

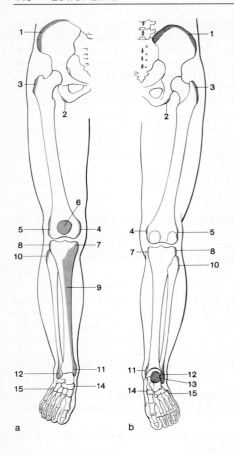

Fig. 165. **Palpable bony points on skeleton of lower extremity** (after *von Lanz-Wachsmuth*)
a View from in front
b View from behind

1 Iliac crest
2 Ischial tuberosity
3 Greater trochanter
4 Medial epicondyle of femur
5 Lateral epicondyle of femur
6 Patella
7 Side of medial condyle of tibia
8 Side of lateral condyle of tibia
9 Medial tibial fascia
10 Head of fibula
11 Medial malleolus
12 Lateral malleolus
13 Tuber calcanei
14 Tuberosity of navicular
15 Tuberosity of fifth metatarsal

– at the *hip bone*: iliac crest, anterior and posterior superior iliac spines, and the ischial tuberosity;
– at the *thigh*: greater trochanter, the two epicondyles of the femur, and the patella;
– at the *leg*: the sides of both tibial condyles, the head of the fibula, the tibial tuberosity, the medial surface of the tibia, and both malleoli; and
– at the *foot*: the tuber clacanei and the tuberosities of the navicular and 5th metatarsal.

The tarsal bones and the metatarsals at the dorsum of the foot, the heads of the metatarsals on the plantar side, and the dorsal surface and sides of the toes are also readily palpable.

For measuring the length of individual skeletal segments of the lower limb, the anterior superior iliac spine, the greater trochanter, the superior margin of the medial tibial condyle, and the medial malleolus are usually used as *measuring points*, which are relatively easy to determine.

2. Cutaneous Vessels and Nerves of the Lower Limb

a) Cutaneous Veins

The venous return of blood takes place in the leg via deep, subfascial veins which course with the arteries and (to a lesser extent) via superficial, epifascially-situated veins (Fig. **166**), which carry off the blood from the skin and subcutaneous tissue (as well as from the deep layers of the foot and the malleolar region).

The cutaneous veins, which possess a thicker vascular wall than deep veins of the same caliber, can be palpated through the skin and can also be visible.

The blood from the superficial venous networks is conveyed via the *great saphenous vein* into the femoral vein and via the *small saphenous vein* into the popliteal vein. Between these two cutaneous veins and the system of deep veins, there are numerous deep anastomoses (clinically called communicating or perforating veins), which pass through the fascia. Valves in the cutaneous veins and the deep anastomoses direct the blood stream into the deep veins at the leg and thigh.

At the foot and in the malleolar region, the preponderant part of the venous connections are free of valves. The valve-bearing anastomoses steer half of the bloodstream to the deep veins and half to the superficial veins.

The veins of the lower limb form a multireticulated, three-dimensional network by means of the numerous connections between superficial veins, between deep veins and between the two systems. Therefore, the ligation of individual veins, as a rule, does no harm. Ligation of the femoral vein, on the other hand, produces a high degree of venous congestion.

If the venous valves in the deep anastomoses are functionally inadequate, the return transport of the blood into the deep veins is necessarily influenced unfavorably. The action of the "muscle pump" is reduced or abolished because the blood now flows back from the subfascial veins into the epifascial veins, where it damms up. This leads to local nutritional disturbances resulting in edema and abscess formations (ulcerations). Varicose veins are particularly frequent in the region of the saphenous veins.

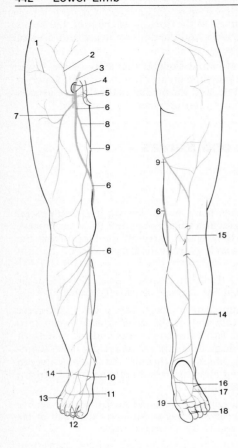

Fig. 166. **Cutaneous veins of lower limb**
a Ventral side
b Dorsal side
  1 Superficial circumflex iliac vein
  2 Superficial epigastric vein
  3 Femoral vein
  4 Saphenous opening bordered by falciform margin
  5 External pudendal veins
  6 Great saphenous vein
  7 Anterior femoral cutaneous vein
  8 Accessory saphenous vein
  9 Femoropopliteal vein
 10 Dorsal venous network of foot
 11 Dorsal venous arch of foot
 12 Dorsal digital veins of foot
 13 Dorsal subcutaneous metatarsal veins
 14 Small saphenous vein
 15 Popliteal vein
 16 Plantar venous network
 17 Plantar venous arch
 18 Plantar digital veins
 19 Plantar metatarsal veins

A closely-meshed venous network, the *venous network of the dorsum of the foot* (Fig. **166 a**), is formed on the surface of the fascia in this region and receives the blood from the deep veins of the dorsum and sole of the foot. In addition, it drains the subcutaneous venous network (absent in the palm of the hand) of the plantar area (Fig. **166 b**).

The longitudinal trunks of the venous network lie predominantly at the sides of the big and little toes, whereas the transverse connections are located especially in the distal region of the metatarsal bones and at the dorsal side of both ankle joints. The lumen of the epifascial vessels is usually wider than that of the deep veins. Direct unions to the superficial venous network of the sole of the foot exist at both margins of the foot and in the interdigital folds between the toes.

The **great saphenous vein** (Fig. **166**) arises from longitudinal veins at the medial side of the dorsum of the foot and receives blood from the venous network of the medial malleolus, *in front of* which it courses to the medial side of the leg. It passes behind the medial condyle of the femur with the saphenous nerve and travels along the anterior surface of the thigh until it reaches the saphenous hiatus, where it ends in the femoral vein (Fig. **204**).

Numerous veins open into the great saphenous vein at the leg and thigh. An *accessory saphenous vein* can come from the medial surface of the thigh; a so-called *anterior femoral cutaneous vein* can carry off blood from the venous network of the lateral anterior surface (distal and middle third). The *superficial epigastric vein* (from the abdominal skin below the navel), the *superficial circumflex iliac vein* (from the skin of the inguinal region), and the *pudendal veins* (from the skin of the external genitalia) usually enter the great saphenous vein near the saphenous hiatus. Occasionally they empty into the femoral vein.

The **small saphenous vein** (Fig. **166b**) arises at the lateral margin of the foot from the dorsal venous network and obtains tributaries in the malleolar region. It courses *behind* the lateral malleolus to the calf, penetrates the fascia cruris, and empties into the popliteal vein between the two heads of the gastrocnemius.

Several transverse connections to the great saphenous vein are generally present in the leg. A superficial anastomosis around the inner side of the thigh (femoropopliteal vein) can unite the small saphenous vein with the great saphenous vein and conduct a more or less large part of the blood along this route to the femoral vein. Deep anastomoses can also exist to the perforating veins or the circumflex femoral vein.

b) Superficial Lymphatic Tracts

As in the arm, *epifascial* and *subfascial lymphatic pathways*, which communicate with each other at the feet, in the region of the popliteal fossa, and in the inguinal area via deep anastomoses, course with the superficial and the deep veins of the lower limb.

The superficial lymphatic vessels pass into the gluteal region and to the posterior side of the thigh after a short course through the fascia lata (Fig. **167 b**) and empty into the deep lymphatic vessels, superficial longitudinal vessels being absent.

The primary bundles of superficial lymphatic vessels of the leg course with both saphenous veins (Fig. **167**).

The superficial lymphatic networks at the dorsum and sole of the foot communicate with each other and with the deep lymphatic pathways.

The lymphatic vessels accompanying the great saphenous vein conduct lymph predominantly from the medial side of the foot, as well as from the skin (the greatest part) of the leg and thigh to the superficial inguinal lymph nodes. The lymph from the lateral side of the foot and from the lateral malleolar region is drained by lymphatic vessels, which course in the leg with the small saphenous vein and either empty into the *popliteal*

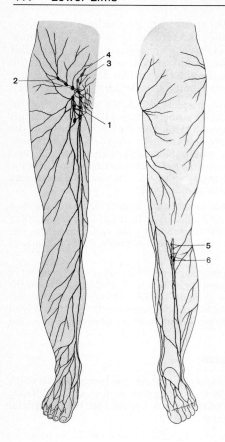

Fig. 167. **Superficial lymphatic tracts of leg and lymph nodes of groin**
Superficial lymphatic pathways and nodes ——
Deep lymphatic pathways and nodes ——
1 Superficial inguinal lymph nodes, longitudinal tract
2 Superficial inguinal lymph nodes, oblique tract
3 Deep inguinal lymph nodes
4 Deep lymphatic tracts to external iliac inguinal nodes
5 Popliteal lymph nodes
6 Superficial popliteal lymph nodes

lymph nodes through the fascia cruris or pass to the epifascial lymphatic pathways along the great saphenous vein. By far the greatest part of the lymph which flows off via the superficial lymphatic pathways is conducted, therefore, directly to the superficial inguinal lymph nodes.

The (7–15) **superficial inguinal lymph nodes** (Figs. **167 a, 204** and **210 a**) lie in the groin on the fascia lata. The group (longitudinal tract) on both sides of the segment near the opening of the great saphenous vein take up lymph from the skin and subcutaneous tissue of almost the entire lower limb, as well as the deep layers of the foot. Lymphatic vessels from the abdominal wall (below the navel), from the caudal segment of the back, from the buttocks, perineum and external genitalia, and in women also from the fundus of the uterus (along the round ligament of the uterus via the inguinal canal) pass to lymph nodes situated along the inguinal ligament (oblique tract).

The lymph nodes of both groups communicate with each other. The distribution of drainage areas for both groups of lymph nodes is variable. Lymph from the leg can also come into nodes of the oblique tract, lymph from the genital regions into medial nodes of the longitudinal tract (or to the superficial inguinal lymph nodes of the opposite side).

Enlarged lymph nodes (e.g. in inflammations in the groin region, tumor metastases) are palpable through the skin, occasionally also visible.

The efferent lymphatic vessels of the superficial inguinal lymph nodes pass through the fascia cribrosa to the deep inguinal lymph nodes.

c) Cutaneous Nerves

Areas of innervation. The regions of innervation of the cutaneous nerves of the lower limb – as in the arm – are irregularly formed. The distribution regions of individual nerves overlap, whereby the nerve fibers for the different sensory qualities, which come from one and the same nerves, behave differently and moreover possess certain individual differences.

The anatomical cutaneous fields, i.e. the technically-demonstrable areas of distribtuion of cutaneous nerves in the subcutaneous tissues, have been described in the section on the arm. Since many cutaneous areas are supplied by two (or more) nerves, the clinically-demonstrable autonomic region of the nerves (in the case of paralysis of the nerves in question) are usually essentially smaller or are completely absent, as in the case of the iliohypogastric and genitofemoral nerves.

The skin of the lower limb has a sensory nerve supply (Fig. **168**) at the **thigh** via the:

– *superior clunial nerves* (dorsal rami of lumbar nerves I–III) in the cranial gluteal region,
– *middle clunial nerves* (dorsal rami of sacral nerves I–III) in the mediocranial segment of the gluteal region,
– *inferior clunial nerves* (from the posterior femoral cutaneous nerve) in the caudal region of the buttocks,
– *lateral cutaneous branch* of the *iliohypogastric nerve* distal to the iliac crest,
– *femoral* (ventral) and *genital* (ventromedial) *rami* of the *genitofemoral nerve* below the inguinal ligament,
– *anterior scrotal (labial) nerves* of the *ilioinguinal nerve* in a field adjacent to the scrotum (the labium majus),
– *posterior femoral cutaneous nerve* at the dorsal side,
– *lateral femoral cutaneous nerve* at the lateral side,

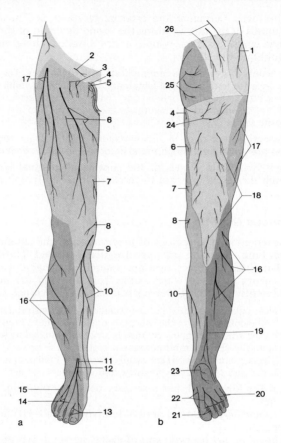

Fig. 168. Cutaneous nerves and anatomical cutaneous fields of lower limb
a Ventral side of leg
b Dorsal side of leg

Regions of innervation
☐ Branches of dorsal rami of lumbar nerves
☐ Branches of dorsal rami of sacral nerves
☐ Branch of lumbar plexus with fibers from anterior ramus of thoracic nerves
☐ Branches of lumbar plexus
☐ Branches of sacral plexus with fibers from lumbar plexus (over lumbosacral trunk)
☐ Branches of sacral plexus

– *anterior cutaneous branches* of the *femoral nerve* at the ventral and ventromedial sides,

– *cutaneous branch* of the *obturator nerve* at the medial side above the knee joint, and

– the *infrapatellar branch* of the *saphenous nerve* (from the femoral nerve) at the medial side below the patella;

at the **leg** via the:

– *lateral sural cutaneous nerve* on the lateral side,

– *medial crural cutaneous rami* of the *saphenous nerve* (from the femoral) on the medial side, and

– *sural nerve* (union of medial sural cutaneous nerve from the tibial nerve with the peroneal communicating ramus from the lateral sural cutaneous nerve) over the Achilles' tendon and at the lateral malleolus;

at the **dorsum of the foot** via the:

– *saphenous nerve* at the medial margin of the foot,

– *medial dorsal cutaneous nerve* (from the superficial peroneal nerve) at the medial side, at the medial margin of the big toe and the facing margins of the 2nd and 3rd toes,

– *intermediate dorsal cutaneous nerve* (from the superficial peroneal nerve) at the lateral side and the facing margins of the 3rd and 4th, as well as the 4th and 5th toes,

– *deep peroneal nerve* at the sides of the 1st and 2nd toes facing each other, and

– *lateral dorsal cutaneous nerve* (from the sural nerve) at the lateral margin of the foot and at the lateral margin of the 5th toe;

at the **sole of the foot** via the

– *medial calcanean branches* (from the tibial nerve) in the heel region,

---

1 Lateral cutaneous ramus ⎱ of iliohypogastric nerve
2 Anterior cutaneous ramus ⎰
3 Branches of femoral ramus ⎱ of genitofemoral nerve
4 Genital ramus ⎰
5 Anterior scrotal nerves of ilio-inguinal nerve
6 Anterior cutaneous rami of femoral nerve
7 Cutaneous ramus of obturator nerve
8 Infrapatellar ramus of saphenous nerve
9 Saphenous nerve
10 Medial crural cutaneous rami of saphenous nerve
11 Dorsal medial cutaneous nerve
12 Dorsal intermediate cutaneous nerve
13 Dorsal lateral digital nerve of the big toe and dorsal medial digital nerve of the 2nd toe

14 Dorsal digital nerves of foot
15 Dorsal lateral cutaneous nerve
16 Branches of lateral sural cutaneous nerve
17 Branches of lateral femoral cutaneous nerve
18 Branches of posterior femoral cutaneous nerve
19 Sural nerve
20 Common plantar digital nerves from lateral plantar nerve
21 Proper plantar digital nerves
22 Common plantar digital nerves from medial plantar nerve
23 Medial calcanean rami from tibial nerve
24 Inferior cluneal nerves
25 Middle cluneal nerves
26 Superior cluneal nerves

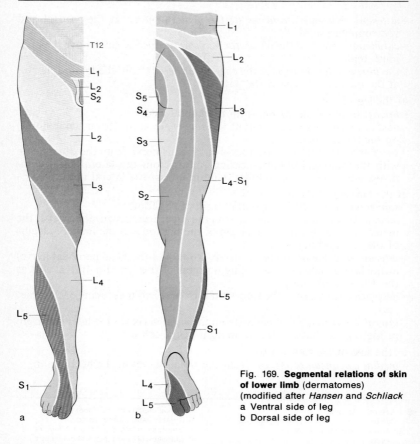

Fig. 169. **Segmental relations of skin of lower limb** (dermatomes) (modified after *Hansen* and *Schliack*
a Ventral side of leg
b Dorsal side of leg

– *medial plantar nerve* (from the tibial nerve) in the medial part and at the $3\frac{1}{2}$ medial toes, and
– *lateral plantar nerve* (from the tibial nerve) in the lateral part and at the $1\frac{1}{2}$ lateral toes.

Segmental relations of the skin of the lower limb (Fig. **169**). The dermatomes of the lower limb arise from somites L2–5 and S1–5. As in the arm, the cutaneous segments are stretched into broad bands of varying width. Dermatomes L5 and S1 reach farthest distally and, like L4, no longer communicate with the corresponding trunk segments. The boundary between lumbar and sacral segments lies at the thigh in an approximately frontal plane, at the leg in a more sagittal plane.

The dermatome schemes of the lower limb completed on the basis of clinical observations and anatomical studies differ considerably in many details. It is undisputed that dermatome L2 is most nearly belt-shaped and is joined distal to L1 (inguinal region). Segment L3 extends particularly on the distal anterior surface of the thigh. A V-shaped cutaneous segment, whose angular summit lies in the skin over the anococcygeal ligament, is assigned to S5 and is surrounded by dermatome S4. Segment S3 lies at the medial side of the proximal thigh and reaches into the gluteal region, whereas the band-shaped area of S2 extends at the dorsal side of the thigh and at the dorsomedial side of the leg. The cutaneous segment L4, which follows L3 distally, passes obliquely from proximolateral to distomedial across the anterior surface of the leg and reaches up to the medial margin of the foot. The skin at the medial part of the dorsum and sole of the foot and the two medial toes belong to segment L5, which also continues forward to the ventrolateral side of the leg. Bands at the dorsal side of the leg and the skin at the heel, at the lateral side of the dorsum and sole of the foot, and at toes III–V belong to the S1 cutaneous segment.

10. Trunk Wall

The **trunk wall** encloses the thoracic and abdominal cavities and is organized segmentally (→ metamerism of body wall, p. 12). The skeleton is formed by the thoracic and lumbar vertebrae, ribs and the sternum. Cranially, the trunk wall ends at the superior thoracic aperture (Fig. **193**); caudally, it is bordered on both sides by the iliac crest and inguinal ligament, ventromedially by the pubic symphysis.

The trunk wall can be divided into the cranial *thoracic wall* and the caudal *abdominal wall*, with the inferior thoracic aperture regarded as the boundary line. Its skeletal border inclines on both sides of the xiphoid process of the sternum across the arches of the ribs and the free ends of the 11th and 12th ribs to the 12th thoracic vertebra.

A subdivision of the trunk wall into anterior, lateral and posterior thoracic and abdominal walls facilitates the topography of the muscles, vessels or nerves in this region. Such a classification, however, remains arbitrary since there are no sharp boundaries at the trunk wall.

A demarcation of the middle region of the dorsal body wall as the *dorsal trunk wall* can be established genetically. Here, on both sides of the median line, the local dorsal muscle anlage, the epimere, develops into the autochthonous musculature of the back. The vertebral column is its supporting structure. All segmental vessels and nerves dispatch a dorsal ramus to the autochthonous back musculature and to the skin covering it, whereas a ventral ramus supplies the ventral (and ventrolateral) trunk wall.

The dorsal side of the trunk is designated in topographical anatomy as the *back*, or *dorsum*. This region of the body thus includes the dorsal body wall and extends from the occiput (superior nuchal line) to the tip of the coccyx. The lateral boundary is not exactly defined.

In the following presentation, the dorsal body wall is treated in its own section (A.). Beyond the true trunk wall, it also includes cranially the adjacent nuchal region (*posterior cervical region*) in the area of the neck and caudally the sacrococcygeal region (*sacral region*). Laterally, the dorsal body wall is bordered on both sides by a perpendicular line at the lateral margin of the autochthonous back musculature (→ erector spinae p. 481).

The term "dorsal body wall" is used here as a genetic (and not as a topographical) concept. In the description of the surface anatomy (B.), the surface topography of the back (and not only the dorsal body wall) is presented so that the muscles which have migrated into the region of the dorsal body wall from the pharyngeal arches and limb muscle anlage can also be discussed.

Correspondingly, in section "C. Ventral Trunk Wall", the true thoracic and abdominal walls are taken into consideration (without including the structures of the dorsal body wall). In this section the ventral body wall – according to its genetic segmentation – and the diaphragm – separating the thoracic and abdominal cavities are described. In section "D. Surface Anatomy of the Anterior Trunk Wall", the topography of surface layer of the thoracic and abdominal walls is discussed.

A. Dorsal Body Wall

1. Vertebral Column

The **vertebral column** forms the *axial skeleton* of the human body. It is a characteristic structural feature of all *vertebrates* and replaces the *notochord* (*chorda dorsalis*), which is formed as an axial organ in early embryonic development. (The vertebrates are a subphylum of the chordates.) In the vertebrate structural plan, the vertebral column lies dorsal to the aorta and – with its principal mass – ventral to the spinal cord, which is enclosed in the vertebral canal.

The vertebral column is an elastic, double S-shaped rod which bears the mass of the body (head, neck, trunk) and the upper limb. It allows extensive movements of the trunk in all planes and thus serves both statics and dynamics. The construction of the vertebral column from numerous individual elements of bone and connective tissue, each of which renders only a small contribution to its mobility, forms the morphological foundation of these two apparently opposite functions.

a) Skeletal Elements of the Vertebral Column

The **vertebrae** are the structural elements of the bony vertebral column. They possess a single basic structure which is adapted in the individual segments of the column to the different static and dynamic requirements.

The organization of the vertebral column is traced back to the segmentation of the somites. During ontogenesis, the vertebral blastema is shifted cranially against the myotomes by half a segment.

Basic Form of a Vertebra

Each vertebra (Figs. **170–174**) consists of two chief parts:
– the short, cylindrical *vertebral body* and
– the thin, bow-like *vertebral arch.*

The vertebral bodies communicate with each other by fibrocartilaginous intervertebral discs, whereas the vertebral arches are connected by articular processes and by ligamentous tracts.

Vertebral bodies. The anterior and lateral margins of both upper and lower surfaces have a pronounced convex curvature, and the posterior margin is slightly retracted. Since the marginal borders form a projecting

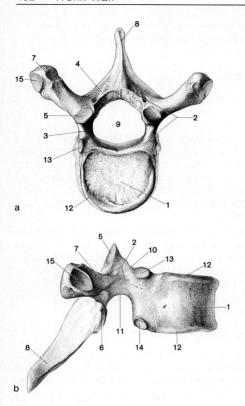

Fig. 170. **Basic structure of vertebra, illustrated by 6th thoracic vertebra**
a Cranial view
b View from right side
 1 Vertebral body
 2 Vertebral arch
 3 Pedicle of vertebral arch
 4 Lamina of vertebral arch
 5 Superior articular process
 6 Inferior articular process
 7 Transverse process
 8 Spinous process
 9 Vertebral foramen
10 Superior vertebral notch
11 Inferior vertebral notch
12 Marginal ridge
3–15 *Typical structural characteristics of thoracic vertebrae*
13 Superior costal fovea
14 Inferior costal fovea
15 Costal fovea of transverse process

ridge at the upper and lower surfaces, the anterior and lateral surfaces of the vertebral bodies are somewhat grooved, and their posterior surface is almost flat.

At the vertical surfaces of the vertebral bodies, a series of foramina is recognizable, through which vascular branches pass. With the exception of the marginal ridges (epiphyses of the vertebral body), the cortex is extraordinarily thin at the upper and lower surfaces and perforated like a sieve. The innumerable fine openings of the spaces of the spongiosa (red bone marrow) are covered on both upper and lower surfaces by a hyaline cartilage closing plate, which unites the osseous vertebral body with the intervertebral disc attaching cranially or caudally.

The spongy trabeculae of the vertebral body are arranged primarily in a vertical and horizontal direction. The organization and thickness corre-

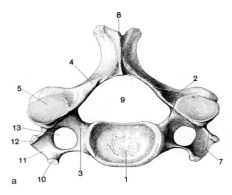

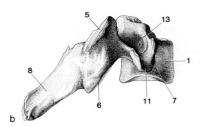

Fig. 171. **Fourth cervical
vertebra**
a Cranial view
b View from right side
1–9 Explanation → Fig. 170
10 Anterior tubercle
11 Sulcus for spinal nerve
12 Posterior tubercle
13 Foramen transversarium

spond to the chief directions and distribution of stress as demonstrated in experimental models. The bodies of presacral vertebrae are adjusted functionally to the axial pressure they are subjected to. They increase in height and surface area from cranial to caudal.

The relative transverse diameter of all vertebral bodies (as compared with the total height of all vertebral bodies) is greater in males than in females.

Two or more vertebral bodies can be fused (synostosed) symmetrically or asymmetrically: fused vertebrae. In the formation of block vertebrae, the vertebral arches are also frequently involved.

Vertebral arches. A root piece, the *pedicle*, and – connected dorsally – a lateral piece form the paired constituents of the vertebral arch, which are joined by the unpaired closing piece, the *lamina*.

The pedicle, which is attached only at the superior half (the dorsolateral corner) of the vertebral body, is thinner and lower than the rest of the arch so that a *superior* and an *inferior vertebral notch* arises at the cranial and caudal margins. The recesses of two adjacent vertebral arches facing

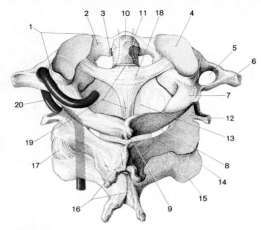

Fig. 172. **Atlas and axis**, dorsocranial view
(Cruciform ligament of atlas preserved, but superior longitudinal band severed)

1 Lateral mass
2 Anterior arch of atlas
3 Fovea dentis
4 Superior articular facet
5 Foramen transversarium
6 Transverse process of atlas
7 Groove for vertebral artery
8 Posterior arch of atlas
9 Posterior tubercle
10 Dens of axis
11 Posterior articular surface of dens

12 Transverse process of axis
13 Body of axis
14 Superior articular process
15 Inferior articular process
16 Spinous process of second and third
   cervical vertebrae
17 Articular capsule
18, 19 *Cruciform ligament of atlas*
18 Transverse ligament of atlas
19 Longitudinal band of cruciform
   ligament
20 Vertebral artery

each other border the *intervertebral foramen* (together with the free surfaces of the vertebral bodies above and below the vertebral arch, the dorsolateral surfaces of the intervertebral disc, and the articular processes articulating with one another). The *intervertebral foramen* (Fig. **182**) is a short canal, the passageway for a spinal nerve leaving the vertebral canal.

The intervertebral foramina are narrow in the region of the cervical vertebrae and relatively wide in the thoracic and lumbar segments. In the lumbar region the intervertebral discs form a greater portion of the boundary than in the cranial segments of the vertebral column. Therefore, prolapse of the disc is found in over 90% of the cases in the lumbar region of the vertebral column [sciatic pain], whereas constriction of the intervertebral foramina owing to exostoses is found predominantly in the cervical region. The spinal nerve passing through the intervertebral foramen is embedded in fat and is accompanied by blood vessels (especially a plexus of veins).

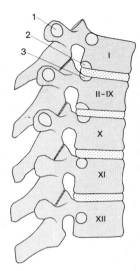

Fig. 173. **Arrangement of articular surfaces on thoracic vertebrae for costovertebral connections**
Scheme
1 Costal facet on transverse process
2 Inferior costal facet
3 Superior costal facet

The lateral piece of the vertebral arch carries two *articular processes*, one directed cranially (*superior articular process*), and the other caudally (*inferior articular process*). The cartilage-covered joint surfaces of these processes (superior and inferior articular facets) articulate with the articular surfaces of the corresponding processes of the preceding or following vertebral arch. From each arch, a strong lateral process projects laterally which is referred to in the cervical and thoracic vertebrae as the *transverse process*. The unpaired end piece of the arch sends out dorsally a median-situated spinous process, which covers the dorsal aspect of the vertebral canal.

If the two halves of the vertebral arch are not fused with one another dorsally, the end piece of the arch is absent (most frequently in the lumbosacral region), and a *spina bifida* exists.

Vertebral canal. Together with the posterior surface of the vertebral body, the vertebral arch borders the *vertebral foramen*. All the vertebral foramina together form the *vertebral canal* which houses the spinal cord. Its wall is completed in the intervertebral regions by intervertebral discs and by ligamentous tracts. The canal is unequally wide in the different regions of the vertebral column; its diameters – corresponding to the position of the thickening of the spinal cord – are greatest in the lower cervical and upper lumbar regions. The curvatures of the vertebral canal correspond to the curvatures of the vertebral column.

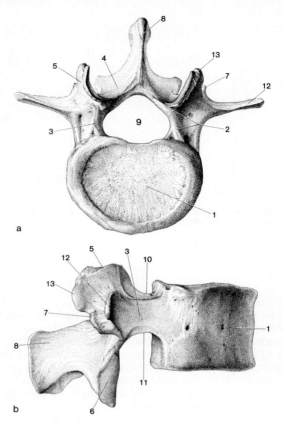

Fig. 174. **Third lumbar vertebra**
a Cranial view
b View from right side

1 Vertebral body
2 Vertebral arch
3 Pedicle of vertebral arch
4 Lamina of vertebral arch
5 Superior articular process
6 Inferior articular process
7 Accessory process

8 Spinous process
9 Vertebral foramen
10 Superior vertebral notch
11 Inferior vertebral notch
12 Costal process
13 Mamillary process

Regional Organization of the Vertebral Column

On the basis of typical variations in the general structure of vertebrae
described above, the following regions of the vertebral column can be

distinguished (Fig. **183 a**):

7 *cervical* vertebrae ⎫
12 *thoracic* vertebrae ⎬ = 24 presacral
5 *lumbar* vertebrae ⎭   vertebrae
5 *sacral* vertebrae   = *sacrum*
4 (3–6) *coccygeal* vertebrae = *coccyx*

The sacral vertebrae are united into a uniform bone, the *sacrum*; the coccygeal vertebrae are fused to form the *coccyx*.

The typical vertebral form is expressed most distinctly in a vertebra located in the middle of its respective region. The *total number of vertebrae* and the boundaries of the individual segments of the vertebral column are not rigidly fixed. The numerical organization of the vertebral column given above with the 33 vertebrae is found, for example, only in about 40% of all individuals. The normal number of 33 vertebrae can be greater or less (inclusion = assimilation of 1st cervical vertebra in the skull, development of up to 6 coccygeal vertebrae or reduction of the coccygeal end of the the vertebral column, etc.). The typical number of 24 presacral vertebra is developed only in about 92% of the cases.

With an increase or decrease in the number of ribs, there is a shifting in the cervicothoracic or thoracolumbar regions; with the fusion of 4 or 6 vertebrae at the sacrum, there are changes in the lumbosacral region. Occasionally, at the border of regions, so-called *transitional vertebrae* appear in which the change of vertebral type has taken place only on one side.

As a relatively frequent variation, the 7th cervical vertebra (more rarely also the 6th) carries a cervical rib unilaterally or bilaterally which can be rudimentary or completely developed and which can articulate with the vertebra or grow together firmly with it. The free ribs – which typically characterize the thoracic vertebrae – can (rarely) be involuted at the true 1st thoractic vertebra. At the vertebra(e) following the typical 12th thoracic vertebra, *lumbar ribs* occasionally appear. Conversely, the 12th thoracic vertabra may not carry a rib and thus belongs to the lumbar vertebral column. Corresponding variations are found (often half-sided) in the lumbosacral and in the sacrococcygeal border regions (e.g., sacralization of a lumbar vertebra, lumbarization of a sacral vertebra).

Forms of Vertebrae in the Different Regions of the Vertebral Column

Cervical vertebrae. In *typical cervical vertebrae III–VII* (Fig. **171**), the vertebral body is proportionately small and approximately rectangular when viewed from above; the vertebral foramen is large and triangular.

The *transverse process* surrounds the *foramen transversarium* since a cervical rib rudiment is fused with it and with the lateral surface of the body as a ventral bar (costal process). The vertebral artery courses craniad in the foramen transversarium of the upper six cervical vertebrae (Figs. **172** and **184**), the vertebral vein often coursing caudad up to the 7th cervical vertebra. The *spinous processes* – inclined slightly caudad and bifid except in the 7th cervical vertebra – increase in length from cranial to caudal. The spinous process of the 7th cervical vertebra is the first of these processes that can be easily palpated through the skin, hence the name *vertebra prominens* (Fig. **188**). (Frequently, however, the spinous process of the 1st thoracic vertebra projects further dorsally.)

The cranial surface of the vertebral body is formed slightly convex in the frontal direction, whereas the caudal surface is slightly concave in the sagittal direction (although it, too, is slightly convex in the frontal direction). In radiograms each side of the superior lateral margin appears as a ridge-like elevation, the *uncus of the vertebral body*. The broad, flat, low articular processes are inclined only a little, the cranial pair facing cranially, dorsally and laterally, and the caudal pair correspondingly facing caudally, ventrally and medially.

The transverse process ends laterally in two small prominences, a ventral and somewhat more medially located *anterior tubercle* and a dorsolateral *posterior tubercle*. Between both tubercles is the groove (*sulcus*) for the *spinal nerve*. The ventral bar of the transverse process is formed exclusively, the dorsal bar predominantly, from the cervical rib rudiment (costal element). The especially well-developed anterior tubercle of the transverse process of the 6th cervical vertebra projects prominently (the anterior tubercle of the 7th cervical vertebra, on the other hand, is reduced or absent) and can be palpated through the skin at the level of the lower margin of the thyroid cartilage. Since the common carotid artery coursing lateral to this tubercle can be pressed against it in an emergency and compressed, the anterior tubercle is referred to as the *carotid tubercle*.

Atlas and *axis*, the first two cervical vertebrae, possess – in connection with the formation of the atlanto-occipital joints – a shape deviating somewhat from the general vertebral structural plan. The atlas, which carries the head, lacks a vertebral body; its structural material has been united with the body of the 2nd cervical vertebra and forms the *dens of the axis* (odontoid process), which projects cranially. Atlas + head rotate around the dens. The atlas and axis, therefore, are rotation vertebrae, in contrast to the remaining vertebrae (flexion vertebrae).

The *atlas* (Fig. **172**) consists of a small *anterior arch* (formed from structural material which, in the other vertebrae, is incorporated into the intervertebral discs) and a more extensive *posterior arch*, which projects dorsally into a small *posterior tubercle*, a rudiment of the spinous process. At the anterior arch, a small *anterior tubercle* projects insignificantly at the ventral surface, and the cartilage-covered *fovea dentis*, a facet for the articulation with the dens, lies on the dorsal surface (Fig. **182**). Anterior and posterior arches are connected with one another by the strong *lateral masses* which project medially. They take up the weight of the head and, on their cranial surface, carry the oval to kidney-shaped articular sockets (*superior articular facets*) for the occipital condyles. Their longitudinal axes converge ventrally.

The round *inferior articular facet* on the lower surface of each lateral mass is flat or slightly concave in the macerated vertebra. They face caudally, medially and somewhat dorsally. The cartilage covering of the joint surface generally forms a low, transversely-placed ridge so that the articulating surface appears moderately convex.

Laterally, the lateral mass continues into the *transverse process*, which is penetrated by the *foramen transversarium*. It projects laterally, can be palpated through the skin behind the angle of the jaw, and is inclined caudally, Directly behind the lateral mass, a transverse groove (*sulcus for the vertebral artery*) cuts into the cranial margin of the dorsal arch. In many cases, it is closed into a foramen. The vertebral artery (Fig. **187**), which comes from the foramen transversarium of the atlas and passes to the foramen magnum, courses in this groove.

The *axis* (Fig. **172**) possesses a vertebral body, vertebral arches and a *dens*, which sits on the vertebral body and ends in a truncated *apex*. The dens possesses oval *anterior* and *posterior articular facets* for articulation ventrally with the fovea dentis of the anterior arch of the atlas and dorsally with the transverse ligament of the atlas (Fig. **182**).

The *superior articular surface* of the atlas, situated lateral to the base of the dens, slopes somewhat laterally and forms a cylindrical indentation of the surface lying transversely. During a rotary movement at the atlanto-axial joint, its convex curvature, which is directed ventrodorsally, causes the inferior articular surface of the atlas to drop minimally (about 2 mm) on the one side anteriorly and on the other side posteriorly. The inferior articular surface of the axis resembles the corresponding surface of the cervical vertebra which follows it. The spinous process is short and bifid.

The **thoracic vertebrae** (Fig. **170**) correspond largely to the illustration on p. 452. Seen from above, the vertebral body is heart-shaped or triangular in appearance and the vertebral foramen round. Characteristic is the formation of the cartilage-covered articular surfaces on the vertebral body and transverse processes for articulation with the free ribs.

Ribs 2–10 are each situated with their rib heads between two vertebrae so that thoracic vetebrae 2–9 carry *superior* and *inferior costal facets* at their superior and inferior margins, each representing half a joint socket (Fig. **173**). The first thoracic vertebra articulates with $1\frac{1}{2}$ ribs and possesses a complete (superior) and a half (inferior) joint socket. The 10th vertebra has only a half socket for the inferior articular facet of the head of the 10th rib. The 11th and 12th thoracic vertebrae each carry a complete articular socket for the corresponding ribs.

The transverse process of the thoracic vertebrae displays a *costal facet* for articulation with the tubercle of the rib. It can be absent on the 11th and 12th vertebrae. The flat joint surfaces of the articular processes face almost frontally, the superior dorsally, the inferior ventrally. The spinous processes are long, the first 10 angled strongly caudad so that they overlap imbricately.

The **lumbar vertebrae** (Fig. **174**) possess well-developed bodies, kidney-shaped in appearance, and triangular vertebral foramina.

In the 5th lumbar vertebra – and also in the 1st sacral vertebra – the anterior surface of the body is higher than the posterior surface. Both vertebral bodies and the intervertebral discs connecting them are wedge-shaped. Thus, for the 5th lumbar vertebra at the relatively movable lumbosacral union, there is the danger that it will slide forward off the cranial surface of the 1st sacral vertebra (spondylolisthesis), which is inclined ventrally about 35° from the horizontal plane.

The lateral process of a lumbar vertebra (*costal process*) is not homologous with the transverse process, but represents a well-developed rib rudiment which is fused with the structural material of the transverse process. As the externally visible remains of the true transverse process, an *accessory process* projects behind the base of the costal process as a small, often indistinct bony tip on the caudal lumbar vertebrae.

The strong spinous processes, flattened on both sides, are directed dorsally. The distance between two spinous processes is relatively large, so that a puncture needle – with the trunk flexed anteriorly – can be easily introduced into the vertebral canal in the lumbar region (→ lumbar puncture, p. 480).

The articular surfaces of the articular processes form sections of a cylindrical surface and stand perpendicular, almost in the sagittal plane. The surface of the caudal articular processes faces externally and is embraced by the concave surface of the cranial process of the next vertebra.

The medial lumbar intertransverse muscles and the long rotatores muscles are attached at the *mamillary process*, a muscular process at the external surface of the superior articular process which is especially developed at the cranial lumbar vertebrae-occasionally also at thoracic vertebrae 10–12.

In the **sacrum** (Fig. **175**), 5 sacral vertebrae, as a rule, are united into an undivided, dorsoventrally-flattened, spade-shaped bone, which is triangular in anterior view. The cranial surface of its broad *base* communicates with the body of the 5th lumbar vertebrae via a wedge-shaped intervertebral disc, whereas caudally its narrow, truncated apex (united synostotically in the elderly) is adjoined to the coccyx. The boundaries of the individual vertebrae are marked on the concave ventral surface (*pelvic surface*) by transverse ridges (*transverse lines*). Transverse processes, rib rudiments and ossified ligamentous tracts, which correspond to the intertransverse and costotransverse ligaments of the thoracic region, are likewise fused and form the *lateral parts* on each side of the sacral body. They carry, at the level of the two and a half upper sacral vertebrae, the *auricular surface*, which forms an amphiarthrosis with the articular surface of the ilium of the same name. The rough, bosselated bony surface of the adjacent, dorsally-situated *sacral tuberosity* serves for the insertion of the interosseous sacro-iliac ligaments.

Owing to the fusion of the vertebrae, rib rudiments and ossified ligaments, 4 T-shaped osseous canals arise on each side at the site of the intervertebral foramina in the region of the upper 4 sacral vertebrae. Sacral nerves I–IV pass through these canals; their ventral and dorsal rami leave the canals via the *anterior* and *posterior sacral foramina*, which lie at both ends of the transverse part of the T and define the lateral border of the united vertebral body. The fused vertebral arches border the caudal continuation of the vertebral canal (*sacral canal*), which is triangular in cross section. Since the arch of the 5th sacral vertebra is largely incomplete and the arch of the 4th sacral vertebra is usually not completely closed, a space arises in the bony posterior wall of the canal, the *sacral hiatus*, which is then practically closed by ligamentous bands, the *superficial posterior sacrococcygeal ligament* (Fig. **181**).

The united spinous processes form a serrated, bony ridge, the *median sacral crest*, on the convex *dorsal surface* of the sacrum. Lateral to it, but still medial to the posterior sacral foramina, there are the paired *intermediate sacral crests* that arise by the fusion of the articular processes. They continue toward the apex into the *sacral cornua* (horns). On each side at the base of the sacrum, an almost frontally-placed cranial articular process, the *superior articular process*, articulates with the inferior articular process of the last lumbar vertebra. The *lateral sacral crest*, which is usually more distinct in the cranial segment, courses lateral to the dorsal sacral foramina. It has arisen from the fusion of the transverse processes, and its small elevations correspond to the accessory processes of the lumbar vertebrae.

The sacrum of the adult generally exhibits distinct *sexual differences* (Fig. **176**). It is longer, narrower and more strongly curved in males than in females.

Coccyx (Fig. **177**). While the first coccygeal vertebra still has vestiges of a vertebral arch, the remaining vertebrae consist only of vertebral body material and become increasing smaller caudally. Dorsally, the cranial surface of the coccyx, which is connected – at least in young people – with the apex of the sacrum by an interarticular disc, stretches towards the sacral cornua in the form of two *coccygeal cornua*, remnants of the cranial articular processes.

The considerable interval on each side between the two processes is bridged over by a *sacrococcygeal articular ligament* (Fig. **181**).

By the 30th year of life, usually the last three, later all, coccygeal vertebrae are synostosed to form the coccyx. However, an articular connection can be found between the 1st and 2nd coccygeal vertebrae which makes a certain mobility of the coccyx possible even beyond 30 when the 1st coccygeal vertebra is united with the sacrum. During birth, the coccyx is withdrawn backward.

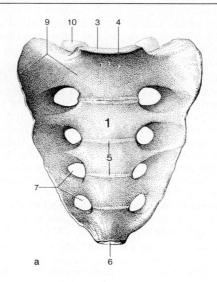

a

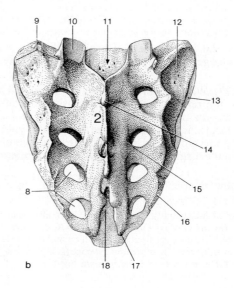

b

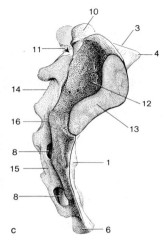

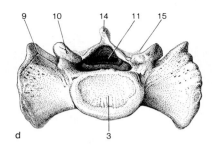

Fig. 175 a–d. **Sacrum**
a Sacrum, ventral view
b Sacrum, dorsal view
c Sacrum, view from right side
d Sacrum, cranial view

1 Pelvic surface
2 Dorsal surface
3 Base of sacrum
4 Promontory
5 Transverse line
6 Apex of sacrum
7 Anterior sacral foramina
8 Posterior sacral foramina
9 Lateral part

10 Superior articular process
11 Sacral canal
12 Sacral tuberosity
13 Auricular surface
14 Median sacral crest
15 Intermediate sacral crest
16 Lateral sacral crest
17 Sacral cornu
18 Sacral hiatus

The **ossification** of the *vertebrae* (Fig. **178**) begins in the 3rd embryonic month (an ossific center in the vertebral body, a perichondral bony center at the base of each vertebral arch), whereby at the cervical and lower lumbar vertebrae the perichondral ossification of the arches appears before the centers in the bodies and not vice versa, as is usual at the other vertebrae. The center of ossification at the base of each arch unites with the ossific center in the vertebral body in the 3rd–5th postnatal year, whereas the ossification zones of the paired arch segments fuse with one another in the 1st–3rd year. The ossification of the cartilaginous marginal ridges takes place from the 12th year onwards. Ossific centers for the apophyses in the processes of the vertebral arches appear around the 12th year. Since they fuse with the vertebrae relatively late (16th–25th year), they can lead to erroneous interpretations of radiograms.

b) Connections of Vertebral Bodies and Arches

The vertebral bodies communicate with each other via *intervertebral discs*, the arches via their own *joints*. Moreover, short and long *tendinous*

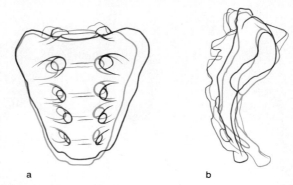

Fig. 176. **Sexual differences of sacrum**
a Ventral veiw
b Lateral view
(contours of male [——] and female [——] sacrum projected over one another)

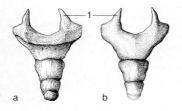

Fig. 177. **Coccyx**
a Ventral view
b Dorsal view
1 Coccygeal cornu

tracts are formed between the vertebral bodies and between the vertebral arches.

The intervertebral discs influence the range of movement of the vertebral column; the joints of the vertebral arches determine especially the direction of movement.

The area responsible for motion between two vertebrae is frequently also designated as a *movement segment*. This includes: the intervertebral discs and their hyaline cartilage attachments, the paired vertebral joints, the paired intervertebral foramina, the corresponding segment of the vertebral canal together with contents, as well as muscles, ligaments, nerves and vessels in the intervertebral region. Especially close topographical and functional relationships exist between the parts of a movement segment so that damage to one part also always affects other parts of a movement segment.

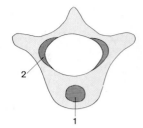

Fig. 178. Vertebral Ossification
1 Central ossific nucleus in vertebral body
2 Perichondral bone at base of vertebral arch

Connections between the Vertebral Bodies

Intervertebral discs (Fig. **180**) unite the bodies of adjacent vertebrae from the 2nd cervical to the sacrum. The height of the avascular and practically aneural discs in the adult amounts altogether to about one-fourth of the presacral vertebral column. Corresponding to the typical curvature of the column, the intervertebral discs are higher anteriorly in the cervical and lumbar segments, but posteriorly in the thoracic region. They increase in their average height and surface area from cranial to caudal.

In the sacrum, the ossification of the discs begins in the 15th year of life and is concluded in the 4th decade. Modified intervertebral discs (without a nucleus pulposus) are present between the sacrum and coccyx and between the coccygeal vertebrae which have not as yet undergone osseous fusion.

The *intervertebral discs* (Figs. **179** and **182**) consist of:
– the *anulus fibrosus*, a fibrous ring (concentrically layered connective tissue lamellae and fibrocartilage) and
– the *nucleus pulposus*, a centrally-located gelatinous nucleus (chondromucoid-gel).

Anulus fibrosus. The outer zone contains firbroblasts (connective tissue cells) lodged between bundles of collagenous fibers and is continuous with an inner zone exhibiting looser tissue with abundant fluid, as well as cartilage cells embedded in a slight amount of ground substance. The bundles of collagenous fibers lie parallel to one another within a lamella and in the opposite direction to those of the following lamella so that a spiral course from vertebral body to vertebral body results. They are anchored at the bony marginal ridges and the hyaline cartilage closing plates of the vertebral bodies. An isolated intervertebral "disc" is thus an artificial product and arises only by transection of the collagenous fibers radiating into the vertebral body.

The *nucleus pulposus* has arisen by the transformation of the hyaline cartilage perichordal cone of the embryonic anlage of the intervertebral disc into a slimy, gelatinous mass with a water content of about 80%. The gelatinous nucleus is subjected to internal pressure. It subjects the surrounding lamellae to pressure from within and swells up when the disc is incised.

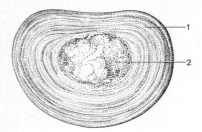

Fig. 179. **Intervertebral disc in region of lumbar verterbral column**
Cranial view
1 Anulus fibrosus
2 Nucleus pulposus

With increasing age (especially pronounced after the 3rd decade), the colloid osmotic pressure of the gelatinous nucleus decreases and the water content diminishes. Deformability and elasticity are reduced. By the end of the 1st decade, cracks regularly appear in the intervertebral discs of the cervical vertebrae – first in the lateral parts of the anulus fibrosus; under the influence of the normal movements of the cervical vertebral column these frequently broaden into continuous, transverse fissures (*uncovertebral fissures*). This does not as a rule, have any pathological significance.

The gelatinous nucleus and fibrous ring act together. The incompressible, but deformable nucleus pulposus is moderately displaceable. It supports the vertebral body like a water cushion, assures an equal distribution of pressure, and keeps the fibrous ring tense. The anulus fibrosus forms a tensile covering which ensures the union of the vertebral bodies and offers resistance to traction and rotation.

Ligaments of the vertebral column (Figs. **180, 182** and **195**). In addition to the intervertebral discs, the vertebral bodies are connected by *anterior* and *posterior ligamentous tracts.*

The *anterior longitudinal ligament* passes from the occipital bone and from the anterior tubercle of the atlas to the sacrum and ends caudally as the *anterior sacrococcygeal ligament*. It is firmly connected with the anterior surface of the vertebral body and is fused with the periosteum at the pelvic fascia of the sacrum.

The weaker dorsal ligamentous band, the *posterior longitudinal ligament*, arises from the clivus, courses along the dorsal surface of the vertebral bodies, and becomes caudally the *deep posterior sacrococcygeal ligament* (Fig. **181**). It is attached at the upper and lower margins of the vertebral bodies and at the intervertebral discs.

Whereas the anterior longitudinal ligament becomes increasingly broader from cranial to caudal, the posterior ligament is distinctly narrower in the caudal region, broadening, however, at the level of the intervertebral discs. In both ligaments the fibers do not traverse the entire length, but extend only over a maximum of 4–5 vertebrae.

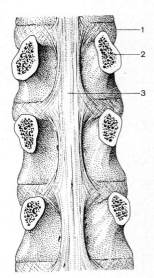

Fig. 180. **Posterior longitudinal ligament in region of lumbar vertebral column**, vertebral arches severed at their roots
1 Intervertebral disc, anulus fibrosus
2 Pedicle of vertebral arch (cut surface)
3 Posterior longitudinal ligament

The column of vertebral bodies, were it freed from the arches, would permit a much larger degree of bending than the complete vertebral column. When the sacrum is fixed, the cranial end can be bent anteriorly or posteriorly to the pelvic level. A stronger forward or backward inclination of this column of vertebral "bodies" is prevented by the posterior or anterior ligamentous tracts. Both ligaments are of critical importance for the maintenance of the characteristic form of the vertebral column since they are stretched by the pressure of the gelatinous nucleus just like the lamellae of the anulus fibrosus.

Connections of the Vertebral Arches

The vertebral arches communicate with one another by joints (*zygapophysial joints*) between the articular processes and by the following ligaments (Figs. **182** and **195**):
– the *ligamenta flava, yellow ligaments* (predominantly elastic "fibers"),
– the *interspinous ligaments* (between the spinous processes),
– the *supraspinous ligaments* (across the tips of the spinous processes from the 7th cervical to the 4th lumbar [rarely up to the sacrum]),
– the *ligamentum nuchae, cervical ligament* (thin tissue plate between the external protuberance and the spine of the 7th cervical vertebra with sparse elastic "fibers" in man), and

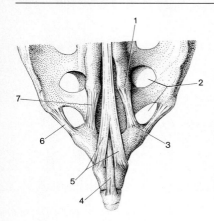

Fig. 181. **Sacrococcygeal connection**, dorsal view
1 Sacral cornu
2 Posterior sacral foramina
3 Coccygeal cornu
4 Deep posterior sacrococcygeal ligament
5 Superficial posterior sacrococcygeal ligament
6 Lateral sacrococcygeal ligament
7 Articular sacrococcygeal ligament

– the *intertransverse ligaments* (weak tendinous tracts in the thoracic region between the transverse processes, in the lumbar region between the accessory processes).

The *lateral sacrococcygeal ligament* extends as a well-developed tendinous tract from the caudal end of the lateral sacral crest to the rudiment of the transverse process of the 1st coccygeal vertebra (Fig. **181**). It can ossify so that a sacrococcygeal foramen (for the ventral ramus of the 5th sacral nerve) is marked off.

Articulations of the vertebral arches are diarthroses, which have arisen as appositional joints. The joint capsule arises at the margins of the articular surfaces of the articular processes (Figs. **172** and **182**). Strengthened by longitudinally-coursing tendinous tracts, it is wide and flaccid at the joints of the cervical vertebrae, narrow and tense at the thoracic and lumbar regions.

In adults primarily in the region of the cervical and middle lumbar vertebral column, in children more or less at all vertebral arch joints, there is a meniscus-like, vascular-rich tissue plate, which is pushed medially between the articular surfaces and communicates with the connective tissue in the intervertebral foramina. A mechanical significance is ascribed to it.

Form and position of the joint surfaces of the articular processes are different in the individual regions of the vertebral column. Correspondingly, the preferred direction and extent of movement also differ.

The articular surfaces are displaced toward one another, and the closing of their surfaces is frequently abolished. The movement deflections between two adjacent vertebrae are relatively slight, but a considerable range of movement can be attained by a summation of individual movements.

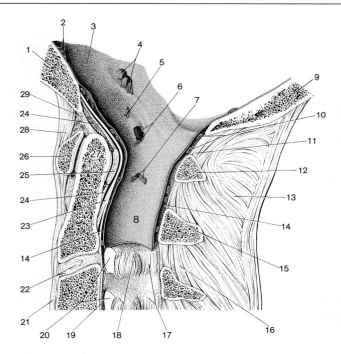

Fig. 182. **Atlanto-occipital joint**, median section in view from left

1 Basilar part of occipital bone
2 Cut surfaces of basilar plexus
3 Cephalic dura mater
4 Glossopharyngeal, vagus and accessory nerves
5 Hypoglossal nerve
6 Vertebral artery and roots of first cervical nerve
7 Roots of second cervical nerve
8 Spinal dura mater, removed caudal to axis (sites of attachment of denticulate ligament not shown)
9 Squama of occipital bone
10 Cut surfaces of transverse anastomoses of posterior internal vertebral venous plexus
11 Posterior atlanto-occipital membrane
12 Posterior arch of atlas
13 Ligamentum nuchae
14 Epidural space (adipose tissue and loose connective tissue not shown)

15 Spinous process of axis
16 Interspinous ligament
17 Ligamenta flava
18 Articular capsules of joints of verterbral arches
19 Posterior longitudinal ligament
20 Intervertebral foramina
21 Anterior longitudinal ligament
22 Intervertebral disc with anulus fibrosus and nucleus pulposus
23 Membrana tectoria
24, 25 *Cruciform ligament of atlas*
24 Longitudinal bands
25 Transverse ligament of atlas
26 Anterior arch of atlas
27 Dens of axis (in froint of and behind joint surfaces covered with cartilage: articular cavity of median atlanto-axial joint)
28 Anterior atlanto-occipital membrane
29 Apical ligament of dens

The articular surfaces of the *cervical vertebrae*, which are slightly inclined toward the horizontal, favor a more varied type of movement and make possible – aside from the movements in the specialized joints of the head – extensive ventral or dorsal flexion, in addition to lateral bending and rotation around the longitudinal axis.

The joint surfaces of the *thoracic vertebra* are placed almost frontally and lie in an oblique plane coursing from ventrocranial to dorsocaudal. They permit an extensive forward flexion, whereas dorsal flexion is restricted by the long, downward-angled spinous processes. A lateral inclination is possible to an extensive degree. The thoracic vertebral column then forms a symmetrically curved arch. A rotation takes place especially in the region of the lower thoracic vertebrae. The predominantly sagittally-aligned articular surfaces of the *lumbar vertebrae* favor extensive rotary movements around a transverse axis and permit limited lateral bending. A rotation around the longitudinal axis, on the other hand, is only possible by a few degrees (also in the case of forward flexion of the trunk).

Ligaments in the region of the vertebral arches (Figs. **182** and **195**). The elastic *ligamenta flava* complete the wall of the vertebral canal between the vertebral arches dorsal to the intervertebral foramina. Like the *interspinous ligaments* and the *supraspinous ligament*, they check an excessive forward bending of the vertebral column. The yellow ligaments are also under tension when the vertebral column is held erect. If the vertebral bodies are separated from the arches, the "arch" of the column is reduced by more than 3 cm.

The *interspinous ligaments* are formed in the region of the cervical vertebral column by anterocranially-directed fibers and extend dorsally into the ligamentum nuchae without a sharp boundary. Both fibrous systems counteract a ventral flexion of the cervical vertebral column. In the region of the thoracic vertebrae, the interspinous ligaments are formed ventrally as thin membranes (without noteworthy mechanical significance), whereas dorsally a longitudinal bundle of fibers, at which tendon fibers of superficial back muscles are attached connects two spinous processes. The longitudinal bundles are stretched by the forward flexion of the vertebral column. In the lumbar region the interspinous ligaments exhibit a posterocranial fibrous course and communicate with the thoracolumbar fascia (fascia of the autochthonous back muscles) and with tendon fibers of the multifidus muscle. In ventral flexion, they retard the movement in the end position; in dorsal flexion, they counteract a dorsal shifting of the cranial vertebrae.

The *supraspinous ligament* consists of fiber tracts which – attached at the spinous processes – pass over several movement segments. It is most strongly formed in the lumbar region, lies superficial to the thoracolumbar fascia, and does not directly communicate with the interspinous ligaments. The ligament is stretched during forward flexion of the vertebral column.

The *ligamentum nuchae*, which in quadruped mammals helps to support the head as a strong, elastic cervical ligament, has little mechanical significance in man under physiological conditions.

Clinical observations indicate, however, that in a whiplash injury, it can absorb part of the force occurring with the extreme ventral flexion of the cervical vertebral column. Traumas of the cervical vertebral column can lead to fractures of the pedicles of the vertebral arches, the articular processes and the vertebral bodies, whereas the laminae, spinous processes and ligamentum nuchae remain uninjured.

Articulation of the Head

The following articular connections exist between the occipital bone of the skull and the vertebral column:
– *atlanto-occipital joint* (paired, articular connection of the kidney-shaped concave superior articular facet of the atlas with the convex occipital condyle of the occipital bone),
– *lateral atlanto-axial joint* (paired, articular connection between the inferior articular surfaces of the atlas and the superior articular surfaces of the axis), and
– *median atlanto-axial joint* (Fig. **182**, unpaired articulation between the anterior or posterior surfaces of the dens of the axis and the fovea dentis of the atlas or the "articular surfaces" of the transverse ligament of the atlas).

The atlanto-axial joints form a functional unit. Because the articulations of the skull, atlas and axis, are subdivided into 6 isolated joint chambers closed off by capsules, the range of movement is restricted, but the precision of movement is enhanced.

Ligaments in the region of the skull, atlas and axis (Fig. **182**). The firm *anterior atlanto-occipital membrane* passes from the anterior arch of the atlas to the basal surface of the occipital bone, its middle part being strengthened by the anterior longitudinal ligament.

The *apical ligament of the dens* courses from the apex of the dens to the anterior margin of the foramen magnum. It can contain remains of the notochord.

The *alar ligaments* originate at the lateral surfaces of the dens and attach at the inner surface of the occipital condyles and the medial margin adjoining the foramen magnum.

The *cruciform ligament of the atlas* (Fig. **172**) consists of longitudinal tracts (*longitudinal fasciculi*), which pass from the posterior surface of the body of the axis to the anterior circumference of the foramen magnum, and a transverse ligament (*transverse ligament of the atlas*). Its fibers insert bilaterally at a roughness on the inner surface of the lateral mass, enclosing the dens dorsally and – except in cases of severe traumatic force (broken neck) – prevent the dens from dislocating and boring into the spinal cord.

The "articular surface" of the transverse ligament of the atlas can exhibit a fibrocartilaginous covering, or cartilage cells can be deposited in the ligament.

The *membrana tectoria*, the broader cranial portion of the posterior longitudinal ligament with shorter fibers from the dorsal surface of the body of the axis, forms the ventral ligamentous boundary of the vertebral canal in the region of the joints of the head.

The *posterior atlanto-occipital membrane*, the "ligamentum flavum" between the atlas and occipital bone, closes the vertebral canal dorsally between the posterior arch of the atlas and the dorsal circumference of the foramen magnum. The relatively thin membrane is penetrated by the vertebral artery (in the cranial cavity), by the suboccipital nerve (toward the deep muscles of the neck) and by a venous plexus.

The lateral atlanto-occipital ligament strengthens the capsule of the atlanto-occipital joint and connects the root of the transverse process of the atlas with the external base of the skull in the region of the jugular process of the occipital bone.

The paired *atlanto-occipital joints* permit nodding forward (up to about 20°) or backward (up to about 30°) and, to a lesser extent, lateral bending of the head. Nodding takes place around a transverse axis which courses behind the external ear through the anterior margin of both mastoid processes. The eccentric skull, resting on the atlas, is balanced by the cervical musculature and the sternocleidomastoid. (In an infant with its still relatively small facial part of the skull, the center of gravity lies behind the axis of rotation and the head tips posteriorly when the musculature is relaxed.)

The longitudinal axes of the joint bodies of the atlanto-occipital articulation converge ventrally. The articular surfaces are like a notch out of a rotary ellipsoid, the large axis of which courses transversely: condylarthrosis. With regard to joint mechanics, the joints of both sides form a unit. The joint capsule is flaccid.

The *extension movement of the head* (dorsal flexion) is hindered by (Fig. **182**):
– the *anterior atlanto-occipital membrane*.

During *forward flexion*, tightening occurs at:
– the *membrana tectoria* and
– the longitudinal tracts (*longitudinal fasciculi*) of the *cruciform ligament of the atlas*.

In the *atlanto-axial joint*, the atlas (and with it, the head) can be rotated toward each side by about 30° around the dens. The *alar ligaments* function as check ligaments, one passing around the dens anteriorly, the other posteriorly, and both tensed.

In the *median atlanto-axial articulation*, anterior and posterior joint compartments communicate with one another by means of a mucous bursa.

c) Statics and Dynamics of the Vertebral Column

The Vertebral Column at Rest

The adult vertebral column is curved during erect posture in the shape of a double S. The curved portion which is concave dorsally is termed a *lordosis*, and that which is convex dorsally a *kyphosis*. Thus, the following are distinguished (Fig. **183 a**):
– the cervical lordosis (from C1 to C6),
– the thoracic kyphosis (from C6 to T9),
– the lumbar lordosis (from T9 to L5), and
– the sacral kyphosis (in the sacral and coccygeal regions).

The sharp bend of the vertebral column at the superior margin of the 1st sacral vertebra, the *promontory*, projects into the entrance of the lesser pelvis and represents an important measuring point for pelvimetry (Fig. **117**).

The vertebral column of the newborn child (Fig. **183 b**) is a rather straight line in the lying position. A dorsal convexity in the thoracic region is only hinted at, whereas there is a slight dorsal concavity in the lumbar region. In the region of the sacrum and coccyx, the *sacral kyphosis* is recognizable. The promontory is already developed in infants, but still relatively flat. In a sitting position, the entire vertebral column forms a convex arch dorsally.

The *cervical lordosis* is formed as soon as the infant begins to lift its head. The cervical vertebral column becomes an elastic rod which carries the head. The center of gravity of the head in the adult lies in front of the atlanto-occipital joint. The head must be held in equilibrium by the dorsal traction girdle of the muscle and tendon apparatuses. Owing to the lordotic curvature, the cervical vertebral column is stressed by axial pressure (from the resultant two forces: body weight and traction girdle).

The *lumbar lordosis* becomes distinct when the infant reaches the end of the 1st postnatal year and is able to walk upright. Its origin is caused by the same factors as the development of cervical lordosis; the eccentric organization of the mass of upper body and abdominal organs, the center of gravity of which lies in front of an erect vertebral column, would lead to an eccentric load on the lumbar vertebrae without the development of a lordotic curvature.

The *thoracic kyphosis* is formed between the two lordotic sections of the vertebral column in the cervical and lumbar regions and represents a curvature opposite to that of the cervical lordosis. It enlarges the thorax dorsally and increases the space necessary for the accommodation of the thoracic organs.

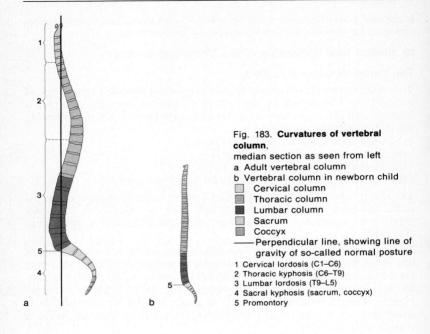

Fig. 183. **Curvatures of vertebral column**,
median section as seen from left
a Adult vertebral column
b Vertebral column in newborn child

☐ Cervical column
▨ Thoracic column
■ Lumbar column
☐ Sacrum
▨ Coccyx
——Perpendicular line, showing line of
　　gravity of so-called normal posture
1 Cervical lordosis (C1–C6)
2 Thoracic kyphosis (C6–T9)
3 Lumbar lordosis (T9–L5)
4 Sacral kyphosis (sacrum, coccyx)
5 Promontory

The cervical vertebral column forms an elastic support for the head; the lumbar vertebral column, which is also dorsally concave carries the upper body as an elastic bony rod and functions as a type of a shock absorber. By the formation of both lordotic curvatures in the cervical and lumbar regions and the opposite kyphotic curvature in the thoracic and sacral regions – in association with the traction girdle – an erect body posture is promoted, although the vertebral column is eccentrically weighted.

The extent of the above-mentioned curvatures of the vertebral column is influenced by the position and condition of the body and depends on constitutional factors. On the basis of the characteristic elasticity caused by its ligamentous apparatus, intervertebral discs and joint structures, the vertebral column, freed of its musculature, strives to reach a certain "natural" curvature, the *balanced* or *characteristic form* of the vertebral column, as soon as the influence of external forces which lead to a deformation stops.

In the course of a day, the vertebral column (in an upright standing or sitting posture over a longer period) becomes about 2 cm shorter since the intervertebral discs are lower (water loss from the gelatinous nucleus?), and the curvatures of the vertebral column increase somewhat (diminution of the individual elasticity of the vertebral column, fatigue of the musculature).

Mild distortions of the vertebral column in the frontal plane (curvatures and counter-curvatures) are physiological. They appear in humans, for example, who regularly prefer the same arm (usually the right) for heavy bodily activity, or result from legs of unequal length (in the case of righthanded people, the left leg is frequently somewhat longer). Pathological lateral curvature of the vertebral column is known as *scoliosis* and is accompanied by severe deformations of the thorax.

The Vertebral Column in Movement

In *ventral flexion* of the whole vertebral column (in the interplay, for example, of the inferior hyoid muscles, the prevertebral cervical muscles, the abdominal musculature, the iliopsoas and the forces of gravity), the thoracic kyphosis is strengthened, whereas the cervical and lumbar lordosis can be equalized up to a straight line. The paired erector spinae muscle is thereby increasingly stretched and can retard the movement. The head, cervical and lumbar vertebral columns can be flexed anteriorly alone or in combination.

In *dorsal flexion* (involving the cooperation of different parts of the erector system), the lordotic curvature of the cervical and lumbar vertebral columns is increased, whereas the thoracic kyphosis is leveled off. Dorsal flexion in the lumbosacral and in the thoracolumbar border regions of the vertebral column, and in the cervical region is particularly favored. Backward flexion of the lumbar vertebral column can be combined with ventral flexion in the cervicothoracic region.

Lateral flexion of the vertebral column (by the iliocostalis, external and internal abdominal obliques of the same side and others) takes place primarily at the same sites as dorsal flexion. If the thoracic vertebral column is involved in lateral flexion, the vertebral column forms a uniformly curved arch. While the abdominal wall is compressed on the flexion side in extreme lateral bending, the musculature on the extensor side is simultaneously extended and actively stretched.

Rotation of the trunk around the longitudinal axis takes place chiefly in the thoracic and cervical regions. Transversospinal traction of one side of the body and spinotransversal muscles of the other, together with portions of the sacrospinal system and the muscle chains of the oblique abdominal muscles, are able to twist the entire vertebral column so far that the chin is almost at right angles to the side (about 80°). By utilizing the range of movement in the inferior ankle and in the hip joints when the feet are fixed, the body can be twisted so far that the face is turned obliquely backward (about 135°).

d) Blood Vessels and Nerves of the Vertebral Column

The *arterial supply of the vertebrae* takes place from *branches of segmental arteries* of the region in question (Figs. **25** and **126**):
- the cervical vertebral column by branches of the vertebral, ascending cervical and deep cervical arteries;
- the thoracic and lumbar vertebral column by branches of the posterior intercostal, lumbar and iliolumbar arteries (last intervertebral foramen); and
- the sacrum by branches of the lateral and median sacral arteries.

In contrast to the skull and brain, which receive blood from separate routes, the blood for the vertebral column and spinal cord arises from the same arteries.

Branches of the periosteal vascular network supply the bones. In the process, anastomotic networks on the anterior surfaces of the vertebral bodies, as well as longitudinal and transverse anastomoses on their posterior surfaces and in the regions of their arches, ensure an extensive collateral circulation. The vessels entering the nutrient foramina supply the bone marrow. The nourishment of the avascular intervertebral discs takes place by diffusion from the spongiosa region of the vertebral body.

Venous blood is carried off from the vertebrae via the valveless *external* and *internal vertebral venous plexuses* (Fig. **184**) and conveyed from there to the vertebral and deep cervical veins (cervical vertebral column), the segmental posterior intercostal and lumbar veins (thoracic and lumbar vertebral column), as well as to the median sacral vein and the lateral sacral veins via the sacral venous plexus (sacrum).

The *anterior external vertebral venous plexus* designates the total of all fine veins at the anterolateral surfaces of the individual vertebral bodies, which are partially covered by the anterior longitudinal ligament. Connections to the anterior internal vertebral venous plexus exist via the *basivertebral veins*.

The *posterior external vertebral venous plexus* lies covered by the autochthonous back musculature as a wide-meshed, primarily longitudinally-directed venous network on each side of the spinous and transverse processes. It communicates cranially with the dural sinus via suboccipital venous networks and emissaries, obtains tributaries from the inner plexus of vertebral veins, and reaches caudally to the sacrum.

Innervation. The posterior surfaces of the vertebral bodies and all remaining wall sections of the vertebral canal, as well as the articular capsules of the joints of the vertebral arches, are supplied by branches of the meningeal ramus of spinal nerves (Fig. **50**), which enters the vertebral canal through the intervertebral foramen.

Pain caused by prolapse of the intervertebral discs is perceived in the region of the richly-innervated posterior longitudinal ligament.

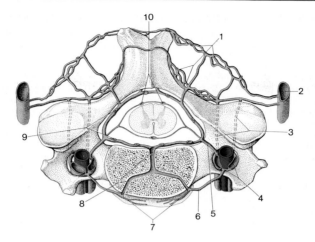

Fig. 184. **Vertebral venous plexus and drainage paths in region of cervical vertebral column,** cranial view (modified after *Clemens*)

1 Posterior external vertebral venous plexus (in two layers in cervical region: near bone and between deep cervical muscles)
2 Deep cervical vein
3 Segmental tributaries to vertebral vein from posterior external vertebral venous plexus
4 Vertebral veins, enclosed vertebral artery
5 Segmental tributary to vertebral vein from internal vertebral venous plexus (intervertebral veins)

6 Segmental tributary to vertebral vein from anterior external vertebral venous plexus
7 Anterior external vertebral venous plexus
8 Basivertebral veins
9 Internal vertebral venous plexus with transverse anastomoses and sagittal connections
10 Posterior spinal veins

2. Vertebral Canal

The vertebral canal (boundary → p. 455) communicates cranially with the cranial cavity via the foramen magnum and extends caudally to the sacral hiatus. It harbors the spinal cord, the roots of the spinal nerves, and the spinal meninges and contains fat and connective tissue, as well as numerous blood vessels.

a) Spinal Meninges

The **tough spinal meninx,** the *dura mater* (Figs. **67** and **182**), forms a tubing made up of predominantly longitudinally coursing connective tissue fibers, which is fixed to bone at the margin of the foramen magnum. It is separated from the wall of the vertebral canal by the *epidural cavity* – whereas the dura and periosteum in the cranial cavity are fused with one another – and ends at the level of the 1st or 2nd sacral vertebra. The caudal continuation of the dural tubing, the *filum of the dura mater*, adjoins the filum terminale of the spinal cord and is attached at the 2nd coccygeal vertebra.

Sack-like processes of the dural tubing pass into the intervertebral foramina and enclose the roots of the spinal nerves. The dura and arachnoid fuse here into a meningeal sheath, which also forms the connective tissue capsule of the spinal ganglion. It continues on the spinal nerves as the epineurium and perineurium.

The anterior and posterior roots of the spinal nerves generally lie close to one another proximal to the spinal ganglion and are covered by a common meningeal sheath. However, they can also pass through the dura separately (thoracic nerves).

In the **epidural space** (*epidural cavity*, Figs. **67** and **182**), loose fibrous connective tissue, fat and the *internal vertebral venous plexus* form a protective cushion. The dural tube is united with the (anterior) wall of the vertebral canal (especially in the cervical and lumbar regions) by connective tissue trabeculae, which permit changes in position, however, during movements of the head and the vertebral column.

Paired, avalvular longitudinal venous plexuses, the *anterior* and the *posterior internal vertebral venous plexus*, course within the epidural space – for the entire length of the vertebral canal – both ventrally (at the posterior surface of the vertebral bodies, partly covered by the posterior longitudinal ligament) and dorsally (at the inner surface of the vertebral arches).

The internal vertebral venous plexuses possess a thin wall with sparse smooth muscle and abundant collagenous fibers. Each of the four longitudinal venous complexes consists of a multiple cross-linked pair of longitudinal veins. The right and left parts of a plexus communicate by transverse anastomoses. The anterior and posterior internal vertebral venous plexuses communicate by sagittal-coursing veins or venous networks, the branches of which curve around the intervertebral foramina. The basivertebral veins empty into the anterior transverse anastomoses; inconstant veins from the vertebral arches and spinous processes drain into the posterior ones. The internal vertebral venous plexuses are fixed in the epidural space by collagenous trabeculae from the periosteum and the dura.

The internal vertebral venous plexuses communicate cranially with the basilar plexus (anterior plexus) and the occipital sinus (posterior plexus), thus offering a drainage possibility for blood from the interior of the skull.

The internal vertebral venous plexus (total capacity in the adult of about 100 ml) takes up venous blood from the spinal cord (spinal branches) and from parts of the vertebral column and carrries it via intervertebral and basivertebral veins to the ventral and the dorsal branches of the segmental vessels (posterior intercostal, lumbar veins), to the vertebral veins, to the sacral venous plexus, and to the external vertebral venous plexus (Fig. **184**).

Internal (and external) vertebral venous plexuses thus are able to deliver blood into both venae cavae. Since the bloodstream in the vertebral venous plexuses and in the azygos system is not directed by venous valves, they represent an important detour in the case of obstructions in the region of the venae cavae or the azygos system, but also of the internal jugular veins. A reflux of blood from the internal vertebral venous plexus into the veins of the spinal cord is prevented by the venous valves of the spinal branches.

Considering the ease in displacement of blood into the extensive, thin-walled networks of the internal vertebral venous plexuses, in which a relatively low blood pressure prevails in comparison to the extravertebral veins, the internal vertebral venous plexuses exert a regulating influence on the physiological variations of cerebrospinal pressure.

Results from animal experiments indicate that the vertebral venous plexuses can be diffusion routes for tumor metastases (e.g. metastases of prostatic carcinoma in the vertebral column).

The **arachnoid of the spinal cord** (Fig. 67) is extremely poor in capillaries and aneural; it spreads out between the surface of the pia and the dura as a delicate connective tissue meshwork. A subdural "space" between the epithelial-lined inner surface of the dura and the epithelial covering of the external layer of the arachnoid is not present in the living under normal conditions. The external layer of the arachnoid lies directly on the dura.

The **pia mater** (Fig. 67) is a vascularized, nerve-rich connective tissue layer and lies on the glial limiting membrane of the spinal cord. It encloses the filum terminale of the spinal cord as the *pial filum terminale*.

The spinal pia mater is not continued on the root filaments (fila radicularia) of the spinal nerve roots as a closed, macroscopically-visible covering, but does form, however, the endoneurium of the individual nerve fibers. The spinal arachnoid accompanies the root filaments and spinal nerve roots through the subarachnoid space and is united with the dura in the above-mentioned meningeal sheath.

The pia mater, which forms a type of "external skeleton" for the spinal cord, communicates on each side with the dura mater by a frontally-placed, connective tissue plate, the *denticulate ligament*. This ligament, which serves as a holding device for the spinal cord, arises (at the level of the 1st cervical to 3rd lumbar segments) at the lateral circumference of the spinal cord between the anterior and posterior roots of the spinal nerves. The free lateral margin is drawn out in the form of a serrated saw-blade; the tips of the teeth are attached at the dura (usually in the middle between the exits of two spinal nerves) and, thus, fix the arachnoid there.

The **subarachnoid space** of the spinal cord (Fig. **67**) communicates cranially with the subarachnoid space of the brain and terminates caudally – like the dural tube – at the level of the 2nd sacral vertebra. The subarachnoid cavity contains cerebrospinal fluid.

Since the arachnoid is continued into the perineural sheaths of the spinal nerves, connections exist between the subarachnoid space and the lymphatic spaces of the spinal nerves, by means of which the cerebrospinal fluid can be discharged.

Lumbar puncture. For the withdrawal of cerebrospinal fluid from the subarachnoid space of the spinal cord, the hypodermic needle is inserted (as a rule) into the subarachnoid space between the spinous processes of the 3rd and 4th or 4th and 5th lumbar vertebrae (generally in the middle of a line which connects the right and left iliac crests), since the spinal cord does not extend so far and the spinal nerve roots avoid the tip of the needle. The distance between the spinous processes (directed straight backward) and the arches of the lumbar vertebrae is considerably greater than in the region of the thoracic vertebral column. Moreover, when fluid is withdrawn near the caudal end of the subarachnoid space, those particles (e.g. cellular elements) which have settled in the fluid are also obtained.

Spinal anesthesia. After a lumbar puncture, an anesthetic solution can be injected into the subarachnoid space to produce a paralysis of the nerve fibers in the spinal nerve roots (motor, sensory and autonomic fibers). The quantity and the specific gravity of the anesthetic permit a certain control of the spinal anesthesia, and by corresponding positioning of the patient the spinal segments can be anesthesized at different levels.

Epidural anesthesia. The injection of an anesthetic solution into the epidural space (e.g. through the sacral hiatus) leads to a paralysis of several spinal nerves near the exit from the dural tube (essentially an extensive nerve block). The localization of the injection site and the volume of the anesthetic injected determine the level and the extent of the anesthesized region.

b) Contents of the Vertebral Canal

The **spinal cord** (Fig. **49**) is about 45 cm long in the adult and ends with the tapered *conus medullaris* at the level of lumbar vertebrae 1–2 (projection site on the anterior trunk wall: somewhat above the middle of a line connecting the navel and apex of the xiphoid process). The conus medullaris continues into the filamentous *filum terminale* (*spinal*) (essentially glial and connective tissue), which can be followed to the posterior surface of the coccyx.

In the embryo, the spinal cord fills up the "vertebral canal" in its entire length. From the 3rd embryonic month onward, however, it grows slower than the vertebral column. The conus medullaris appears, therefore, to move further craniad as time progresses (so-called *ascent* of the spinal cord). In the 6th fetal month, it lies at the level of the 1st sacral vertebra, and at birth it is at the level of L3.

In the adult, the *roots of the spinal nerves*, which originally pass almost horizontal (at the level of their segment of origin) to the intervertebral foramina, therefore, course (approximately from the 5th cervical) first obliquely and then more and more steeply downward for an increasingly longer distance in the vertebral canal in order to reach the corresponding intervertebral foramen. Caudal to the 1st lumbar vertebra, the anterior and posterior *roots* of the caudal spinal nerves – closely crowded around the filum terminale – pass downward and form the *cauda equina*.

Spinal nerves. The 31 pairs of *spinal nerves* each arise from the union of the *anterior* and *posterior roots* into the *spinal nerve trunk* within the intervertebral foramen (Figs. **50** and **185**). The spinal nerve roots "originate" from the spinal cord with more or less numerous root filaments (*Fila radicularia*) in longitudinal series (one dorsal and two to three ventral). Directly proximal to the site of union, the posterior root is thickened into the *spinal ganglion*, which contains the cell bodies of the pseudo-unipolar sensory nerve cells of the posterior root fibers. The anterior root is purely motor, the posterior root sensory, and the spinal nerve consequently mixed.

Since the spinal nerve exiting between the atlas and occipital bone is designated as the 1st cervical nerve, the following are normally distinguished (Fig. **49**):
- 8 *cervical nerves,*
- 12 *thoracic nerves,*
- 5 *lumbar nerves,*
- 5 *sacral nerves,* and
- 1 *coccygeal nerve.*

The dorsal root of the 1st cervical nerve can be absent. When it is present, the 1st cervical ganglion is found on the posterior arch of the atlas in the sulcus of the vertebral artery. The spinal ganglia from C2–L3 lie in the intervertebral foramina, the ganglia of the caudal lumbar nerves in the region bordering the vertebral canal, and the sacral ganglia completely in the sacral canal.

3. Organization and Innervation of the Autochthonous Back Musculature

The musculature situated in the back region and arranged in several layers, as can be seen from their innervation, has developed only in part at the location and is thus *genuine* or *autochthonous back musculature*. It is designated in its totality as the *erector spinae muscle*. This *deep* back musculature is overlapped by *superficial* back muscles ($\rightarrow$ p. 186). Muscles of the shoulder girdle and the free limbs (*spinohumeral muscles*) have secondarily shifted their origin to the vertebral column. A derivative of the *branchiomeric musculature*, the trapezius, has been displaced from

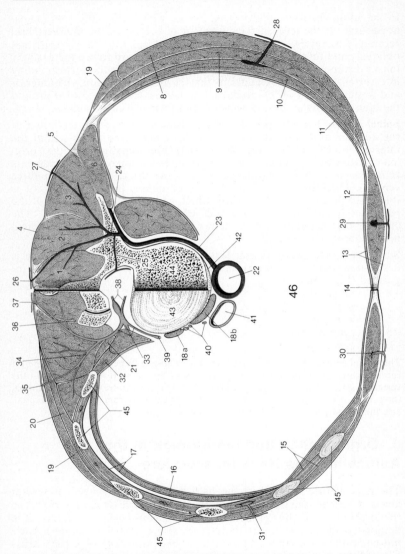

Fig. 185. **Transverse section through abdominal wall**, cranial view (after *Pernkopf*)
Schematic layered section: on right side through intervertebral disc (between L1 and
2), on left side through vertebral body of L2. (vessels and nerves only exemplified;
right joint of vertebral arch between L1 and 2, spinous process, supraspinous
ligaments, interspinal and posterior longitudinal ligaments illustrated, but not labelled)

cranially onto the back. Tracts of the ventral trunk musculature have also reached the back, the serratus posterior muscles having been pushed between the spinohumeral and the autochthonous back muscles as *spinocostal muscles*. Finally, the *anterior intertransverse muscles*, which extend as serial homologs of the intercostal muscles ventral to the erector spinae – between the rib rudiments of the cervical and lumbar vertebrae, are also back muscles of ventral origin.

The *autochthonous back musculature* (Fig. **185**) lies directly on the axial skeleton. It is – in contrast to the remaining somatic musculature – innervated by *dorsal rami of spinal nerves*. The muscles of this system play a role in all movements of the vertebral column, either by active contraction or by passive decrease in tonus (e.g. forward flexion of the vertebral column using the force of gravity or by contraction of the ventral trunk musculature). Furthermore, the erector spinae play an essential role in securing the upright body position (distortion of the vertebral column, e.g. as the result of a diseased debility of the musculature).

The *thoracolumbar fascia* is the **fascia of the erector spinae.** Formed in the thoracic-lumbar region, it is a fascial covering comparable to the group fasciae of the limb musculature. In the region of the back of the neck, the

1–3 *Erector spinae*
1 Medial tract (spinalis)
2 Longissimus
3 Iliocostalis
4, 5 *Thoracolumbar fascia*
4 Superficial layer
5 Deep layer
6 Quadratus lumborum
7 Psoas major
8 External abdominal oblique
9 Internal abdominal oblique
10 Transversus abdominis
11 Parietal peritoneum and transversalis fascia
12 Rectus abdominis
13 Sheath of rectus abdominis
14 Linea alba
15 Intercostals: external, internal, innermost
16 Costal part of diaphragm
17 Parietal pleura and endothoracic fasica
18 Right crus of lumbar part of diaphragm
18a Lateral band
18b Medial band
19 Latissimus dorsi
20 Serratus posterior inferior
21 Lumbar intertransverse muscles
22 Aorta
23 Lumbar artery
24 Dorsal branch of lumbar artery

25 Spinal branch of dorsal branch
26 Medial cutaneous branch of dorsal branch
27 Laterial cutaneous branch of dorsal branch
28 Lateral cutaneous branch of lumbar artery
29 Superior epigastric artery with anterior cutaneous branch
30 Anterior cutaneous ramus of eighth intercostal nerve
31 Lateral cutaneous ramus of eighth intercostal nerve
32 Subcostal nerve in quadratus lumborum
33 Lumbar nerve with dorsal, ventral and communicating rami
34 Lateral twig of dorsal branch
35 Lateral cutaneous branch of dorsal branch
36 Medial twig of dorsal branch
37 Medial cutaneous branch of dorsal branch
38 Ventral root, dorsal root of lumbar nerve
39 Sympathetic trunk
40 Azygos vein, greater and lesser splanchnic nerves
41 Inferior vena cava
42 Anterior longitudinal ligament
43 Intervertebral disc between L1 and 2 (cut surface)
44 Second lumbar vertebra (cut surface)
45 Ribs XII–VII
46 Abdominal cavity

nuchal fascia covers the superficial layers of the erector spinae and separates them from the superficial back muscles covering them, which have migrated to the back. Individual muscle fasciae envelop the short, deeply situated nuchal muscles.

The **thoracolumbar fascia** (Fig. **185**) covers the erector spinae with its superficial layer and encloses ventrally the lumbar part of the lateral tract of autochthonous back musculature with its deep layer. Both layers are united lateral to the iliocostalis. They enclose the erector spinae in an osteofibrous canal, which is delimited medially by the spinous processes and vertebral arches, laterally by the transverse and costal processes, as well as a dorsomedial section of the thoracic wall or – in the lumbar region – by the deep layer of the thoracolumbar fascia. Dorsally, the superficial fascial layer attached to the spinous processes shuts off the canal.

The *superficial layer*, the thoracolumbar fascia in the true sense (Fig. **198**), is attached at the spinous processes of the thoracic, lumbar and sacral vertebrae, as well as at the iliac crest. It is fused in its caudal part with the aponeurosis of the latissimus dorsi and serratus posterior inferior; in the sacral region it is grown together with the common tendon of insertion of the longissimus and iliocostalis and therefore strikingly firm here. Cranially, the superficial fascial layer can be followed to the level of the serratus posterior superior; laterally, it is attached at the angle of the ribs on the other side of the point of insertion of the iliocostalis.

The *deep layer* of the thoracodorsal fascia spreads out dorsal to the quadratus lumborum, between the 12th rib, the costal processes of the lumbar vertebrae and the iliac crest. At the same time, it forms the medial portion of the aponeurotic origin of the transversus abdominis muscle.

The **nuchal fascia** (Fig. **198**) lies beneath the trapezius and rhomboids and covers the semispinalis capitis and splenius muscles. Medially, the generally weak, matted connective tissue plate is fused with the ligamentum nuchae; laterally, it communicates with the fascia of the levator scapulae and, via this fascia, with the superficial lamina of the cervical fascia.

The **erector spinae** originates at the sacrum with its caudal bundles, at the ligaments situated there and at the iliac crest. The cranial muscles of the system are attached at the occiput.

The original metameric organization of the true back musculature has been preserved in man (and mammals) only in the deep layer. Superficial muscle tracts extend over several segments. A true separation into delimited individual muscles and organization by fasciae is found only in the nuchal region. Otherwise, usually only the artificially prepared tracts present coherent muscle systems. In the thoracic region of the vertebral column (kyphotic curvature), the muscle mass is less.

At the erector spinae two tracts are distinguished traditionally: a *medial* tract, which is confined to the channel formed by the spinous processes and transverse processes, and a *lateral* longitudinal tract, which has been extended to the iliac crest and the ribs. This organization corresponds to a different *innervation* of both muscle tracts *via medial or lateral branches of the dorsal rami of spinal nerves.*

a) Medial Tract of Erector Spinae

The medial tract of the autochthonous back musculature – if the three deep nuchal muscles are disregarded – consists of a relatively weak *spinal* and a well-developed *transversospinal* system (Fig. **186 a**).

Spinal System

The fibers of the spinal system pass from vertebral spine to vertebral spine (**interspinal muscles**: paired, unisegmental, absent in the middle region of the thoracic vertebral column) or pass over at least one vertebra (**spinalis muscle**: between C2 and L2).

The **spinalis muscle** forms a thin bundle between the vertebral spines and the longissimus and is developed, as a rule, only in the thoracic region (*spinalis thoracis* from T2 to L2 [3]) and in the nuchal region (*spinalis cervicis* from C2 to T2). The 5th cervical and 9th thoracic vertebrae usually remain free.

As a rare variant, muscle bundles course from the spines of the cervical and cranial thoracic vertebrae to the external occipital protuberance (*spinalis capitis*).

Transversospinal System

The muscle bundles of the **transversospinal muscle** course from the transverse processes to the spinous processes of cranially situated vertebrae. The more superficial the muscle tracts, the more vertebrae are passed over.

The metameric **rotator muscles** (rotatores) form the deepest layer of this system.

The *rotatores breves muscles* pass from the root of a transverse process to the vertebral arch and to the base of the spinous process of the next higher vertebra. The *rotatores longi muscles* cover the short rotators. They possess the same origin and insertion sites but pass over one vertebra. The rotator muscles are clearly delineated at the thoracic vertebral column (*rotatores thoracis*), but can also be differentiated in the cervical and in the lumbar regions: *rotatores cervicis* and *lumborum.*

The **multifidus**, the layer of the transversospinal system situated superficial to the rotators, is strongly developed, especially in the lumbar region.

The origin of the multifidus extends from C4(5) to S4, the insertion taking place at the spines of C2 to L5. Of the muscle bundles pennated in varying arrangements, the deeper-situated pass over 2 vertebrae between their origin and insertion, and the superficial bundles over 3–5 vertebrae.

The **semispinalis** forms the most superficial layer of the transversospinal system. It is generally absent in the lumbar region. Its fibers pass over at least 5, usually 6–7 vertebrae. The head portion of the muscle (*semi-spinalis capitis*) passes over the atlanto-occipital joint to the squamous part of the occipital bone near the midline and cooperates – depending on the synergists concerned – in the powerful rotary movements or in the stabilization and strong dorsal flexion of the head.

If the semispinalis capitis is transected in the laboratory and both end pieces are turned back, the spine of the axis becomes visible as a prominent center for muscle tracts (Fig. **187**), which insert at this process (right and left semispinalis cervicis) or originate there (obliquus capitis inferior and rectus capitis posterior major).

The *semispinalis thoracis* passes from the transverse processes of T7(6)–T11(12) to the spines of the last 2 cervical and the first 3(4) thoracic vertebrae. The *semispinalis cervicis* arises at the transverse processes of T2(3) and T6(7) and inserts at the spinous processes of C2–6. Thoracic and cervical semispinalis muscles frequently form a unit. As with the multifidus, the muscle fibers of the same slips of origin are distributed over several attachment slips.

The *semispinalis capitis*, which completely covers the cervical portion of the muscle, arises largely from the blastema which forms the lateral tract of the autochthonous back musculature. It is, therefore, not only innervated by medial, but also by lateral twigs of the dorsal spinal nerve branches. The muscle bundles originate from the transverse processes (the cranial bundle more from the root of the transverse process and the lateral surface of the inferior articular process) of vertebrae C3–T6 (8) and insert at the occiput below the superior nuchal line (Fig. **187**). The muscle is complex pennate and incompletely organized into a

▶

Fig. 186. Autochthonous muscles of the back
a Muscles of medial tract and posterior intertransverse muscles
b Muscles of lateral tract, except posterior intertransverse and obliquus capitis superior muscles
  (only portions of muscular systems or individual segmental muscles represented)

1–7 *Transversospinal system*
1 Insertion bundles
2 Origin bundles
3 Rotatores (longus and brevis)
4 Multifidus
5 Semispinalis thoracis
6 Semispinalis cervicis
7 Semispinalis capitis
8, 9 *Spinal system*
8 Interspinalis (lumborum, thoracis, cervicis)
9 Spinalis (thoracis, cervicis)
10 Medial lumbar intertransverse muscle
11 Posterior cervical intertransverse muscle
12, 13 *Spinostransversal system*

12 Splenius capitis
13 Splenius cervicis
14–20 *Sacrospinal system*
14 Iliocostalis cervicis
15 Iliocostalis thoracis
16 Iliocostalis lumborum
17 Longissimus capitis
18 Longissimus cervicis
19 Longissimus thoracis
20 Common aponeurosis of origin of sacrospinal system
21 Levatores costarum (longus and brevis)

Innervation:

▢▢▢ ▨▦ Medial (in the case of 7 also lateral) branches of dorsal rami of corresponding spinal nerves

▢▢▨▢ Lateral branches of dorsal rami of corresponding spinal nerves

▨ Lateral branches of dorsal rami (in addition to branches of ventral rami) of corresponding spinal nerves

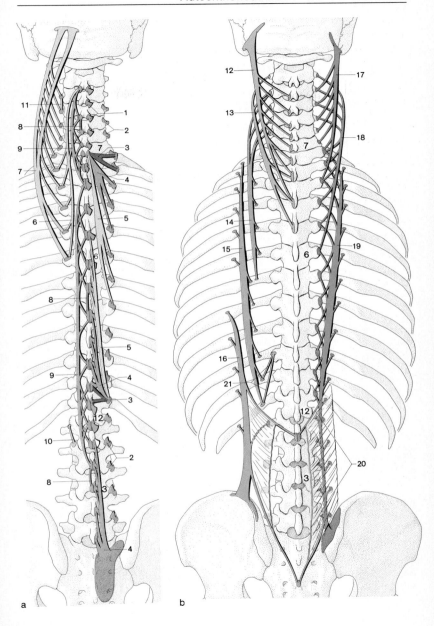

a

b

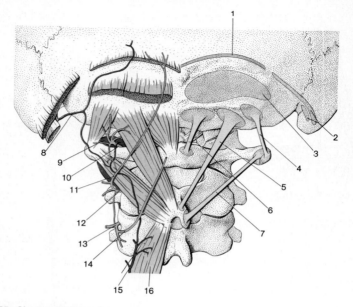

Fig. 187. **Short nuchal muscles**
Arteries and nerves of nape of neck
(Terminal branches of arteries and nerves not shown)

1–3 *Muscle origins or attachment areas* for:
1 Trapezius
2 Splenius capitis and (under it) longissimus capitis
3 Semispinalis capitis
4 Obliquus capitis superior
5 Rectus capitis posterior major
6 Rectus capitis posterior minor and alar ligament
7 Obliquus capitis inferior

8 Occipital artery
9 Vertebral artery
10 Suboccipital nerve (dorsal branch of first cervical nerve)
11 Greater occipital nerve
12 Dorsal ramus of second cervical nerve
13 Dorsal ramus of third cervical nerve
14 Third occipital nerve
15 Deep cervical artery
16 Semispinalis cervicis

Innervation:
☐ Accessory nerve and ventral rami of cervical nerves (II), III and IV
☐ Medial branches of dorsal rami of corresponding spinal nerves
☐ Lateral branches of dorsal rami of corresponding spinal nerves

narrower medial and a fibrous-rich lateral bundle, both of which possess an intermediate tendon (the medial tract sometimes two).

b) Lateral Tract of Erector Spinae

The lateral tract consists of the unisegmental *posterior intertransverse* and *obliquus capitis superior muscles* and the *sacrospinal* and *spinotransversal system* (Fig. **186 b**).

The **posterior cervical intertransverse muscles** (Fig. **186 a**) each pass from the posterior tubercle of a cervicle transverse process to the next following or to the transverse process of the 1st thoracic vertebra. Only the *medial part* belongs to the autochthonous back musculature; the directly adjacent *lateral part* is innervated by the ventral ramus of the corresponding cervical nerve.

The **thoracic intertransverse muscles** are formed as simple muscular bundles usually only between the processes of vertebrae T10–L1.

The **medial lumbar intertransverse muscles** connect the accessory process with the mamillary process of the following lumbar vertebra (Fig. **186 a**).

The medial and lateral lumbar intertransverse muscles situated most caudally pass almost horizontally from the iliac tuberosity of the ilium in a ventral direction to the accessory and costal processes of L5. Both muscles counteract a sliding off of L5 anteriorly and secure the sacroiliac joint.

Sacrospinal System

The sacrospinal muscle system forms the main part of the lateral tract of the autochthonous back musculature. It extends laterally from the region of the vertebral column and at the upper margin of the ilium finds a new surface of origin, in addition to the origin and insertion sites at the ribs. Only the caudal origin of the muscle appears homogeneous. It forms a powerful tendinous plate which is attached at the spines of the lumbar vertebrae, at the dorsal surface of the sacrum and at the dorsomedial portion of the iliac crest and is fused with the thoracolumbar fascia. The muscular part of the system, on the other hand, is separated into the *lateral iliocostalis* and the *medial longissimus* (Fig. **185**). The lateral cutaneous rami of the dorsal branches of the thoracic nerves traverse between the two muscle bundles.

The **iliocostalis** (Fig. **186 b**) can be differentiated more or less distinctly into a lumbar, a thoracic and a cervical segment. In principle, the points of origin arise medially, whereas the attachment bundles are attached laterally. The lateral displacement of origins (iliac crest, ribs) and insertions (costal processes, ribs, posterior tubercle of transverse processes of cervical vertebrae = most laterally situated segment of the respective rib rudiments) increases the lever force of the muscle for lateral bending.

The *iliocostalis lumborum*, which arises at the tendinous plate described above and at the iliac crest (here fleshy), inserts at the angles of the 6th (to 9th) caudal ribs. Medial to this attachment site, the slips of origin of the *iliocostalis thoracis* arise, which insert at the costal angles of ribs I–VII(VI). The bundles of origin of the *iliocostalis cervicis* comes from the angles of ribs 3(4) to 7 and insert at the posterior tubercles of cervical vertebral processes 3(4) to 6.

The **longissimus** (Fig. **186 b**) extends from the sacrum to the occiput, yet is grouped in the official nomenclature as lumbar and thoracic parts of the *longissimus thoracis*, to which the *longissimus cervicis* and *longissimus capitis* are attached cranially. The muscle lies medial to the iliocostalis and has been displaced in the adult for the most part over the transversospinal muscles of the medial tract. Just as in the case of the iliocostalis, the bundles of origin come from the medial side, and the insertion slips go laterally (e.g. origin from the common tendinous plate, insertion at the ribs; origin from the transverse processes of the upper thoracic vertebrae, insertion at the rib homologs of the cervical vertebrae = posterior tubercle of the transverse processes). The longissimus, however, is more complicated in structure than the iliocostalis. In the thoracolumbar part, additional medial insertions (transverse processes of the thoracic vertebrae, accessory processes of the lumbar vertebrae) and accessory medial bundles of origin (transverse processes of thoracic vertebrae) are still added. The muscle tracts are attached, therefore, both at the ribs and at the vertebral column. The cephalic part of the longissimus inserts far lateral to the mastoid process and thus can effect rotary movements of the head toward the same side.

The *longissimus thoracis* arises together with the iliocostalis lumborum by means of a strong tendinous plate from the lumbar spines, the sacrum, the posterior margin of the ilium and the posterior sacroiliac ligaments. So-called accessory points of origin come from the transverse processes of the 6 caudal thoracic vertebrae and the mamillary process of the first two lumbar vertebrae. In the thoracic region the medial insertion takes place at the transverse processes of all thoracic vertebrae, and the lateral insertion is medial to the costal angles of ribs 2–12. In the lumbar portion of the vertebral column, the fiber bundles insert at the corresponding homolog, the medial bundles at the accessory process of lumbar vertebrae I to IV (as well as at the mamillary process of L5), and the lateral insertion slips at the costal processes of L1–4 (as well as at the deep layer of the thoracodorsal fascia).

The *longissimus cervicis* arises from the transverse processes of the upper 6 thoracic vertebrae and usually obtains additional origin bundles from the root of the transverse processes of C3–6(7). The tendons of insertion attach at the posterior tubercles of the transverse processes of C2–5.

The *longissimus capitis* arises – medial to the slips of origin of the cervical portion of the longissimus – from the transverse processes of vertebrae C3–T3. Its fibers form a slender, more sagittally placed muscle bundle, which attaches to the mastoid process of the temporal bone (Fig. **187**).

Spinotransverse System

This muscular system consists only of the **splenius**, which covers and winds around the cranial segment of the erector spinae as a broad muscular aponeurosis. It arises in the middle of the body at the ligamentum nuchae and the spines of the upper thoracic vertebrae, yet is associated with the lateral tract of the autochthonous back musculature since it is innervated by lateral twigs of the dorsal branches of the spinal nerves. The muscle is separated in its course and attachment, less distinctly at its origin, into the *splenius capitis* and *splenius cervicis*. The muscular tracts of both parts of the muscle pass from medial to lateral (the neck part to the transverse processes of the upper cervical vertebrae, the head part to the mastoid process and to the squama of the occipital bone) and turn toward the same side.

The *splenius capitis* comes from the ligamentum nuchae (from C3) and from the spines of C7 and T1–3 and attaches at the mastoid process and at the superior nuchal line. The *splenius cervicis* arises from the spinous process of T3–5(6) and the supraspinous ligament and curves around the semispinalis capitis and the longissimus capitis dorsolaterally. It inserts with two strong slips at the posterior tubercle of the transverse process of the atlas and axis and with a weak, often absent slip at the posterior tubercle of C3.

c) Levatores Costarum and Anterior Intertransverse Muscles

The so-called rib elevators, the levatores costarum, are innervated (chiefly) by the dorsal branches of the spinal nerves and may thus be legitimately discussed with the autochthonous back muscles. The anterior intertransverse muscles, on the other hand, as serial homologs of the intercostal muscles, are of ventral origin. Since they act – by means of the vertebral arch joints – exclusively on the cervical or lumbar vertebral column, they are – notwithstanding their genetic relation – described here.

The **levatores costarum** (Fig. **186 b**) are supplied by a lateral twig of the lateral rami of the dorsal branches of the spinal nerves and are regarded as derivatives of the lateral tract. They pass downward from the transverse processes of the last cervical and upper 11 thoracic vertebrae to the next or second next rib.

The *levatores costarum*, however, can also contain material from the external intercostal muscles, as the supplementary innervation from the intercostal nerves observable at various points makes clear. For a long time, these muscles were regarded as derivatives of the external intercostal muscles.

The *short levatores costarum* are unisegmental and insert medial to the costal angle of the following caudal rib. The *long levatores costarum* pass more steeply downwards and skip over a rib. They are usually found only in the cranial and caudal portions of the thorax.

The function of the small, thick muscle tracts is not yet clearly defined. They probably are not so much rib elevators as extensors and lateral benders of the vertebral column.

The **anterior intertransverse muscles** are separated from the posterior intertransverse muscles by the ventral ramus of the corresponding spinal nerve which also innervates them. Like all short muscles of the vertebral column, they regulate and synchronize movements in the respective vertebral arch joints when movements of the total or partial vertebral column are elicited by the long tracts of the back musculature. In the case of unilateral contraction, they cooperate in the lateral flexion of the vertebral column.

The *anterior cervical intertransverse muscles* unite the anterior tubercles of two cervical transverse processes. The muscle can be absent between the atlas and axis.

The *lateral lumbar intertransverse muscles* spread out with a ventral portion between the costal processes of two consecutive lumbar vertebrae and a dorsal portion between the accessory and costal processes. The muscle located farthest caudad unites the costal process of the 5th lumbar vertebra with the iliac tuberosity ($\rightarrow$ p. 489).

d) Short Nuchal Muscles

Four (paired) independent, unisegmental muscles which are bounded by fascia, *short* or *deep nuchal muscles* (Fig. **187**), lie deep between the axis and occiput near the bone. They cooperate in the fine adjustment of head posture and in differentiated head movements.

The organization of this musculature occurred in phylogenesis parallel to the organization of the joints of the head, which in man led to 6 isolated articular compartments.

Innervation: Of the short nuchal muscles, the obliquus capitis inferior and the two straight head muscles (recti capitis posterior major and minor) are innervated by medial branches of the dorsal ramus of the 1st and 2nd cervical nerves and are therefore parts of the medial muscle bundle. The obliquus capitis superior, supplied by lateral twigs from the dorsal ramus of the 1st cervical nerve, belongs to the lateral tract.

The **rectus capitis posterior major** passes laterally from the spine of the axis cranial to the middle third of the inferior nuchal line.

The short **rectus capitis posterior minor** (the most cranially-situated interspinal muscle) arises at the posterior tubercle of the atlas and inserts medial to the previously-mentioned muscle below the inferior nuchal line.

The **obliquus capitis superior**, the most cranially-situated posterior intertransverse muscle, passes steeply upward from the dorsal bar of the transverse process of the atlas to the inferior nuchal line and attaches lateral and somewhat above the insertion of the rectus capitis posterior major.

The **obliquus capitis inferior** arises at the spinous process of the axis and attaches at the transverse process of the atlas. It forms the lower margin of a triangular fossa (medial border: rectus capitis posterior major; lateral border: obliquus capitis superior), in the depth of which there can be found the vertebral artery and dorsal ramus of the 1st cervical nerve (=suboccipital nerve), which supplies the 4 deep nuchal muscles.

The *rectus capitis lateralis* belongs to the anterior cervical intertransverse muscles, which extend between the anterior tubercles of two adjacent cervical vertebrae. The *rectus capitis anterior* is a prevertebral cervical muscle. Both are thus derivatives of the ventrolateral trunk musculature. However, they should also be discussed here since they also act on the atlanto-occipital joint and recently have been grouped as suboccipital muscles with the 4 deep nuchal muscles mentioned above.

The **rectus capitis lateralis** arises as a typical anterior cervical intertransverse muscle from the anterior tubercle of the transverse process of the atlas, passes to the occiput, and inserts at the jugular process, which sometimes projects lateral to the condyle as the paramastoid process.

The **rectus capitis anterior** takes its origin at the lateral mass of the atlas and at the root of the transverse process; it attaches at the basilar part of the occipital bone, lateral to the pharyngeal tubercle.

Innervation of the rectus capitis lateralis and rectus capitis anterior: from the ventral ramus of cervical nerves I and II.

4. Action of the Autochthonous Back Musculature on the Vertebral Column and Joints of the Head

a) Action of Erector Spinae on the Vertebral Column

In movements of the vertebral column, the different systems of autochthonous back muscles on both sides cooperate as synergists and antagonists. The contraction, however, can remain limited to definite segments of the long muscular tracts and to a certain number of short muscles so that, besides movements of the total vertebral column, movements in individual regions are also possible.

Dorsal flexion takes place through bilateral contraction of the erector spinae and leads to an extension of the vertebral column; the decrease in tonus results in *ventral flexion* when the body is held erect.

Lateral flexion is produced by the unilateral contraction of the erector spinae. For a lateral movement of the trunk, the lateral tract of the autochthonous back musculature possesses an especially favorable lever action. The back muscles of the opposite side inhibit and control this movement by a corresponding reduction of their tension. Lateral bending can be combined with a rotary movement.

Rotation toward the opposite side is effected by the muscles of the transversospinal system. The rotatores muscles have an especially favorable potential for action during this process since they course only slightly inclined against the axis of rotation. The splenius turns toward the same side. Its spinotransversely-coursing fibers form a muscular chain, for example, with the transversospinal muscle tracts of the other side, which is continued ventrally into the external abdominal oblique muscle. (The oblique abdominal muscles play an essential part in the rotation of the trunk.) Thus, there arises on each side of the body a muscular tract which encircles the trunk in a helical line and reaches from the head to the margin of the pelvis.

The *maintenance of the characteristic form of the vertebral column* in the erect body position is likewise ensured to an essential degree by the autochthonous musculature of the back. (The ligamentous apparatus alone does not suffice for this task.) It forms a complicated bracing system, the individual tracts of which are interdependent. The fact that each transverse process is connected by means of muscles tracts with a series of spinous processes and, conversely, that each spinous process is united with several transverse processes already indicates the extent and strength of this bracing.

b) Action of Muscles on the Joints of the Head

Extensive and (or) powerful head movements are produced by the contraction of the long muscles inserting at the head. The suboccipital muscles, whose action is confined to the joints of the head, make small, precisely synchronized movements of the head possible, independent of the position of the vertebral column.

The recti capitis posteriores of both sides are essentially involved in the *nodding of the head* as a finely graduated dorsal flexion of the head. The long nuchal muscles (semispinalis capitis, longissimus capitis, splenius capitis) are primarily responsible for holding the head upright and strong dorsal flexion in association with the sternocleidomastoid (the muscles of both sides of the body). The rectus capitis anterior helps to bend the head forward when both sides contract. Its torque, however, in comparison with the action of the longus capitis and the hyoid muscles, is slight (in an upright position the influence of gravity suffices when the nuchal muscles are relaxed).

The *lateral bending of the head* is carried out as a fine movement by the short nuchal muscles of one side, especially the rectus capitis lateralis. Powerful lateral movements are caused particularly by the sternocleidomastoid, the splenius capitis and the longissimus capitis. The rotary component of the splenius and longissimus muscles is counteracted in the process by the opposing rotary action of the sternocleidomastoid.

Rotary movements of the head are carried out by the rectus capitis posterior major and obliquus capitis inferior. They pass over the atlantoaxial joint and are able to rotate the atlas and, with it, also the head toward the same side. A stronger rotary movement is accomplished by the longissimus capitis and splenius capitis (toward the same side), as well as the sternocleidomastoid and the part of the trapezius originating from the occiput (toward the opposite side). The tendency of these muscles to bring about a simultaneous lateral bending of the head is counteracted by the nuchal muscles of the other side.

5. Blood Vessels and Nerves of the Dorsal Body Wall

The **blood vessels and nerves of the dorsal body wall** are arranged according to a simple basic pattern. The *vascular supply* of the autochthonous back muscles and the skin is provided by the *dorsal branches of the segmental vessels*, and the *innervation* takes place via *dorsal rami of the spinal nerves*. The cranial portion of the dorsal body wall, the nuchal region, exhibits peculiarities with regard to its vascular and nervous supply.

The spinohumeral and spinocostal muscles displaced onto the back are supplied by ventral branches of the spinal nerves, the trapezius by the accessory nerve. The blood vessels of the limb muscles pushed onto the back are branches of the limb vessels (subclavian and axillary arteries and veins).

Arteries. The *dorsal branches* arise in the thoracic and lumbar portions of the dorsal body wall from the segmental *posterior intercostal arteries* (Figs. **25** and **26**), the *subcostal artery* and from the *lumbar arteries* (Fig. **185**). Corresponding dorsal branches arise at the neck from the *deep cervical artery* and in the sacral region from the *lateral sacral artery* (Fig. **126**).

The *dorsal branches* dispatch a *spinal branch* through the intervertebral foramen to the wall and contents of the vertebral canal, ramify in the autochthonous back musculature, and divide into a *medial cutaneous* and a *lateral cutaneous branch* (Fig. **189**).

The **veins** accompany the arterial branches; the dorsal branches transport blood from the back musculature and skin of the back and empty into the segmental veins of the dorsal body wall (posterior intercostal and lumbar veins).

Intervertebral veins, which communicate with the internal venous plexus of the vertebrae and receive *spinal branches* from the spinal cord and its membranes, empty into the vertebral vein in the neck region and into dorsal branches of the segmental veins in the thoracic and lumbar regions.

Nerves. The *dorsal ramus* of each spinal nerve gives off (through the intervertebral foramen) a *meningeal branch* to the wall of the vertebral canal and to the dura, divides into a medial and lateral branch (to the medial and lateral tracts of the autochthonous muscles of the back), and ends (in principle) in the skin as *medial cutaneous* and *lateral cutaneous branches* (Figs. **185** and **189**).

Vessels and nerves of the back of the neck. The back of the neck represents the cranial portion of the back which lies above the line: acromion – spinous process of the 7th cervical vertebral – acromion and which extends to the external occipital protuberance and to the superior nuchal line (lateral border: line from the mastoid process to the acromion).

The nuchal region no longer exhibits the metameric arrangement of the *blood vessels* so clearly as the dorsal trunk wall. The segmental arteries arise from the *vertebral* and *deep cervical arteries*. Moreover, branches of the *occipital, transverse cervical, superficial cervical* and *ascending cervical arteries* pass to the nuchal musculature, as well as partly to the skin.

Variations from the typical branching pattern of the *branches of the dorsal spinal nerves* described for the back are to be observed in cervical nerves I–III. In addition, the *lesser occipital nerve*, still a derivative of the ventral branches of the spinal nerve, passes from the cervical plexus to the skin of the nuchal region and the occiput.

Arteries. The **vertebral artery** arises from the convex side of the vascular arch as the 1st branch of the subclavian artery (Fig. **193**), enters the foramen transversarium of the 6th cervical vertebra, and passes craniad through the foramina of the remaining cervical transverse processes (Fig. **172**). At the atlas it courses medially in the sulcus of the vertebral artery behind the lateral mass, pierces the posterior atlanto-occipital membrane, the dura, and the arachnoid into the subarachnoid space, and arrives in the cranial cavity via the foramen magnum. Both vertebral arteries unite on the clivus at the level of the posterior margin of the pons into the unpaired *basilar artery*.

The *vertebral artery* gives off extracranial *spinal branches* (through the intervertebral foramen to the spinal nerves and spinal ganglia) and *muscular branches* (to the deep cervical muscles). At the anterior and posterior circumference of the foramen magnum, it dispatches a *meningeal branch* (*anterior, posterior*) both to the dura mater and to the diploë of the posterior cranial fossa respectively. From the *intracranial part*, the *posterior spinal artery* (posterior longitudinal trunk in, or in the vicinity of, the dorsolateral sulcus of the spinal cord with tributaries from the spinal branches) and the *anterior spinal artery* (after union with the vessel of the same name on the opposite side, an unpaired longitudinal trunk in the medial ventral fissure of the spinal cord) pass to the spinal cord in the vertebral canal as recurrent vessels. Numerous anastomoses exist between the two dorsal longitudinal trunks and the anterior spinal artery.

If the vertebral artery is damaged, the site of the injury must always be ligated proximally and distally because of the intracranial and the extracranial connections of the right and left vertebral arteries (basilar artery, spinal arteries).

The **deep cervical artery** originates from the costocervical trunk (Fig. **193**). It courses between the transverse processes of the 7th cervical and the 1st thoracic vertebra to the semispinalis capitis and to the deep nuchal muscles (Fig. **187**). It gives off *spinal branches* to the vertebral canal.

The **occipital artery** (from the external carotid) passes below the posterior belly of the digastric to the sulcus of the occipital artery at the inner side of the mastoid process (Fig. **187**) and courses beneath the splenius capitis to the occiput. It perforates the trapezius (or reaches the surface at its lateral margin) and ramifies at the scalp (*occipital branches*, Fig. **189**), whereby it anastomoses with branches of the superficial temporal and posterior auricular arteries.

The occipital artery sends branches to the sternocleidomastoid and to the nuchal muscles, among others. It gives off a *mastoid branch* (through the mastoid foramen) to the diploë and to the dura mater of the posterior cranial fossa, as well as a variable *auricular branch* to the posterior surface of the pinna.

Veins. The blood from the nuchal region is transported into the external jugular vein by superficial veins and flows off into the brachiocephalic vein via two strong veins in the depth of the back of the neck: the *vertebral* and *deep cervical veins*. Both veins anastomose with the *occipital vein* and the *suboccipital venous plexus* (venous network between the atlas and occiput connected by emissary veins with the confluens of the sinuses and the sigmoid sinus in the cranial cavity).

The **vertebral vein** accompanies the vertebral artery (as a plexus of communicating veins) and receives segmental tributaries (intervertebral veins) from the vertebral canal (Fig. **184**). It exits from the 6th (more rarely the 7th) foramen of the transverse process and receives the deep cervical vein usually in front of its entry into the brachiocephalic vein.

The **deep cervical vein** courses with the artery of the same name beneath the semispinalis capitis and carries blood from the posterior external vertebral venous plexus (Fig. **184**).

Nerves (Fig. **187**). The 1st cervical nerve generally contains only motor fibers. Its dorsal ramus is designated as the **suboccipital nerve**. It passes in the suboccipital triangle below the vertebral artery across the posterior arch of the atlas and gives off branches to the short nuchal muscles, the longissimus capitis and the semispinalis capitis.

The very large dorsal ramus of the 2nd cervical nerve known as the **greater occipital nerve** is predominantly sensory. Accompanied by branches of the occipital artery, its twigs supply an extensive area of skin at the back of the head which can reach up to the crown.

The greater occipital nerve bends around the obliquus capitis inferior, penetrates the semispinalis capitis (motor fibers to the head part of the long back muscles), and passes through the tendon of origin of the trapezius – or below the lateral margin of the muscle – into the subcutaneous tissue somewhat beneath the superior nuchal line.

The dorsal ramus of cervical nerve III can likewise send a somewhat stronger cutaneous branch, the *third* (*tertius*) *occipital nerve*, to the occiput, where it communicates with the greater occipital nerve.

Suboccipital puncture. A puncture needle can be inserted between the occipital bone and the posterior arch of the atlas through the posterior atlanto-occipital membrane (palpable with some slight resistance at this site), the dura, and the arachnoid into the subarachnoid space, which is enlarged here to form the cerebellomedullary cistern. By this procedure, cerebrospinal fluid can be removed or air can be injected for the filling of the ventricular system (via the openings of the 4th ventricle). In order to avoid damaging the vertebral artery, the puncture must be made as close to the median plane as possible.

B. Surface Anatomy of the Back

1. Surface Relief of the Back and Palpable Bony Points

On the dorsal side of the back with the body held upright, the *dorsal furrow* can be recognized in the midline passing downward from the spinous process of C7 to the sacrum (Fig. **188**). The subcutaneous connective tissue here is fixed at the spinous processes, the skin therefore being drawn inward, whereas on both sides of this furrow the longitudinal swelling of the erector spinae is evident. In the sacral region, the furrow is broadened into the *sacral triangle*. The base of this triangular recess is formed by a line uniting the two posterior superior iliac spines (in the region of these spines the skin is fixed to the periosteum). The gluteus maximus bulges on both sides of the lateral margins of this triangle, the apex of which is directed caudally and is continued into the *gluteal cleft*. Especially in women, the skin over the 5th lumbar vertebra is perceptibly drawn in so that on the whole a diamond-shaped depression, *Michaelis's rhomboid*, is formed. (The superior, lateral boundary of this rhomboid forms the transition between the tendinous and fleshy parts of the erector spinae).

In the normal female pelvis, the vertical diameter of the rhomboid is only a little greater than the horizontal (= distance of both sacroiliac joints).

From the form of the rhomboid, the obstetrician can draw conclusions on the width of the lesser pelvis or can recognize a deformation.

Palpable bony points (Fig. **188**). In the midline, the external occipital protuberance and the vertebral spines from C7(6) downward are distinctly palpable, although strong forward flexion of the trunk is required at the level of the thoracic and lumbar vertebral columns. In this body position, moderate scolioses are recognizable. Since the spine of the scapula and the acromion can be palpated through the skin, the position and mobility of the shoulder blade can be estimated.

In slender, powerfully-built men, the marginal contours of the superficial back muscles (especially the latissimus dorsi, trapezius) and tendon sheath of the trapezius can be visible.

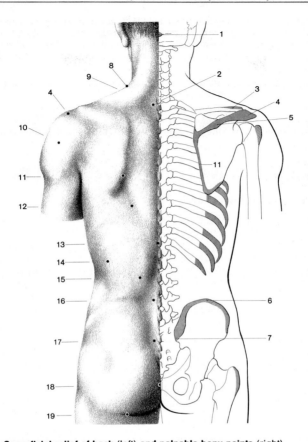

Fig. 188. **Superficial relief of back** (left) **and palpable bony points** (right)

1 External occipital protuberance
2 Spinous process of
   seventh cervical vertebra
3 Clavicle
4 Acromion
5 Spine of scapula
6 Iliac crest
7 Posterior superior iliac spine
8 Cranial marginal outline of trapezius
9 Rhomboidal tendon sheath of trapezius
10 Bulge of deltoid
11 Medial marginal outline of scapula
12 Caudal marginal outline of trapezius
13 Posterior median furrow
14 Marginal outline of latissimus dorsi
15 Longitudinal bulge of erector spinae
16 Michaelis's rhomboid
17 Sacral triangle
18 Gluteal cleft
19 Gluteal furrow

The skin of the back is quite firm, yet easily movable in general owing to the loose subcutaneous tissue. In the nuchal region, where the subcutaneous tissue is very firm and fat lobules are compartmentalized by connective tissue trabeculae into individual units of variable dimensions, a transverse swelling arises when the head is flexed dorsally.

Inflammatory processes in the nuchal region (furuncle, carbuncle) consequently produce very painful tensions.

The *crease lines* of the skin are approximately transverse in the nuchal region, above the scapula, and in the lumbar region. In the area of the dorsal trunk wall situated between them, they are slightly oblique, sloping downward from medial to lateral (Fig. **71**).

2. Cutaneous Vessels and Nerves of the Back

a) Cutaneous Arteries and Veins

The **cutaneous arteries** of the back (Fig. **189**) are terminal branches of the *segmental dorsal branches*. They arise in the cervical region from the deep cervical artery, in the dorsal trunk wall from the posterior and lumbar intercostal arteries, and in the sacral region from the lateral sacral artery. Each dorsal branch ramifies (in principle) into two main branches (Fig. **26**). The *medial cutaneous branch* passes into the subcutaneous tissue beside the series of spinous processes; the *lateral cutaneous branch* arrives at the subcutaneous tissue lateral to the erector spinae (Fig. **185**).

In the scapular region, cutaneous branches of the transverse cervical and suprascapular arteries replace the lateral cutaneous branches missing here.

Cutaneous veins accompany the corresponding arterial branches and communicate via dorsal branches with the posterior external vertebral venous plexus and the

1 Third occipital nerve
2 Greater occipital nerve
3 Posterior ramus of great auricular nerve
4 Lesser occipital nerve
5 Medial cutaneous branches of dorsal rami of cervical nerves
6 Lateral supraclavicular nerves
7 Cutaneous branches of dorsal rami of thoracic nerves
8 Dorsal branches of lateral cutaneous rami of intercostal nerves
9 Lateral cutaneous branch of iliohypogastric nerve
10 Superior clunial nerves
11 Middle clunial nerves
12 Occipital branches of occipital artery and vein
13 Cutaneous branches of deep cervical artery and vein
14 Cutaneous branches of superficial cervical artery
15 Acromial network (inflow and outflow via suprascapular and thoraco-acromial arteries and veins)
16 Cutaneous branches of suprascapular and circumflex scapular arteries and veins
17 Cutaneous branches from dorsal branches of posterior intercostal arteries and veins
18 Subcutaneous venous network of back (incompletely shown)
19 Dorsal branches of lateral cutaneous branches of posterior intercostal arteries and veins
20 Dorsal branches of lateral cutaneous branches of lumbar artery and vein
21 Lateral cutaneous branches of dorsal branches of lumbar arteries and veins
22 Cutaneous branches of superior gluteal artery and vein
23 Cutaneous branches of "dorsal branches" of lateral sacral arteries and veins

▶

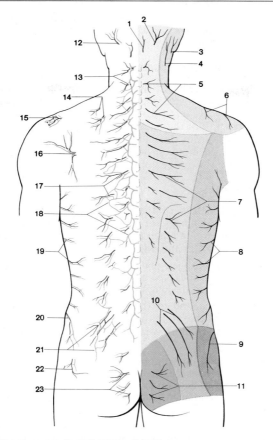

Fig. 189. **Cutaneous vessels and nerves of back**
Schematic representation of cutaneous arteries and veins (left side) and cutaneous
nerves and anatomical cutaneous fields (right side)
(· · · Boundary line between supply regions of medial and lateral cutaneous branches of
dorsal rami of thoracic nerves).
☐ Dorsal rami of cervical nerves
☐ Dorsal rami of thoracic nerves
☐ Dorsal rami of lumbar nerves
☐ Dorsal rami of sacral nerves
☐ Ventral rami of cervical nerves (cervical plexus)
☐ Ventral rami of thoracic nerves (intercostal nerves)
☐ Ventral rami of lumbar nerves (lumbar plexus)

segmental veins. Just as in the anterior trunk wall, a wide-meshed *subcutaneous venous network* is developed upon the fascia; it communicates with branches of the segmental veins (Fig. **189**).

b) Superficial Lymphatic Tracts

Lymphatic drainage (Fig. **210**) of the superior nuchal region takes place (partly via *occipital lymph nodes* located at the level of the superior nuchal line) to the deep cervical lymph nodes. From the inferior nuchal region and the thoracic portion of the back, the lymph is carried to the axillary lymph nodes, whereas from the caudal part of the dorsal trunk wall, it travels to the superficial inguinal lymph nodes. The lymphatic drainage pathways, moreover, also go beyond the midline.

c) Cutaneous Nerves

The **innervation** of the skin of the back takes place by the terminal branches of the *dorsal rami of the spinal nerves, medial cutaneous* and *lateral cutaneous rami*, which reach the subcutaneous tissue together with the blood vessels (Figs. **185** and **189**).

The medial twigs course obliquely above the multifidus and arrive at the sub-cutaneous tissue near the spinous processes. The lateral branches pass through the muscle layer usually between the longissimus and iliocostalis.

In the back of the neck and in the region of the scapula, the lateral cutaneous branches are absent; in the lower part of the back, on the other hand, the medial rami are more weakly developed or are not demonstrable in dissection.

The lateral branches of the dorsal rami of the three cranial lumbar and sacral nerves pass as *superior* and *middle clunial nerves* to the skin of the buttocks (Fig. **168 b**). The dorsal ramus of both caudal lumbar and sacral nerves, as well as the coccygeal nerve possesses no lateral cutaneous branches.

Segmental relations of the skin (Fig. **57 b**). Each dorsal ramus of a spinal nerve supplies with its cutaneous branches a band-shaped area of the skin, which is continued as the trunk wall – along a medial convex line proceeding through the inferior angle of the scapula – with a break in the supply region of the corresponding ventral ramus. At the neck and on the shoulder, the innervation areas of the branches of the cervical plexus no longer supplied segmentally are continued ventrally. The segmentally-innervated cutaneous regions follow one another from cranial to caudal (from C2–Co 1). Of course, each of these skin areas is innervated uni-segmentally with regard to pain sensation, whereas the fibers for pressure, touch, etc. of the respective segmental nerves overlap to neighboring segments.

Head's zones. The cutaneous regions innervated unisegmentally with regard to pain sensation correspond to Head's zones. Increased sensitivity to pain (hyperalgia) appearing there can indicate the disorder of an internal organ to the physician. A hyperalgia in zones T7 and T8 at the left side of the vertebral column, for example, points to a gastric ulcer.

C. Ventral Trunk Wall

1. Thoracic Wall

The **skeleton of the thoracic wall** (Fig. **193**) consists dorsally of the *thoracic vertebral column*, laterally and ventrally of 12 *ribs* (*costae*) attaching ventrally on each side of the *breast bone*, the *sternum*. These skeletal elements together form the *thorax*. The *intercostal spaces* are closed and braced by the *intercostal muscles*.

On this *deep layer*, which still exhibits the metameric organization of the body wall, muscles spread out from the region of the back, abdomen and upper limb. They form the *middle layer* of the throacic wall and are discussed with the corresponding groups of muscles.

In the *superficial layer*, which is formed by the skin, subcutaneous tissue and the *thoracic fascia* (*pectoral fascia*), the *mammary glands* (seen topographically) have developed as organs of the subcutaneous tissue.

a) Skeletal Elements of the Thorax

The *ribs* consist of a long, bony dorsal segment, the *costal bone*, which articulates with the thoracic vertebrae, and a short, cartilaginous ventral section, the *costal cartilage*.

Ribs I–VII (rarely VIII) reach the sternum directly as *true ribs*. Ribs VIII–XII are designated as *false ribs*. The 8th, 9th and 10th ribs communicate only indirectly with the sternum; the ends of their costal cartilages adjoin the cartilage of the next higher rib and form the *rib arch* (*costal arch*). Ribs XI and XII (also rib X in about 70% of the cases) end freely and are movable in the thoracic wall, embedded in the thoracic musculature: *floating ribs*.

Ribs I and XII are the shortest (the latter can vary considerably in length), and the 7th is the longest. The costal cartilages increase in length from the 1st to the 7th ribs, then become shorter again.

Whereas the cartilage of ribs I–III continues approximately in the direction of the bony ribs (the first costal cartilage is extremely short), the following costal cartilages exhibit an angulation of the ventral portion cranially which increases more strongly up to the 10th rib: *costal cartilage angle*. The site of the angle always lies within the cartilage piece, never at the cartilage-bone border.

Frequently, a transverse articular connection (*interchondral joint*) exists between the cartilages of the 6th and 7th ribs (more rarely between the 5th and 6th, or 7th and 8th).

Ribs II–IX show a threefold curvature. The *curvature surface* produces the lateral bulging of the thorax. Owing to the *curvature edge*, the ventral end of the rib is lower than the vertebral end by up to 2 vertebrae. Through the *torsion* of the ribs around their longitudinal axes, the external surface of the ribs – especially pronounced in the case of the upper ribs – faces at the vertebral end somewhat caudad, at the ventral end slightly craniad.

The 1st rib is strongly flattened in a craniocaudal plane. Surface curvature and torsion are absent, whereas the marginal curvature is very pronounced and causes the arched form of the rib. In the 12th rib there is a surface curvature, but the marginal curvature is very slight and torsion is absent.

The *bony ribs* (Fig. **190**) are distinguished by:
- the *head of the rib*, which articulates with the thoracic vertebrae;
- the *neck of the rib*, the upper margin of which can be tapered off into the *crest of the neck*; and
- the *body of the rib*, which begins at the *costal tubercle* and turns back ventrally at the *costal angle*.

At ribs 2–10(11), the *articular surface of their heads* (Figs. **190 a, c** and **195**) is divided by a *ridge* into two facets (articulation with the corresponding costal foveae of two vertebrae). The neck is attached to the head of the rib dorsolaterally (at the 1st rib laterally). The rib body continues first in the direction of the neck and turns back ventrally only at the rib angle, which lies more and more laterally in the ribs that follow caudally. In the 1st rib, the rib angle coincides with the costal tubercle. In ribs 1–10, this tubercle bears the cartilage-covered *articular facet* for articulation with the transverse process of the thoracic vertebrae, whereas at ribs 11 and 12, it is only weakly developed.

With respect to the first 10 ribs, the inner surface of the body – up to about the level of the axillary line – is hollowed out along the lower margin by the *costal groove*, in which the intercostal vessels take their course. The lower margin of the body of the ribs is tapered off accordingly in the region near the vertebrae.

Above the surface of the 1st rib, the clavicular vessels course in two shallow grooves, the *groove for the subclavian artery* (dorsolateral) and the *groove for the subclavian vein* (ventromedial). Between the two grooves there is an elevation, the *scalene tubercle*, for the attachment of the scalenus anterior muscle and dorsal to it a roughness for the insertion of the scalenus medius. The external surfaces of ribs 2–9 – near the bone-cartilage border – each bear a slight elevation for the slips of origin of the serratus anterior, which is particularly distinct at the 2nd rib and termed there the *tuberosity for the serratus anterior*.

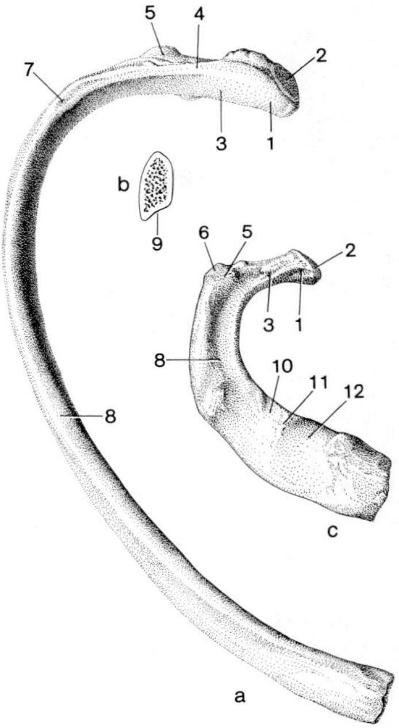

Fig. 190. **Bony ribs**
a Seventh rib, cranial view
b Seventh rib, cross section at costal
  angle
c First rib, cranial view
1 Head of rib
2 Articular surface of head of rib
3 Neck of rib
4 Crest of neck
5 Costal tubercle
6 Articular surface of tubercle
7 Costal angle
8 Body of rib
9 Costal groove
10 Groove for subclavian artery
11 Tubercle for scalenus anterior
12 Groove for subclavian vein

According to most authors, supernumerary ribs (cervical ribs, lumbar ribs) are much more frequent (about 6%) than a decrease in the number of ribs. Cervical ribs which are completely developed to any extent seem to occur only somewhat less than 1% of the European population. In this case, brachial vessels and the brachial plexus cross the cervical rib and can be affected (e.g. when carrying a heavy backpack).

The **sternum** (Figs. **191** and **193**) in the adult consists of three bony parts:
– the short, broad *manubrium*;
– the long, narrow *body*; and
– the *xiphoid process*, which usually has cartilaginous ends and is often bifid or perforated.

The manubrium and body communicate by the *manubriosternal synchondrosis*, the body and xiphoid process by the *xiphosternal synchondrosis* (Fig. **194**).

In the connective tissue of the superior cartilaginous joint (fibrocartilaginous disc with the layer of hyaline cartilage at the bony border), a transverse fissure filled with synovial fluid appears in over 30% of the

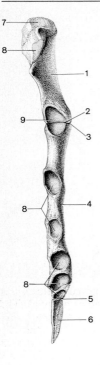

Fig. 191. **Sternum**, view from right side
1 Manubrium of sternum
2 Manubriosternal synchondrosis
  (symphysis)
3 Sternal angle
4 Body of sternum
5 Xiphosternal synchondrosis
6 Xiphoid process
7 Clavicular notch
8 Costal notches
9 Costal notch II

cases. Termed the *manubriosternal symphysis*, it is ossified in 10% of the cases at 30 years of age. The xiphosternal synchondrosis is also transformed into a synostosis, as a rule, after the age of 40.

The manubrium possesses an indentation on its cranial margin, the *jugular notch*, which is palpable through the skin. A laterally-situated, paired indentation, the *clavicular notch*, serves for articulation with the clavicle. The *costal notches* (for $1\frac{1}{2}$ ribs at the manubrium, $5\frac{1}{2}$ ribs at the body) receive the 7 sternal ribs, of which the 1st is connected by a synchondrosis, whereas the remaining ribs articulate with the sternum. The manubrium and body are frequently joined at an angle: *sternal angle*. The 2nd rib can be palpated and identified through the skin lateral to this transverse ridge, whereas the sternal end of the 1st rib is covered by the clavicle. Similar transverse bony ridges are formed between corresponding costal notches of the sternal body by the synostotic fusion of the bony plates of the juvenile sternum, which are developed from several ossific centers.

The spongiosa of the sternum contains red bone marrow which – since the sternum lies directly beneath the skin – can be removed by sternal puncture for diagnostic purposes.

Ossification: The ossification of the *ribs* begins at the end of the 2nd embryonic month and proceeds from the vertebral end toward the sternum. The ventral portion of the rib anlage remains cartilaginous. The costal cartilages can calcify postnatally and are then visible in radiograms. Their calcification begins at the 1st rib, the extent of calcium deposition increasing from cranial to caudal. The calcification can already be far advanced in a 25-year-old or, in exceptional cases, largely lacking even in a 60-year-old. At the cartilage-bone border of the rib, an uncalcified, more radiolucent narrow segment is always preserved (danger of being mistaken for a rib fracture). The epiphyses at the heads of the ribs and the costal tubercles appear at the age of puberty and fuse with the bony ribs usually between the ages of 20 and 25.

The union of the ossific centers originating in the cartilaginous *sternum* (6th to 10th fetal month and in early infancy, Fig. **192 b**) begins around puberty and is concluded around the 25th year. Occasionally, the union is incomplete: sternum multipartitum.

If, during ontogenesis, the complete fusion of the two cartilaginous sternal ridges which form the sternum (Fig. **192 a**) does not occur, holes appear (danger of an injury to the heart in the case of a sternal puncture). In rare cases, a continuous longitudinal fissure is present: congenital sternal fissure.

The **thorax** (Fig. **193**) encloses the *thoracic cavity*. Viewed ventrally, it looks like a truncated cone; the lateral contour resembles an oval. The thoracic cavity is kidney-shaped in cross section. The column of vertebral bodies projects dorsally into the thoracic cavity. The portion of the ribs near the vertebrae course first obliquely dorsolaterally and turn back ventrally at the *costal angle*. Thus, a longitudinal groove, the *pulmonary sulcus*, which broadens caudally, arises on both sides of the column of

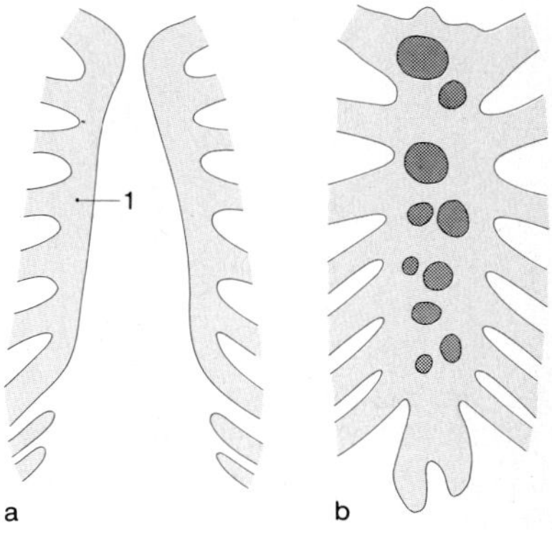

Fig. 192. **Development of sternum**
a Sternal bars (middle of second embryonic month) not yet fused
b Ossific centers in sternum (7th postnatal month)
1 Sternal bar

a   b

vertebral bodies and receives the dorsal part of the lung. The lungs thus lie not only ventrally, but also lateral to the vertebral column (better weight distribution in connection with the upright gait).

The **intercostal spaces** are wider ventrally than dorsally, wider between the upper ribs (especially between ribs 3 and 4, as well as 4 and 5) than

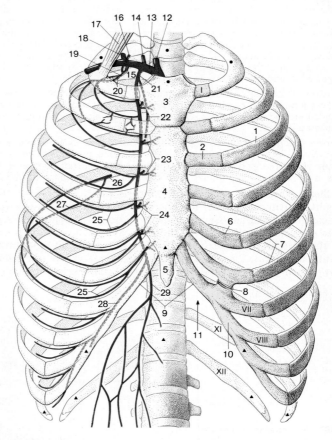

Fig. 193. **Thorax**, ventral view
Internal thoracic artery and branches (right side)

I–VII	True ribs	● Superior thoracic aperture (thoracic inlet)
VIII–XII	False ribs	▲ Inferior throacic aperture (thoracic outlet)
XI, XII	Floating ribs	

between the lower ribs. Intercostal spaces I–V(VI) are closed ventrally by the sternal margin, the following 4(3) spaces by the costal cartilages, whereas the two caudal spaces lack a ventral closure.

The heart-shaped **superior thoracic aperture** (*thoracic inlet*) is bordered by the 1st thoracic vertebra, the 1st pair of ribs, and the upper margin of the manubrium. The inlet plane lies obliquely; the cranial sternal margin lies in a mid-position at the level of the 2nd thoracic vertebra.

The transversely-oval **inferior thoracic aperture** is markedly wider and enlarges from dorsal to ventral. It is surrounded by the 12th thoracic vertebra, the free ends of the 12th and 11th ribs, the rib arches, and the caudal end of the sternum.

In the barrel-shaped thorax of the newborn child, the sagittal diameter is relatively greater than in the adult, yet always absolutely smaller than the transverse diameter. The inclination of the ribs is slight. In the adult they course more steeply downwards. The *angle of the rib arches* (*infrasternal angle*) has decreased, and the inferior thoracic aperture is relatively narrower than in the infant. In females, the thorax is not only absolutely shorter, but also proportionately narrower than in males.

In the elderly, the thorax is flattened, the ribs slope steeply downward, and the rib angle is very acute. Individual variations of the thorax are frequent (narrow-chested and broad-chested individuals).

Scoliosis of the vertebral column is accompanied by corresponding deformations of the ribs and the thorax. In severe cases, a considerable displacement of the thoracic organs occurs, with strong restrictions in the functioning of the heart and lung. The thorax is more or less rigid and fixed in the expiration position.

◀ 1 Bony rib
2 Costal cartilage
3 Manubrium of sternum
4 Body of sternum
5 Xiphoid process
6 Costal cartilage angle
7 Intercostal space
8 Interchondral joint (opened)
9 Infrasternal angle
10 Costal arch
11 Pulmonary sulcus
12 Right common carotid artery
13 Right subclavian artery
14 Vertebral artery
15 Costocervical trunk
16 Deep cervical artery

17 Scalenus anterior
18 Thyrocervical trunk
19 Highest intercostal artery
20 Posterior intercostal arteries I, II
21 Internal thoracic artery
22 Pericardiacophrenic artery
23 Sternal branches
24 Perforating branches
25 Anterior intercostal branches, anastomose with posterior intercostal arteries (26) and collateral branches (27)
26 Posterior intercostal artery
27 Collateral branch
28 Musculophrenic artery
29 Superior epigastric artery, anastomoses with inferior epigastric artery

b) Connections of the Ribs

Sternocostal connections (Fig. **194**). The 1st rib (and sometimes also the lower sternal ribs) are united continuously with the sternum by a synchondrosis, the remaining eight articulating at the *sternocostal joints*. The cavity of the 2nd sternocostal joint is frequently (that of the 3rd or 5th joint more rarely) bisected by an *intra-articular sternocostal ligament*. From the perichondrium of the ribs, the *radiate sternocostal ligaments* spread into the joint capsule, and on the ventral side of the sternum they are interlaced with chiefly intersecting fibrous tracts to form the *sternal membrane*. The corresponding fibrous system on the dorsal side of the sternum is more weakly developed. Longitudinal coursing fibers from the cartilage of the 6th and 7th ribs to the xiphoid process are referred to as the *costoxiphoid ligaments*.

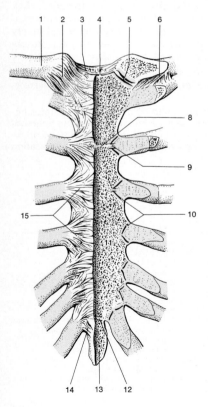

Fig. 194. **Sternum and sternal connections,** ventral view
(Medial clavicular joint and sternocostal unions of left side opened by frontal saw cut)

1 Sternal end of clavicle
2 Anterior sternoclavicular ligament
3 Interclavicular ligament
4 Jugular notch
5 Articular disc in sternoclavicular joint
6 Costoclavicular ligament
7 Manubrium of sternum
8 Manubriosternal synchondrosis
9 Intra-articular sternocostal ligament
10 Sternocostal joints
11 Body of sternum
12 Xiphosternal synchondrosis
13 Xiphoid process
14 Costoxiphoid ligaments
15 Radiate sternocostal ligaments

Costovertebral connections (Figs. **195** and **196**). The ribs articulate with the thoracic vertebral bodies by means of their heads (joints of the heads of the ribs) and with the transverse processes by means of their tubercles, except for the 11th and 12th ribs (costotransverse joints).

In the *joints of the heads of the ribs*, the heads of the 1st, 11th and 12 ribs articulate with the costal facets of the corresponding thoracic vertebral body, whereas the superior and inferior costal facets of two successive thoracic vertebral bodies and the intervertebral disc form the joint socket for ribs 2–10.

In these joints, the articular cavity is divided into two compartments by an *intra-articular ligament* which is fixed at the crest on the head of the rib. On the ventral side, the *radiate costal ligament* strengthens the joint capsule, whose fibers pass from the head of the ribs to the two vertebral bodies and the intervertebral disc.

The *costotransverse joints* connect the costal tubercles of ribs I–X with the transverse process of the corresponding thoracic vertebra.

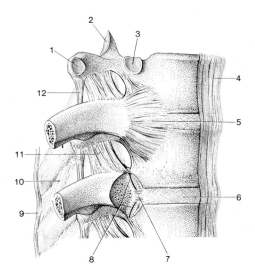

Fig. 195. **Union of vertebrae and ribs**, view from right side and somewhat ventral (Head of lower rib sawed off obliquely, joint of head of rib opened)

1 Costal facet of transverse process	7 Intra-articular ligament of head of rib
2 Superior articular process	8 Articular surface of head of rib
3 Superior costal facet	9 Supraspinous ligament
4 Anterior longitudinal ligament	10 Interspinous ligament
5 Radiate costal ligament	11 Superior costrotransverse ligament
6 Intervertebral disc	12 Intertransverse ligament

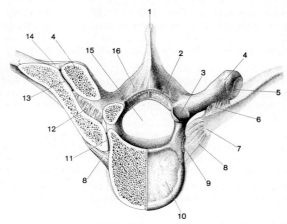

Fig. 196. Connections of sixth thoracic vertebra with right sixth rib and left seventh rib, cranial view

1 Spinous process
2 Ligamentum flavum (severed)
3 Superior articular process
4 Transverse process (right cut surface)
5 Costal facet of transverse process
6 Superior costotransverse ligament
7 Head of rib
8 Radiate costal ligament

9 Superior costal facet
10 Vertebral body (right half cut surface)
11 Joint of head of rib
12 Costotransverse ligament
13 Costotransverse joint
14 Lateral costotransverse ligament
15 Vertebral foramen
16 Lamina of vertebral arch

Ribs II–V(VI) carry out a conical rotation in these joints, whereas the costal tubercles of ribs 7–10 slide dorsally and cranically on the flat articular surfaces of the transverse processes.

The transversely-directed fibrous tracts of the *lateral costotransverse ligament*, which passes from the apeⱼ of the transverse process to the costal tubercle, lie on the posterior surfaces of the joint capsules.

Two additional ligaments play an essential role in guiding movements at the costovertebral joints: the *costotransverse ligament* fills the gap between the neck of the rib and the transverse process (*costotransverse foramen*) and courses from the dorsal side of the neck of the rib to the verntral surface of the corresponding transverse process; the *superior costotransverse ligament* suspends the neck of the rib from the transverse process of the next higher vertebra.

The movements at the costal joints are presented in the discussion of the mechanics of respiratory movements (→ p. 528).

c) Organization and Innervation of the Autochthonous Thoracic Musculature

The **autochthonous thoracic musculature** (Fig. **197**) consists of:
- the *external* and *internal intercostal muscles* in the intercostal spaces.
- the *subcostal muscles*, which are segmented off from the internal intercostal muscles and have expanded secondarily into neighboring segments as unisegmental muscles, and
- the *transversus thoracic* (sternocostalis) muscle, the cranial continuation of the transversus abdominis formed from the myotomes of somites T2–T6.

Innervation of the autochthonous thoracic musculature: intercostal nerves (ventral rami of thoracic nerves).

The *serrati posteriores*, which have pushed dorsally over the autochthonous back musculature, likewise belong genetically to the ventral trunk musculature. Although they have shifted their origin to the vertebral column, they are supplied by ventral rami of the thoracic nerves.

The **external intercostal muscles** (Figs. **185** and **199**) form the superficial layer of the intercostals. They extend into all the intercostal spaces from the costal tubercle to the bone-cartilage border of the ribs. Their fibers course obliquely from behind and above to forward and below (like the fibers of the external abdominal oblique). Between the costal cartilages, they are replaced by fibrous tracts of connective tissue (*external intercostal membrane*).

The **internal intercostal muscles** (Figs. **185** and **199**) are covered in all intercostal spaces by the external intercostal muscles. Their fibers – approximately at right angles to the external intercostal muscles – pass from dorsal caudal to ventral cranial (like the fibers of the internal abdominal oblique, which are attached caudally without a sharp border). Ventrally, the internal intercostals extend to the sternum, dorsally only up to the costal angle. In the region of the dorsal ends of the ribs, the bundles of muscle fibers are replaced by the tendinous *internal intercostal membrane*.

The deep layer of the internal intercostal muscles is separated off by the intercostal vessels and nerves as the innermost intercostal muscle (*intercostalis intimus*). The portion of the internal intercostal muscle situated between the rib cartilages is also referred to as the intercartilaginous muscle.

The **subcostal muscles** exhibit the same direction of fibers as the internal intercostal muscles. They appear only in the caudal region of the thorax in the vicinity of the rib angle and pass over 1–2 ribs. Each muscle belly – in spite of the expansion into at least two intercostal spaces – is innervated by only one intercostal nerve.

The **transversus thoracis**, likewise a derivative of the internal intercostal muscles, arises on the inner side of the thorax at the lateral margin of the sternum in the lower part of its body and at the xiphoid process. The

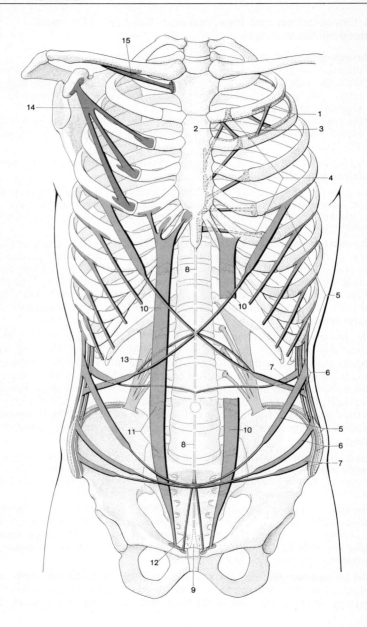

insertion takes place at costal cartilages II–VI (near the bone-cartilage border). Only the caudal bundles of fibers pass in a transverse direction; the superior muscular tracts course obliquely upward. The cranial part of the muscle is often transformed into tendon.

Action of the intercostal muscles. The intercostal muscles brace the intercostal spaces against the pressure changes in the pleural cavity during inspiration and expiration. The external intercostal and intercartilaginous muscles elevate the ribs, thus cooperating in inspiratory movements of the thorax. The portions of the internal intercostal muscles situated between the bony ribs, on the other hand, lower the ribs and help in expiration. The contraction of the muscle bundles of the transversus thoracis draws the rib cartilages downward. These muscle bundles play a role in expiration ($\rightarrow$ respiratory mechanics, p. 528).

The **serratus posterior superior** (Fig. **198**) arises with a thin, but strong aponeurosis from the spines of the last two cervical and the first two thoracic vertebrae. It courses obliquely caudad and inserts with 4 fleshy slips at ribs 1–4 lateral to the costal angle – and thus also lateral to the attachment of the iliocostalis muscle. The muscle possesses a favorable leverage for elevation of the ribs and cooperates in inspiration.

The **serratus posterior inferior** (Fig. **198**) originates from the spines of the last two thoracic and the first two lumbar vertebrae. It inserts with short tendons at ribs 9–12, lateral to the costal angle.

The aponeurosis of origin of the muscle is fused with the thoracolumbar fascia and the tendinous plate of the latissimus dorsi. The 4 broad muscle bellies, which partly overlap one another, are completely covered by the latissimus dorsi and course obliquely laterally and cranially, almost in a transverse direction to their site of attachment.

The serratus posterior inferior counteracts a narrowing of the inferior thoracic aperture (traction of the diaphragm) and thus cooperates in inspiration.

◀ Fig. 197. **Muscles of thoracic and abdominal wall**

1 External intercostal
2 Internal intercostal (= intercartilagineus muscle between costal cartilages)
3 Internal intercostal (between bony ribs)
4 Transversus thoracis
5 External abdominal oblique
6 Internal abdominal oblique
7 Transversus abdominis

8 Linea alba
9 Adminiculum of linea alba
10 Rectus abdominis
11 Tendinous intersections
12 Pyramidalis
13 Quadratus lumborum
14 Pectoralis minor
15 Subclavius

Innervation:

☐ Nerve to subclavius
■ Medial and lateral pectoral nerves
▦ Ventral rami of thoracic or lumbar nerves
☐ Ventral rami of thoracic nerve XII; and lumbar nerves I–III

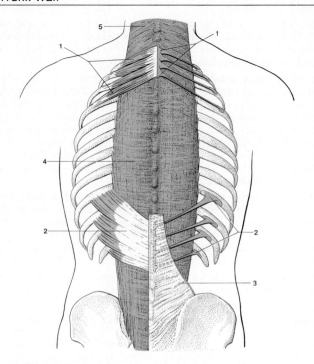

Fig. 198. **Serrati posteriores muscles and thoracolumbar fascia**
1 Serratus posterior superior
2 Serratus posterior inferior
3 Aponeurosis of origin of latissimus dorsi, interwoven with superficial layer of thoracolumbar fascia
  (severed on right side, not shown on left)
4 Superficial layer of thoracolumbar fascia
5 Nuchal fascia

d) Intercostal Vessels and Nerves

For the supply of the deep layer and also part of the superficial layer of the thoracic wall, each intercostal space contains segmental conduction pathways, usually in the following craniocaudal sequence (Figs. **25–27** and **199**):

– an *intercostal vein*, which forms a venous arch between the azygos system and the internal thoracic veins (subclavian vein);

– an *intercostal artery*, which as a collateral connects the thoracic aorta – in the 1st and 2nd intercostal spaces the costocervical trunk

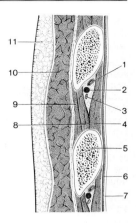

Fig. 199. **Section through thoracic wall somewhat behind axillary line**, ventrolateral view
Intercostal vessels and nerve (collateral rami not shown)
1 Posterior intercostal vein
2 Posterior intercostal artery
3 Intercostal nerve
4 Innermost intercostal muscle
5 Bony rib
6 Endothoracic fascia
7 Parietal pleura
8 Internal intercostal muscle
9 External intercostal muscle
10 Serratus anterior
11 Subcutaneous connective tissue

(subclavian artery) – with the internal thoracic artery (subclavian artery); and

– an *intercostal nerve*, which innervates the autochthonous thoracic or abdominal musculature, the skin of the dorsolateral and ventral trunk wall, as well as the parietal pleura and parietal peritoneum.

The corresponding segmental vessels at the lower margin of the 12th rib, the *subcostal artery* and *vein* and the *subcostal nerve*, travel in the abdominal wall.

Arteries. The arterial arch of each intercostal space consists of a *posterior intercostal artery* coursing from dorsal to ventral and a partial ventral segment, the *anterior intercostal ramus*, anastomosing with it (Fig. **193**).

The *posterior intercostal arteries I* and *II* (for the 1st and 2nd intercostal spaces) arise from the highest intercostal artery (costocervical trunk).

The *posterior intercostal arteries III–XI*, as well as the *subcostal artery*, originate at the posterior wall of the aorta.

The right intercostal arteries pass dorsal to the esophagus, thoracic duct and azygos vein above the right anterolateral surface of the vertebral body; on the left side, they course dorsal to the hemiazygos veins or accessory hemiazygos vein. In front of the heads of the ribs, the vessels of both sides cross dorsal to the sympathetic trunk and give off the *dorsal branch* in the costocervical region (to the back musculature and skin), which in turn dispatches the *spinal branch* through the intervertebral foramen (to the spinal meninges), as well as *medial* and *lateral cutaneous branches* through the autochthonous back musculature.

Embedded in the endothoracic fascia, the main trunk of each intercostal artery reaches the costal groove and passes ventrally – first between the internal and external intercostal muscles, then into the internal intercostal muscle (Fig. **199**). In the region of the midaxillary line, the artery leaves the protection of the rib and courses ventrally along the lower margin of the rib into the anterior segment of the intercostal space to anastomose with the anterior intercostal branch.

The main branch of the intercostal artery gives off a thin *collateral branch* at the costal angle which passes ventrally along the upper margin of the following rib and likewise anastomoses with an anterior intercostal branch (Fig. **193**). A *lateral cutaneous branch* leaves the main branch at the lateral wall of the thorax and divides into two twigs, one directed anteriorly and the other posteriorly (Fig. **185**). In females, the *lateral mammary branches* passing to the mammary gland (from the lateral cutaneous branches) are especially pronounced.

The caudal intercostal arteries which accompany the false ribs pass over the arches of the ribs and course with their terminal sections – like the subcostal artery – into the muscular wall of the abdomen between the transversus abdominis and the internal abdominal oblique.

The *anterior intercostal branches* (usually two per intercostal space, Fig. **193**) complete the segmental arterial arch when they anastomose with the posterior intercostal arteries and their collateral branch. They arise from the internal thoracic artery (for the upper 5–6 intercostal spaces) and its lateral terminal branch, the musculophrenic artery (for the lower intercostal spaces).

In the case of stenosis of the **Isthmus aortae**, the collateral circulation developed by means of the transverse connections between the aorta and the internal thoracic artery can provide the blood supply for the trunk and lower limb.

Veins. In arrangement and course, the intercostal venous arches correspond largely to the intercostal arteries and are composed of *posterior* and *anterior intercostal veins*. They lie (usually) cranial to the corresponding intercostal artery and course up to the midaxillary line completely protected in the costal groove (Fig. **199**).

The *posterior intercostal veins* empty on the right side into the azygos vein and on the left into the hemiazygos vein or accessory hemiazygos vein (Fig. **27**).

From the 1st intercostal space, the blood is conducted via the *highest intercostal vein* into the brachiocephalic vein (or vertebral vein). Posterior intercostal veins II–IV (on the right side only II and III) unite into the *superior intercostal vein*, which enters the azygos vein on the right side and, the brachiocephalic vein on the left.

The *anterior intercostal veins* empty into the internal thoracic veins.

Lymphatic vessels. Segmental lymphatic tracts accompany the intercostal vessels (Fig. **29**). The discharge of lymph takes place dorsally via the *intercostal lymph nodes* (in the vicinity of the heads of the ribs) into the thoracic duct, ventrally via the *parasternal lymph nodes* (along the internal thoracic vessels) into the thoracic duct (left) or the right lymphatic duct (right) or into the respective venous angle.

Nerves. The segmental nerves of the thoracic wall, the *intercostal nerves*, are the ventral branches of the thoracic nerves. The branching pattern of the thoracic nerves corresponds largely to that of the intercostal arteries.

After branching off from the spinal nerve, the *intercostal nerve* still courses for some distance in the endothoracic fascia, just beneath the parietal pleura. It enters the internal intercostal muscle at the costal angle where the muscle "begins" – and thus somewhat earlier than the vessels – and passes ventrally (Fig. **199**) along the lower margin of the rib (thus not protected by the bone).

Only the branch for the external intercostal muscle (in the corresponding segments with the lateral twigs for the serratus posterior muscles [C8–T4 and T9–T11]) courses between the external and internal intercostal muscles. The intercostal nerve itself adjoins the intercostal vessels which separate the two layers of the internal intercostal muscle. It gives off motor branches to the two layers of the internal intercostal muscle, if necessary, to the subcostalis and transversus thoracis, and supplies sensory innervation to the parietal pleura.

The *lateral cutaneous branch* (Figs. **185** and **209**) passes between the slips of origin of the serratus anterior – at about the midaxillary line – to the skin of the lateral thoracic wall and ramifies into an anterior and a posterior branch. The sensory terminal branch of the intercostal nerve reaches the ventral thoracic skin beside the sternum as the *anterior cutaneous branch*. Both cutaneous branches give off *mammary branches* (*lateral, medial*) to the skin of the mammary gland.

The ventral ramus of the 1st thoracic nerve dispatches the greatest part of its fibers to the brachial plexus (Fig. **58**). The relatively weak 1st intercostal nerve lacks a lateral cutaneous branch. The posterior branch passes as the *intercostobrachial nerve* from the lateral cutaneous ramus of the 2nd (occasionally also the 3rd) intercostal nerve to the limb (to the medial brachial cutaneous nerve).

The 7 caudal intercostal nerves leave the thoracic region and pass to the abdominal wall (the 10th to the region of the navel). They provide motor innervation to the abdominal musculature, sensory innervation to the abdominal skin and peritoneum.

Puncture of the pleural cavity: Since the intercostal vessels lie protected in the costal groove to about the middle of the axillary line, they are not particularly exposed in their dorsolateral course to stabbing wounds of the thoracic wall, but they can be affected if the ribs are fractured. Therefore, punctures of the pleural cavity should be undertaken in the 5th–7th intercostal space dorsal to the axillary line if possible. The intercostal nerve not covered by the rib generally avoids the needle. Because of its relatively long course near the pleura before entering into the muscle layer, it can be irritated by an inflammation of the pleura (pleurisy).

e) Endothoracic Fascia and Internal Thoracic Vessels

The **endothoracic fascia** is primarily loose connective tissue, which lines the wall of the pleural cavity – except the mediastinum – and which continues into the connective tissue of the mediastinum at the sternum and vertebral column (Figs. **199** and **210 b**). The endothoracic fascia is designated, therefore, as the subserous layer of connective tissue of the parietal pleura in the region of the thoracic wall, pleural cupola (cervical pleura), and diaphragm.

The subserous connective tissue of the cervical pleura communicates with the connective tissue of the neck, particularly the deep cervical fascia. Connective tissue tracts, which are more or less distinctly adlimited (from the vertebral column, from the fascial coverings of the scalene muscles, from the neurovascular sheaths of the neck, from the region of the esophagus and trachea), and occasionally a tendinous tract of the scalenus anterior radiate into this section of the endothoracic fascia called the *suprapleural membrane* and cooperate in bracing the cervical pleura against the traction of the lung.

The portion of the endothoracic fascia situated between the diaphragmatic pleura and the diaphragm is designated as the *phrenicopleural fascia*.

The endothoracic fascia spreads at the thoracic wall between the costal pleura and the ribs and between the fascia of the intercostal muscles and the transversus thoracis, the *thoracic fascia*. The intercostal vessels and nerves course dorsally in the endothoracic fascia. Ventrally, the internal thoracic vessels lie embedded in the fascia cranial to the 3rd rib before they are forced out of the fascia by the transversus thoracis muscles.

Injury to the parasternal region can lead to an opening of the vessels and to hemorrhaging into the pleural cavity.

Internal thoracic vessels. The **internal thoracic artery** (Fig. **193**) arises at the concave side of the subclavian artery and passes downward in the endothoracic fascia – about 1 cm lateral to the marign of the sternum – behind the rib cartilages, but in front of the costal pleura. It is underlaid by the transversus thoracis caudal to the 3rd rib and divides in the 6th intercostal space into two terminal branches, the *musculophrenic* and *superior epigastric arteries*.

After a short course, the *internal thoracic artery* gives off the *pericardiacophrenic artery*, which accompanies the phrenic nerve to the diaphragm between the mediastinal pleura and the pericardium and which dispatches branches to the pericardium. In addition, it sends *anterior intercostal branches* into the upper 5–6 intercostal spaces, where they anastomose with the posterior intercostal arteries and their collaterals.

Small branches pass as *thymic branches* to the thymus, as *mediastinal branches* into the anterior mediastinum and to the mediastinal pleura, and as inconstant *tracheal* and *bronchial branches* to the trachea and bronchi. *Sternal branches* supply the sternum and the transversus thoracis. *Perforating branches* penetrate the thoracic wall in the upper 5 intercostal spaces, ramify on the anterior surface of the sternum, in the pectoralis major, and in the skin, and dispatch *medial mammary branches* to the mammary gland. As a frequent variant, the *lateral costal branch* leaves the internal thoracic artery behind the 1st costal cartilage, passes obliquely downward at the inner surface of the anterior thoracic wall, and is united with the intercostal arteries.

As a lateral terminal branch of the internal thoracic artery, the *musculophrenic artery* travels along the costal slips of origin of the diaphragm and gives off *anterior intercostal branches* to the lower intercostal spaces, in addition to branches to the diaphragm, as well as to the origins of the lateral abdominal muscles. The medial terminal branch, the *superior epigastric artery*, leaves the thoracic cavity in the vicinity of the sterno-costal triangle (Larrey's cleft → p. 527) and passes downward in the rectus sheath.

The *superior epigastric artery* anastomoses in the rectus abdominis with the terminal branches of the inferior epigastric artery (from the external iliac artery) so that a collateral circulation can be established in the event of a slow occlusion of the aorta.

The **internal thoracic veins** correspond in their course to the internal thoracic artery. Their branches are the companion veins of the arterial branches. Cranial to the 3rd rib, the internal thoracic vein is single, courses medial to the artery, and flows into the brachiocephalic vein. The superior epigastric veins receive the *subcutaneous veins of the abdomen* from the abdominal skin (Fig. **209**).

The anastomoses at the posterior wall of the rectus abdominis between the inferior epigastric veins, which flow into the external iliac vein, and the superior epigastric veins, which drain into the internal thoracic vein, can be of clinical importance. In the case of occlusion of the inferior vena cava, blood from the lower half of the body can arrive at the superior vena cava by means of this collateral route.

2. Diaphragm

The dome-shaped **diaphragm** (Figs. **200** and **201**) forms both the floor of the thoracic cavity and the roof of the abdominal cavity. The closed, musculotendinous partition represents a peculiarity of mammals. It has become the most important respiratory muscle. The muscle material is derived phylogenetically from cervical myotomes 3–5 and is innervated by the phrenic nerve from the cervical plexus (C4 [3, 5]).

Muscle origin and central tendon. The muscle arises ring–shaped at the inferior thoracic aperture. The muscle fibers pass upward in an arch and radiate into a central tendinous plate, the *central tendon*. The concavity faces the abdominal cavity and is directed ventrocaudally.

The muscular diaphragm comprises three parts: *lumbar, costal* and *sternal*.

The *lumbar part* is the most strongly developed. It consists of a *right* and a *left crus*, each of which possesses a medial and a lateral portion.

The former labelling of these parts as *medial crus* and *lateral crus* facilitated the description and comprehension of the structure of the right and left halves of the lumbar part of the diaphragm. This terminology will be retained here – although it is no longer the official nomenclature.

The *medial crus* arises from the bodies of lumbar vertebrae 1–3 (on the right side also L4). The inner margins of the medial crura of both sides border the *aortic opening (aortic hiatus)*, which is surrounded by a

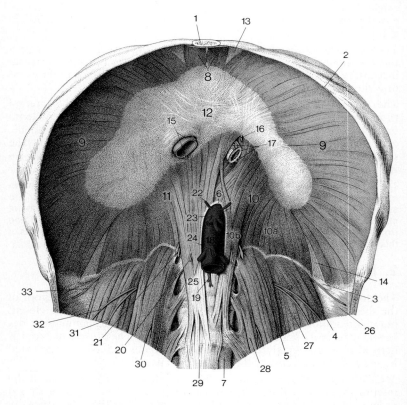

Fig. 200. **Diaphragm**, view of abdominal surface

tendinous arch, the *median arcuate ligament*, and thus is not compressed, but enlarged during contraction of the diaphragm. The aorta and, behind it, the thoracic duct course through this hiatus. Cranial to this point of passage, a muscular tract splits off from the crura, which is usually stronger from the right medial crus, somewhat weaker from the left; the two bundles of fibers cross each other. It is predominantly the fibers of the right crus and its fiber bundle crossing to the left, however, which are involved in delimiting the *esophageal hiatus*, which – shifted insignificantly to the left of the median plane – lies above the aortic hiatus. The esophagus is united movably with the muscular border of the passageway by loose connective tissue. The muscle fibers of both medial diaphragmatic crura course toward the posterior margin of the middle lobe of the central tendon.

The esophageal hiatus, through which the esophagus, as well as the anterior and posterior trunks of the vagus nerve pass, is constricted by contraction of the diaphragm. The entrance of the greater splanchnic nerve, on the right side together with the azygos vein and on the left with the hemiazygos vein, demarcates a narrow lateral portion of the medial diaphragmatic crus at the level of L2 or L3. It was formerly referred to as a separate "intermediate crus".

The *lateral crus* of the lumbar part possesses a bipartite origin. The medial portion comes from the lateral surface of the 1st and 2nd lumbar vertebral bodies and from a tendinous arch passing to the costal process

1 Sternum (cut surface)
2 Costal arch
3 Twelfth rib
4 Lateral arcuate ligament
5 Medial arcuate ligament
6 Median arcuate ligament
7 Fourth lumbar vertebra
8–14 *Diaphragm*
8 Sternal part
9 Costal part
10, 11 Lumbar part
10 Left crus of lumbar part
10a Lateral band of left crus
10b Medial band of left crus
11 Right crus of lumbar part
12 Central tendon
13 Muscle-poor area between costal and sternal parts (Larrey's cleft; sternocostal triangle)
14 Muscle-poor area between lumbar and costal parts (Bochdalek's triangle; vertebrocostal trigone)
15–21 *Structures passing through diaphragm*
15 Inferior vena cava and phrenico-abdominal ramus of right phrenic nerve in foramen for inferior vena cava

16 Phrenico-abdominal ramus of left phrenic nerve through esophageal opening, lumbar part or central tendon
17 Esophagus, as well as anterior and posterior vagal trunks in esophageal opening
18 Aorta in aortic opening
19 Thoracic duct in aortic opening
20 Azygos vein and greater splanchnic nerve (usually) through medial crus
21 Sympathetic trunk and (usually also) lesser splanchnic nerve between median and lateral crura
22–25 *Branches of abdominal aorta*
22 Right inferior phrenic artery
23 Celiac trunk
24 Superior mesenteric artery
25 Right renal artery
26 Transversus abdominis
27 Quadratus lumborum
28 Psoas major
29 Anterior longitudinal ligament
30 Genitofemoral nerve
31 Ilio-inguinal nerve
32 Iliohypogastric nerve
33 Subcostal nerve

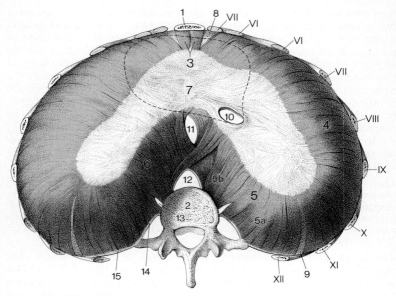

Fig. 201. **Diaphragm**, view of thoracic surface (after *Pernkopf*)
Limit of coalesced surfaces of diaphragm and pericardium (----)

VII–XII cartilaginous or bony ribs (cut surface)
 1 Sternum (cut surface)
 2 First lumbar vertebra
3–9 *Diaphragm*
 3 Sternal part
 4 Costal part
5, 6 Lumbar part
 5 Right crus of lumbar part
 5a Lateral band of right crus
 5b Medial band of right crus
 6 Left crus of lumbar part
 7 Central tendon
 8 Muscle-poor area between sternal and
   costal parts (Larrey's cleft; sternocostal
   triangle)

 9 Muscle-poor area between costal and
   lumbar parts (Bochdalek's triangle;
   vertebrocostal trigone)
10–13 *Openings in diaphragm*
 10 Foramen for inferior vena cava
 11 Esophageal opening
 12 Aortic opening, framed by median arcuate
   ligament
 13 Opening between medial and lateral bands
   of left crus for passage of sympathetic
   trunk and lesser splanchnic nerve
 14 Medial arcuate ligament, bridges over
   psoas major
 15 Lateral arcuate ligament, bridges over
   quadratus lumborum

of the 1st or 2nd lumbar vertebra. This arch bridges over the psoas muscle
as the *medial arcuate ligament* (*psoas arcade*). The lateral portion originates from the *lateral arcuate ligament*, a tendinous arch which extends
over the quadratus lumborum to the 12th rib from the lateral process of
the 1st or 2nd lumbar vertebra (*quadratus arcade*). The muscle fibers of
the lateral crus, which is thin and flat in contrast to the medial crus,
course steeply upward to the central tendon.

Through a gap between the medial and the lateral crura the sympathetic trunk passes together with the lesser splanchnic nerve, provided this nerve does not pass with the greater splanchnic nerve through the medial crus.

The *costal part* arises in steps from the inner surface of the cartilage of the 6 caudal ribs, alternating with the slips of origin of the transversus abdominis. The costal muscle bundles form the main part of the muscular dome of the diaphragm and insert at the lateral and anterior margins of the central tendon.

The *sternal part* is narrow and thin. Its fibers come from the dorsal side of the xiphoid process; individual fibers also come from the aponeurosis of the transversus abdominis. It attaches at the anterior margin of the middle lobe of the central tendon.

The *central tendon* is somewhat V-shaped in cranial view. A smaller middle lobe is directed ventrally, and a more extensive lateral lobe is directed dorsolaterally on each side. The right lateral lobe is perforated at the posterior margin near its base by the *foramen for the vena cava*, through which the inferior vena cava and the phrenico-abdominal branch of the right phrenic nerve traverse. The usually oblong opening is surrounded by immobile, intertwined tendinous bundles, which fix the vascular wall so that the vascular lumen is held permanently open. The middle lobe of the central tendon and the basal portion of both lateral lobes have grown together with the pericardium; the foramen for the vena cava is still included in the fused surface. The curvature of the diaphragm is somewhat depressed (heart saddle) at this site so that a right and a left dome can be distinguished. Below the right dome, which is about 1/2–1 intercostal space higher than the left dome, is the liver, and below the left dome is the stomach.

Apart from respiration, the **position of the diaphragm** is influenced by age, sex, and body type. Moreover, it is dependent upon body position: in a supine posture, the domes of the diaphragm are located about 2 cm higher than in an upright posture. In small children, the right dome is projected at the 8th or 9th thoracic vertebra, after the 7th year at the 9th–10th; the left dome lies lower by about half a vertebra. In males, respiratory movements can carry the right dome of the diaphragm upward to the level of T8 and downward to T11. In females, the diaphragm usually lies somewhat lower (except during pregnancy). With increasing age, the domes of the diaphragm gradually sink somewhat lower.

With respect to the thorax, the right dome of the diaphragm in the cadaver and also during deep expiration in the living resides at the level of the 4th intercostal space, the left at the level of the cartilage-bone border of the 5th rib (Fig. **202**). The heart saddle reaches the level of the middle of T10. During contraction of the diaphragm, the domes are leveled off

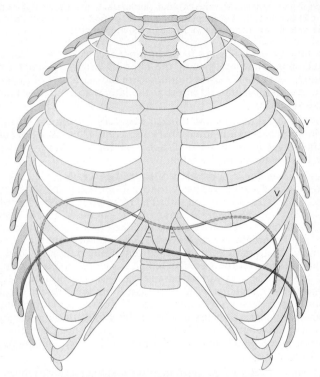

Fig. 202. **Positions of ribs and diaphragm during deep expiration (———) and deep inspiration (——)**

and strongly lowered. During deep inspiration, the right dome can be drawn down to the level of the upper margin of the 6th rib (at the bone-cartilage border), and the left dome to the 6th intercostal space. The heart saddle then lies at the level of the lower margin of T11.

Since the ribs are lifted during inspiration and the apex of the xiphoid process ascends simultaneously to about the level of T10, the heart saddle can lie lower during deep inspiration than the origin of the sternal part. During maximal muscle contraction and simultaneous elevation of the thorax, the fibers of the sternal portion of the diaphragm must, therefore, course downward from their origin toward the heart saddle. The anterior portion of the central tendon is then lowered so far that it lies below the apex of the xiphoid process, and the heart descends into the epigastric space. The "eversion" of the sternal part during deepest inspiration is caused by the traction of the contracting anterior muscle slips of the costal part, the musculotendinous arch of which is so leveled off that it pulls the sternal part and the ventral part of the central tendon downward like a sling. The traction of the lumbar crura directed dorsocaudally levels off the curvature of the diaphragm in general.

Sites of muscle-poor areas of the diaphragm (Figs. **200** and **201**). Between the lumbar and costal parts of the diaphragm, a triangular site frequently remains free of muscles (*Bochdalek's triangle*) and is adjoined by the superior pole of the kidney. A similar, small triangular muscular gap between the costal and sternal parts is known as *Larrey's cleft*. In both of these muscle-free regions of the diaphragm, the pleura and peritoneum lie closely adjacent so that pathological processes can easily migrate through them.

Since the diaphragm projects relatively far into the thoracic space, a perforating injury of the thoracic wall (bullet or stab wound) – especially if it occurs during the expiration phase – can involve both the pleural and the abdominal cavities and the organs situated there, depending upon the direction of the wound canal.

Vascular and nerve supply of the diaphragm. The *arterial supply* takes place on the thoracic side of the diaphragm via the *pericardiacophrenic* and *musculophrenic arteries* (branches of the internal thoracic artery), as well as via the *superior phrenic arteries* (small branches of the aorta to the lumbar part of the diaphragm). The *inferior phrenic arteries* ramify at the abdominal surface; they arise from the abdominal aorta in the aortic hiatus (Fig. **200**) and anastomose with branches of the intercostal arteries and the pericardiacophrenic artery.

The *venous drainage* is provided by the companion veins of the arteries mentioned.

The *lymphatic drainage* takes place in the thoracic region via *superior phrenic lymph nodes* (behind the xiphoid process and the bone-cartilage border of the 7th rib), *lateral pericardial lymph nodes* (between the pericardium and mediastinal pleura), *parasternal lymph nodes* (along the internal thoracic vessels) and via *posterior mediastinal lymph nodes* (in the posterior mediastinum). In the abdominal region, lymphatic vessels pass from the diaphragm to *inferior phrenic lymph nodes* (at the crura of the lumbar part) and to *lumbar lymphatic nodes* (in front of and beside the abdominal aorta and inferior vena cava). Yet, the diaphragm forms no true lymphatic sheath. Lymph from the fundus of the stomach and from the diaphragmatic surface of the liver also arrives at the mediastinal lymph nodes (cancerous metastases can take this route).

Innervation. The diaphragm is supplied by the predominantly motor *phrenic nerve*. The right phrenic nerve reaches the diaphragm at the foramen of the vena cava, and the left behind the apex of the heart. Sensory fibers (Fig. **200**) on the right side pass through the foramen of the vena cava and on the left side through the esophageal hiatus, the lumbar part, or the central tendon as *phrenicoabdominal branches*. They spread out in the peritoneum up to the gallbladder and pancreas (in diseases of the liver and gallbladder, pain can radiate into the right shoulder, and in diseases of the pancreas into the left shoulder).

Diaphragmatic herniae. Considering the complicated ontogenesis of the diaphragm (with contributions from the transverse septum, pleuroperitoneal folds, meso-esophagus and the body wall), it is understandable that congenital diaphragmatic defects can appear (particularly in the region of Bochdalek's triangle, more often on the left than on the right side). If the muscularization of the diaphragm does not occur at a local site, "congenital" diaphragmatic herniae arise, which are usually recognizable only a few years after birth. Acquired, nontraumatic diaphragmatic herniae appear in the region of the esophageal hiatus. Diaphragmatic ruptures (traumatic diaphragmatic "herniae") arise by direct violence (e.g. stabbing) or as a result of contused abdominal injuries.

In all of these cases, the abdominal viscera can be displaced into the thoracic space. In herniae, the hernial sac consists of a thin membrane formed from peritoneum and pleura. The lungs can be compressed, the mediastinum and heart displaced so that a weak or fatal impediment in respiration and circulation can result. In herniae in the region of the esophageal hiatus, the diaphragm can be drawn tent-like into the thoracic space; the cranial portion of the stomach lies in the thoracic cavity and is constricted by the diaphragm at the place of entrance (sliding hernia). In para-esophageal herniae, the stomach entrance remains at the typical site, but the fundus of the stomach is pushed forward into the thoracic cavity next to the esophagus.

3. Respiratory Mechanics

Abdominal breathing and *thoracic (costal) breathing* can be distinguished, which combine with one another: *mixed respiration. Abdominal respiration* predominates only in the infant; it is the exclusive type of respiration up to the 3rd year of life. During pregnancy, *costal respiration* becomes more important.

In *abdominal respiration*, the thoracic cavity is extended caudally by the contraction of the diaphragm (Fig. **202**). With the termination of muscular contraction, the diaphragm relaxes and ascends in height, because the elastic elements of the lungs, which were stretched during inspiration, exert a traction and pull the diaphragm upwards. The abdominal viscera also rise on account of the tension of the abdominal musculature.

In *thoracic respiration*, the ribs are elevated and the thoracic cavity is enlarged not only in the craniocaudal, but also in the sagittal and frontal directions. Especially the scalene muscles ($\rightarrow$ p. 730) function in inspiration during regular respiration, assisted by the external intercostal and intercartilaginous muscles of the upper intercostal spaces, as well as the serratus posterior superior. In deep inspiration, the caudal external intercostal muscles also participate. If the muscles mentioned relax at the end of the inspiration phase, the thorax tries to reverse the deformation forced upon it by the enlargement and strives for a middle position between extreme rib elevation and depression (balanced position). Beyond this position, the internal intercostals and the transversus thoracis produce another depression of the ribs, which can be strengthened by a contraction of the abdominal musculature.

The abdominal muscles play an essential role in spasmodic expiration when the glottis is closed, e.g. when speaking, singing, coughing and sneezing (the initially closed glottis is abruptly opened).

A *paralysis of the intercostal muscles* should not influence normal respiration very much. However, sucking (paralysis of the external intercostals) and blowing (paralysis of the internal intercostals) are impeded.

The enlargement of the thoracic cavity during costal respiration is made possible by the shape of the ribs, their position, and the manner of their connection with the vertebral column and sternum. Owing to the oblique position of the ribs toward the vertical plane, the apex of the rib is carried upward and forward during rib elevation. Space gained in the sagittal direction is the greater, the longer the rib and the more oblique its initial position. Since the neck of the rib, around whose longitudinal axis the rotary movement (from the 7th rib down it is a sliding movement) takes place, is positioned obliquely to the median plane from the 2nd rib on, the apices of the ribs must also be carried toward the side during elevation of the ribs. The enlargement of the thoracic cavity laterally is especially pronounced at the middle and the lower ribs. The sternum, with which the sternal ribs – and indirectly also ribs 8–10 – are united, is displaced cranially and ventrally when the ribs are elevated, thereby adjusting the sternal angle. The sternum coordinates, as it were, the movement of the bony ribs, whose apices – in the case of free endings – would be led into different positions considering the variable lengths of the ribs and the unequal oblique position of their necks.

This adjustment of divergent movements of the ends of the bony ribs is possible owing to the deformability of the costal cartilages. The angles of the costal cartilages are thereby increased, the rib cartilage torqued, and a rotary movement takes place at the sternocostal joints. Because of these inspiratory deformations tensions appear in the thoracic skeleton and in the ligamentous apparatus. They are the basic reason why the thorax – after the relaxation of the inspiratory-active muscles – strives after a balanced position to equalize these tensions, and a depression of the ribs takes place – at first, even without muscular activity.

The inspiratory enlargement of the thorax is accompanied by an extension of the vertebral column, whereas expiration produces a flexion of it. These movements are reflexive, but can be voluntarily modified.

4. Abdominal Wall

At the abdominal wall, the following layers are distinguished (from outside inward):
– a *superficial layer*, formed of skin, subcutaneous connective tissue

(partly with considerable deposits of fat), and superficial abdominal fascia (as part of the general body fascia);

– a *middle layer*, consisting of deformable musculotendinous plates between the lower thoracic and upper pelvic margins, an inner abdominal fascia (*transversalis fascia*), which borders the deep middle layer, and the lumbar vertebral column (as the only skeletal support of the abdominal wall); and

– a *deep layer*, formed by a subserous connective tissue, quite strong in places, and by the parietal peritoneum, the lining layer of the peritoneal cavity.

In contrast to the thoracic wall which, owing to the bony thorax, has a permanent form determined by the skeleton, the abdominal wall obtains its typical structural and functional properties chiefly from the middle musculotendinous layer (true abdominal wall). It is able to adapt itself, on the one hand, to the alternating degree to which the abdominal space is filled and, on the other hand, can exert pressure on the abdominal contents. The abdominal musculature cooperates in expiration and plays a decisive additional role as the power plant of trunk movements. With the exception of the extension of the vertebral column, in which it is only passively concerned, it carries out all movements of the thoracic and lumbar vertebral columns – together with the muscles of the erector spinae.

a) Abdominal Fascia

The **superficial abdominal fascia** (Figs. **203** and **206**) covers the musculotendinous plate of the external abdominal oblique muscle. It continues cranially into the pectoral fascia, caudally into the fascia lata on the thigh. In the region of the linea alba, the superficial abdominal fascia is connected firmly with the aponeurosis of the external oblique and with the inguinal ligament at the inguinal furrow.

At the external inguinal ring, the fascia in males continues into the spermatic cord and, together with the aponeurosis of the external abdominal oblique, forms a covering, the *external spermatic fascia* (Fig. **206**), which is situated superficial to the cremasteric fascia and the cremaster muscle. In females, delicate connective tissue tracts of the superficial abdominal fascia are attached to the round ligament of the uterus, which passes through the inguinal canal to the labium majus.

The laterocranial border of the external inguinal ring is formed by bundles of collagenous fibers of the superficial abdominal fascia (*intercrural fibers*), which pass, oblique and superficial to the aponeurosis, above the pointed lateral end of the aponeurotic cleft (Fig. **204**).

The caudal continuation of the superficial abdominal fascia, rich in elastic networks, is designated as the *fundiform ligament of the penis* (Fig. **123**). It arises from the superficial abdominal fascia cranial to the symphysis, embraces the corpus cavernosum penis from both sides with two crura – placed superficial to the suspensory ligament of the penis – and radiates into the scrotum.

The **internal abdominal fascia** (*transversalis fascia*, Figs. **185, 203** and **206**) covers the inner surface of the muscular and aponeurotic wall of the abdominal cavity, as well as the abdominal surface of the diaphragm. It is strengthened in the region of the navel as the *umbilical fascia* and continues dorsally on the quadratus lumborum as a thin fascial layer. At the medial margin of this muscle, it communicates with the psoas fascia. Caudally, the transversalis fascia is attached at the inguinal ligament, where it merges into the iliac fascia. Above the inguinal ligament, at the medial margin of the internal inguinal ring, the inner abdominal fascia is strengthened by longitudinal tracts, the *interfoveolar ligament*. At the internal inguinal ring, the fascia evaginates through the inguinal canal and covers the spermatic cord, epididymis and testis as the *internal spermatic fascia* (Figs. **204–206**).

The transversalis fascia is firmly and immovably connected with the subserous connective tissue of the peritoneum. Therefore, it also remains beneath the arcuate line dorsal to the rectus abdominis and does not pass into the ventral layer of the rectus sheath with the aponeurosis of the transversus abdominis.

b) Organization and Innervation of the Abdominal Musculature

The **abdominal musculature** (Fig. **197**) consists of the *lateral* (broad) and *anterior* (straight) *abdominal muscles*, as well as the *deep* (posterior) *abdominal muscle* (quadratus lumborum). It is a part of the ventral trunk musculature. The metameric organization has disappeared.

The *innervation* takes place via ventral branches of thoracic nerves 5–12 and lumbar nerves 1 and 2.

In the description of the muscles, the segmental nerves supplying them are indicated parenthetically after the muscle's name.

The flat, broad abdominal muscles merge on the ventral side into large, flat tendinous plates, the fibers of which interlace at the midline and unite with fibers of the opposite side. Thus, a median "longitudinal band" arises, which passes from the xiphoid process to the pubic symphysis, the *linea alba* (Figs. **185** and **203–205**). It is strengthened at its caudal portion on the ventral side by a triangular expansion (*adminiculum lineae albae*), which is fixed at the upper margin of the pubic symphysis.

The linea alba consists predominantly of crisscrossed collagenous fibers, which are supplemented by longitudinally-coursing fibers in the cranial and caudal portions. In the region of the umbilicus, it exhibits a circular opening, the *umbilical anulus* (Fig. **203 b**), the margin of which is strengthened by circular bundles of fibers.

Lateral Abdominal Muscles

The lateral abdominal muscles and their aponeuroses are layered in three strata. From the outside inward they are: the external abdominal oblique, the internal abdominal oblique, and the transversus abdominis.

The **external abdominal oblique** (T5–12 [L1]) is the most extensive of the three broad abdominal muscles (Figs. **185** and **105**). Its fleshy origin arises from the external surface of the 8 caudal ribs with partly overlapping slips of origin, which alternate cranially with the slips of origin of the serratus anterior and caudally with those of the latissimus dorsi. The muscle inserts at the iliac crest, inguinal ligament, pubis and linea alba.

The bundles of muscle fibers course slightly divergent from posterosuperior to antero-inferior (like the fibers of the external intercostals). The first bundle passes only a bit obliquely, whereas the most caudal courses steeply downward. The transition in the tendinous plate occurs parallel to the lateral margin of the rectus in a rather straight line, which somewhat cranial to the anterior superior iliac spine bends sharply in a right angle or acute angle to the upper margin of the edge of the ilium. In this way, a *muscular edge* is formed, which is often recognizable through the skin (Fig. **204**) and is usually distinctly emphasized in antique sculptures.

The dorsocaudal bundles of fibers of the external abdominal oblique have fleshy insertions at the external lip of the ventral two-thirds of the iliac crest. They bulge over the iliac crest as long as the muscle is not stretched, thus covering the upper margin of the pelvis, and form the *inguinal swelling* (Fig. **207**).

In most humans, more frequently in females than in males, the latissimus dorsi does not adjoin the external abdominal oblique directly. Between the anterior and posterior margins of both muscles there is a triangular field, the *lumbar triangle*, bordered caudally by the iliac crest. The muscular abdominal wall at this site is formed solely by the internal abdominal oblique and the transversus abdominis. Here, abscesses originating at the vertebral column and migrating along the iliac crest can escape outward; in rare cases, lumbar herniae (inferior) also appear here.

The **internal abdominal oblique** (T8–12, L1, 2) arises from the thoracolumbar fascia, the intermediate line of the iliac crest, and the lateral half of the inguinal ligament. Its fibers course fan-like – partly perpendicular to the muscle bundles of the external abdominal oblique – to their attachment at the lower margin of the thorax (ribs [9]10–12) and to a ventral tendinous plate, which cuts into the rectus abdominis. In the linea alba, the tendon fibers of the aponeurosis of the internal oblique are interlaced with the tendon fibers of the external abdominal oblique (Fig. **203**) and continue into the aponeurosis of the external oblique of the opposite side. Thus, a continuous musculotendinous oblique girdle of the abdominal wall is formed, which binds the oblique muscles of both sides into a working unit.

The dorsal bundles of fibers of the internal abdominal oblique rise steeply upward and insert fleshy at the lower margin of costal cartilages (IX) X–XII. They continue cranially into the internal intercostal muscles without a sharp boundary. The farther ventrally the muscle fibers of the internal abdominal oblique arise at the iliac crest, the less steep is their ascent. The bundles of fibers course approximately horizontally from the anterior superior iliac spine; from the inguinal ligament they pass obliquely downward (Fig. **204**). In the caudal region, it is very difficult to distinguish the internal oblique from the transversus abdominis. The connective tissue layer, in which the nerves course and which separates the two muscle plates cranially, ends at the level of the anterior superior iliac spine; the anterior cutaneous branch of the iliohypogastric nerve and the ilio-inguinal nerve travel on the ventral surface of the internal abdominal oblique.

The internal oblique and the transversus abdominis give off fiber bundles, which accompany the spermatic cord in males as the **cremaster muscle** and surround the testis like a sling (Figs. **204** and **206**). The muscle is able to pull the testis somewhat upward in the scrotum. In females, sparse muscle fibers can course to the external inguinal ring with the round ligament of the uterus.

Innervation of cremaster: genital branch of the genitofemoral nerve.

The **transversus abdominis** (T5–12, L1, 2) adjoins the transversus thoracis caudally. It arises from the inner side of the cartilage of the ribs VII (VI, V) to XII, from the costal processes of the lumbar vertebrae (via the deep layer of the thoracolumbar fascia), from the internal lip of the iliac crest and from the lateral portion of the inguinal ligament. Its fibers travel approximately horizontally – perpendicular to the straight abdominal muscle – and go over into a crescent-shaped, laterally-convex line, the *arcuate line* (*linea semilunaris*), in the aponeurosis (Fig. **205**).

The aponeurosis of the transversus abdominis is involved in the formation of the rectus sheath (Figs. **185** and **203**). At the linea alba, its fibers communicate intimately with the fibers of the aponeurosis of the internal abdominal oblique.

Anterior Abdominal Muscles

The **rectus abdominis** (T[5,6]7 – T12[L1]) passes on both sides of the anterior midline as a relatively narrow muscular band from the sternal ends of ribs 5–7, frequently also from the xiphoid process, to the superior margin of the pubis and attaches at the pubic crest and the symphysis (Fig. **205**). Fibers radiate from the oval tendon of attachment of the muscle, across the midline into the *suspensory ligament of the penis* (*clitoris*), which passes as the caudal continuation of the linea alba from the symphysis to the dorsal surface of the penis (clitoris).

The rectus abdominis is organized into 4–5 muscle bellies by 3–4 irregularly-scattered *tendinous intersections* (Fig. **197**), which course transversely and do not always penetrate the entire thickness of the muscle. The individual muscle bellies can contract separately without the contractive effect being cancelled by a stretching of the neighboring sections.

Two of these inscriptions lie above the navel, one resides at the level of the navel, and the inconstant 4th tendinous intersection is at the level of the arcuate line. The subdivision of the muscle represents a pseudometamerism since each muscle belly contains material from different myotomes.

The tendinous insertions have fused ventrally with the anterior layer of the rectus sheath and medially with the linea alba. Therefore, the muscle, e.g. in lateral bending of the trunk, cannot be withdrawn from its paramedian position. Owing to the fusion, obliquely-directed traction forces in the direction of the rectus abdominis can undergo a change in direction.

The **pyramidalis** (T12) is a small, variably developed muscle which is absent in about 20% of the cases. It passes between the aponeuroses of both oblique abdominal muscles or in the rectus sheath from the pubic symphysis to the linea alba, which it can tense.

The **rectus sheath** represents a muscular compartment, by means of which the rectus abdominis is fixed in its position and directed in its contraction (Figs. **185** and **203**). It consists of an *anterior* and a *posterior layer* or *lamina*.

The anterior lamina is purely tendinous. It is formed by the fusion of aponeurosis of the external oblique, the ventral lamina of the aponeurosis of the internal oblique and, below the navel (more precisely, below the arcuate line), also the caudal portion of the aponeurosis of the trans-versus abdominis (Figs. **204** and **206**). The dorsal aponeurotic layer of the internal abdominal oblique and the cranial two-thirds of the aponeurosis of the transversalis abdominis, together with the transversalis fascia, form the posterior layer of the rectus sheath. Below the navel, the dorsal layer of the aponeurosis of the internal oblique ends at a more or less distinctly bordered arched line, the *arcuate line* (Fig. **205**). Caudal to it, the aponeurosis of the transverse abdominis is attached to the anterior layer of the rectus sheath so that in the caudal third the posterior wall of the rectus sheath is formed only by the transversalis fascia.

Deep (Posterior) Abdominal Muscle

The **quadratus lumborum** (T12, L1–3) extends lateral to the lumbar vertebral column between the iliac crest (internal lip) and the 12th rib. It is covered dorsally by the deep layer of the thoracolumbar fascia and at its anterior surface by a continuation of the transversalis fascia.

The ventral fibers of the muscle pass from the iliac crest to the 12th rib (Fig. **200**). The fiber bundles of the dorsal portion attach to the 12th rib, as well as to the costal processes of the first four lumbar vertebrae. Intermediate fibers course from the costal processes to the 12th rib.

c) Statics and Dynamics of the Abdominal Wall

The tendinous fibers of the broad abdominal muscles are interlaced in the linea alba and are continued into the aponeuroses of the muscles of the

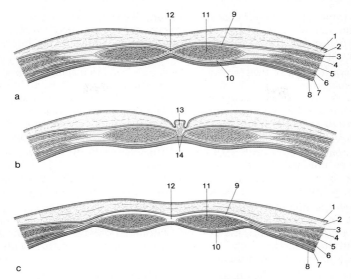

Fig. 203. **Schematic cross sections through anterior abdominal wall**
Rectus sheath
a Cranial to umbilicus
b At level of umbilicus
c Caudal to arcuate line

 1 Skin
 2 Subcutaneous connective tissue
 3 Superficial abdominal fascia (investing
   layer of external oblique)
 4 External oblique
 5 Internal oblique
 6 Transversus abdominis
 7 Transversalis fascia

 8 Peritoneum
 9 Anterior layer } of rectus sheath
10 Posterior layer
11 Rectus abdominis
12 Linea alba
13 Umbilical papilla
14 Umbilical ring

contralateral side. Thus a transverse (transversus abdominis) and an oblique (abdominal obliques) girdle arise. The rectus abdominis braces the anterior, and the quadratus lumborum the posterior abdominal wall. The covering of the rectus abdominis by the rectus sheath formed from the aponeurouses of the broad abdominal muscles brings the rectus muscle into a close functional relationship with these muscles.

The *abdominal musculature* can:
– *act* on the *contents of the abdominal cavity*.
– *be involved in expiration* (depression of the thorax, elevation of the diaphragm through pressure on the abdominal contents), and
– *carry out movements of the trunk.*

The tonus of the abdominal musculature determines the tension of the abdominal wall. It is controlled reflexly and is adjusted to changing external and internal influences (body position, filling of the intestinal tract, etc.).

The contraction of the *transversus abdominis* leads to a *constriction of the abdominal viscera*. By the additional exertion of the rest of the abdominal muscles (as well as the diaphragm and the musculature of the pelvic floor), intra-abdominal pressure is increased: *abdominal muscular pressure* (evacuation of the intestine, emptying of the bladder; expulsion of the fetus at birth; strengthened or aggravated expiration, abrupt coughing).

The contraction of both *recti muscles* (together with the exertion of the oblique muscles of both sides) makes possible a *forward flexing of the trunk*, also against resistance or when lying down; with a fixed upper body, it brings about an elevation of the anterior margin of the pelvis.

The *oblique* and the *straight abdominal muscles* of the same side can carry out a *lateral bending of the trunk* together with the *quadratus lumborum*. For a *rotary movement*, the external abdominal oblique of one side and the internal abdominal oblique of the other side work together (with the autochthonous trunk musculature).

The *quadratus lumborum* can draw the 12th rib downward.

d) Weak Sites of the Abdominal Wall

The construction of the abdominal wall from deformable musculotendinous plates provides the prerequisite for the various functions of the abdominal musculature, a reinforcing of the abdominal wall by skeletal elements taking place only to a limited extent. Moreover, a muscular covering is absent at the extensive aponeuroses in the region of the linea alba, which is up to 2.5 cm wide cranial to the navel, and in a band situated lateral to the rectus abdominis. At the navel, the site of passage of the embryonic umbilical vessels surrounded by an umbilical ring is filled postnatally by a connective tissue plug (*umbilical papilla*, Fig. **203 b**); the structural contents of the inguinal "canal" penetrate the abdominal wall throughout life. Below the inguinal ligament, the femoral vessels pass through the vascular compartment (lacuna vasorum), the medial portion of which is occluded only in part by fascial layers (transversalis fascia, iliac fascia, femoral ring).

Wall regions in which only aponeuroses, fasciae or other connective tissue structures form the foundation of the abdominal wall, but especially "openings", which are imperfectly sealed off mechanically, are weak sites, *points of least resistance*. At these sites, gaps (*herniae*) can appear due to embryonic malformation and/or acute or chronic elevation of intra-abdominal pressure. Especially endangered are the cranial portions of the linea alba, the navel, as well as regions of the inguinal canal and femoral canal.

An *external hernia* is defined as a protrusion of viscera (or parts of viscera) through a gap in the abdominal wall (*hernial orifice*) into a pathologically formed cavity (*hernial sac*) which is lined by parietal peritoneum. The intra-abdominal elevation in pressure can have various causes (e.g. chronic cough, chronic constipation, heavy bodily work). The development of a hernia is facilitated by a weak abdominal wall (e.g. divergence of recti muscles after several pregnancies [diastasis recti], postoperative scars).

Epigastric hernia. In this type of hernia, the hernia sac arises in the cranial portion of the linea alba (e.g. in diastasis recti or in a defect of the linea alba).

Umbilical hernia. In a congenital umbilical hernia, the physiological omphalocele does not completely involute. The thin hernial sac consists of peritoneum and amnion.

An acquired umbilical hernia in the new born child arises before the umbilical papilla is developed and before the umbilical wound has closed. The hernial sac, therefore, consists only of peritoneum and delicate connective tissue; it is not covered with skin. In both forms of umbilical herniae, there is the danger of an inflammation of the peritoneum (peritonitis). In infancy, the still soft umbilical papilla can give way under increased abdominal pressure (continuous crying), and a skin-covered hernial sac can form. The acquired umbilical hernia in the adult occurs especially in women in which the umbilical ring has enlarged after several pregnancies. This ring is the hernial orifice in all forms of umbilical herniae.

e) Hernial Orifices in the Inguinal Region

The **inguinal ligament** passes from the anterior superior iliac spine to the pubic tubercle and forms the caudal boundary of the ventral abdominal wall (Figs. **123** and **204**).

The inguinal ligament is not a uniformly-shaped, typical ligament. The lateral part of the bow-shaped connective tissue band is a strengthened, taut fibrous tract of the *iliac fascia* which encloses the iliopsoas. The angled medial crus of the inguinal ligament is formed by the caudal margin of the aponeurosis of the external abdominal oblique. The bundles of fibers of the lateral portion partly continue into the medial section and partly split off from the ligament of the *iliopectineal arch* bordering the muscular compartment.

The superficial abdominal fascia, which merges caudally into the fascia lata of the thigh, is connected with the external surface of the inguinal ligament. The transversalis fascia is attached at the inner side of the ligament.

Inguinal Canal

The anterior abdominal wall is perforated above the inguinal ligament by the **inguinal canal** (Figs. **204** and **206**). It courses obliquely from dorsal, lateral and cranial to ventral, medial and caudal and reaches a length of 40 mm or more, although the abdominal wall here is only 6–8 mm thick. The inguinal canal maintains a lumen only after the removal of its contents, i.e. when the spermatic cord in males or the round ligament of the uterus in females is removed by dissection.

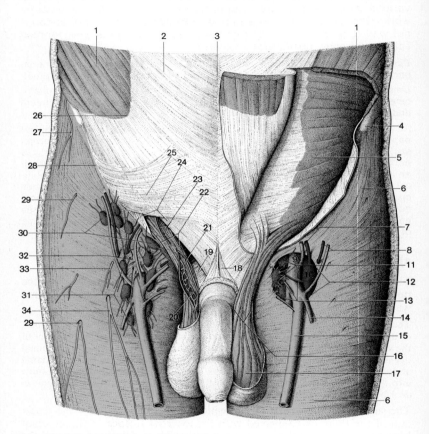

Fig. 204. **Anterior abdominal wall**, ventral view
Groin region and saphenous opening
(Superficial abdominal fascia and cremasteric fascia removed.
Spermatic cord opened on right side; external oblique severed on left side and retracted medially; cribriform fascia dissected off and deep inguinal lymph nodes depicted)

The *spermatic cord* – a fascial funnel of the transversalis fascia embedded in the cremaster muscle and the internal spermatic fascia – contains the ductus deferens and the artery of the ductus deferens accompanying it, the testicular artery, the pampiniform plexus, and the autonomic nerve plexus of the testicular plexus (Fig. **123**).

The inguinal ligament and the *reflected ligament* form the *floor of the inguinal canal*. The reflected ligament arises from the caudal fibers of the aponeurosis of the external abdominal oblique (lateral crus), which turn inward at the level of the inguinal ligament and course to the linea alba and to the pubic bone (posterior to the pubic tubercle) behind the medial portion of the inguinal ligament. Thus, an oblique groove is formed which leads medially downward and receives the spermatic cord.

The *roof of the inguinal canal* is formed by the caudal margin of the internal oblique and transversus abdominis. Fiber bundles are also given off to the spermatic cord (cremaster muscle) or to the round ligament of the uterus.

The *anterior wall* consists of the aponeurosis of the external abdominal oblique; the *posterior wall* is formed by the transversalis fascia and its strengthening tracts.

The *external (superficial) inguinal ring* (Fig. **123**) forms the external "opening" of the inguinal canal. It lies lateral to the pubic tubercle and is covered by the superficial abdominal fascia and the aponeurosis of the external oblique, which continues on the spermatic cord as the *external spermatic fascia*. The external inguinal ring itself can be seen as a slit-like

1 External oblique
2 Anterior layer of rectal sheath
3 Linea alba
4 Anterior superior iliac spine
5 Internal oblique
6 Fascia lata
7 Superficial epigastric artery and vein
8 Superficial circumflex iliac artery and vein
9 Femoral vein
10 Femoral artery
11 Deep inguinal lymph nodes
12 Falciform margin, arched margin of saphenous opening
13 External pudendal arteries and veins
14 Accessory saphenous vein
15 Great saphenous vein
16 Cremaster
17 Internal spermatic fascia
18 Adminiculum of linea alba
19 Reflected ligament
20 Testicular artery and pampiniform plexus
21 Ductus deferens and artery of ductus deferens
22 Genital branch of genitofemoral nerve (medial) and ilio-inguinal nerve (lateral to spermatic cord)
23 Cremasteric artery and vein
24 Medial and lateral crura of aponeurosis of external oblique
25 Intercrural fibers
26 Muscle edge
27 Lateral cutaneous branch of iliohypogastric nerve
28 Inguinal ligament
29 Branches of lateral femoral cutaneous nerve
30, 31 Superficial inguinal lymph nodes
30 Oblique tract
31 Longitudinal tract
32 Cribriform fascia, connective tissue closing plate of saphenous opening
33 Femoral branch of genitofemoral nerve
34 Anterior cutaneous branches of femoral nerve

opening only after removal of the superficial abdominal fascia and after severance of the aponeurosis of the extenal oblique. The medial margin is formed by the *medial crus*, which is not marked off from the remaining aponeurosis. The lateral contour of the margin is formed by the *lateral crus*, whose fibers make up the medial portion of the inguinal ligament and are turned partially inward (i.e. the most caudal fibers) to form the reflected ligament. Both crura are connected by *intercrural fibers* (from the superficial abdominal fascia), which border the external inguinal ring laterocranially.

The *internal (deep) inguinal ring* becomes visible when the transversalis fascia is removed at the posterior surface of the anterior abdominal wall. In this way, the margin of the fascial funnel, which evaginates into the inguinal canal and covers the spermatic cord as the *internal spermatic fascia*, is dissected free.

Inguinal Fossae

The *lateral inguinal fossa* (Figs. **205** and **206**) marks the position of the deep inguinal ring at the posterior surface of the ventral abdominal wall covered by the peritoneum. This fossa is separated from the medial inguinal fossa by the *lateral umbilical fold*, a peritoneal fold which is formed by the inferior epigastric vessels.

The inferior epigastric artery and vein run cranially "up" the inter-foveolar ligament (i.e. between the "ligament" and the peritoneum) and pass through the posterior layer of the rectus sheath at the dorsal surface of the rectus abdominis. In the lateral inguinal fossa, the peritoneum can still exhibit rudimentary remains of the embryonic processus vaginalis. The *interfoveolar ligament* represents a reinforcement of the transversalis fascia; it passes in a craniocaudal direction near the medial margin of the internal inguinal ring, parallel to the margin of the rectus. It can be accompanied, or in part replaced, by fine, longitudinal bundles of fibers of the transversus abdominis, the tendons of which insert at the pubic tubercle or radiate into the reflected ligament.

The *medial inguinal fossa* (Figs. **205** and **206**) is bordered medially by the *medial umbilical fold*, in which the *medial umbilical ligament* (= obliterated umbilical artery) passes to the navel. The mediocaudal margin of the fossa is strengthened by a fibrous plate, the *falx inguinalis [conjoined tendon]*. The fibers of the falx originate from the aponeurosis of the transversus abdominis and the rectus sheath. They pass obliquely caudad at the lateral margin of the rectus and attach at the pecten of the pubis.

The medial inguinal fossa corresponds to the external inguinal ring at the ventral surface of the anterior abdominal wall. The abdominal wall here is largely free of muscle and is formed predominantly by the transversalis fascia and its strengthening tracts. Only the variable fiber bundles of the

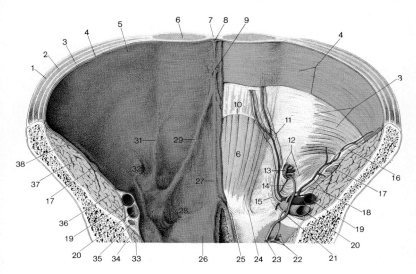

Fig. 205. **Anterior abdominal wall**, dorsal view
(Peritoneum removed from right side)

 1 External oblique
 2 Internal oblique
 3 Transversus abdominis and semilunar line
 4 Transversalis fascia (removed below umbilicus on right side)
 5 Parietal peritoneum
 6 Rectus abdominis
 7 Linea alba
 8 Ligamentum teres of liver
 9 Umbilicus
10 Arcuate line (rectus sheath)
11 Inferior epigastric artery and vein
12 Border of deep inguinal ring
13 Internal spermatic fascia (served at exit of fascial funnel from transversalis fascia) envelopes, among other things, ductus deferens, testicular vessels; genital branch of genitofemoral nerve on medial wall of funnel depicted, but not labelled)
14 Cremasteric artery
15 Interfoveolar ligament
16 Inguinal ligament
17 Femoral nerve
18 Deep circumflex iliac artery and vein
19 External iliac artery

20 External iliac vein
21 Pubic branch of inferior epigastric artery (severed)
22 Obturator artery and vein, obturator nerve
23 Ductus deferens
24 Falx inguinalis
25 Adminiculum of linea alba
26 Urinary bladder (cut open in midline)
27 Median umbilical fold, formed by median umbilical ligament (= obliterated urachus)
28 Supravesical fossa
29 Medial umbilical fold, peritoneal fold formed by medial umbilical ligament (= obliterated umbilical artery)
30 Medial inguinal fossa
31 Lateral umbilical fold, peritoneal fold formed by inferior epigastric vessels
32 Lateral inguinal fossa
33 Obturator internus
34 Obturator fascia
35 Rosenmüller's lymph node
36 Psoas major
37 Iliacus
38 Iliac fascia

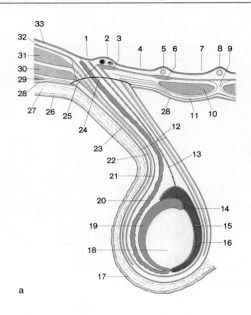

a

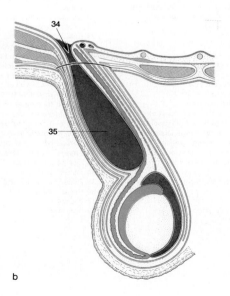

b

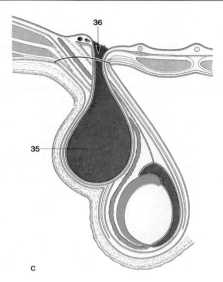

c

Fig. 206. **Schematic sections through inguinal canal and spermatic cord**
a Coverings of spermatic cord and testis
b Lateral (indirect or oblique) acquired inguinal hernia
c Medial (direct or straight) inguinal hernia

 1 Lateral inguinal fossa
 2 Lateral umbilical fold, peritoneal fold formed by inferior espigastric artery and vein
 3 Interfoveolar ligament
 4 Medial inguinal fossa
 5 Medial umbilical fold, peritoneal fold formed by medial umbilical ligament (=obliterated unbilical artery)
 6 Falx inguinalis
 7 Supravesical fossa
 8 Median umbilical fold, formed by median umbilical ligament (=obliterated urachus)
 9 Adminiculum of linea alba
10 Rectus abdominis
11 Anterior layer of rectus sheath
12 Spermatic cord
13 Vestigial processus vaginalis
14, 15 Tunical vaginalis of testis
14 Parietal layer
15 Visceral layer
16 Scrotal cavity

17 Dartos
18 Testis
19 Epididymis
20 Ductus deferens
21 Internal spermatic fascia
22 Cremaster and cremasteric fascia
23 External spermatic fascia
24, 25 External and internal ''opening'' of inguinal canal
24 Superficial inguinal ring
25 Deep inguinal ring
26 Skin
27 Subcutaneous connective tissue
28 Superficial abdominal fascia
29 External oblique
30 Internal oblique
31 Transversus abdominis
32 Transversalis fascia
33 Peritoneum
34 Hernial opening in lateral inguinal fossa
35 Hernial sac
36 Hernial opening in medial inguinal fossa

interfoveolar muscle appear as muscular consituents of the wall. The medial inguinal fossa thus becomes the weakest site of the abdominal wall, which can give way under increased intra-abdominal pressure and become a hernial orifice (medial inguinal hernia).

The triangular area situated between the two medial umbilical folds is bisected in the midline by the *median umbilical fold*. This peritoneal fold contains the *median umbilical ligament*, the obliterated urachus. The fossae located above the urinary bladder and bordered laterally by the medial umbilical folds are referred to as the *supravesical fossae*.

Inguinal herniae can emanate both from the lateral and from the medial inguinal fossa. The hernial orifice thus always lies cranial to the inguinal ligament (in the case of a femoral hernia it always lies below the inguinal ligament). *Lateral inguinal herniae* (= indirect or oblique inguinal herniae) and *medial inguinal herniae* (= direct or straight inguinal herniae) can be distinguished.

In *lateral inguinal herniae* (Fig. **206 b**), the orifice lies in the lateral inguinal fossa, i.e. lateral to the inferior epigastric artery. Lateral inguinal herniae are pushed forward in the inguinal canal, the hernial sac laying inside of the spermatic cord. They can be "congenital" or acquired.

In "congenital" inguinal herniae, the processus vaginalis is not obliterated. As a result of increased intra-abdominal pressure by the abdominal musculature, the abdominal viscera push forward after birth into the peritoneal outpocketing and enlarge it.

Medial inguinal herniae (Fig. **206 c**) are always acquired. They evaginate the peritoneum and the transversalis fascia of the medial inguinal fossa and pass through the abdominal wall in a straight direction. The hernial orifice thus lies medial to the inferior epigastric vessels. In both medial and lateral inguinal herniae, the hernial sac bulges in the region of the external inguinal ring.

f) Vessels and Nerves of the Abdominal Wall

Arteries. The arterial supply of the abdominal wall involves, among others:
– segmental arteries: the 5 caudal *posterior intercostal arteries*, the *subcostal artery*, and the *lumbar arteries* (Fig. **25**);
– an arterial longitudinal system: the *superior* (Figs. **185** and **193**) and *inferior epigastric* (from the external iliac artery, Fig. **205**) *arteries*, which anastomose with one another in the rectus abdominis muscle; and
– a muscular branch: the *ascending branch* of the *deep circumflex iliac artery* (from the external iliac artery, Fig. **126**), which passes upward

between the transversus abdominis and internal abdominal oblique in the border region of the ventral and lateral abdominal wall (and is endangered during operative opening of the abdominal cavity by oblique or transverse incisions with a lateral line of incision).

The *posterior intercostal arteries VII – XI* pass over the costal arches, course obliquely downward – like the *subcostal artery* – in the ventral abdominal wall between the transversus abdominis and internal oblique, and enter the rectus abdominis.

They give off *lateral cutaneous branches* to the side and ventral branches to the abdominal skin near the midline.

The *lumbar arteries* continue the series of segmental arteries caudally as paired segmental arteries (the 5th pair, *lowest lumbar artery*, arises from the median sacral artery).

The main branch of the lumbar artery (Fig. **185**) arrives in the muscular abdominal wall dorsal to the psoas (for the three cranial lumbar arteries also dorsal to the quadratus lumborum), where it courses between the transversus and internal oblique and in the axillary line gives off a twig to the skin of the lateral body wall. Ventral cutaneous branches are absent (the ventral abdominal skin is supplied by the intercostal arteries, the subcostal artery, and by branches of the epigastric arteries).

The lumbar arteries anastomose ventrally with branches of the inferior epigastric artery, cranially with the intercostal arteries, caudally with the iliolumbar and deep circumflex iliac arteries, and with one another. In the case of slow occlusion of the caudal end of the aorta, they can be enlarged into functionally sufficient collateral connections between the aortic "stump" and the external iliac artery (and thus also – retrograde – the internal iliac artery).

The **inferior epigastric artery** courses dorsally upward "on" the interfoveolar ligament, penetrates the rectus sheath, and passes cranially on the posterior surface of the rectus abdominis.

The *pubic branch* courses to the symphysis and is connected by means of a lateral branch, the *obturator branch*, with the pubic branch of the obturator artery (Fig. **126**). The *cremasteric artery* (Figs. **204** and **205**) arises in the vicinity of the deep inguinal ring, passes into the scrotum with the spermatic cord, and supplies the cremaster muscle. In females, the *artery of the round ligament of the uterus* accompanies the same ligament to the labium majus.

The inferior epigastric artery supplies the rectus abdominis and the lateral abdominal muscles. It anastomoses above the navel with the superior epigastric artery, the terminal branch of the internal thoracic artery, and thus connects the external iliac artery with the subclavian artery. The segmental arteries are also connected here.

In a *puncture* of the abdominal cavity, injuries to the inferior epigastric artery can be avoided if the puncture is placed at the border to the lateral third of a line connecting the navel and anterior superior iliac spine (usually on the left side since the sigmoid colon is avoided, whereas the cecum might be damaged on the right side). An alternative point of puncture is halfway between the pubic symphysis and the navel in the midline.

Veins. The blood from the abdominal wall can be carried off via the *companion veins* of the arteries. In addition, connections exist between the deep and the superficial veins of the abdominal wall (e.g. inferior and superficial epigastric veins), and there are numerous anastomoses between the drainage areas of the superior and inferior venae cavae so that extensive collateral pathways can be readily formed between both venae cavae in the case of drainage obstruction.

The *lumbar veins* open directly into the inferior vena cava and via a longitudinal anastomosis, the *ascending lumbar vein*, into the azygos vein on the right side and the hemiazygos vein on the left side, which also receive the *posterior intercostal veins* (Fig. 27). The ascending lumbar vein communicates caudally with the common iliac vein. The *inferior epigastric* (usually doubled) and the *deep circumflex iliac veins* drain into the external iliac vein (Fig. 205), whereas the *superficial epigastric vein* and the *external pudendal veins* empty into the great saphenous vein or into the femoral vein (Fig. 166 a).

The *inferior vena cana anastomoses with* the branches of the *superior vena cava*:
– by means of the ascending lumbar veins,
– via the lumbar veins and the vertebral venous plexus,
– by the connections of the inferior and superior epigastric veins at the dorsal surface of the rectus abdominis, and
– via the superficial epigastric vein, which communicates with the thoraco-epigastric veins (Fig. 209).

The *hepatic portal vein* communicates with the superficial and the deep veins of the abdominal wall in the vicinity of the navel via fine venous branches, the *para-umbilical veins* (Fig. 209), which course in the ligamentum teres (round ligament of the liver). In a blockage of the portal vein, blood can flow through para-umbilical veins craniad to the superior vena cava and caudad to the drainage area of the inferior vena cava via the enlarged and tortuously coursing veins of the abdominal wall (caput medusae).

The **lymphatic pathways** from the deep layers of the abdominal wall accompany the blood vessels. They convey lymph to the *parasternal lymph nodes* (along the internal thoracic vessels), via the *inferior epigastric lymph nodes* (along the inferior epigastric vessels) to the *external* and *common iliac lymph nodes* (along the iliac vessels) and also to the *lumbar lymph nodes* (lateral to the aorta and inferior vena cava), as well as directly to the lumbar lymph nodes – from the muscle layers of the posterior abdominal wall.

Nerves. The lateral abdominal muscles are supplied by the *caudal intercostal nerves*, by the *subcostal nerve*, and by the two long cranial branches of the lumbar plexus, the *iliohypogastric* and *ilio-inguinal nerves* (Fig. 200). The anterior abdominal muscles generally receive only the ventral rami of thoracic nerves (T7–12). The quadratus lumborum is innervated mainly by short branches of the lumbar plexus (T12, L1–3).

The unisegmental lateral lumbar intertransverse muscles receive short muscular branches from the "roots" of the lumbar plexus.

Sensory branches of the nerves of the abdominal wall innervate the parietal layer of the peritoneum.

The *caudal intercostal nerves* pass over the costal arches with the vessels of the same name and – like the subcostal nerve – course between the transversus and internal oblique. They give off muscular branches to the lateral abdominal muscles and dispatch *lateral cutaneous rami* (Figs. **185** and **209**) in the serrated line between the origins of the serratus anterior and the external abdominal oblique. The ventral terminal branch of the caudal intercostal nerves enters the rectus sheath, innervates the muscle, and sends the *anterior cutaneous ramus* to the skin.

The *iliohypogastric* and *ilio-inguinal nerves* often arise as a common stem at the lateral margin of the psoas, course laterally on the anterior surface of the quadratus lumborum behind the kidney, proceed between transversus and internal oblique (to which they give off muscular branches), and pass ventrally above the iliac crest parallel to one another.

D. Surface Anatomy of the Anterior Trunk Wall

1. Surface Relief of the Anterior Trunk Wall and Palpable Bony Points

The **surface relief** óf the *thoracic wall* (Fig. **210**) in well-built males is determined on the ventral surface by the contours of the pectoralis major and is shaped in the lower lateral region by the serrated line which separates the alternating origins of the serratus anterior and the external obique (Gerdy's line). Between the clavicular portion of the large breast muscle and the deltoid, the skin is depressed below the middle of the clavicle (in slender individuals) to form the infraclavicular fossa (Mohrenheim's fossa). At the lower margin of the thorax, the origin of the rectus abdominis protrudes on each side of the midline.

A contracted sternalis muscle, developed as a variant, can be visible through the skin as a longitudinal swelling at the margin of the sternum and can fill the anterior median furrow (partially).

The skin, which is generally very movable, is fixed in the thoracic region at the sternal membrane. Here, in males, a more or less well developed terminal hairiness can appear, which can extend laterally into the axilla and which continues caudally onto the abdominal skin.

In females, the surface relief of the thoracic wall is essentially determined by the size, shape and position of the mammary glands.

The *soft tissue relief of the abdominal wall* in very slender, well-developed males exhibits the two longitudinal swellings of the rectus abdominis separated by a median groove and the transverse furrows caused by the tendinous insertions. The transition of the muscle belly of the external oblique into its aponeurosis can appear as a *muscular edge* somewhat cranial to the anterior superior iliac spine (Figs. **204** and **210 a**). When the lateral abdominal musculature is relaxed, the external oblique bulges over the iliac crest as an *inguinal swelling*.

In most individuals – especially in females with less prominent musculature and relatively higher deposits of subcutaneous fat – the amount and distribution of the fat deposits determine the surface appearance of the abdominal wall.

In the subcutaneous tissue, several connective tissue layers can be represented, between which fat is deposited to a variable extent. These connective tissue plates are attached somewhat more firmly to one another in the median plane and are connected with the rectus sheath so that a shallow, median longitudinal furrow also arises below the navel in obese individuals, which fills up caudally toward the *mons pubis*.

At the *navel* (*umbilicus*), subcutaneous fat is absent. The skin has fused with the *umbilical papilla* and sunk in to form the *umbilical fossa* (Fig. **203b**). In slender individuals, the umbilicus lies somewhat below the middle between the xiphoid process and the pubic symphysis, at about the level of the upper margin of the 4th lumbar vertebra.

The *direction of the cleavages* of the skin at the anterior abdominal wall courses slightly oblique from laterocranial to mediocaudal (Fig. **71**). (In incisions made in the direction of the cleavage lines, the margins of the wound usually fit together well.)

The *hairiness* of the mons pubis ends in females with a horizontal boundary line, whereas in males it can extend in the midline up to the umbilicus and go over into the thoracic hair.

At the *thoracic wall*, the clavicle, jugular notch of the sternum. sternal angle, ribs and costal arches represent the **palpable bony points** (Fig. **207**) which permit an easy orientation.

Only the 1st rib, which is covered by the clavicle, is not palpable. It is better to count the ribs in the bony portion since the cartilages of ribs 6–10 lie relatively close together. The sternal angle marks the level of the sternal insertion of the 2nd rib.

At the caudal border of the *abdominal wall*, the anterior superior iliac spine and the iliac crest can be identified without difficulty.

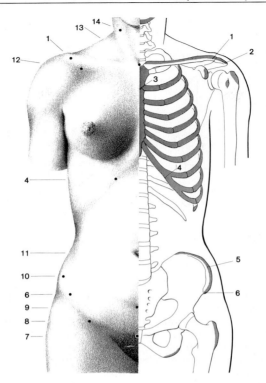

Fig. 207. **Surface relief of female anterior trunk wall** (right side) **and palpable bony points** (left)

1 Acromial end of clavicle
2 Acromion
3 Sternal angle
4 Costal arch
5 Iliac crest
6 Anterior superior iliac spine
7 Transverse line at upper margin of mons pubis

8 Inguinal furrow
9 Transverse abdominal furrow
10 Inguinal swelling
11 Umbilicus
12 Clavipectoral triangle (Infraclavicular fossa)
13 Jugular notch of sternum
14 Bulge of sternocleidomastoid

Organization of the trunk wall (Fig. **208**). A "coordinate system" is used to *subdivide the trunk wall*. It consists of palpable parts of the skeleton (sternum, ribs, spinous process of vertebra) and of perpendicular lines which course through easily definable segments of the thoracic wall. With the help of this system, projection points of inner organs or certain conditions can be localized on the thoracic wall.

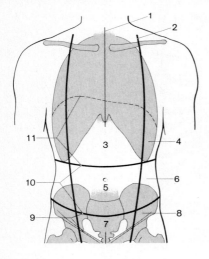

Fig. 208. **Regional organization of abdominal wall**
1 Anterior median line
2 Midclavicular line
3 Epigastric region
4 Hypochondriac region
5 Umbilical region
6 Lateral (lumbar) region
7 Pubic region
8 Inguinal region
9 Inferior abdominal region
10 Middle abdominal region
11 Superior abdominal region

The following longitudinal lines are employed:
– the *anterior median line*, the vertical line in the middle of the anterior surface of the trunk;
– the *posterior median line*, the vertical line in the middle of the back;
– the *midclavicular line*, the vertical line through the middle of the clavicle – the designation *mammary line*, which is used in clinics, is less precise (particularly in women because of the different development of the breasts and their variable position);
– the *midaxillary line*, the vertical line *midway* between the anterior and posterior axillary folds (the *anterior axillary line* courses perpendicularly through the caudal end of the anterior axillary fold; the *posterior axillary line* runs correspondingly perpendicularly through the attachment of the posterior axillary fold at the back); and
– the *scapular line*, the vertical line through the inferior angle of the scapula when the arm is hanging down normally.

Regional organization of the abdominal wall. Two horizontal lines, which course through the deepest point of the 10th rib and the highest point of the two iliac crests, separate the abdominal wall into three segments: *superior*, *middle*, and *inferior abdominal regions*. Longitudinal lines at the lateral margin of both recti abdominis muscles divide each of these abdominal regions into an unpaired median field and two paired fields.

The following regions are distinguished:
– at the superior abdominal region: medially, the *epigastric region*, and laterally, the *right* and *left hypochondriac regions*;

- at the middle abdominal region: medially, the *umbilical region*, and laterally, the *right* and *left lateral* (lumbar) *regions*;
- at the inferior abdominal region: medially, the *pubic* (hypogastric) *region*, and laterally, the *right* and *left inguinal regions*.

The middle of a line connecting the anterior superior iliac spine with the umbilicus (*McBurney's point*) frequently corresponds to the projection point of the base of the vermiform appendix on the anterior abdominal wall. The apex of this organ can be projected at *Lanz's point*, i.e. the point occupying the right third of a line connecting the two anterior superior iliac spines. Since the position and length of the appendix varies considerably, the significance of these two points as characteristic pain sites in an inflammation of the appendix is strongly limited, of course.

2. Cutaneous Vessels and Nerves of the Anterior Trunk Wall

a) Cutaneous Arteries

At the *lateral trunk wall*, the posterior intercostal arteries, the subcostal artery, and the lumbar arteries each give off a *lateral cutaneous branch*, which divides into an anterior and a posterior branch (Figs. **26** and **209**).

Branches of the lateral thoracic artery ramify in the skin of the anterior axillary fold; branches of the thoracodorsal artery divide in the skin of the axillary fossa. These cutaneous branches communicate with one another and with the lateral cutaneous branches.

The deltoid branch of the thoraco-acromial artery likewise dispatches branches to the subcutaneous tissue between the pectoralis major and the deltoid and to the skin over the infraclavicular fossa.

The superficial circumflex iliac artery, which arises from the femoral artery somewhat distal to the inguinal ligament and courses laterally nearly parallel to the inguinal ligament, supplies the skin of the inguinal region.

The cutaneous arteries of the *anterior trunk wall* penetrate the fascia near the midline. *Perforating branches* from the internal thoracic artery ramify in the skin of the chest, whereas the ventral abdominal skin is supplied by anterior cutaneous branches, which are terminal branches of posterior intercostal arteries VII–XI and the subcostal artery.

Cutaneous branches to the anterior abdominal wall also come from the superficial epigastric artery, which arises from the femoral artery somewhat below the inguinal ligament (Figs. **204** and **209**) and passes cranially in the subcutaneous tissue to about the level of the umbilical fossa. Fine twigs to the abdominal skin come from the deep arteries, the superior and inferior epigastric arteries. Small *inguinal branches* from the external pudendal arteries (from the femoral artery) supply the skin in the region of the external inguinal ring.

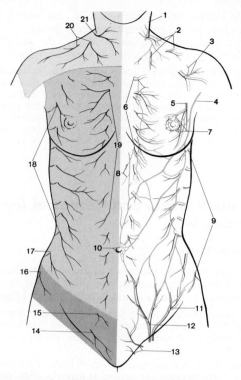

Fig. 209. Cutaneous vessels and nerves of anterior trunk wall
Schematic depiction of cutaneous arteries and veins on left side of body, of cutaneous nerves and anatomical cutaneous fields on right side

▢ Ventral rami of cervical nerves (cervical plexus)
▨ Ventral rami of thoracic nerves (intercostal nerves)
▧ Ventral rami of lumbar nerves (lumbar plexus)

1 Anterior jugular vein
2 Cutaneous branches of superficial cervical artery and accompanying veins
3 Branches of thoraco-acromial artery and vein
4 Thoraco-epigastric vein
5 Lateral thoracic artery and vein with lateral mammary branches
6 Perforating branches with medial mammary branches and accompanying veins
7 Areolar venous plexus
8 Subcutaneous abdominal veins
9 Lateral cutaneous branches of posterior intercostal and lumbar arteries and veins
10 Para-umbilical veins
11 Superficial circumflex iliac artery and vein
12 Superficial epigastric artery and vein

13 Branches of external pudendal arteries and veins
14 Anterior labial nerves of ilio-inguinal nerve
15 Anterior cutaneous branch ⎫ of iliohypogastric
16 Lateral cutaneous branch ⎬ nerve
17 Lateral cutaneous branch of subcostal nerves
18 Lateral cutaneous branches of intercostal nerves with lateral mammary branches
19 Anterior cutaneous branches of intercostal nerves with medial mammary branches
20 Medial and intermediate supraclavicular nerves
21 Transverse cervical (colli) nerve

b) Cutaneous Veins

From the well-developed *subcutaneous venous network of the anterior trunk wall* (Fig. **209**), the blood is carried off by the *companion veins* of the cutaneous arteries into the intercostal veins, the internal thoracic vein, and the lumbar veins, as well as into the axillary vein (via the lateral thoracic, thoracodorsal or thoraco-acromial veins) and into the femoral vein (via the superficial epigastric and superficial circumflex iliac veins which usually enter the great saphenous vein at the saphenous hiatus).

At the chest wall, there are additional drainage possibilities into the anterior jugular and cephalic veins.

In an obstruction of the venous return in the abdominal cavity, the usually weak *thoraco-epigastric veins* can become enlarged and obtain considerable clinical significance. They exit from the subcutaneous venous network of the abdominal wall and convey the blood directly or indirectly into the axillary vein. By means of anastomoses with the superficial epigastric vein, which empties into the femoral vein (usually via the great saphenous vein), a collateral pathway exists between the venae cavae, which becomes enlarged if there is an *obstruction in the drainage of the inferior vena cava*. In a *blockage of the hepatic portal vein*, portal blood can be discharged via the para-umbilical veins and the thoraco-epigastric or superficial epigastric veins into the drainage area of both the superior and inferior venae cavae.

c) Superficial Lymphatic Pathways

Lymph drainage (Fig. 210) from the thoracic wall and the part of the abdominal wall situated above the umbilicus takes place mainly via the *pectoral axillary lymph nodes* (at the lower margin of the pectoralis minor), whereas that from the region caudal to the navel occurs via the *superficial inguinal lymph nodes* (in the inguinal region).

Connections exist, moreover, to intercostal and parasternal lymph nodes (also across the midline).

d) Cutaneous Nerves

The **cutaneous innervation** of the lateral and anterior trunk walls (Fig. **209**) is largely taken over by the ventral branches of the thoracic nerves (intercostal nerves, subcostal nerve). They provide *lateral* and *anterior cutaneous branches*.

The cutaneous branches to the lateral trunk wall arise from intercostal nerves II–XI and the subcostal nerve; the anterior cutaneous branches in the thoracic region come from the cranial six intercostal nerves and at the abdominal wall from intercostal nerves VII–XI and the subcostal nerve.

The *lateral cutaneous branches* pass into the subcutaneous tissue approximately at the axillary line between the slips of origin of the serratus anterior and external oblique and branch off (often already before entering the fascia) into an anterior and a posterior ramus.

The *anterior cutaneous branches* penetrate the thoracic fascia near the sternal margin; at the abdominal wall they are usually doubled, whereby one branch perforates the rectus abdominis and the other penetrates the aponeurosis after passing along the lateral margin of the rectus.

Branches from the cervical plexus, the *medial* and *intermediate supraclavicular nerves*, pass below the platysma and over the clavicle to the skin of the clavicular region and the area of the cranial thoracic wall (up to the level of ribs 3 – 4).

The skin above and medial to the external inguinal ring is supplied by the *anterior*

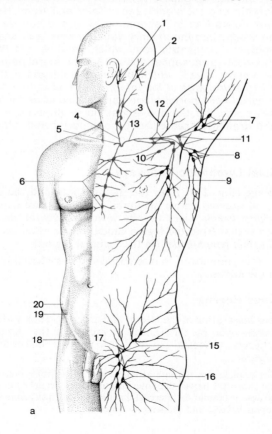

a

cutaneous branch of the *iliohypogastric nerve*; a small cutaneous area above the symphysis is supplied by the *ilio-inguinal nerve*.

Segmental relations of the skin and **Head's zones.** The ventral rami of

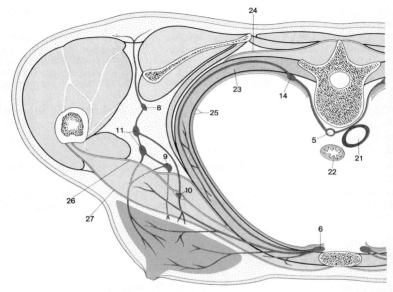

Fig. 210. **Lymphatic pathways of trunk wall**

a Superficial lymphatic pathways of ventral trunk wall and
   nape of neck
   Superficial lymphatic pathways and lymph nodes ———
   Deep lymphatic pathways and lymph nodes ——

b Lymphatic tracts of mammary gland (shown in a schematic
   transverse section after Pernkopf; ribs in thoracic wall not
   depicted)

1 Mastoid lymph nodes
2 Occipital lymph nodes
3 Deep cervical lymph nodes
4 Jugular trunk
5 Thoracic duct
6 Parasternal lymph nodes
7 Lateral axillary lymph nodes
8 Subscapular axillary lymph nodes
9 Pectoral axillary lymph nodes
10 Interpectoral axillary lymph nodes
11 Central axillary lymph nodes
12 Apical axillary lymph nodes
13 Subclavian trunk
14 Intercostal lympn nodes
15, 16 Superficial inguinal lymph nodes

15 Oblique tract
16 Longitudinal tract
17 Lymphatic drainage via deep inguinal
   lymph nodes to external iliac lymph nodes
18 Inguinal furrow
19 Muscle edge
20 Inguinal swelling
21 Aorta
22 Esophagus
23 Deep layer of thoracic wall (ribs and
   intercostal muscles)
24 Thoracolumbar fascia
25 Parietal pleura and endothoracic fascia
26 Clavipectoral fascia
27 Pectoral fascia

nerves T2–12 and L1 supply cutaneous areas (Fig. **57a**) with their cutaneous branches: these areas are approximately belt-like at the thoracic wall and at the epigastric region, slightly sloping toward the midline below the umbilicus.

The segmental areas of innervation at the thoracic wall are not identical with the intercostal spaces.

The 1st intercostal nerve, which lacks a lateral cutaneous ramus, does not possess an autonomic cutaneous region. The dermatome adjoining cutaneous segment T2 cranially is innervated (almost exclusively) by fibers of the cervical plexus (supraclavicular nerves) from spinal cord segment C4. Between segmental zones C4 and T2, there is thus a segmental gap (*hiatus*) since the sensory fibers of the missing segments pass to the upper limb.

The fibers for touch and temperature perception overlap on adjacent segments; only the fibers for pain sensation show no overlapping and are distributed within only one segment. These unisegmentally-innervated dermatomes correspond to Head's zones.

A series of heart disorders can produce hyperalgesia in dermatomes T2–8 on the left side of the body.

In certain dermatomes of the abdominal skin, "crossed" segmental hyperalgesias can appear, for example, in diseases of the gastro-intestinal or urogenital tract.

3. Female Breast

a) Form and Position of the Female Breast (Mammary Gland)

The female breast, *mammary gland* (Fig. **211**), lies within the subcutaneous tissue. It consists of *glandular tissue*, connective tissue and fat. The 15–20 *conical glandular lobes* and the fat tissue are gathered by a common connective tissue stroma into the *body of the mammary gland*. The connective tissue plates and cords (retinacula) of this stroma organizes the subcutaneous fat into individual compartments. The firmness of the breast is determined by the filling and the bracing of these compartments, and the form is determined by their arrangement and expansion.

Form and size, to a limited extent also position of the organ, are influenced in addition by a multitude of factors (e.g. age, nutritional state, structural body type, hormone balance, posture, functional condition, number of pregnancies, duration of nursing).

In a supine position, the breast of the sexually mature female appears as a (usually) hemispherical protrusion at the level of the ribs 3–6 supported by the thoracic fascia, with which it is movably connected by loose connective tissue. The connective tissue tracts, which course from the

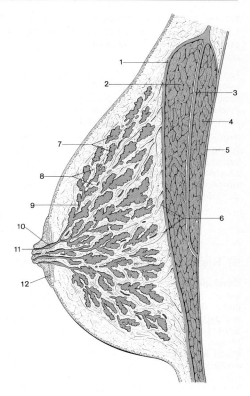

Fig. 211. **Sagittal section through female breast (mammary gland)** Pectoral fasciae, medial view of cut surface

 1 Pectoral fascia
 2 Pectoralis major
 3 Clavipectoral fascia
 4 Pectoralis minor
 5 Fascia of intercostal muscles (external thoracic fascia)
 6 Suspensory ligaments of breast
 7, 8 Body of mammary gland
 7 Parenchyma
 8 Fat bodies
 9 Lactiferous duct
10 Lactiferous sinus
11 Lactiferous duct
12 Radial and circular smooth muscle

dermis layer of the gland to the thin displaceable layer of the thoracic fascia, are known as the *suspensory ligaments of the breast*.

The mammary gland can extend laterally over the lower margin of the pectoral major to the serratus anterior (axillary lobe). The inferior half of the gland is more rounded. In young, nulliparous women (not having borne children), it should merge into the thoracic wall without a fold (Fig. **207**).

After the first child, the breast is usually somewhat more flaccid and sags more distinctly in a standing posture. After several pregnancies and in the elderly, the connective tissue anchoring the gland to the thoracic fascia often loosens, and the sagging of the breast becomes quite pronounced (*pendulous breast*).

The conically-formed *nipple* lies in the center of the likewise strongly pigmented *areola*, which is somewhat below the middle of the breast. The erectile nipple (numerous sensory nerve endings, complicated system of smooth muscle cells and elastic fibers) faces slightly upward. The excretory ducts of the mammary gland and free sebaceous glands open on it.

In the skin of the areola there are sweat glands, as well as sebaceous glands, which open partly free, partly into the hair follicles of fine, small hairs. In the marginal zone of the areola 10–15 apocrine *areolar glands* (of Montgomery) form a ring of small, rounded papillae. Their secretion moistens the nipple and the lips of the infant and contributes to the airtight closure during the sucking action.

The nipple can be very low (*flat nipple*). The excretory ducts of the mammary gland can also open into a small fossa (*pitted nipple*). In both cases, the postnatal proliferation of mesenchyme has not occurred, or not to a sufficient degree, so that the developmental stage attained at the end of fetal development is more or less preserved. In the case of a flat nipple, nursing is usually possible, whereas a pitted nipple represents an absolute hindrance to nursing.

b) Histology of the Mammary Gland

Development of the mammary gland. A *milk stripe* (longitudinally-coursing, striated epithelial thickening at the ventrolateral trunk wall) can be recognized at the end of the 1st embryonic month as the first primordium of the mammary gland; by the 2nd month, it forms the *milk ridge*. Shortly after its origin, the milk ridge undergoes involution in humans with the exception of a small area in the breast region. From this circumscribed epithelial thickening, the anlage of the mammary gland, about 20 epithelial cords, appear in the 5th fetal month; they grow into the underlying mesenchyme and undergo branching. The glandular field, from which only partly-canalized epithelial cords extend toward the end of fetal development, broadens into a small fossa situated in the skin. The nipple generally develops only after birth: connective tissue advances toward the depressed glandular field, raises it to the level of the surrounding skin, and finally causes a nipple to emerge from the areola.

In the region of the milk ridge, additional portions can persist, and accessory nipples can develop: *polythelia* (most frequent in the axillary region). When non-involuted portions of the milk ridge develop into supernumerary mammary glands, it is referred to as *polymastia*.

At birth, the mammary gland consists of the lactiferous ducts, which invaginate into the connective tissue. They continue towards the epithelium as lactiferous sinuses before narrowing again into funnel shapes and opening onto the glandular field, which is often still a foveate depression.

In the 1st month of life, the terminal portions of the lactiferous ducts form the so-called *witches' milk* under the influence of maternal hormones.

During childhood, the lactiferous ducts in both sexes undergo further development very slowly. The degree and length of branching increase moderately. At puberty, the epithelial portion of the gland – especially in girls – proliferates considerably along with the development of the connective tissue stroma, which encloses the lactiferous ducts and borders the glandular lobes.

The **inactive** (nonlactating) **mammary gland** of the sexually-mature female consists of 15–20 branched, tubulo-alveolar glands – corresponding to the number of lobes – of the apocrine type, which lie in the subcutaneous tissue. They are ensheathed in cell-rich and capillary-rich connective tissue, which is embedded in the compact fibrous stroma. Fat cells can infiltrate it and form the quantitatively-dominant fat bodies of the gland.

The changes during the ovarian cycle are mild and reversible (insignificant budding and enlargement of the lactiferous ducts, secretion of a small amount of fat-poor fluid). The completion of the mammary gland into a functional gland takes place only during pregnancy.

Active (lactating) **mammary gland**. Already in the 2nd month of pregnancy, the lactiferous ducts begin to send out buds under the influence of estrogen and to undergo further branching. They become completely canalized and after the middle of pregnancy, stimulated by progesterone, form countless alveoli (simple cuboidal epithelium) from lateral and terminal buds. The connective tissue of the glandular body is repressed; the lobular organization of the strongly vascularized organ becomes clearly evident. The enlargement of the breast can be recognized macroscopically.

From the 8th month of pregnancy, the mammary gland, under the influence of prolactin, forms *colostrum* (yellowish, fat-containing fluid with colostrum corpuscles = wandering cells and cellular debris, in contrast to mature milk which is protein-rich, but poor in fat and carbohydrates). The secretion of milk begins a few days after birth. The groups of alveoli secrete alternately. The delivery of milk is caused by sucking and is accelerated by the contraction of the myoepithelial cells which surround the alveoli and lactiferous ducts. (The tactile stimulus of sucking induces the secretion of oxytocin [neurohormonal reflex], which causes the myoepithelium to contract).

During *weaning* (*ablactation*), milk retention occurs. The extended alveoli can tear. For the most part, they involute. Wandering cells phagocytize the milk remnants and remove them (mainly via the lymph pathways). The loose connective tissue around the lactiferous ducts and the compact fibrous stroma increase, and the organ is transformed into an inactive mammary gland.

Mammary gland after menopause. The lactiferous ducts are only partially preserved, in places obliterated or cystically enlarged (possibility of pathological changes). The typical lobular organization of the organ is lost. The adipose tissue can increase considerably in mass so that the breast becomes larger.

The **male breast** shows principally the same structure as the inactive female gland, but remains small ($\emptyset$ about 1.5 cm, thickness 0.5 cm).

Under the increased influence of female sex hormones, e.g. in hormonal fluctuations at the time of puberty, the male breast becomes enlarged (*gynecomastia*) and secretion can be observed.

c) Vessels and Nerves of the Mammary Gland

Arteries (Fig. **209**). The arterial blood supply of the mammary gland is taken over by *perforating branches* of the internal thoracic artery with *medial mammary branches* from intercostal spaces 2–4 (to the medial, superior portion of the organ); two *lateral mammary branches* from the lateral thoracic artery (to the lateral region of the gland); and *lateral mammary branches* from intercostal arteries 2–5 (especially to the deep portion of the breast). Branches of all three vascular trunks mentioned supply the nipple.

Veins. Superficial veins (Fig. **209**) communicate with a plexus (*areolar venous plexus*) located in the region of the areola and are usually distinctly visible through the skin during pregnancy and lactation. They bring blood to the internal and lateral thoracic veins, partly also to the veins of the abdominal wall, and communicate with the deep veins which convey the blood to the intercostal veins.

The **lymphatic vessels** of the mammary gland (Fig. **210**) are of particular importance as pathways for spreading cancerous metastases. Lymphatic vessels course from a *superficial* (subcutaneous) and a *deep network*, which anastomose with each other. Lymph is thus conveyed:

- *to the axilla* (about 75% of the lymph in a healthy gland); to the pectoral axillary lymph nodes (at the lower margin of the pectoralis minor on the superior digitations of the serratus anterior, partly via *paramammary lymph nodes* at the lateral margin of the gland) and from there (or directly) to the *central axillary lymph nodes* (on the inferior surface of subscapularis; in the case of metastatic spread into the pectoral and the central axillary lymph nodes frequently involving irritation of the intercostobrachial nerve), to the *apical axillary lymph nodes* (cranial to the pectoralis minor, along the subclavian vein) or to the *deep cervical lymph nodes* situated above the clavicle (supraclavicular);
- *through the pectoralis major* to the small lymph nodes between the two breast muscles (*interpectoral axillary lymph nodes*) and from there to the central and the apical axillary lymph nodes;
- *through the thoracic wall* to the *parasternal lymph nodes* (along the internal thoracic vessels), partly also across the midline to the opposite side and along the lateral cutaneous branches and posterior intercostal arteries to the *intercostal lymph nodes* (in the vicinity of the heads of the ribs).

A metastatic spread of mammary carcinoma via lymph pathways can also take place through the diaphragm to the lymph nodes of the epigastric region.

The **sensory innervation** takes place via *lateral* and *medial mammary branches* of intercostal nerves (Fig. **209**), the secretory fibers coming from the perivascular plexus.

11. Head

The **head** is distinguished from the trunk in its basic structural plan by *peculiarities* of organ systems concentrated at the rostral pole of the body. The large sense organs (olfactory, visual, balance and hearing organs) which mediate contact with the environment and the openings for the respiratory and digestive tracts are localized here.

The olfactory organ is described in the "Nasal Cavity" section because of its topographical relationship to this passageway. The eye, as well as the vestibular and auditory organs, on the other hand, are treated as exceptions to the otherwise topographical organization of this book and are discussed in volume 2 in the chapter "Central Nervous System" on account of their close functional connection to this system.

In mammals, the consumption and breaking down of food, which is usually in coarse particles, necessitate an efficient masticating apparatus (upper and lower jaw, teeth, masticatory muscles, jaw articulation). For respiration, the trachea must always be kept open, i.e. the wall of the entry orifice (nares) needs to be reinforced by parts of the skeleton. The embryologically-determined crossing of the respiratory and digestive pathways in the region of the pharynx ($\rightarrow$ p. 758) results in a construction which is an important prerequisite for the acquisition of articulated speech. The specific development of the facial musculature makes possible a highly efficient mimetic organ of expression. Finally, the shape of the head is essentially determined by its function as the carrier of the brain.

A. Skull

The **skull** (*cranium*) is the bony foundation of the head. Since muscles at the skull – in comparison to the trunk and limbs – are attached only to a slight extent, its soft tissue covering remains relatively thin. The skeleton of the head defines largely the *external shape of the head* and, apart from the skull base, is accessible for external study by palpation. Individual differences in the shape of the head are generally based on differences in the shape of the skull.

The *soft tissue covering* is unequally thick in the different regions of the head. It is relatively thick in the region of the masseter muscle, the lips and below the orbit of the eye, whereas it is very thin at the forehead, above the zygomatic arch and at the scalp.

These differences can be put to use in a reconstruction of the physiognomy using only the bony skull. For this purpose, plasticine borders are marked at appropriate heights in the different regions and their surfaces connected. This procedure has often been used successfully in legal medicine for identification purposes.

On the basis of genetic and topographical aspects, two parts of the skull can be distinguished: **neurocranium** and **viscerocranium** (Fig. **212**). The *neurocranium* forms a closed protective capsule for the brain while at the same time enclosing the labyrinth organ and the middle ear. The bones of the neurocranium are united immovably with one another and with the viscerocranium by sutures or cartilaginous joints. Apart from the joints between the auditory ossicles, there is only a single articular connection between the bones of the skull, the *temporomandibular* (jaw) *joint*.

The *viscerocranium* (facial skeleton) consists of the *nasal skeleton* and the *jaw skeleton*. The bones of the neurocranium and the nasal skeleton are designated as *cranial bones*, and the elements of the jaw skeleton as *facial bones*.

The organs in the head lie close to one another, the bones of the skull frequently having positional relationships to several organs. The roof of the orbit, for example, forms also the floor of the anterior cranial fossa. The palate is both the floor of the nasal cavity and the roof of the oral cavity.

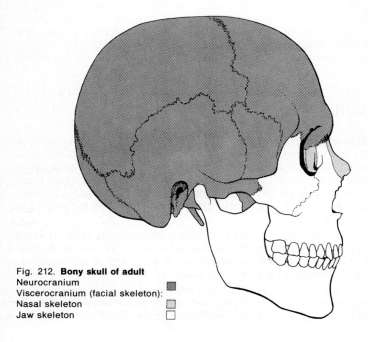

Fig. 212. **Bony skull of adult**
Neurocranium
Viscerocranium (facial skeleton):
Nasal skeleton
Jaw skeleton

These close proximities can lead to the spreading of pathological processes from one region to another, e.g. from the teeth to the jaw cavity, from the middle ear cavity to the posterior cranial fossa or – by the vascular route – from the facial soft parts to the cranial meninges.

The bony skull is composed of diverse and unequal parts, yet it represents a constructive unit (→ pp. 568 and 646).

1. Structural Plan of the Head

During the early phase of embryogenesis, the human head – in contrast to the segmental organization of the body wall – shows no metameric structures in the dorsal region. This *rostrocaudal part of the head*, to which the anlagen of the olfactory, visual, and labyrinth organs also belong is a regionally specialized formation. It has not arisen from the trunk and it also does not correspond to any structural part of the trunk. Only at the "*head-trunk border*" does material from the most rostral trunk somites transform into mesenchyme and contribute to the construction of the occipital region.

In the *ventral (visceral) region of the head*, a segmental organization appears during early embryonic development which is absent in this form at the trunk, branchiomerism (→ p. 13). It can be traced back to the serially-organized pharyngeal pouches and the visceral arches lying between them.

Three parts contribute to the structure of the head:
– *rostrodorsal region*, a new formation in vertebrates,
– *primary trunk material (spinal region)* with metameric arrangement
  (→ variations in the atlanto-occipital region, p. 574), and
– a *ventral (visceral) region* with branchiomeres.

2. Review of Skull Development

In the skull, elements of different morphological value are sealed together into a uniform whole. The shaping of this complex organ is determined equally by local, regionally-limited growth processes and by the formative power of the environment (influence of brain, masticatory apparatus, etc). Without a basic knowledge of phylogenetic and ontogenetic development, the morphology of the cranium can only be inadequately understood. The following discussion of the morphogenesis of the skull is intended to provide an understanding of the composition of the skull beyond a mere formal description.

The skull develops within the mesenchyme which surrounds the central nervous system: from cartilaginous anlagen, *endocranium* (Fig. **213**), and from covering (membrane) bones, *exocranium*. The cartilaginous pri-

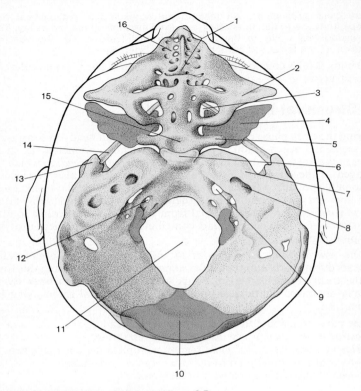

Fig. 213. **Chondrocranium of fetus** of 100 mm C.R.,
view of interior of skull base (superior aspect)
Endochondral ossification in squamous part of occipital bone
("supra-occipital" bone) and in greater wing of sphenoid (ala
temporalis)

1 Nasal capsule
2 Ala orbitalis (anlage of lesser wing)
3 Optic foramen
4 Greater wing (ossified ala temporalis)
5 Still cartilaginous root of ala
  temporalis
6 Dorsum sellae
7 Otic capsule
8 Internal acoustic meatus

9 Jugular foramen
10 Squama of occipital bone
   ("supra-occipital" bone)
11 Foramen magnum
12 Hypoglossal canal
13 Tegmen tympani
14 Meckel's cartilage
15 Hypophysial fossa
16 Lamina cribrosa

mordia ossify during ontogenesis as replacement bones and are enlarged by incremental bone; only in the nasal skeleton are the cartilaginous skeletal elements preserved as nasal cartilages.

In the *neurocranium* both the base of the skull (basicranium) with the otic capsule and a narrow bar (tectum), which embraces the medulla oblongata dorsally, originate from a cartilaginous precursor, i.e. as *replacement bones*. The roof of the skull and parts of its lateral wall are formed in connective tissue, i.e. as *membrane bones*.

Processes preformed in cartilage likewise extend from the center of the basicranium. The temporal wings of the chondrocranium become the greater wings of the sphenoid of the osseous skull, and the orbital wings become the lesser wings of the sphenoid (Fig. **213**). The processes grow around most cranial nerves and border their exit sites.

The temporal wing is originally a visceral cartilage element, part of the 1st pharyngeal arch. It becomes detached from the visceral region in connection with the enlargement of the brain and is attached to the neurocranium. Thus, a new, *secondary* cranial base arises in the middle of the basicranium and encloses structures in the cranial cavity which were originally located outside ot the skull (e.g. trigeminal ganglion).

In the *facial skeleton*, the bones of the jaw skeleton and individual elements of the nasal skeleton (lacrimal, nasal, vomer) are developed as *membrane bones*.

In the viscerocranium, a cartilage bar is established embryonically as a constituent of the 1st pharyngeal arch (mandibular arch) (primary lower jaw = Meckel's cartilage, Figs. **213** and **214**). Lateral to it, the definitive lower jaw, the mandible, is formed as a membrane bone. A (secondary) jaw articulation (appositional joint) is then formed by the secondary apposition of the mandible at the squamous part of the temporal bone. The greatest part of Meckel's cartilage completely degenerates. Its posterior articular portion is separated off and incorporated into the sound-conducting apparatus of the middle ear as the malleus (Fig. **214**). The incus is likewise developed from the dorsal end of the mandibular arch.

The 2nd pharyngeal arch (hyoid arch) gives rise to the third auditory ossicle, the stapes, from its proximal portion. The rest of the arch forms, first of all, a long cartilaginous bar (Reichert's cartilage), which ossifies in its superior portion and fuses with the temporal bone as the styloid process. The middle piece regresses to form the stylohyoid ligament, and the distal part ossifies as the lesser horn of the hyoid bone. Occasionally, the entire hyoid arch can ossify in the adult.

Variations in the Number of Skull Bones

The **number of skull bones** in humans is not absolutely constant. First of all, it is dependent upon age. The two frontal bones, as a rule, fuse in the second year of life into a single, sutureless bone. Between the ages of 16 and 18, the sphenoid fuses with the occipital to form the basi-occipital bone. As a variant, the two frontal bones can occasionally remain separated in the adult by a suture (metopism).

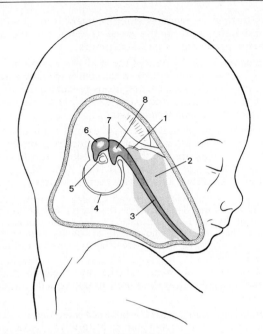

Fig. 214. **Primary and secondary jaw articulation in
embryo** of 62 mm C. R.

1 Secondary jaw articulation
  (temporomandibular joint)
2 Mandible (dentary)
3 Meckel's cartilage
4 Tympanic ring, later tympanic
  part of temporal bone

5 Stapes
6 Incus
7 Incudomallear joint (=primary
  jaw articulation)
8 Malleus

Not every supernumerary bone in the adult skull is the remnant of an original
independent element. Frequently, additional *sutural* (*wormian*) *bones* occur in
sutures between the margins of the large, flat bones of the cranium (Fig. **215**).
They represent irregularities in the ossification of very extensive osseous territories
and have no phylogenetic significance.

Proportions and Symmetrical Relationships of the Head and Skull

Just as the individual parts of the body are differently proportioned
during different developmental phases, so the functionally-different parts
of the head also exhibit age-related, varying proportions. The brain
develops early ontogenetically and grows rapidly, whereas the masti-

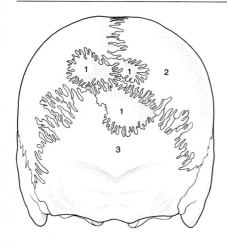

Fig. 215. **Sutural bones between parietal and squama of occipital**
1 Sutural bones
2 Parietal bone
3 Squamous part of occipital bone

catory apparatus at first lags behind in growth, correlative to its later functional deployment. Hence, the neural portion of the head greatly outstrips the facial part in the earlier developmental phases. A comparison of the skull of the newborn child with that of the adult (Figs. **216** and **217**) illustrates these proportional differences.

In a lateral projection of the surface area of the skull, the facial portion in the newborn child occupies about one-sixth of the surface, whereas in the adult it is over one-third (Fig. **216**). Body weight increases postnally about 20 times, brain weight around 6.5 times. Thus, brain weight after birth lags behind in rate of growth. Of course, the brain has already reached about 80% of its final weight by the end of the 2nd year. In the 6th year, the growth of the brain has almost ceased.

The growth of the face and the jaw depends largely on the development of the teeth and is thus closely correlated with the emergence of the deciduous teeth, their replacement by permanent teeth, and the appearance of additional teeth. As a result, the jaw skeleton experiences a considerable burst of growth after completion of brain growth, that is after the 6th year of life – especially at puberty.

Insignificant lateral asymmetries regularly exist in the head and skull. They can be determined accurately by comparison of individual trajectories measured on both sides of the head and as slight distortions of the longitudinal axis of the face. A completely symmetrical face, which can be constructed photographically by the artificial union of two right or two left facial halves, appears boring from an esthetic viewpoint. Works of art from all eras have always taken this phenomenon into account. In about 60% of the cases, the right half of the face is distinguished by a somewhat greater mass. The reason for facial asymmetry lies essentially in random variants of growth.

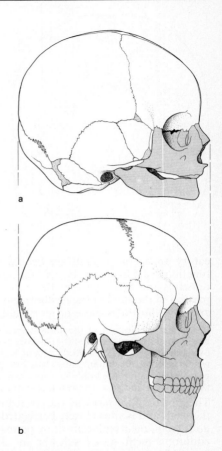

Fig. 216. **Proportions and proportional differences of neurocranium and viscerocranium during postnatal development**
a Skull of newborn child
b Adult skull brought to same length
Neurocranium ☐
Viscerocranium ▨

b

Alterations in dentition (loss of teeth in the upper jaw) can lead secondarily to transformations of the maxillary sinus, which in turn influence the proportions of the face.

Right-left asymmetries of the brain, which are functionally significant, occur regularly and perhaps also play a causal role in the origin of skull asymmetries.

Structural Factors of the Skull

The shape of the skull is influenced by mutually-dependent factors, for example, the shape and size of the brain, the development of the masti-

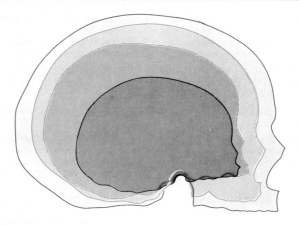

Fig. 217. **Skull growth during postnatal development** (after *Merkel* and after *Hasselwander*)
Skull outlines drawn superimposed, skull oriented on upper margin of zygomatic arch
Skull outline of a newborn child ——
        a one-year-old ——
        a seven-year-old ——
        an adult ——

catory apparatus, the sense organs of the head, and the respiratory passages. The cranium can be perceived as a passive framework which is constructed among the head organs on which it is spatially dependent and which, at the same time, must form a constructive whole. The total picture of the skull is a compromise between the different factors.

The morphology of the brain produces a surface pattern (relief) at the inner wall of the cranial cavity which is a rough negative of the configuration of the brain. The forces (masticatory pressures, muscle traction) exerted by the masticatory apparatus influence the external relief of the skull. The direction and extent of the forces acting from the inside and outside are not identical, however, and affect the skull differently. For the fine tuning which results in a uniform total construction of the skull, pneumatization (formation of accessory cavities containing air) plays a decisive role.

Enlargement of the cranial volume in early childhood (hydrocephalus = water on the brain) causes a balloon-like distension of the skull so that most sutures remain open. A decrease in cranial volume (microcephaly, bird-headed malformation) leads to the formation of a greatly flattened calvarium with a receding forehead and premature suture closings. In both cases, the skull adapts to the given conditions and does not follow special morphogenetic laws.

In the complete absence of the cerebrum (anencephaly), only the base of the skull exhibits an approximately normal development; the roof of the cranium is absent. Complex disturbances in very early developmental stages (disorders in determination) are responsible for the defects in these cases.

Influences of the musculature on the form of the skull affect particularly the formation of the finer surface relief and the development of the supporting basic construction of the skull.

Deficiency or paralysis of the masticatory muscles can result in deformations and asymmetries of the bones.

Deviations from the norm in the shape of the skull can be produced by irregularities in suture closure, especially by premature sutural synostosis. In almost all such cases, the variations in shape results from genuine malformations which are already determined before the development of the skeletal tissue.

In premature sutural synostosis of the frontal bone, the bone protrudes like a keel since the lateral frontal eminences are absent. In contrast to the parietal region, the frontal region is considerably narrowed (trigonocephaly). This malformation is always coupled with an anomaly of the olfactory lobe. Premature closure of the coronal suture leads to the formation of a steeple or tower skull (oxycephaly, special form of acrocephaly). In this case, the growth in width of the skull is disturbed, the cranium growing in height and toward the occiput.

3. Skeletal Elements of the Skull

In systemic anatomy, the **skull** (*cranial*) **bones**, represented by elements of the neurocranium and nasal skeleton, are distinguished from the **facial bones** which comprise the jaw skeleton (Fig. **212**). The skeletal elements connecting the tympanic membrane and inner ear are grouped together as the **auditory ossicles**. The following organization of the human skull thus results (→ Table **4**).

a) Bones of the Neurocranium

The **occipital bone** (Figs. **218**, **219**, **235** and **236**) is a large bone which arises from the fusion of membrane and cartilage bone anlagen.

The *occipital bone* in the adult consists of four parts:
- the *basilar part*, basal and in the middle, located directly in front of and below the medulla oblongata;
- two *lateral* (condylar) *parts*, which adjoin the basilar part laterally; and
- the *squamous part*, which unites the two lateral parts as an unpaired, dorsal middle piece.

Portions of the occipital bone surround the *foramen magnum*, which connects the cranial cavity with the vertebral canal (structural contents → p. 616).

Table **4** Organization of the human skull

Cranial bones			
Neurocranium		*Nasal Skeleton*	
Occipital	mc	Ethmoid	c
Sphenoid	mc	Inferior Nasal Concha	c
Temporal	mc	Nasal	m
Parietal	m	Lacrimal	m
Frontal	m	Vomer	m
		in addition, the nasal cartilages	
Facial bones			
Jaw Skeleton			
Maxilla	m	Hyoid	c
Palatine	m		
Zygomatic	m		
Mandible	m		
Auditory Ossicles			
Malleus	c		
Incus	c		
Stapes	c		

Explanation: m = membrane (covering) bone;
c = cartilage (replacement) bone;
mc = mixed bone

The *basilar part* forms the anterior margin of the foramen magnum. At its anterior surface, it merges into the *spheno-occipital synchondrosis* (Fig. **252 d**).

The cartilaginous joint ossifies in the 16th–18th year. The occipital and sphenoid fuse into a uniform bone, the *basilar*.

The superior (cerebral) surface of the basilar part, together with the posterior surface of the dorsum sellae (sphenoid), forms the *clivus*, upon which parts of the brainstem (medulla oblongata and pons) lie. The lateral margins of the basilar part participate in the boundary of the *petro-occipital fissure*, which is closed by fibrocartilage. The inferior (basal) surface of the basilar part contains in its middle the *pharyngeal tubercle* (Fig. **274**), which serves for the attachment of the tendinous bands of the pharyngeal constrictor (pharyngeal raphe). Moreover, the basal surface customarily shows a ridge-like configuration, which corresponds to the insertions of the longus capitis and rectus capitis anterior muscles.

The two *lateral parts* (located on both sides of the foramen magnum) communicate rostrally with the temporal bone. On their inferior surface, they bear articular processes (*occipital condyles*) for the atlas. The articular surfaces have an oblong ovoid shape and are more strongly curved

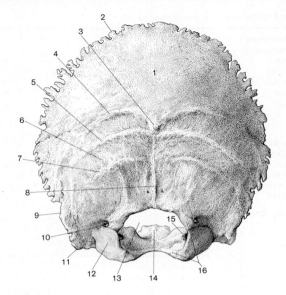

Fig. 218. **Occipital bone**, view from behind and below

1 Squamous part of occipital bone
2 Lambdoidal margin
3 External occipital protuberance
4 Highest nuchal line
5 Superior nuchal line
6 Nuchal plane
7 Inferior nuchal line
8 External occipital crest

9 Mastoid margin
10 Condylar fossa and condylar canal
11 Jugular process
12 Occipital condyle
13 Foramen magnum
14 Basilar part of occipital bone
15 Hypoglossal canal
16 Lateral (condylar) part of occipital bone

from behind forward than in a transverse direction. The longitudinal axes of the condyles of both sides converge anteriorly. Behind each condyle, there is a depression, the *condylar fossa*, into which an inconstant venous channel (*condylar canal*) can open. "Above" the condyle, the lateral part is penetrated by the exit canal of the hypoglossal nerve (*hypoglossal canal*).

At the anterolateral margin, the lateral part is drawn out into the *jugular process*. Medial to it, the jugular notch is situated which borders the *jugular foramen* together with the petrous portion of the temporal bone (penetrating conduction paths→ p. 616). The notch is frequently divided into an anterior and a posterior half by a bony peg, the *intrajugular process*.

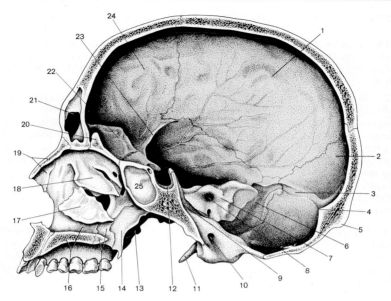

Fig. 219. **Median section of skull**, medial view

1 Parietal bone
2 Squamous part of occipital bone
3 Groove for transverse sinus
4 Internal occipital protuberance
5 External occipital protuberance
6 Groove for sigmoid sinus
7 Petrous part of temporal bone
8 Opening and internal
 acoustic meatus
9 Clivus
10 Hypoglossal canal
11 Styloid process of temporal bone
12 Hypophysial fossa
13 Lateral plate of pterygoid process
14 Medial plate of pterygoid process

15 Palatine bone
16 Maxilla
17 Inferior nasal concha
18 Middle nasal concha,
 dorsocranial to it, superior
 nasal concha
 (not labelled)
19 Nasal bone
20 Crista galli
21 Frontal sinus
22 Orbital part of frontal bone
23 Lesser wing of sphenoid
24 Squamous part of frontal bone
25 Sphenoidal sinus

The *paramastoid process* can project from the jugular process as a more less distinct elevation in the direction of the transverse process of the atlas. It can be interpreted as a transverse process of an occipital vertebra, the structural components of which were not completely integrated into the occipital bone.

The *squamous portion of the occipital bone* has the form of a triangle. The base forms the posterior margin of the foramen magnum; the apex faces upward and is inserted between the two parietal bones. The squama is split so that a superior and an inferior squama can be distinguished (Fig.

252 d). At their boundary, the *external occipital protuberance* arises that marks the border between the cranial roof (occipital plane) and cranial floor (nuchal plane). The border between membrane and cartilage bones lies above the protuberance, that is, in the region of the superior squama. The nuchal plane forms the attachment surface for the nuchal musculature.

On the internal relief, the *internal occipital protuberance* corresponds situationally to the external occipital projection. Here, the *groove for the superior sagittal sinus* meets with the *groove for the transverse sinus*, both bony channels taking up the corresponding blood conduits. The tentorium cerebelli attaches at the superior and inferior margins of the groove for the transverse sinus, whereas the falx cerebelli attaches at both margins of the groove for the superior sagittal sinus. The insignificant falx cerebelli arises below the internal occipital protuberance from a bony ridge which passes to the posterior margin of the foramen magnum and – provided it is more strongly developed – is referred to as the *internal occipital crest*.

A cross-shaped relief, the *cruciform eminence*, formed by the two grooves and the bony ridge arises on the internal surface of the squama. Four fossae are delimited by it. The two fossae above the groove for the transverse sinus border on the occipital lobe of the cerebrum; the two fossae below this groove form the floor and the posterior wall of the posterior cranial fossa, which houses the cerebellum and the medulla oblongata.

Since the externally-palpable external occipital protuberance simultaneously marks the position of the internal occipital protuberance, it represents an important orientation point for brain topography.

The *superior* and *inferior nuchal lines* are distinguished on the external surface of the inferior squama. They are caused by muscular attachments and exhibit quite variable individual differences. The *highest nuchal line* (origin of the trapezius muscle) is clearly molded on the superior squama.

At the apex of the occipital squama, a transverse bony suture can be present which borders the *interparietal bone*. This suture is usually not identical with the border between membrane and cartilage bones, but rather lies above it. Variations and supernumerary ossific centers in the region of the upper part of the occipital squama are very common.

Variations in the atlanto-occipital region. In early development, material (head somites) belonging originally to the trunk region is included in the occipital region ($\rightarrow$ p. 563). During phylogenesis, the head-trunk border shifts caudally, and variants occasionally appear in this transition region. The area around the foramen magnum, for example, can assume more or less the shape of a vertebra similar to the atlas: *manifestation of an occipital vertebra*.

The hypoglossal canal can be divided by a bar, the margin of the foramen magnum thickened, or the paramastoid process can become distinctly prominent as the equivalent of a transverse process. In extreme cases, the entire region of the foramen magnum can assume the shape of an atlas.

The *assimilation of the atlas* (Fig. **220**) is to be distinguished from the manifestation of an occipital vertebra. In these cases, the first, normally free vertebra is secondarily fused with the occiput (atlanto-occipital synostosis). The occiput thus receives a "cervical vertebra" in addition.

In both cases, the first free vertebra has the shape of an axis. In individual cases, the question whether it is the manifestation of an occipital vertebra or an assimilation of the atlas can often be decided only by counting the number of free vertebrae. The assimilation of the atlas can occur unilaterally or bilaterally.

Unilateral assimilation of the atlas can be the cause of specific forms of torticollis. By asymmetry and distortion, a narrowing of the vertebral canal or the intervertebral formamina can occur and – as a result of this – neurological symptoms can be manifested.

The **sphenoid bone** (Figs. **219**, **221**, **222** and **236**) adjoins the occipital bone anteriorly, fuses with it in the 16th–18 year to form the *basilar bone*, and forms the middle portion of the skull base.

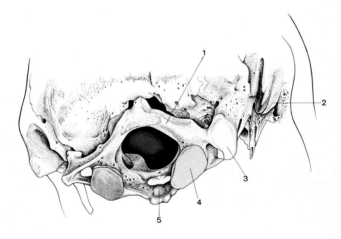

Fig. 220. **Assimilation of atlas** into adult skull,
view from behind and below
Transverse process of atlas on right
side forms bony union with
occipital bone

1 Posterior arch of atlas
2 Mastoid process
3 Transverse process of atlas
4 Inferior articular facet of atlas
5 Facet for dens

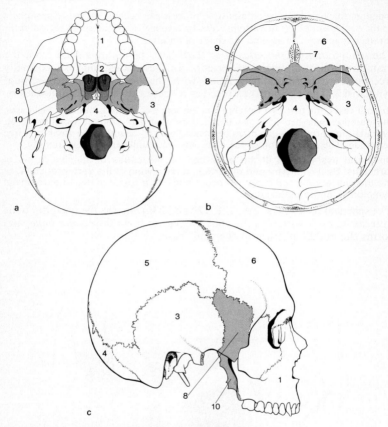

Fig. 221. Incorporation of sphenoid bone into osseous construction of skull
a View from below (inferior aspect)
b View from inside (superior aspect)
c Lateral view

1 Maxilla
2 Palatine bone
3 Temporal bone
4 Occipital bone
5 Parietal bone

6 Frontal bone
7 Ethmoid bone
8 Greater wing ⎫
9 Lesser wing ⎬ of sphenoid bone
10 Pterygoid process ⎭

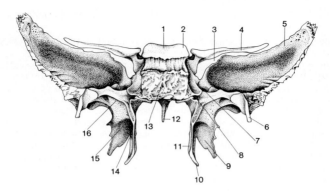

Fig. 222. **Sphenoid bone**, posterior view

1 Dorsum sellae
2 Posterior clinoid process
3 Superior orbital fissure
4 Lesser wing
5 Greater wing, cerebral surface
6 Sphenoidal spine
7 Foramen rotundum
8 Pterygoid canal

9 Lateral plate of pterygoid process
10 Pterygoid hamulus
11 Medial plate of pterygoid process
12 Sphenoidal rostrum
13 Body of shenoid
14 Pterygoid notch
15 Pterygoid fossa
16 Scaphoid fossa

The *sphenoid* consists of an unpaired *middle piece* and three paired *processes*. The following are distinguished:
- *body*,
- *lesser wing*, which extends laterally from the anterior portion of the body;
- *greater wing*, which spreads out laterally and anteriorly from the posterior portion of the body; and
- the *pterygoid process*, which is directed downward and borders laterally the posterior openings of the osseous nasal cavity.

The sphenoid bone cannot be seen completely on the external surface of the skull since it is concealed for the most part by the nasal and jaw skeleton. Between the parietal, temporal and frontal bones, the greater wing forms a (small) part of the lateral wall of the skull. The greater and lesser wings also participate significantly in bordering the bony wall of the orbit (Fig. **242**). Particularly complicated relationships result from the extended position of the sphenoid, its varied regional connections, and its numerous nerve and vascular passages.

The sphenoid is developed essentially by endochondral ossification in the orbito-temporal region of the chondrocranium. Moreover, a membrane bone, the ptery-goid, fuses with the medial lamina of the pterygoid process of the sphenoid. The middle region of the chondrocranium ($\rightarrow$ p. 565) exhibits a central basal portion and two lateral pairs of wings, the orbital wings in front, the temporal wings behind (Fig. 213).

The sphenoid complex ossifies first as posterior and anterior sphenoids (Fig. 252d). To each of these parts belong a pair of wings and a basal part. The posterior sphenoid arises from a primary paired basal ossification (basisphenoid) and the early ossification of the temporal wings. In the ossified condition, these are called greater wings. The anterior sphenoid arises from three ossific loci in the base, which fuse early into the presphenoid. In the ossified state, the anterior wings (orbital wings) are referred to as the lesser wings. The lateral lamina of the pterygoid process ossifies as cartilage bone from the greater wing. Finally, in the large bones of the sphenoid there are cartilage bones, the sphenoidal conchae (ossicles of Bertini), which are still paired and which form the rostral end of the sphenoidal sinus. They segment off from the posterior part of the cartilaginous nasal capsule and fuse with the presphenoid at the time of puberty. Secondary cartilage appears in the pterygoid.

Presphenoid and basisphenoid remain separated by a cartilaginous joint, the intersphenoidal synchondrosis (Fig. 252 d), which always lies below the anterior margin of the hypophysial fossa. The fusion of the basisphenoid and presphenoid into a uniform sphenoidal body already begins prenatally.

The *body of the sphenoid* possesses a superior (cerebral) surface, two lateral surfaces, an anterior surface, and an inferior surface.

The *cerebral surface* is united in front with the lamina cribrosa of the ethmoid bone by the *spheno-ethmoidal suture*. The level anterior portion, the *jugum sphenoidale*, is marked off behind by a transverse ridge, the *(pre)chiasmatic groove*, which connects right and left optic canals. Directly behind this groove there is the *sella turcica ("Turkish saddle")*, which occupies the middle part of the cerebral surface. It usually begins anteriorly with the *tuberculum sellae* (pommel of the "saddle"), situated in the midline, and sinks in to form the *hypophysial fossa* (the seat of the the "saddle"). The sella turcica, together with the hypophysial fossa, is bordered posteriorly by the transverse *dorsum sellae* (back of the "saddle"), which projects on both sides as the *posterior clinoid process*.

A small projection, the *middle clinoid process*, can be formed on each side of the tuberculum sellae.

The posterior surface of the dorsum sellae – after ossification of the spheno-occipital synchondrosis – continues into the cerebral surface of the basilar part of the occipital bone and with it forms the *clivus*.

At both *lateral surfaces* of the sphenoid, the slightly S-shaped, tortuous *carotid groove* courses for the intracranial portion of the internal carotid artery. This groove begins posteriorly, close to the front of the apex of the petrous portion of the temporal bone, and is bordered laterally by a pointed osseous cone, the *lingula sphenoidalis*. It ascends slightly forward at the side of the sella turcica and terminates between the anterior clinoid process and the sella turcica (or the middle clinoid process).

At the *anterior surface* of the body of the sphenoid, there is a bony ridge in the median plane, the *sphenoidal crest*, which is continued downward into the *rostrum sphenoidale* – at the border to the inferior surface. The crest is adjoined by the perpendicular plate of the ethmoid, and the rostrum by the vomer. The paired *sphenoidal sinus* opens on both sides of the sphenoidal crest, its anterior and inferior walls being formed by a thin, triangular bony plate, the *sphenoidal concha*. It borders from lateral and below the paired *apertures of the sphenoidal sinus*. The sphenoidal sinus possesses a variable shape and is often only of the size of a pea. Yet, the sphenoidal sinus can also pneumatize neighboring bones beyond the body of the sphenoid. The *septum of the sphenoidal sinus* usually lies distinctly asymmetrical.

The base of the human skull is bent like a kyphosis. The extent of the bending can be determined by the sphenoidal-clivus angle (angle between a tangent drawn at the inner surface of the clivus and a tangent drawn at the jugum sphenoidale). The vertex of the angle in the adult lies above the hypophysial fossa. The plane of the clivus is also of significance for the determination of the relative position of the viscerocranium to the neurocranium. The slope of the jaw skeleton in relation to the base if the skull is fundamentally independent of the specific flexion of the base. In the human, this "prebasial kyphosis" has about the same dimension as the true flexion of the base ("sellar kyphosis"). The true sellar kyphosis of the base is unique to man and is especially correlated with the enormous development of the cerebrum.

The *lesser wing of the sphenoid* arises on each side of the body with two roots, which contain the *optic canal* between them. The free end of the wing facing laterally is usually connected with the greater wing by a connective tissue tract. Occasionally, however, a bony fusion of both wings also occurs here. A space, the *superior orbital fissure*, remains between the lesser and greater wings for the passage of cranial nerves III, IV, V_1, VI and the superior ophthalmic vein (Fig. **241**). The anterior margin of the lesser wing adjoins the frontal bone (at the *sphenofrontal suture*) and in the root region also borders on the ethmoid. The posterior, medial corner of the lesser wing projects medially as the *anterior clinoid process*. The superior surface forms the posterior portion of the anterior cranial fossa. The inferior surface of the wing forms a part of the orbital roof.

The *greater wing of the sphenoid* arises bilaterally from the posterior part of the body of the sphenoid. The root portion is penetrated by two nerve openings, in front by the *foramen rotundum* (maxillary nerve) and behind by the *foramen ovale* (mandibular nerve). Lateral and posterior to the foramen ovale, the *foramen spinosum* (middle meningeal artery) is located in the greater wing.

At the greater wing, the inner surface (*cerebral surface*) is slightly hollowed out. It forms the floor of the middle cranial fossa and receives the apex of the temporal lobe of the cerebrum. Posterolaterally, it runs out into a sharp tip, the *sphenoidal spine*, immediately in front of which lies the *foramen spinosum*. The lateral margin of the cerebral surface makes sutural contact (Fig. **226**) with the frontal bone (*sphenofrontal suture*), with the parietal bone (*sphenoparietal suture*) and with the squama of the temporal bone (*sphenosquamosal suture*). The posterior margin adjoins the pyramidal portion of the temporal bone from the front and bounds the *sphenopetrosal fissure* laterally, the *foramen lacerum* medially.

The *external surface* of the greater wing is intricately structured and can be divided into *orbital, temporal* and *maxillary surfaces*.

The *orbital surface* (Fig. **227**) forms a large part of the wall of the orbit. Its superior margin communicates laterally with the frontal bone (*frontal margin*), whereas it ends free medially and borders the *superior orbital fissure* from below. The sharp-edged lower margin of the orbital surface, together with parts of the maxilla and zygomatic bones, border the *inferior orbital fissure*, through which the infra-orbital artery and nerve arrive at the floor of the orbit from the pterygopalatine fossa. The serrated lateral margin (*zygomatic margin*) passes downward anterior to the frontal margin and makes contact with the zygomatic bone.

The *temporal surface* (Fig. **226**) faces laterally and forms a part of the lateral wall of the skull (temporal plane). It curves at the *infratemporal crest* into the inferior surface of the greater wing of the sphenoid (site of origin of the pterygoid muscle), which lies horizontally. This area of the temporal surface located at the external base of the cranium forms the roof of the *infratemporal fossa*. At the lower surface of the greater wing, a shallow *groove* for the cartilaginous part of the *auditory tube* is evident at the posterior margin, lateral to the pterygoid process.

The small *maxillary surface* situated medial to the orbital surface connects with the pterygoid process anteriorly and is turned toward the maxillary bone. The foramen rotundum opens on it.

The *pterygoid process* originates with two roots, between which the sagittally directed *pterygoid canal* (for the vessels and nerves of the pterygoid canal) courses, and passes downward in the lateral wall of the choanae. The pterygoid canal opens (below the maxillary surface) into the pterygopalatine fossa. Shortly after its origin, the pterygoid process splits into *medial* and *lateral plates*, which bound a longitudinal groove, the *pterygoid fossa* (origin of the medial pterygoid muscle) on their dorsal side. Below this fossa the two plates spread apart and form a wedge-shaped notch, the *pterygoid notch*, in which the pyramidal process of the palatine bone is inserted.

In the root region of the posterior border of the *medial plate* there is a depression, the *scaphoid fossa*, which serves as the site of origin of the levator veli palatini muscle. Inferiorly, the medial plate is prolonged into a hook, the *pterygoid hamulus*, which possesses a notch, the *groove of the pterygoid hamulus*. The tendon of the tensor veli palatini winds around this groove.

At the base of the pterygoid process, a thin bony lamina, the *vaginal process*, projects medially from the medial plate and adjoins the pterygoid process of the vomer. The vaginal process and the inferior surface of the sphenoid form a groove which opens toward the median plane.

The *lateral plate* ends rounded below. In the middle of its posterior margin it can carry a bony process (*pterygospinous process*) which occasionally fuses with the sphenoidal spine and then encloses the *pterygospinous foramen*. The pterygospinous process represents an ossification of the *pterygospinous ligament*, which is regularly present and which passes from the lateral plate to the sphenoidal spine between the medial and lateral pterygoid muscles.

The **temporal bone** (Figs. **223–226, 235** and **236**) forms a part of both the basicranium and the lateral wall of the skull. It encloses the inner ear, the middle ear and parts of the external acoustic meatus. By means of the zygomatic arch, the temporal bone participates in anchoring the upper jaw and contains itself the socket for the articulation of the jaw. It forms the protective covering for numerous nerves and vessels and provides a ligamentous attachment for the movable fixation of the hyoid bone.

The different components of the *temporal bone* unite only shortly before birth into a uniform large bone consisting of the following parts:
– the *petrous part*, which encloses the middle ear and lies at the base of the skull;

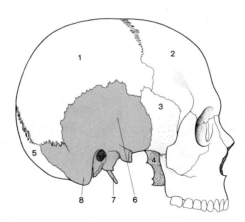

Fig. 223. **Incorporation of temporal bone into osseous construction of skull** (zygomatic arch resected)

1 Parietal bone	5 Occipital bone
2 Frontal bone	6 Squamous part ⎫
3 Greater wing ⎫ of sphenoid bone	7 Styloid process ⎬ of temporal bone
4 Lesser wing ⎭	8 Mastoid process ⎭

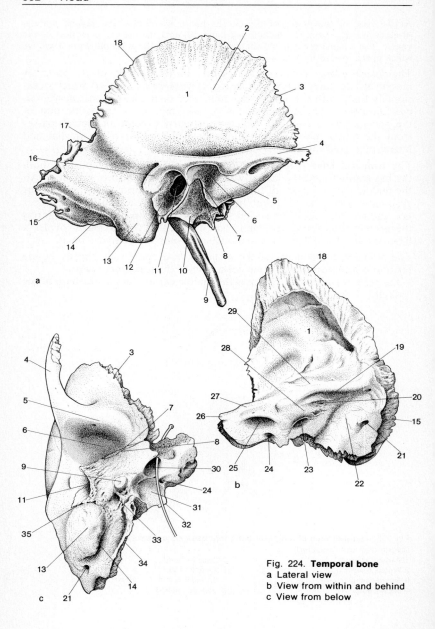

Fig. 224. **Temporal bone**
a Lateral view
b View from within and behind
c View from below

- the *tympanic part*, which forms the floor and the anterior and posterior walls of the external acoustic meatus; and
- the *squamous part*, which forms the lateral wall of the skull between the sphenoid and occipital bones and which articulates at its basal surface with the articular head of the mandible.

The otic capsule (Fig. 213), preformed in cartilage, ossifies from several loci and is then designated as the petrous portion of the temporal bone. It is attached early to the upper end of the hyoid arch which ossifies as endochondral bone of visceral origin and becomes the styloid process.

Two membrane bones are fused with these cartilage bones. The sqamous part arises as membrane bone in the lateral wall of the skull. A rostrally-directed process is involved in the formation of the zygomatic arch and carries the socket for the jaw articulation. The tympanic part is originally a membrane bone of the primary lower jaw (of Meckel's cartilage). It surrounds the external acoustic meatus and a part of the tympanic cavity from below and thus helps to form a middle ear capsule enclosed in bone.

The *petrous part* of the temporal bone lies free at the external and the internal base of the skull, whereas the tympanic and squamosal parts are visible at the lateral wall of the skull. The lateral part of the petrous portion, however, reaches the free external surface of the cranium posteriorly between the squamous portion and the occipital bone and forms the *mastoid process* behind the external acoustic meatus. The squamous part also participates in its construction, an independent "mastoid portion" being nonexistent.

In the newborn child, the petrous part forms only a relatively small area at the postero-inferior corner of the external wall of the skull (Figs. 252a, d). During childhood, this region gradually develops into the mastoid process, the anterior portion of which is derived from the squamous part. The point of contact of

1 Squamous part
2 Temporal surface
3 Sphenoidal margin
4 Zygomatic process
5 Articular tubercle
6 Mandibular fossa
7 Petrosquamous fissure
8 Petrotympanic fissure
9 Styloid process or root of styloid process
10 Sheath of styloid process (vaginal process)
11 External acoustic foramen
12 Tympanic part
13 Mastoid process
14 Mastoid notch
15 Occipital margin
16 Suprameatal spine
17 Parietal notch
18 Parietal margin
19 Groove for superior petrosal sinus
20 Subarcuate fossa
21 Mastoid foramen
22 Groove for sigmoid sinus
23 External opening of vestibular aqueduct
24 External opening of cochlear canaliculus
25 Foramen and internal acoustic meatus
26 Apex of petrous part
27 Superior margin of petrous part
28 Posterior surface of petrous part
29 Arcuate eminence
30 Probe in carotid canal
31 Jugular fossa
32 Intrajugular process
33 Stylomastoid foramen
34 Posterior margin of petrous part
35 Tympanomastoid fissure

the two genetically different components can persist as the *squamosomastoid suture*.

The *mastoid process* borders on the parietal bone with its superior margin (*parietomastoid suture*) and on the occipital bone with its posterior margin (*occipitomastoid suture*). The mastoid process is pneumatized from the *tympanic cavity* and contains the *mastoid air cells* (→ Vol. 2, Fig. **164**). The sternocleidomastoid, splenius capitis and longissimus capitis muscles attach at the lateral aspect of the mastoid process. The *mastoid notch* (origin of the posterior belly of the digastric muscle) lies medial to the apex of the process. Still further medially there is the *groove for the occipital artery*. At the cerebral surface of the mastoid process, a deep *fossa for the sigmoid sinus* courses.

Through the *mastoid foramen*, a hole near the posterior margin of this bony fossa, the mastoid emissary vein carries blood from the sigmoid sinus externally into the occipital vein.

Pyramidal part of temporal bone. The portion of the petrous part situated medially and in front of the mastoid process, together with the tympanic part and the styloid process, forms the pyramidal portion of the temporal bone. It projects into the cranial cavity with one edge, the *superior margin of the petrous part*.

The superior border of the pyramidal portion is directed from postero-lateral to anteromedial toward the *apex of the pyramid (apex of the petrous part)* and forms the border between the middle and posterior cranial fossae. The superior margin separates an anterior surface (*anterior surface of petrous portion*), which faces toward the inferior side of the temporal squama from a posterior surface (*posterior surface of petrous part*), which is directed toward the cerebellum. The inferior surface (*inferior surface of petrous part*) is part of the external base; the lateral surface does not lie free, but merges into the mastoid process. The apex of the pyramidal portion and the posterior margin of the greater wing of the sphenoid border the *foramen lacerum*, which continues laterally into the sphenopetrosal fissure. The foramen lacerum and the fissure extending from it closed at the nonmacerated skull by fibrocartilage (*sphenopetrosal synchondrosis*).

At the *anterior surface of the pyramid* near its apex there is an indentation for the trigeminal ganglion (*trigeminal impression*). Above the facial canal, the greater petrosal nerve passes through the thin bony lamellae at the *hiatus of the canal for the greater petrosal nerve* and courses in the *groove for the greater petrosal nerve* to the foramen lacerum (Fig. **241**). The parallel *groove for the lesser petrosal nerve* begins somewhat lateral and inferior to the above-mentioned groove at the *hiatus of the canal for the lesser petrosal nerve* and carries the lesser petrosal nerve (from the glosso-pharyngeal nerve) to the sphenopetrosal fissure or the foramen ovale. In the lateral region of the anterior surface near the superior border of the

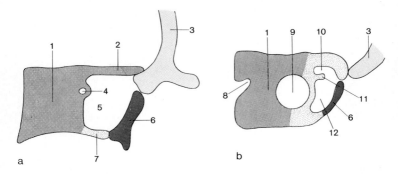

Fig. 225. Temporal bone, semischematic cross section perpendicular to longitudinal axis of petrous part of temporal bone, posterior view
Section b lies rostral to section a

1 Petrous part of temporal bone
2 Tegmen tympani
3 Squamous part of temporal bone
4 Facial canal
5 Tympanic cavity
6 Tympanic part of temporal bone
7 Floor of tympanic cavity
8 Internal acoustic meatus
9 Carotid canal
10 Semicanal for tensor tympani
11 Septum of musculotubal canal
12 Semicanal for auditory tube

petrous portion there is a rounded elevation, the *arcuate eminence*, caused by the superior semicircular canal of the vestibular system. The part attaching laterally forms the roof of the tympanic cavity (*tegmen tympani*).

The *groove for the superior petrosal sinus* passes along the upper border of the pyramid. At the posterior margin of the posterior surface courses the *groove for the inferior petrosal sinus*. Both longitudinal grooves contain the venous blood channel of the same name. The *margin of the posterior part of the petrous temporal*, which marks off the posterior against the inferior pyramidal surface, communicates with the basilar part of the occipital bone via the fibrocartilaginous *petro-occipital synchondrosis*. In this cartilaginous joint, the *jugular notch* leaves a space in the petrous temporal which borders the *jugular foramen* together with the notch of the occipital bone (occipital notch).

The jugular notch can be subdivided by the *intrajugular process*, which touches the process of the occipital bone (occipital process) and bisects the *jugular foramen*.

At the *posterior surface* of the pyramid, the *internal acoustic meatus* commences with the *internal acoustic foramen*, through which pass the facial and vestibulocochlear nerves, as well as the labyrinthine vessels.

The *floor* (*fundus*) *of the internal acoustic meatus* is divided by a transverse bony ridge, the *transverse crest*. Above the ridge, a section designated as the *area of the facial nerve* lies medially (and anteriorly), at which the facial canal begins;

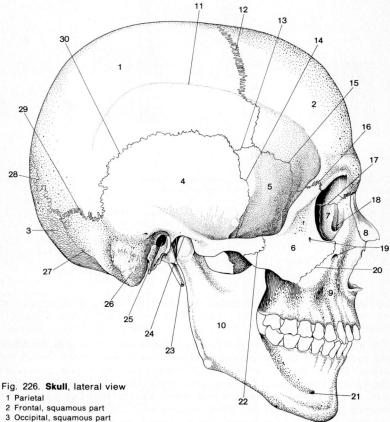

Fig. 226. **Skull**, lateral view
 1 Parietal
 2 Frontal, squamous part
 3 Occipital, squamous part
 4 Temporal, squamous part
 5 Greater wing of sphenoid,
   temporal surface
 6 Zygomatic
 7 Lacrimal
 8 Nasal
 9 Maxilla
10 Mandible
11 Inferior temporal line
12 Coronal suture
13 Sphenoparietal suture
14 Sphenosquamosal suture
15 Sphenofrontal suture
16 Frontozygomatic suture
17 Frontolacrimal and frontomaxillary
   sutures
18 Fossa for lacrimal sac
19 Zygomaticofacial and infra-orbital
   foramina
20 Zygomaticomaxillary suture
21 Mental foramen
22 Temporozygomatic suture
23 Styloid process of temporal
24 Temporomandibular joint
25 External acoustic opening
26 Mastoid process
27 Occipitomastoid suture
28 Lambdoidal suture
29 Parietomastoid suture
30 Squamosal suture

laterally, there is the *superior vestibular area* for the passage of the fibers of the utriculo-ampullary nerve. The medial half below the transverse crest takes in the *cochlear area* with the *spiral foraminous tract*, the point of passage for the fibers to the cochear ganglion. Lateral to it, the openings for the passage of the fibers of the saccular nerve lie in the *inferior vestibular area.* Still further laterally (and posteriorly), there is the *solitary foramen (foramen singulare)* for the posterior ampullary nerve.

Lateral to, and somewhat above, the internal acoustic foramen, the *external aperture* of the *aqueduct of the vestibule* is concealed by a small osseous squama. By means of this opening, the blind-ending endolymphatic duct with its endolymphatic sac arrives at the cranial cavity.

Lateral to the internal acoustic foramen, near the upper border of the posterior pyramidal surface, lies the *subarcuate fossa*, which is considerably deeper in the fetus and child than in the adult. It pushes forward against the concavity of the anterior semicircular canal and is of significance only insofar as the dura is firmly attached here also in the adult.

The *inferior pyramidal surface* is part of the external basicranium. It forms the floor of the tympanic cavity and the musculotubal canal. In the middle of the inferior surface the *carotid canal* begins. In front of it and somewhat lateral to it, lies the external opening of the *musculotubal canal* which opens at the anterior wall of the tympanic cavity.

The carotid canal first ascends perpendicularly in the temporal pyramid, then bends sharply medially and anteriorly and courses horizontally to its opening at the apex of the pyramid. At the bending site, fine *caroticotympanic canaliculi* begin, and carry nerves of the same name from the sympathetic carotid plexus to the tympanic cavity.

The musculotubal canal is a double canal. Through the incompletely delimited upper half of the canal passes the tensor tympani; the auditory (pharyngotympanic) tube lies in the larger, lower compartment.

Behind the external opening of the carotid canal, the *jugular fossa*, a dome-shaped space in front of and above the jugular foramen, receives the superior bulb of the internal jugular vein. In the middle of the fossa, a fine canal (*mastoid canaliculus*) begins and transmits the auricular ramus of the vagus nerve to the tympanomastoid fissure and thus into the region of the external ear.

In the spine-like dividing ridge between the jugular fossa and the external opening of the carotid canal, lies the small *petrosal fossa*, which receives the inferior ganglion of the glossopharyngeal nerve. The *tympanic canaliculus*, which transmits the tymphanic nerve (initial part of the lesser petrosal nerve) and the inferior tympanic artery to the middle ear cavity, begins at the base of this fossa. Medial to the petrosal fossa, the perilymphatic duct exits from the petrous temporal at the *external aperture of the cochlear canaliculus* (*aqueduct of the cochlea*).

Lateral to the jugular fossa, the *styloid process* is fused with the pyramidal base. Between this process and the mastoid process, there is the opening of the facial canal (*stylomastoid foramen*).

In the newborn child, the *tympanic part* of the temporal bone consists only of a ring (*tympanic anulus*), open above (Figs. **214** and **252 d**), in which the tympanic membrane is spanned. The free ends of the bony anulus, the *greater* (anterior) and *lesser* (posterior) *tympanic spines*, rest on the undersurface of the temporal squama, which closes the gap with an indented marginal segment (*tympanic notch*) and completes the ring.

In the course of postnatal development, the tympanic anulus grows out into a groove, open above, which embraces the medial portion of the external acoustic meatus from below, behind and in front. The osseous groove is completed by the squamous part as the bony *external acoustic meatus*, the external opening of which is designated as the *external acoustic foramen*. The medial end of the external acoustic meatus is closed by the tympanic membrane, which is stretched in a shallow sulcus (*tympanic groove*). The bony external acoustic meatus is separated from the mastoid process situated posterior to it by a furrow filled with connective tissue (*tympanomastoid fissure*). The auricular ramus of the vagus nerve passes through it from the mastoid canaliculus.

With its lower margin the tympanic part forms the *sheath of the styloid process* and covers the root of this process. Medially, the tympanic part fuses with a bony plate growing out from the petrous part as the *floor of the tympanic cavity*. The anterosuperior margin of the bony groove formed by the tympanic part in the region of the external acoustic meatus communicates with the squamous part at the *tympanosquamous fissure*. Further medially, a process of the tegmen tympani protrudes obliquely downward between the squamous and tympanic parts up to the external base of the skull. In this way two furrows originate here, the *petrosquamous fissure* (closed at the inner side, usually bony later) and in front of it the *petrotympanic fissure*. The latter conducts the chorda tympani, a branch of the facial nerve, from the tympanic cavity to the external base of the skull.

The *squamous part* can be divided into the squama proper and a more basal portion which is connected with zygomatic arch at the *temporozygomatic suture* and forms the socket of the jaw articulation.

With its sphenoidal margin the disc-shaped squama borders anteriorly on the greater wing of the sphenoid (*sphenosquamous suture*); with its parietal margin it borders upwards on the parietal bone (*squamous suture*). In the notch between the posterior margin of the temporal squama and the superior margin of the mastoid process (*parietal notch*) is inserted the mastoid angle of the parietal.

The external surface of the squamous part of the temporal bone (*temporal surface*) forms a portion of the field of origin of the temporalis muscle. On it, above the external acoustic foramen, a shallow groove (*groove for the middle temporal artery*) passes upward for the vessel of the same name. The *cerebral surface* of the squama is turned toward the cranial cavity.

With its branches the middle meningeal artery has embossed its surface with *arterial grooves.*

At the basal part of the squama, the *zygomatic process* projects anteriorly and forms the *zygomatic arch* together with the temporal process of the zygomatic bone. At the base of the zygomatic process, a cylindrical bony projection (*articular tubercle*) lies on the lower surface. Behind it, the articular socket of the jaw joint (*mandibular fossa*) is spread out. The true *articular surface* is covered with fibrocartilage, which is continued on the articular tubercle.

Interior spaces of the temporal bone. The temporal bone contains the membranous labyrinth, as well as canals for vessels and nerves. The corresponding spaces in the bone are roughly a negative image of these structures and will be discussed in connection with the sense organs. References is made here to some general relationships.

The temporal bone harbors two different systems of spaces. The labyrinth organ is enclosed in the petrous portion. Secondarily, the space system of the middle ear (tympanic cavity and tube) is embedded in the temporal bone. It lies outside of the petrous part, but below the squamous part and medially in front of the tympanic part. The connection between the middle ear space and the interior of the labyrinth capsule takes place via two windows (*fenestrae*) at the medial wall of the tympanic cavity: the *vestibular* (oval) *window*, to which the footplate of the stapes is attached, and below it the *cochlear* (round) *window*, which is closed by the secondary tympanic membrane.

The canals in the petrous portion can be characterized in the following abbreviated form:

The *carotid canal* transports the internal carotid artery and the internal carotid plexus into the cranial cavity.

The *caroticotympanic canaliculi* convey sympathetic nerve fibers as caroticotympanic nerves from the internal carotid plexus to the tympanic plexus.

The *facial canal* begins at the area of the facial nerve in the internal acoustic meatus, courses laterally forward up to the *genu of the facial canal* below the hiatus of the canal for the greater petrosal nerve. Here the sensory geniculate ganglion of the facial nerve is situated and here the greater petrosal nerve carrying parasympathetic fibers leaves the facial trunk. The facial canal bends around laterally and backwards at the genu in an acute angle. It courses in the medial wall of the tympanic cavity, from which it is separated only by a thin, occasionally incomplete bony lamella, so that pathological processes can spread from the tympanic cavity. Below the lateral semicircular canal, the facial canal passes downward in the arch and opens at the stylomastoid foramen in the external base of the skull between the mastoid process and the styloid process.

The *musculotubal canal* is divided incompletely by the *septum of the musculotubal canal* into an upper semicanal (*semicanal for the tensor tympani muscle*) and a lower semicanal (*semicanal for the auditory tube*). The musculotubal canal opens with both semicanals at the anterior wall of the tympanic cavity. It lies directly in front of the carotid canal.

The tympanic nerve (from the glossopharyngeal nerve) and the inferior tympanic artery course in the *tympanic canaliculus*. The canal begins at the petrosal fossa and opens into the tympanic cavity. Its continuation is the canal of the lesser petrosal nerve, which ends at the anterior surface of the pyramid.

The *canaliculus of the chorda tympani*, which contains the chorda tympani and the posterior tympanic artery, begins in the facial canal just above the stylomastoid foramen and opens into the tympanic cavity. It continues into the "anterior chordal canal" which courses through the petrotympanic fissure.

In the *mastoid canaliculus* the auricular ramus of the vagus nerve passes from the jugular fossa to the tympanomastoid fissure.

The *vestibular aqueduct*, a narrow canal for the endolymphatic duct, leads from the vestibule of the osseous labyrinth to the external aperture at the posterior pyramidal surface.

The *cochlear aqueduct*, which encloses the perilymphatic duct, begins at the scala tympani and opens with the external aperture at the inferior surface of the pyramid in front of the jugular fossa.

The paired **parietal bones** (Figs. 219, 226, and 234) cover a considerable part of the cranial roof and lateral wall between the frontal and occipital bones. The bones possess four margins which form four angles.

The *anterior (frontal) margin* forms the *coronal suture* with the frontal bone. The *superior (sagittal) margin* meets the parietal bone of the opposite side in the midline at the *sagittal suture*. The *posterior (occipital) margin* joins the squamous portion of the occipital bone at the *lambdoidal suture*. The *inferior (squamous) margin* forms the *squamous suture* with the squamous portion of the temporal bone and is attached in the region of the antero-inferior angle (*sphenoidal angle*) usually to the greater wing of the sphenoid by the *shenoparietal suture*.

The sphenoidal angle is drawn out more acutely and longer than the *frontal angle* (anterosuperiorly), the *occipital angle* (posterosuperiorly) and the *mastoid angle* (postero-inferiorly). On the whole, the parietal bone is arched like a dish. The part of the *external surface* projecting widest externally is designated as the *parietal eminence*, which is more strongly pronounced in the newborn child and infant than in the adult.

In the vicinity of the sagittal margin, the bone can be penetrated by a *parietal foramen* for the parietal emissary vein which connects the superior sagittal sinus with the superficial temporal vein (Fig. 237).

Below the parietal eminence, two curved lines course transversely over the external surface: *superior* and *inferior temporal lines*. The lower line marks the upper border of the field of origin of the temporalis muscle. The superior temporal line serves for the attachement of the temporalis fascia.

At the *inner surface* of the parietal bone, depressions (*digital impressions*) corresponding to the cerebral convolutions (gyri) and elevations (*cerebral juga*) corresponding to the cerebral sulci are recognizable. At the superior margin, the *groove for the superior sagittal sinus* has been imprinted for the blood vessel of the same name. Lateral to it, there are small osseous pits (*granular pits*), into which project villus-like processes of the arachnoid. Distinctly recognizable *arterial grooves* stem from branches of the middle meningeal artery (from the maxillary artery). They pass obliquely backward and upward from the antero-inferior angle. At the inner side of the mastoid angle, there is a short portion of the *groove for the sigmoid sinus* for the sinus of the same name.

The **frontal bone** (Figs. **219, 226–228, 234** and **236**) forms the anterior end of the cranial cavity and the largest part of the roof of the orbit. It is also part of the upper border of the nasal cavity.

At the *frontal bone* the following are distinguished:
– the *frontal squama*, which completes the cranium anteriorly:
– the two *orbital parts*, which form the roof of the orbit and the floor of the anterior cranial fossa on each side; and
– the *nasal part*, the unpaired middle section between the two orbital parts.

The frontal arises bilaterally as pure membrane bones. The two frontal bones are originally separated by a suture (*frontal suture*) which lies in the continuation of the sagittal suture (Fig. **252b**). Osseous fusion of the suture usually occurs in the 2nd year of life. As a variant, the suture can persist in the adult (metopism). In cases of the abnormal enlargement of the cranial cavity (e.g. congenital widening of the subarachnoid space, hydrocephalus), metopism regularly occurs. The frontal suture and the sagittal suture together form a cross with the coronal suture.

The steep position of the frontal squama is caused by the development of the frontal lobes of the cerebrum and is, therefore, an essential characteristic of the human skull. In the mammalian series, a progressive erection of the "sloping" forehead can be recognized. In humans, the anterior pole of the forehead no longer lies behind, but above the nasal cavity. The individual curvature of the forehead, however, not only depends on this steep position, but also is caused by the pneumatization of the squama.

The *frontal squama* communicates at its upper margin (*parietal margin*) with the parietal bones by means of the *coronal suture*. Laterally and below, the additional surface for the greater wings of the sphenoid adjoins this suture at the *sphenofrontal suture*. It extends to the posterior margin of the orbital part where, at the inner base of the skull in direct continuation of the greater wing, the lesser wing of the sphenoid is attached medially.

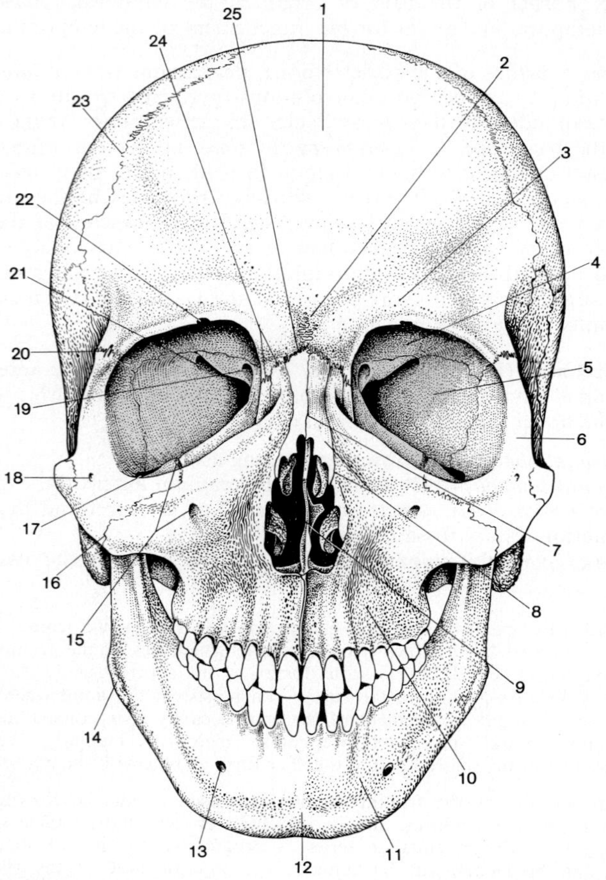

Fig. 227. **Skull**, anterior view

1 Frontal, squamous part
2 Glabella
3 Superciliary arch
4 Orbital part of frontal bone
5 Greater wing of sphenoid, orbital surface
6 Zygomatic
7 Internasal suture
8 Nasal bone and nasomaxillary suture
9 Bony nasal septum
10 Maxilla
11 Mandible
12 Mental protuberance
13 Mental foramen
14 Angle of mandible

15 Infra-orbital foramen and infra-orbital groove
16 Zygomaticomaxillary suture
17 Inferior orbital fissure
18 Zygomaticofacial foramen
19 Optic canal
20 Frontozygomatic suture
21 Superior orbital fissure
22 Supra-orbital notch
23 Coronal suture
24 Frontomaxillary (medial) and frontolacrimal (lateral) sutures
25 Frontonasal suture

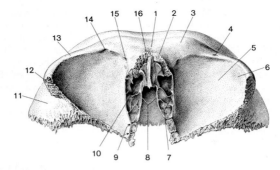

Fig. 228. **Frontal bone**, view from below

1 Glabella
2 Nasal margin, lower border of nasal
   part of frontal bone
3 Superciliary arch
4 Supra-orbital foramen
5 Orbital part, orbital surface
6 Fossa for lacrimal gland
7 Ethmoidal air cells
8 Ethmoidal notch

9 Recesses for ethmoidal foramina
10 Opening of frontal sinus
11 Temporal surface
12 Zygomatic surface
13 Supra-orbital margin
14 Supra-orbital notch
15 Frontal notch
16 Nasal spine

The *external surface* of the frontal squama is slightly arched with *frontal eminences* projecting on both sides of the midline. Below it – but at some distance from the upper margin of the orbit (the *supra-orbital margin*) – the variably formed *superciliary arch* passes bow-shaped from medial to lateral. Between both superciliary arches there is a flattened area, the *glabella*.

The superciliary arch might be interpreted as the remains of a supra-orbital swelling (torus supra-orbitalis) appearing in primates and primitive humans. It is probably a reinforced supporting pillar of the facial skeleton which absorbs the force generated by the masticatory muscles.

The medial half of the *supra-orbital margin* exhibits two notches: a *frontal notch* located medially and a *supra-orbital notch* somewhat further laterally. Both notches can also be formed individually as *foramina*. By means of the supra-orbital notch, the lateral branch of the supra-orbital nerve (from the ophthalmic nerve) arrives at the skin of the forntal area; the medial ramus of the supra-orbital nerve passes through the frontal notch. The nerves are accompanied by corresponding vascular branches from the ophthalmic artery. Laterally, the supra-orbital margin is continued into the *zygomatic process*, which projects laterally at the lower margin of the squama. It communicates with the zygomatic bone via the *frontozygomatic suture*. The lateral contour of the margin of the zygomatic process is continued into the *temporal line*. It limits the lateral surface of the frontal squama (*temporal surface*).

On the cerebral surface of the squama (*internal surface*), the *groove for the superior sagittal sinus* courses in the midline. Its margins come together and pass downward as an undivided ridge (*frontal crest*) which serves for the attachment of the falx cerebri. A blind pit (*foramen cecum*) lies at the lower end of the crest near the border of the ethmoid bone and functions as an attachment site for the dura mater. The inner surface of the squama exhibits *digital impressions, cerebral ridges* and several vascular grooves running vertically, which serve for the frontal branch of the middle meningeal artery laterally and for the anterior meningeal artery medially.

The *orbital parts* form the roof of both orbits, which are slightly curved toward the cerebral side. Their medial margins, together with the posterior margin of the nasal part, border a deep notch (*ethmoidal notch*) in which the ethmoid bone with the cribriform plate is inserted. The posterior margin of each orbital part adjoints the greater and lesser wings of the sphenoid at the sphenofrontal suture. At the medial wall of the orbit (from back to front) the orbital part adjoins the orbital plate of the ethmoid at the fronto-ethmoidal suture and at the upper margin of the lacrimal bone it borders the frontolacrimal suture.

The surface of the orbital part facing the orbit (*orbital surface*) possesses laterally a shallow depression (*lacrimal fossa*) for the lacrimal gland. Medially and anteriorly at the roof of the orbit, there is the *trochlear pit* to which a connective tissue sling (trochlea) is attached. The trochlea can also be anchored by means of a small bony process (trochlear spine) which sometimes develops at the lateral margin of the pit. The connective tissue loop contains a tubular cartilaginous pulley around which the tendon of the superior oblique turns back toward the eyeball at a sharp angle.

In the fronto-ethmoidal suture are two holes (*anterior* and *posterior ethmoidal foramina*). By means of the anterior foramen, the anterior ethmoidal nerve (from the nasociliary, a branch of the ophthalmic) and the anterior ethmoidal artery and vein (from the ophthalmic artery and superior ophthalmic vein) arrive at the anterior cranial fossa from the orbit. They pass from there into the nasal cavity via the cribriform plate of the ethmoid. The posterior ethmodial nerve (also from the nasociliary) passes through the posterior ethmoidal foramen to the mucous membrane of the ethmoidal air cells.

The *nasal part* of the frontal bone is drawn out in the midline into a pointed process (*nasal spine*). On each side, the roughened anterior surface (*nasal margin*) articulates with the nasal bone (*nasofrontal suture*) and, immediately lateral to this, with the frontal process of the maxillary bone (*frontomaxillary suture*).

At the inferior surface, the frontal bone exhibits pit-like indentations (*ethmoidal pits*) in the narrow band between the lateral margin of the ethmoidal notch and the orbital roof (medial margin of the orbital plate). These overlap corresponding pits of the ethmoid bone and form the superior covering of the ethmoidal labyrinth. Further forward on the pit-like surface are the paired *openings into the frontal sinus.*

The development of the frontal sinuses varies considerably in different individuals. The paired *frontal sinus* usually extends far into the squama and into the superciliary arch, but can (rarely) also pneumatize the roof of the orbit. Both frontal sinuses are separated by a *septum* and often show strong lateral asymmetry.

b) Bones and Cartilage of the Nasal Skeleton

The **ethmoid** (Figs. **229, 230** and **245**) arises as unpaired cartilage bones in the cartilaginous nasal capsule. In a frontal section, the T-shaped *middle piece* and paired *lateral pieces* can be distinguished.

The *ethmoid* consists of:
- the vertically-placed *perpendicular plate*, the perpendicular part of the T;
- the *cribriform plate*, the horizontal arm of the T; and
- the paired *ethmoidal labyrinths*, which are the lateral parts lying between the nasal and orbital cavities and enclosing the *ethmoidal air cells.*

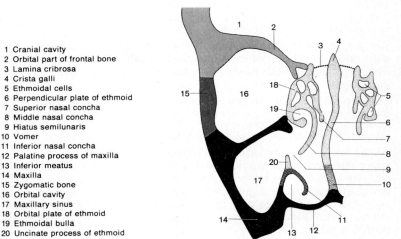

1 Cranial cavity
2 Orbital part of frontal bone
3 Lamina cribrosa
4 Crista galli
5 Ethmoidal cells
6 Perpendicular plate of ethmoid
7 Superior nasal concha
8 Middle nasal concha
9 Hiatus semilunaris
10 Vomer
11 Inferior nasal concha
12 Palatine process of maxilla
13 Inferior meatus
14 Maxilla
15 Zygomatic bone
16 Orbital cavity
17 Maxillary sinus
18 Orbital plate of ethmoid
19 Ethmoidal bulla
20 Uncinate process of ethmoid

Fig. 229. **Schematic frontal section through nasal skeleton**, anterior view
Orbital and nasal cavities, maxillary sinus

Ethmoid bone	☐	Maxilla	■
Vomer	▦	Zygomatic bone	▨
Inferior nasal concha	▨	Frontal bone	▨

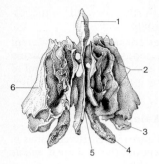

Fig. 230. **Ethmoid bone**, anterior view
1 Crista galli
2 Ethmoidal labyrinth
3 Uncinate process
4 Middle nasal concha
5 Perpendicular plate
6 Orbital plate

The *cribriform plate* is inserted in the ethmoidal notch of the frontal bone. The osseous plate shows numerous holes, passages for the olfactory nerves from the olfactory mucosa to the olfactory bulb. In the median plane, the *crista galli* projects into the cranial cavity from the ethmoidal plate and serves as an attachment site for the falx cerebri.

The foramen cecum lies in the frontal bone in front of the crista galli, occasionally also between the ethmoidal plate and the frontal bone. Paired, wing-like processes (*wings of the crista galli*) can extend to the frontal bone from the crista galli and surround the foramen cecum from the sides.

The *perpendicular plate* continues the crista galli below the ethmoidal plate and forms the posterior, superior part of the osseous nasal septum. The perpendicular plate rarely lies in the median plane; usually it resides on one side or the other.

The perpendicular plate borders on the sphenoidal crest of the body of the sphenoid posteriorly, on the vomer postero-inferiorly, and on the cartilage of the nasal septum inferiorly. Anterosuperiorly, the plate is inserted behind and below the nasal spine of the forntal bone; at the anterior margin the nasal bones lie on it.

At the *lateral part*, the *orbital plate* (lamina papyracea), which is often paper-thin, bounds the ethmoidal labyrinth from the orbit. The *ethmoidal cells* are air-filled, sinous spaces which communicate with the true nasal cavity and are lined with mucous membrane. The *anterior* and the *middle ethmoidal air cells* open into the nasal cavity between the middle and inferior nasal conchae; the *posterior ethmoidal cells* open above the middle concha.

The open ethmoidal cells are closed by adjacent bones (especially above the nasal part of the frontal bone, behind by the anterior surface of the body of the sphenoid, in front by the lacrimal bone). Between the upper margin of the orbital plate and the frontal bone, the anterior and posterior ethmoidal foramina are notched on each side.

At the medial side of the ethmoidal labyrinth, two *nasal conchae* (*superior* and *middle nasal conchae*) project into the nasal cavity from the lateral part of the ethmoid.

The conchae arise ontogenetically as mucosal swellings. Initially, cartilaginous conchae are formed in them as delicate lamellae which always go out from the lateral part of the ethmoid bone. The *inferior nasal concha* is already segmented off from the ethmoid before the conclusion of ossification and ossifies independently.

Occasionally, the ethmoid also gives rise to a rudimentary *supreme nasal concha*.

The superior nasal concha roofs over the *superior nasal meatus*, while the middle nasal concha covers the *middle nasal meatus*.

A large ethmoidal cell (*ethmoidal bulla*, Fig. **245**), concealed by the middle nasal concha, protrudes into the middle nasal meatus and compresses from above the wide opening of the maxillary sinus in the isolated maxilla. The opening of the maxillary sinus is bridged over anteriorly and inferiorly by a process of the ethmoid (*uncinate process*) which passes obliquely backward and downward as a thin, hook-shaped bony plate from the anterior margin of the lateral part of the ethmoid bone and ends free. Together with the ethmoidal bulla, the uncinate process borders a crescent-shaped opening in the lateral wall of the osseous nasal cavity. Termed the *hiatus semilunaris*, this aperture provides access from the middle nasal meatus to the frontal and maxillary sinuses, as well as to the ethmoidal air cells located in front of the ethmoidal bulla.

The independent **inferior nasal concha** (Figs. **219, 229** and **245**) is larger than the other conchae and exhibits a rounded anterior end and a pointed posterior end. Its superior margin is sharply bent laterally and projects into the opening of the maxillary sinus as the *maxillary process*. At the anterior end, the short *lacrimal process* juts upward to the lacrimal bone. As the *ethmoidal process*, the posterior end reaches the apex of the uncinate process.

The **nasal bone** (Figs. **226** and **242**) is a small, quadrangular membrane bone in the upper part of the bridge (dorsum) of the nose. Both nasal bones join one another in the midline at the *internasal suture* (Fig. **227**). They border superiorly on the frontal bone at the *frontonasal suture* and laterally on the frontal process of the maxillary bone at the *nasomaxillary suture*. The free inferior margin becomes part of the border of the bony *external nasal opening* (*piriform aperture*).

The anterior ethmoidal nerve courses in a longitudinal groove (*ethmoidal groove*) on the inferior surface of the nasal bone.

The **lacrimal bone** (Figs. **226** and **242**) is inserted as a small membrane bone between the frontal, ethmoid and maxilla at the boundary of the orbit and facial surface. Its inferior margin on its inner aspect has contact with the inferior concha. At the upper surface a vertical ridge (*posterior lacrimal crest*) marks off the narrow "facial part" from the broader "orbital part". This ridge, together with a corresponding anterior lacrimal crest at the maxillary bone, borders the *lacrimal groove* and the *fossa* for the lacrimal sac and the nasolacrimal duct.

A hook-shaped bony process, the *lacrimal hamulus*, encloses the lacrimal sac laterally and anteriorly.

The **vomer** (Figs. **229** and **243**), an unpaired membrane bone, forms the lower portion of the osseous nasal septum.

The vomer arises at the lower margin of the cartilaginous nasal septum from two obliquely positioned lamellae which fuse with one another. The initially V-shaped bone – in frontal section – assumes the figure of a Y in the course of ontogenesis since the bending point of the two lateral parts develops into a thick plate. The two lateral parts of the bony anlage, on the other hand, lag behind in growth and change into two small, wing-shaped processes.

The vomer, as an irregularly shaped, quadrangular bony plate, borders inferiorly on the nasal crest of the maxilla and palatine bone. At the superior margin of the vertically-placed bony plate, the two *alae* (wings) *of the vomer* spread apart and enclasp the rostrum sphenoidale.

Laterally, the alae of the vomer extend on each side to the vaginal process at the root of the pterygoid process and (in front of it) the sphenoidal process of the palatine bone. The bony groove bordered by the vaginal process and the inferior surface of the sphenoidal body is closed by the ala into the *vomerovaginal canal*, through which a branch of the sphenopalatine artery courses.

The anterior margin of the vomer slopes obliquely forward. It communicates posterosuperiorly with the perpendicular plate of the ethmoid, antero-inferiorly with the cartilaginous part of the nasal septum. The free posterior margin of the vomer likewise passes obliquely from posterosuperiorly to antero-inferiorly and separates the two *posterior nasal openings (choanae)* from one another.

The **nasal cartilage** is preserved in the adult as the uncalcified remains of the chondrocranium. It forms the skeleton in the anterior part of the external nose and a part of the nasal septum antero-inferiorly. In front of the nasal bone, the *lateral nasal cartilage* lies on the bridge of the nose as part of the former cartilaginous lateral wall of the nasal capsule. In the region of the ala of the nose, the isolated *greater* and *lesser alar cartilages* are attached. The *nasal septum cartilage* sends out a process (*posterior [sphenoidal] process*) of varying length between the ethmoid and the vomer (Fig. **243**).

c) Bones of the Jaw Skeleton

The paired **maxilla** (Figs. **229**, **231** and **235**) is a central structural element of the viscerocranium. It borders on the orbit and nasal cavity, forms the largest portion of the roof of the oral cavity and receives the roots of all the maxillary teeth on each side.

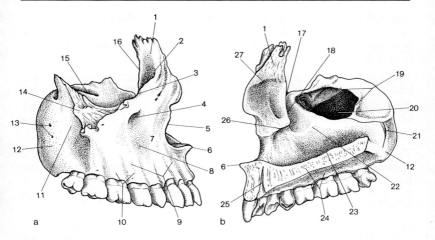

Fig. 231. **Maxilla** a lateral view b Medial view

1 Frontal process
2 Anterior lacrimal crest
3 Infra-orbital margin
4 Infra-orbital foramen
5 Nasal notch
6 Anterior nasal spine
7 Body of maxilla
8 Canine fossa
9 Alveolar processes
10 Alveolar juga
11 Infratemporal surface
12 Tuber of maxilla
13 Alveolar foramina
14 Zygomatic process

15 Infra-orbital groove, continues as
   infra-orbital canal
16 Lacrimal margin
17 Lacrimal notch
18 Groove for nasolacrimal duct
19 Opening of maxillary sinus
20 Maxillary sinus
21 Greater palatine canal
22 Nasal surface
23 Nasal crest
24 Palatine process
25 Incisive canal
26 Conchal crest
27 Ethmoidal crest

In the maxilla, two originally independent membrane bones are united, the upper jawbone in the narrow sense and the *premaxilla (incisive, intermaxillary)*. They fuse during early embryonic development into one unit. The remains of a *premaxillary (incisive) suture* (Fig. **252d**) can occasionally be preserved. The original premaxillary region includes that part of the maxilla in which the two upper incisors take root.

Malformations which appear as facial clefts (harelips) never occur at the border of the premaxilla and the true maxillary bone, but rather lie in the region of the premaxilla.

The *maxilla* consists of a large *middle piece*, or body, and four *processes* emanating from it:

The irregularly-shaped *maxillary body* is pneumatized and harbors the *maxillary sinus*.

The *frontal process* passes steeply upward between the nasal bone (*naso-maxillary suture*) and the lacrimal bone (*lacrimomaxillary suture*) and is attached to the nasal part of the frontal bone by the *frontomaxillary suture* (Fig. **227**).

The massive *zygomatic process* passes laterally from the maxillary body and borders on the zygomatic bone at the *zygomaticomaxillary suture*.

The *alveolar process* is the downward continuation of the anterior surface of the maxillary body and bears the *dental alveoli* for one-half of the maxillary teeth.

The *palatal process* passes from the body of the maxilla medialward as a horizontal osseous plate and communicates in the median plane with the palatal process of the other maxilla via the *median palatine suture* and at the posterior margin with the palatine bone via the *transverse palatine suture*.

Four surfaces are distinguished at the *body of the maxilla*. The *anterior surface* borders on the lower margin of the orbit (*infra-orbital margin*) and continues laterally, without a sharp boundary, into the zygomatic process. The bow-shaped medial margin of the anterior surface (*nasal notch*) forms the lateral and lower boundary of the piriform aperture, ending rostrally as the *anterior nasal spine*. Forward and upward, the "facial surface" of the maxillary body is continued into the *frontal process* and downward into the *alveolar process*. The *infra-orbital foramen*, the site of exit of the infra-orbital nerve (from the maxillary nerve) and the infra-orbital artery, lies below the infra-orbital margin. Near the alveolar process, the anterior surface is depressed to form the *canine fossa*, the field of origin of the levator anguli oris muscle.

The *orbital surface* of the body of the maxilla forms the largest part of the floor of the orbit (Fig. **242**). Its posterior margin is directed toward the greater wing of the sphenoid, with which it borders the inferior orbital fissure. Posteriorly, the medial margin possesses a contact surface to the orbital process of the palatine bone (*palatomaxillary suture*); anteriorly, it communicates first with the orbital surface of the ethmoid (*ethmoidomax-illary suture*) and then with the lacrimal bone (*lacrimomaxillary suture*).

The *infra-orbital groove* passes anteriorly along the floor of the orbit from the inferior orbital fissure (Fig. **227**). It is closed as the *infra-orbital canal* between the floor of the orbit and the roof of the maxillary sinus and opens with the *infra-orbital foramen* at the surface of the face.

The bony process, which transforms the groove into a canal, arises from the zygomatic process of the maxilla. Occasionally, the *infra-orbital suture* which runs from the beginning of the canal at the floor of the orbit to the infra-orbital foramen can be preserved.

Fine osseous canals lead from the infra-orbital groove and canal to the dental alveoli and carry nerve branches (middle and anterior superior alveolar rami from the maxillary nerve) to the maxillary teeth (except the last two molars).

The *infratemporal surface*, the posterior surface of the maxillary body, lies behind the zygomatic process. Toward the anterior surface it is marked off by the infrazygomatic crest, which is continued on the facial surface from the lower margin of the zygomatic process.

The body of the maxillary bone is distended in the region of the infratemporal surface to form the *tuber of the maxilla*. Some holes (*alveolar foramina*) and the canals (*alveolar canals*) emanating from them conduct branches of the infra-orbital nerve (posterior superior alveolar rami) to the molar teeth. Near the medial margin of the posterior surface, the *greater palatine groove* is evident; it is complemented by the groove of the same name on the palatine bone and becomes the *greater palatine canal*, which passes from the *pterygopalatine fossa* to the hard palate. The canal transmits the greater palatine nerve (a branch of the pterygopalatine nerves with sensory fibers from the pterygopalatine nerve and secretory fibers from the pterygopalatine ganglion) and the descending palatine artery (from the maxillary artery).

The tuber of the maxilla and the pterygoid process are in close contact lateral to the greater palatine groove. They are separated only by a narrow opening, the *pterygomaxillary fissure* (Figs. **242** and **246**).

The medial surface (*nasal surface*) of the body of the maxilla forms the lateral wall of the nasal cavity. It contains the large opening of the maxillary sinus (*maxillary hiatus*), which is strongly compressed by adjacent bones (uncinate process of the ethmoid, inferior nasal concha, palatine bone). The *maxillary sinus* (Fig. **242**) fills nearly the entire body of the maxilla. Its deepest point lies at the level of the first molar tooth.

Since the opening is found high above the floor of the sinus, fluids effused into the maxillary sinus have no unrestricted outlet.

In front of the maxillary hiatus, the groove for the nasolacrimal duct (*lacrimal groove*) passes downward at the nasal surface. This groove, which begins at the floor of the orbit with a recess (*lacrimal notch*), forms the lateral wall of the *nasolacrimal canal*. The canal is closed off medially by the lacrimal bone and the lacrimal process of the inferior nasal concha. The widened entrance, the *fossa of the lacrimal sac* (Fig. **242**), lies at the medial wall of the orbit, close to the floor between the posterior lacrimal crest of the lacrimal bone and the *anterior lacrimal crest* of the frontal process of the maxilla.

At the transition to the frontal process, a bony ridge (*conchal crest*) slopes slightly toward the nasal notch at the anterior portion of the nasal surface and gives attachment to the inferior nasal concha. Parallel to it on the medial surface of the frontal process is the *ethmoidal crest*, which serves for the attachment of the anterior end of the middle nasal concha.

The free margin (*alveolar arch*) of the *alveolar process* is curved like a bow and contains 8 *dental alveoli* (Fig. **274**). The roots of the teeth correspond to bulging prominences on the external surface (*alveolar juga*). The individual alveoli are separated by *interalveolar septa*. In multirooted teeth, fine *interradicular septa* lie within the alveoli.

The *palatine processes* of both maxillae form the anterior two-thirds of the hard palate. At the medial margin where the palatal processes of both sides are united by the *median palatine suture*, the *nasal crest* rises toward the nasal cavity. This ridge, which runs out anteriorly into the *anterior nasal spine*, is adjoined from above by the vomer (behind) and by the cartilaginous nasal septum (in front).

The bony palate is perforated in the region bordering the premaxilla and the maxilla proper by the *incisive canal*. It begins paired at the floor of the nasal cavity and opens at the roof of the oral cavity (with 2–4 fine *incisive foramina*) into the uniform *incisiva fossa*, which is closed by an epithelial cone. The nasopalatine nerve (from the maxillary nerve) traverses this canal from the nasal cavity to the palate. At the posterior margin of the palatal process of the maxilla – extremely lateral, near the alveolar process – is the *greater palatine foramen*, whose medial and posterior borders are formed by the horizontal plate of the palatine bone.

Through this opening, the greater palatine nerve passes from the canal of the same name. Together with branches of the greater palatine artery (from the descending palatine artery), its branches travel forward to the inferior surface of the palate within *palatine grooves* which are limited by small bony ridges (*palatine spines*).

The **palatine bone** (Fig. **232** and **244**), as a paired membrane bone, consists of two plates which form an angle of about 60° open medially. The vertical plate (*perpendicular plate*) participates in the structure of the posterior part of the lateral nasal wall, while the *horizontal plate* forms the posterior third of the hard palate. The bone fills the gap between the maxilla and the pterygoid process of the sphenoid.

At the back the *perpendicular plate* borders the pterygopalatine fossa medially with its external surface (*maxillary surface*); with the greater palatine groove, it completes the groove of the maxilla into the canal of the same name; at the front it covers a large part of the hiatus maxillaris from behind.

Lesser palatine canals (usually two, for the nerves of the same name) leave the greater palatine canal, penetrate the pyramidal process and open at the *lesser palatine foramina* on the horizontal plate.

At its upper end the perpendicular plate splits into two processes (orbital and sphenoidal) situated one behind the other and separated by a V-shaped notch (*sphenopalatine notch*). The *orbital process* (anterior) is united with the maxilla, ethmoid and sphenoid. Its free upper surface

1 Maxillary opening and maxillary sinus
2 Ethmoidal crest
3 Orbital process
4 Sphenopalatine notch
5 Sphenoidal process
6 Nasal surface and perpendicular plate
7 Conchal crest
8 Pyramidal process
9 Horizontal plate
10 Nasal crest
11 Palatine process
12 Body of sphenoid
13 Sphenopalatine foramen
14 Medial plate of pterygoid process
15 Inferior nasal concha

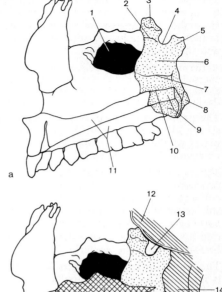

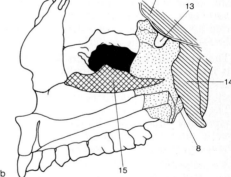

Fig. 232. **Incorporation of palatine bone in lateral wall of nasal cavity**, medial view
a Relative position of palatine bone to maxilla
b Relative position of palatine bone to sphenoid, maxilla and inferior nasal concha

| Palatine | ⬚ | Sphenoid | ▨ |
| Maxilla | ☐ | Inferior nasal concha | ⬚ |

forms a small part of the floor of the orbit (posteromedial). The *sphenoidal process* (posterior) adjoins the body of the sphenoid and the vaginal process at the root of the pterygoid process.

Between the vaginal process of the sphenoid and the sphenoidal process of the palatine bone is a fine canal (*palatovaginal canal*) through which the pharyngeal ramus passes from the pterygopalatine ganglion to the pharyngeal mucosa.

The *sphenopalatine notch* is transformed into the *sphenopalatine foramen* by the body of the sphenoid. It transmits the posterior superior nasal rami from the pterygopalatine ganglion and the sphenopalatine artery, the branches of which pass into the mucous membrane of the nasal cavity and the paranasal sinuses.

At the medial surface of the perpendicular plate (*nasal surface*), two parallel ridges course approximately horizontally, a *conchal crest* (about in the middle) and an *ethmoidal crest* (at the base of the orbital process), to which the posterior ends of the inferior and the middle nasal conchae are fixed.

The postero-inferior end of the perpendicular plate is prolonged into a strong *pyramidal process* that is inserted between the medial and lateral plates of the pterygoid process in the pterygoid notch. It delimits the pterygoid fossa downward.

The *horizontal plate* of the palatine bone borders anteriorly on the palatal process of the maxilla (*transverse palatine suture*). Its medial margin is connected with the horizontal plate of the palatine bone of the opposite side at the *median palatine suture*. At the *nasal surface*, it juts up as the *nasal crest*, which ends posteriorly with the *posterior nasal spine*. On the inferior surface (*palatine surface*), a transverse ridge (*palatine crest*) can be formed near the posterior margin.

The **zygomatic bone** (Figs. **226**, **227** and **235**), as a paired membrane bone, is inserted between the maxilla, temporal and frontal. Of the two processes, the *temporal process* adjoins the zygomatic process of the temporal squama at the *temporozygomatic suture* and forms the *zygomatic arch*. The strong *frontal process* communicates with the frontal bone (*fronto-zygomatic suture*) and with the greater wing of the sphenoid (*sphenozygomatic suture*). At the zygomatic process of the maxilla, a broad area of contact exists at the *zygomaticomaxillary suture*.

A small protuberance, the *marginal tubercle*, occasionally projects at the posterior margin of the frontal process and serves as an attachment site for fibers of the aponeurotic temporalis fascia.

Of the three surfaces of the zygomatic bone, the *lateral surface* is turned anterolaterally, whereas the *temporal surface* is directed toward the temporal fossa. The *orbital surface* forms a large part of the lateral wall of the orbit.

At the lateral wall of the orbit, the zygomatic nerve (from the maxillary nerve) passes into the orbital surface of the zygomatic bone at the *zygomatico-orbital foramen*. The bony canal divides and transmits the zygomaticofacial nerve through the *zygomaticofacial foramen* situated at the lateral surface and the zygomaticotemporal nerve through the *zygomaticotemporal foramen* at the temporal surface.

The **mandible** (Figs. **226**, **227** and **233**) is the only freely movable skull bone.

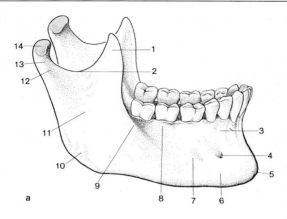

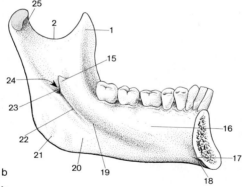

Fig. 233. **Mandible**
a Lateral view
b Left half of mandible, medial view

1 Coronoid process
2 Mandibular notch
3 Alveolar juga
4 Mental foramen
5 Mental protuberance
6 Base of mandible
7 Body of mandible
8 Alveolar part
9 Oblique line
10 Angle of mandible
11 Ramus of mandible
12 Condylar process
13 Neck of mandible

14 Head of mandible
15 Lingula
16 Sublingual fovea
17 Mental spine
18 Digastric fossa
19 Mylohyoid line
20 Submandibular fovea
21 Pterygoid tuberosity
22 Mylohyoid groove
23 Mandibular foramen
24 Mandibular canal
25 Pterygoid fovea

It arises lateral to Meckel's cartilage as paired membrane bones that are originally united syndesmotically at the mental symphysis, synostosis occurring during the first year of life.

After the fusion of both anlagen, the mandible forms a horseshoe-shaped, unpaired skeletal portion consisting of a horizontal *body* and an ascending *ramus* on each side. The mandibular body and ramus first form a relatively obtuse angle (150° in the newborn child), which in the adult approaches more of a right angle (100–130°).

After a total loss of teeth in the mandible and the disappearance of the dental alveoli, the angle increases again to values of more than 130°.

At the *body of the mandible*, the tooth-bearing *alveolar part* rests on the well-developed lower part (*base of the mandible*). The *external surface* of the base displays the *mental protuberance* in front. Both basal corners of this three-sided field are designated as the *mental tubercle*. The development of a chin and the synostosis of the mandibular symphysis are characteristics of the human skull.

These specifically human developments are evidently connected with the broadening of the whole skull, corresponding to the enlargement of the telencephalon. The broad, stretched arch of the lower jaw apparently requires an additional reinforcement at its weakest point, the chin region.

The depressed region of origin of the mentalis muscle (*fossa mentalis*) lies lateral to the mental tubercle. The *mental foramen*, which transmits the mental nerve (terminal branch of the inferior alveolar nerve from the mandibular nerve) and the mental artery (from the inferior alveolar artery), opens lateral to this field below the 1st or 2nd premolar tooth. The *oblique line* passes obliquely upward in the lateral region of the mandibular body and goes over into the anterior margin of the mandibular ramus.

At the *inner surface* of the body of the mandible in the region of the symphysis is the *mental spine* (origin of the genioglossus muscle above and the geniohyoid below). The anterior belly of the digastric attaches in the chin region at a more or less distinctly defined fossa (*digastric fossa*) near the lower margin. Somewhat above and lateral to it is a flat recess (*sublingual fovea*) containing the sublingual gland. In the posterior half of the mandibular body, the *mylohyoid line* can be distinguishable on the inner surface as an oblique, posteriorly-ascending line of origin of the mylohyoid muscle. Immediately below it, at the transition to the jaw angle is situated the *submandibular fovea* for the submandibular gland.

The *alveolar part* of the mandibular body ends with a parabola-shaped, arched free margin (*alveolar arch*), which contains the *dental alveoli* for the mandibular teeth.

As in the maxilla, the alveoli of the mandible are separated by *interalveolar septa* and subdivided in multirooted teeth by *interradicular septa*. Bulges (alveolar juga) are prominent on the external surface of the alveolar part; they are caused by the roots of the teeth.

The *mandibular ramus* arises from the body of the mandible at the *angle of the jaw (mandibular angle)*. The jaw angle, which projects backward and downward, can exhibit roughnesses on its external and internal surfaces for muscular attachments: on the outside the *masseteric tuberosity* for the masseter muscle and on the inside the *pterygoid tuberosity* for the medial pterygoid muscle.

The ramus divides at its upper end into an anterior pointed muscular process (*coronoid process*), at which the tendon of the temporalis muscle inserts, and a posterior articular process (*condylar process*), which bears the articular *head* and slender *neck of the mandible*. Between the two processes in the *mandibular notch* through which the masseter nerve (from the mandibular nerve) and the vessels of the same name pass to the masseter muscle.

The *pterygoid fovea*, the site of insertion of a head of the lateral pterygoid muscle, lies directly below the articular head at the anterior surface of the condylar process.

An opening on the inner side of the madibular ramus, the *mandibular foramen*, leads into the *mandibular canal*, which passes within the mandible up to the mental foramen. This bony canal conveys the inferior alveolar nerve and the vessels of the same name.

The *lingula of the mandible*, a small bony projection to which the sphenomandibular ligament is attached, somewhat overlaps the mandibular foramen in front. From this opening, the *mylohyoid groove*, a furrow for the mylohyoid nerve (from the mandibular nerve), passes obliquely downward to the mandibular body along the inner surface of the mandibular ramus.

The total construction of the mandible consists of a continous compact bony trabecula, the "basal arch" (Fig. 251), passing from the articular head across the ramus and body to the chin; on this arch there are areas for muscular insertions (coronoid process, angle of mandible) and for the teeth (alveolar processes). In the toothless jaw of infants, these areas are lacking or are very weak (coronoid process). When teeth are lost in the elderly, the alveolar part undergoes involution. The angle of the jaw and the muscular processes disintegrate from the margins and then project more sharply.

The **hyoid bone** lies above the larynx and below the root of the tongue. In a systemic classification, it is grouped along with the facial bones. Functionally, however, it belongs to the locomotor apparatus of the neck and is therefore discussed there (→ p. 725).

4. Cranium

a) Cranial Roof and Lateral Wall

The **roof of the cranium** (*calvaria*, Fig. 234) is made up of plates of bones (frontal squama, parietal, upper part of occipital squama) that are curved in the longitudinal and transverse directions. The degree of curvature and thus the height of the cranium are an expression of brain size.

In the adult, the roof of the skull in the occipital region is wider than in the frontal area. In the relatively large cranium of the newborn child, the external occipital protuberance and the parietal and frontal tuberosities project so that the outline of the cranium appears pentagonal (Fig. 252 b).

The membrane bones of the skull roof arise separately and grow toward each other. The coupling of individual bones to one another has not yet been completed in the newborn child so that closed connective tissue intervals (*fontanelles*) remain at the corners of the bones (Fig. 252). The rhomboid-shaped *large* anterior (*frontal*) *fontanelle* lies between the upper angles of the parietal and frontal bones; between the apex of the occipital squama and the posterior, upper angle of the parietal bone, the triangular, *small* posterior (*occipital*) *fontanelle* is located.

Since both fontanelles are easily palpable through the scalp of the newborn child and are clearly distinct in their shape (anterior fontanelle: quadrangular; posterior fontanelle; triangular), they permit, during childbirth, a directional orientation in respect to the child's head and an estimation of its position in the mother's pelvis.

The *sphenoidal fontanelle* lies between the antero-inferior angle of the parietal and the superior margin of the greater wing of the sphenoid. Between the lower margin of the parietal, temporal squama and occipital squama, the still-cartilaginous petrous part of the temporal pushes against the surface of the skull. This zone (*mastoid fontanelle*) is thus the basis of closed gaps of the skull wall which lack fibrous tissue.

The anterior fontanelle remains open into the 2nd postnatal year, whereas the occipital and sphenoidal fontanelles already close shortly after birth.

After closure of the fontanelles, the *cranial sutures* form a characteristic design (Fig. 252). Between the frontal and the two parietal bones, the *coronal suture* courses transversely across the roof of the skull and is joined behind by the *sagittal suture*, which is situated between the two parietals. At the posterior end of the sagittal suture, the two portions of the *lambdoidal suture*, which course obliquely, separate the parietal bones from the occipital squama. These sutures are developed as *serrated sutures*. At the lateral wall, the short *sphenoparietal suture* replaces the sphenoidal fontanelle. The squamous part of the temporal bone adjoins the inferior margin of the parietal bone in a convex, upward line and forms the *squamosal suture*. The superior margin of the temporal squama overlaps the inferior margin of the parietal bone. Toward the occipital bone, the squamous suture merges into the suture between the parietal and mastoid process of the temporal bone (*parietomastoid suture*).

The roof of the skull is covered over by a uniform, tough periosteum (*pericranium*). In a child, the external periosteum adheres relatively loosely to the bone and can be lifted off by trauma (subperiosteal bleeding, cephalic hematoma).

The inner side of the calvaria is likewise lined by periosteum. In the course of development, it fuses with the dura mater into a (macroscopically) uniform, strong layer. When the skull cap (cranial vault) is removed during autopsy, the bones in the adult are easily detached from the dura. In children, the separation of the bones from the dura is hardly possible, since the external layer of connective tissue is still osteogenic tissue and therefore remains firmly united with the newly-deposited, exterior bone. Prior to the closure of the cranial suture while the skull bones are still movable, the dura plays an important role as a uniform supporting and bracing system of the cranial roof.

The roof of the skull is approximately 5 mm thick, of which the compact external osseous layer, the *external lamina* (external table), comprises 1.5 mm and the equally compact *internal lamina* (internal table) comprises 0.5 mm. The two layers enclose a spongy osseous material (*diploë*) between them, the interstices of which contain red bone marrow.

The bony skull roof is elastically deformable to a limited extent. In circumscribed trauma, the internal table can splinter while the external table remains intact.

Numerous *diploic veins* (Fig. **237**) pass through the diploë in broad canals (*diploic canals*); they communicate on the one hand with venous channels of the inner skull and on the other empty into veins of the external soft parts of the head via four venous trunks (*frontal diploic vein, temporal diploic veins, occipital diploic vein*).

The diploic veins are additional drainage paths for the blood in the cranial veins in the case of stagnation. They also have significance as pathways for the spread of infections from the soft parts of the head to the interior of the cranium.

The internal relief of the calvaria is determined by the adjacent soft parts. Most distinct are the *arterial grooves* on the parietal and squama of the occipital bones caused by branches of the middle meningeal artery. The venous sinuses of the interior of the skull produce impressions on the inner wall (e.g. the grooves for the superior sagittal, transverse and sigmoid sinuses). In addition to the groove of the superior sagittal sinus, pit-like depressions (*granular pits*) are found which exhibit varying degrees of individual development. They are produced by tuft-like outgrowths of the arachnoid (*arachnoid granulations*) which originate from about the 3rd year onward and (usually) increase with age. Impressions of sulci (*cerebral ridges*) and convolutions (*digital impressions*) in humans are only weakly expressed at the roof of the skull, in contrast to the base.

The **lateral wall of the skull** (*temporal plane*) is formed by the parietal (below the superior temporal line), the frontal squama (behind the temporal line), the greater wing of the sphenoid and by the squamous part of the temporal bone. At the external base of the skull, it is bordered by the infratemporal crest of the greater wing of the sphenoid and by the zygomatic arch. The temporal plane is depressed below the inferior line into the *temporal fossa*, the region of origin of the temporalis muscle. Toward the base, the temporal fossa is continous with the infratemporal fossa.

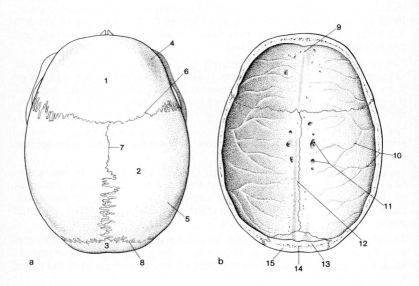

Fig. 234. **Calvaria**
a External view
b Internal view

1 Frontal bone
2 Parietal bone
3 Occipital bone
4 Frontal eminence
5 Parietal eminence
6 Coronal suture
7 Sagittal suture
8 Lambdoidal suture
9 Frontal crest
10 Arterial grooves
11 Granular pits
12 Groove for superior sagittal sinus
13 Internal table
14 Diploë
15 External table

b) External Base of the Skull

At the **external base of the skull** (*external basicranium*, Fig. **235**), the jaw skeleton is attached to the cranium anteriorly and conceals it thoroughly. In the middle and in the posterior region, the cranium is freely accessible for observation from below.

Close behind the center of the skull base lies the foramen magnum, which is flanked on both sides by the articular processes for the atlas (occipital condyles). The condylar canal (for the condylar emissary vein) opens directly below the condyle. Lateral to, and above, the articular process opens the hypoglossal canal. The jugular foramen lies between the lateral part of the occipital bone and the temporal pyramid. The styloid process and, dorsolateral to it, the mastoid process are visible on the temporal bone. Behind the root of the styloid process, lies the stylomastoid foramen.

In the nuchal region, the occipital squama adjoins the foramen magnum. Its configuration is expressed by the external occipital protuberance and the paired supreme nuchal line, superior nuchal line and inferior nuchal line.

Between the anterior margin of the foramen magnum and the posterior margin of the palate, the skull base is formed in the middle by the bodies of the occipital and sphenoid bones. The inferior side of the occipital carries the pharyngeal tubercle, at which the pharynx is fixed by means of the pharyngeal raphé (Fig. **274**). Lateral to the basilar part of the occipital, the foramen lacerum is recessed between the apex of the temporal pyramid and the root of the pterygoid process. At the lower side of the temporal bone, the carotid canal begins at the petrous part; laterally, the mandibular fossa and the articular tubercle adjoin the squamous part. Directly behind the articular fossa and in front of the external acoustic meatus are openings of the petrosquamous and petrotympanic fissures (exit of the chorda tympani).

The pterygoid processes adjoin the posterior margin of the palatine bone laterally. With their medial and lateral plates, they border the pterygoid fossa, which opens posteriorly. Above the posterior margin of the palatine are the choanae the posterior openings into the nasal cavity which are separated from one another by the free margin of the vomer. The medial plate of the pterygoid process with the pterygoid hamulus, the horizontal plate of the palatine and the vomer provide the bony borders of the choanae. Lateral to the root of the pterygoid process, the basicranium is formed by the greater wing of the sphenoid, which projects posteriorly as the sphenoidal spine. In the greater wing, the foramen spinosum (for the middle meningeal artery) lies posterolaterally; somewhat further medially and rostrally is the foramen ovale (for the mandibular nerve). Laterally, at the body of the sphenoid is attached the horizontal part of the lower surface of the greater wing, which bends back along the infratemporal crest into the vertical temporal surface, i.e. into the lateral wall of the skull. Between the pterygoid process and the maxilla, the pterygomaxillary fissure leads into the pterygopalatine fossa (Figs. **242** and **246**).

The anterior portion of the skull base is formed by the hard palate which is bounded by the dental arch of the maxilla. The transverse palatine suture, which separates the palatine process of the maxilla from the horizontal plate of the palatine, courses approximately at the border of the posterior quarter of the palatal surface. The incisive fossa, into which the incisive canal opens with 2–4 foramina (Fig. **274**), is located in the anterior portion of the palate, where remnants of an intermaxillary (incisive) suture can be visible. In the posterolateral region of the hard palate are the greater palatine foramen and, behind it, the lesser palatine foramen, the openings for the palatine nerves and arteries.

c) Internal Base of the Skull

The **internal base of the skull** (*internal basicranium*, Figs. **236**, **238** and **241**) forms the floor of the *cranial cavity*. From anterior to posterior, three *cranial fossae* can be distinguished: *anterior*, *middle* and *posterior*, which follow one another in steps declining toward the occiput. The anterior cranial fossa lies highest, the posterior lowest. The configuration of the internal base of the skull is the negative image of the base of the brain.

In the anterior cranial fossa lie the olfactory and frontal lobes of the cerebrum. The middle cranial fossa contains in its central region the basal portion of the midbrain and the hypophysis; in its lateral region the temporal lobes of the cerebrum project strongly basally. The posterior cranial fossa supports the cerebellum.

The border between the anterior and middle cranial fossae is formed laterally by the posterior margin of the lesser wing of the sphenoid, medially by the posterior margin of the jugum sphenoidale. The middle

---

13 Jugular fossa
14 Foramen magnum
15 External occipital protuberance
16 Superior nuchal line
17 Inferior nuchal line
18 Occipital condyle
19 Mastoid process
20 Stylomastoid foramen
21 Opening of external acoustic meatus

22 External opening of carotid canal
23 Styloid process of temporal bone
24 Foramen lacerum
25 Lateral plate of pterygoid process
26 Medial plate of pterygoid process
27 Lesser palatine foramen
28 Greater palatine foramen
29 Transverse palatine suture
30 Median palatine suture

►

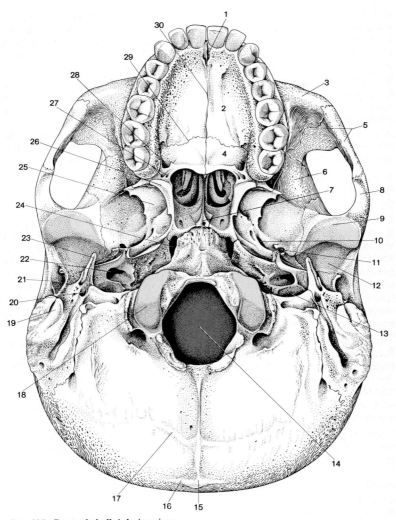

Fig. 235. **Base of skull**, inferior view

1 Incisive fossa ⎫
2 Palatine process ⎬ of maxilla
3 Zygomatic process ⎭
4 Horizontal plate of palatine bone
5 Zygomatic bone
6 Greater wing of sphenoid

7 Vomer
8 Zygomatic process of temporal bone
9 Articular tubercle
10 Foramen ovale
11 Foramen spinosum
12 Mandibular fossa

and posterior fossae are separated laterally by the upper edge of the temporal pyramid and in the middle by the dorsum sellae. This boundary is completed by the tentorium cerebelli, a dural plate which extends between the cerebellum and occipital lobes of the cerebrum and contains an opening (tentorial notch) in the middle for the brain stem.

The *floor of the anterior cranial fossa* is formed by the orbital parts of the frontal, the cribriform plate of the ethmoid, the jugum sphenoidale and the lesser wings of the sphenoid. The crista galli, which projects from the cribriform plate of the ethmoid, and the foramen cecum located in front of it are attachment sites for the falx cerebri, which projects between the two cerebral hemispheres. The cribriform plate is penetrated by the openings for the olfactory nerves and the anterior ethmoidal vessels.

The *floor of the middle cranial fossa* is formed in the middle by the body of the sphenoid and laterally by the greater wing of the sphenoid, parts of the temporal squama and the anterior surface of the temporal pyramid.

In the middle part of the middle cranial fossa, the (pre)chiasmatic groove is located rostrally, at the anterior margin of the sella turcica. This shallow transverse groove, which leads laterally into the optic canal (for the optic nerve) contains the chiasmatic cistern, a dilatation of the subarachnoid space. The optic chiasma lies above the depression. In the sella turcica, the tuberculum sellae, the hypophysial fossa for the reception of the hypophysis, and the tuberculum sellae follow in sequence from anterior to posterior. The carotid groove (for the internal carotid artery) courses at the lateral surface of the body of the sphenoid.

The junction between the central and lateral regions of the middle cranial fossa contains the trigeminal ganglion and the initial sections of the three trigeminal branches within the *cavum trigeminale* (Meckel's cavity). This "nerve chamber" is covered by periosteum and is separated from the cranial cavity by a dural plate. This portion of the bony skull (the spout or mouth of the middle cranial fossa) is not shaped by the brain, but by the nerve chamber.

The root portion of the greater wing is already penetrated in the region of the nerve chamber by the foramen rotundum (for the maxillary nerve), behind it and somewhat laterally by the foramen ovale (for the mandibular nerve) and posteriorly by the foramen spinosum (for the middle meningeal artery). Further laterally is the cavity for the temporal lobes of the cerebrum. At the inner surface of the greater wing of the sphenoid and the temporal squama are impressions for the branches of the middle meningeal artery.

The superior orbital fissure (for cranial nerves III, IV, VI, V_1 and the superior ophthalmic vein) between the greater and lesser wings connects the middle cranial fossa with the orbital cavity. The foramen lacerum, closed by fibrocartilage, is recessed between the greater wing and the

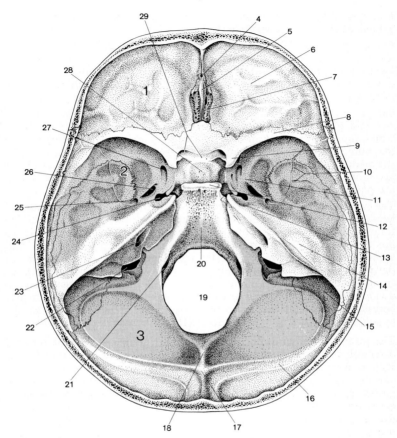

Fig. 236. **Base of skull**, superior aspect

1 Anterior cranial fossa
2 Middle cranial fossa
3 Posterior cranial fossa
4 Foramen caecum
5 Crista galli
6 Orbital part of frontal bone
7 Lamina cribrosa
8 Lesser wing of sphenoid
9 Anterior clinoid process
10 Arterial grooves
11 Greater wing of sphenoid
12 Dorsum sellae
13 Trigeminal impression
14 Petrous part of temporal bone
15 Groove for sigmoid sinus

16 Groove for transverse sinus
17 Internal occipital protuberance
18 Internal occipital crest
19 Foramen magnum
20 Clivus
21 Hypoglossal canal
22 Jugular foramen
23 Opening of internal acoustic meatus
24 Foramen lacerum
25 Foramen spinosum
26 Foramen ovale
27 Foramen rotundum
28 Hypophysial fossa in sella turcica
29 Optic canal and chiasmatic groove

pyramid. Above it, the internal carotid artery arrives at the carotid groove at the body of the sphenoid.

On the anterior surface of the petrous temporal, the grooves of the greater and lesser petrosal nerves course as shallow channels to the foramen lacerum or sphenopetrosal fissure. The anterior semicircular canal of the inner ear produces a swelling on the lateral portion of the anterior surface of the pyramid. The tegmen tympani lies anterolateral to it.

The *floor of the posterior cranial fossa* is formed by the clivus, by the pyramid of the temporal bone and by the occipital bone. The clivus, which supports the pons and medulla oblongata, borders on the foramen magnum with its posterior margin. The foramen magnum is traversed by the medulla oblongata, the vertebral and spinal arteries, as well as by the accessory nerve. The groove for the inferior petrosal sinus passes along the posterior margin of the petrous temporal.

The jugular foramen forms a recess in the petro-occipital synchondrosis between the petrous temporal and the lateral portion of the occipital. The following pass through this foramen (in sequence from anteromedial to posterolateral): inferior petrosal sinus, glossopharyngeal, vagus and accessory nerves, as well as the internal jugular vein. The nerve compartment situated anteromedially is faintly marked off from the venous compartment by the intrajugular processes. A connective tissue septum divides the jugular foramen between cranial nerves IX and X, but not between nerves and veins. At the base of the occipital condyle, the hypoglossal canal (for cranial nerve XII) perforates the occipital bone.

The internal configuration of the occipital squama shows the internal occipital protuberance and the cruciform eminence. Its perpendicular limb is formed by the groove for the superior sagittal sinus and the variable internal occipital crest; its transverse limb is produced by the paired grooves for the transverse sinus. The cerebellar hemispheres occupy both of the lower fossae marked off by it, whereas the two upper fossae lying above the posterior cranial fossa contain the occipital lobes of the cerebrum.

In the angle formed by the cerebral surface of the mastoid process and the posterior surface of the temporal pyramid, the groove for the sigmoid sinus is engraved in the wall of the posterior cranial fossa (Fig. 236). Medial to it, the internal acoustic meatus begins at the posterior surface of the petrous temporal with the internal auditory foramen (entrance for cranial nerves VII, VIII and the labyrinthine artery). The aperture of the aqueduct of the vestibule (exit of the endolymphatic duct, which terminates at the endolymphatic sac beneath the dura) follows posterolaterally.

Near the upper edge of the temporal pyramid, the subarcuate fossa lies lateral to the internal acoustic meatus. In this region the dura is solidly anchored to the bone.

d) Cranial Meninges

The **cranial meninges** (Fig. **237** and **238**) fill the space between the inner side of the skull and the surface of the brain (→ also pp. 153 ff.). From the outside to the inside they are as follows:

– *dura mater*, which in the cranium has fused with the periosteum;
– *arachnoid*, which fits closely against the dura everywhere; and
– *pia mater*, which covers the brain surface as a delicate connective tissue layer and sinks into all sulci and recesses.

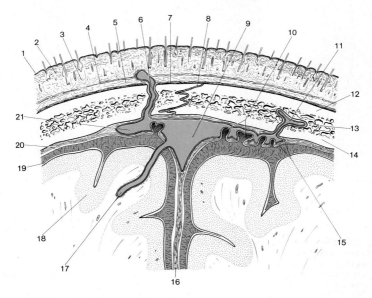

Fig. 237. **Scalp and calvaria**, cross section
Meninges and superior sagittal sinus

1–5 *Scalp*

1, 2 *Skin*

1 Epidermis (with hair)
2 Dermis
3 Subcutaneous connective tissue
4 Galea aponeurotica
5 Subaponeurotic cleft, allows free movement of above layers
6 Parietal emissary vein in parietal foramen
7 Pericranium
8 Sagittal suture
9 Superior sagittal sinus
10 Arachnoid granulations
11 Diploic vein in diploic channel
12 External table of parietal bone
13 Diploë
14 Internal table of parietal bone
15 Periosteal ("outer") and meningeal ("inner") layer of cephalic dura mater.
16 Falx cerebri
17 Superior cerebral vein
18 Cerebral cortex
19 Cephalic pia mater
20 Arachnoid and subarachnoid space
21 Lateral lacuna of superior sagittal sinus

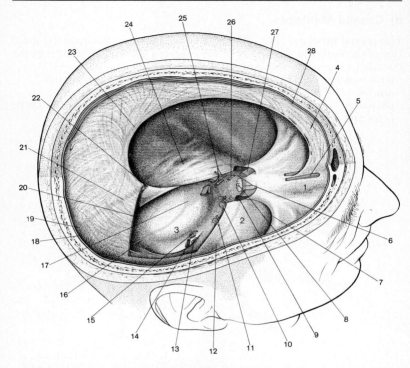

Fig. 238. **Falx cerebri and tentorium cerebelli, venous sinuses of dura**, intracranial course of cephalic vessels and nerves, oblique view from above

1 Anterior cranial fossa
2 Middle cranial fossa
3 Posterior cranial fossa
4 Falx cerebri
5 Olfactory bulb and tract
6 Cavernous sinus and intercavernous sinus
7 Sphenoparietal sinus
8 Hypophysial stalk
9 Internal carotid artery
10 Trigeminal nerve
11 Facial and vestibulocochlear nerves
12 Superior petrosal sinus
13 Glossopharyngeal, vagus and accessory nerves
14 Vertebral artery
15 Hypoglossal nerve
16 Inferior petrosal sinus
17 Opening of sigmoid sinus into superior bulb of jugular vein
18 Occipital sinus
19 Confluence of sinuses
20 Tentorium cerebelli, cut margin
21 Straight sinus
22 Great cerebral vein
23 Inferior sagittal sinus
24 Sigmoid sinus
25 Abducens (behind) and trochlear (in front) nerves
26 Oculomotor nerve
27 Optic nerve
28 Superior sagittal sinus

In clinics, the uniform dura-periosteal layer is often designated as the *pachymeninx* and contrasted with the other two meninges, the *leptomeninx,* an organization that corresponds to their functional relationships since the dura is more closely related to the skull bones and the leptomeninx to the brain. Also, in pathological processes, the pachymeninx and leptomeninx react differently.

Cranial Dura

At the **cephalic dura,** the periosteal and meningeal layers can still be distinguished microscopically in the adult and are often designated as "external" and "internal" layers of the dura. In the region of the venous conduits, they are separated. At the foramen magnum, both layers withdraw from one another and border the epidural cavity of the vertebral canal.

In children, the dura adheres firmly to the periosteal layer at the cranial bones; in adults, on the other hand, it is easily detached (→ p. 609). A firm anchoring to bone is preserved only at the foramen cecum and the crista galli, as well as in the subarcuate fossa on each side at the posterior surface of the temporal pyramid.

On the whole, the cephalic dura forms a protective capsule around the brain. It dispatches septa-like processes, especially the falx cerebri and falx cerebelli, between the large cranial parts which prevent their displacement.

The *falx cerebri* penetrates between the two cerebral hemispheres and extends nearly to the corpus callosum. It originates at the crista galli, at the foramen cecum and at the margins of the groove of the superior sagittal sinus (up to the internal occipital protuberance). It contains the superior sagittal sinus in its superior margin, the inferior sagittal sinus in its lower free margin, and has grown together with the tentorium cerebelli.

The narrow *falx cerebelli* forms a lower continuation of the falx cerebri below the tentorium cerebelli and lies between the two cerebellar hemispheres. In its posterior margin it encloses the occipital sinus.

The *tentorium cerebelli* projects between the cerebellum and the occipital lobes of the cerebrum. It is attached on each side at the margins of the groove of the transverse sinus and at the superior edge of the temporal pyramid. Near the apex of the petrous temporal, it passes over the trigeminal impression to the posterior clinoid process and reaches the anterior clinoid process rostrally. Toward the midline, the tentorium ascends slightly. Behind, in the median plane, the ridge of the tentorium meets the falx cerebri and encloses the straight sinus. The medial margins of the tentorium border a triangular notch (*tentorial notch*), the floor of which is formed by the dorsum sellae. The brain stem passes through this opening, which connects the cerebellar space with the cerebral space.

The *diaphragma sellae* (Fig. **263**) stretches over the sella turcica as a horizontal dural plate between the clinoid processes and separates the hypophysial fossa from the rest of the cranial cavity. The diaphragma – near its posterior margin – is penetrated by a wide opening for the hypophysial stalk. At its margin, the dura passes into the arachnoid, which rests on the upper surface of the hypophysis. The hypophysial fossa itself is covered by periosteum which communicates by loose connective tissue with the connective tissue capsule of the hypophysis. Thus, the hypophysis lies outside of the dura.

The dura and (especially) its septa brace the vault of the skull and secure it against external forces (masticatory musculature). Therefore, the septa consist predominantly of tendinous, stout bundles of collagenous fibers which course mostly arched and tangential in the falx cerebri.

Vessels and Nerves of the Dura Mater

The **arteries of the dura mater** (*meningeal arteries*) course between the dura and the bone. In addition to the dura, they supply especially the flat bones of the skull (red bone marrow).

The *anterior meningeal artery* leaves the anterior ethmoidal artery in the anterior cranial fossa and supplies a small region beside the crista galli.

The *middle meningeal artery* from the maxillary artery enters the middle cranial cavity via the foramen spinosum (Fig. **241**). It gives off a usually weak anastomosis to the lacrimal artery and divides into anterior and posterior branches (*frontal* and *parietal branches*). The site of division can lie just above the foramen spinosum or also higher up in the region of the parietal bone. The frontal branch courses steeply upward, while the parietal branch passes almost horizontally backward.

Ruptures of the middle meningeal artery lead to epidural bleeding. If the trunk of the artery is injured, the hematoma spreads out directly above the plane of the zygomatic arch. Hematomas from the anterior branch can extend in the direction of the parietal (crown) from the posterior frontal and the anterior temporal regions. Hematomas from the parietal branch lie above the ear. Epidural hematomas produce compression symptoms at the brain.

The *middle meningeal artery* gives off the *anastomotic branch*, which is usually weak and which arrives at the orbit through the superior orbital fissure and is connected with the lacrimal artery, a branch of the ophthalmic artery. Occasionally, the anastomosis is so strongly developed that the middle meningeal artery appears to arise from the ophthalmic artery or the latter is formed as a branch of the middle meningeal artery.

The *posterior meningeal artery* (usually from the ascending pharyngeal artery) enters the cranial cavity (as a rule) through the jugular foramen and supplies a small area in the medial region of the posterior cranial fossa.

The **venous blood conduits of the dura** (*dural sinuses*, Figs. **238, 240** and **278**) form a system of "collecting veins" which receives the blood from the cerebral veins and which also communicates with the diploic veins. The blood drains directly or indirectly into the internal jugular vein, to a lesser extent also into the venous plexus of the vertebral column.

By means of the occipital diploic vein and emissary veins, blood from the transverse and sigmoid sinuses can arrive at the external jugular vein and thus into the subclavian vein.

The valveless dural sinuses extend with rigid walls between the meningeal and periosteal layer of the dura or between the two layers of the dural septum. In this way, the lumen is always held open, and an unhindered flow of blood from the interior of the cranium is guaranteed. The sinus wall is free of muscle and consists of an endothelium and the fibrous connective tissue of the pachymeninx. The venous blood conduits of the cephalic dura correspond in their anlage to the epidural venous plexuses in the vertebral canal.

Four dural sinuses course in the median plane and are therefore unpaired: superior and inferior sagittal sinuses, straight sinus and occipital sinus. The unpaired intercavernous sinus forms an anterior and a posterior transverse portion between the cavernous sinuses of both sides. All the other blood vessels are paired.

The *superior sagittal sinus* travels toward the occiput from the crista galli in the upper convex margin of the falx cerebri and opens – in common with the straight and occipital sinuses – into the transverse sinus. This union is designated as the *confluence of the sinuses*.

Lateral protrusions (*lateral lacunae*, Fig. **237**) of the superior sagittal sinus are invaginated by arachnoid granulations and receive superficial cerebral veins.

The *inferior sagittal sinus* passes backward in the lower concave margin of the falx cerebri and opens into the straight sinus together with the great cerebral vein.

The *straight sinus* courses into the confluence of the sinuses at the line of fusion of the falx cerebri with the tentorium cerebelli. It receives the superior cerebellar veins, in addition to the inferior sagittal sinus and the great cerebral vein.

The *occipital sinus* lies in the posterior margin of the falx cerebelli and unites the confluence of the sinuses with the venous plexus at the foramen magnum, which communicates with the epidural dorsal veins in the vertebral canal.

The *transverse sinus* (usually larger on the right) passes from the confluence into the groove of the transverse sinus laterally and continues into the *sigmoid sinus*, which courses at the inner side of the mastoid process in an S-shaped arch to the jugular foramen and opens into the bulb of the superior jugular vein.

In the region of the groove for the sigmoid sinus, the inner bony table of the temporal bone is often very thin. The mastoid process is pneumatized from the tympanic cavity. Infectious processes can spread from the mastoid air cells to the sigmoid sinus and produce a thrombosis of a sinus.

The *cavernous sinus* lies lateral to the sella turcica as an irregularly-shaped blood space traversed by connective tissue cords. An anterior and a posterior *intercavernous sinus* connect the cavernous sinus on both sides so that a "venous" ring arises which surrounds the hypophysis.

The intercavernous and cavernous sinuses are covered by the diaphragma sellae and the lateral continuation of the diaphragma.

In the lateral wall of the cavernous sinus are found (in a sequence from superior to inferior) the oculomotor, trochlear and ophthalmic nerves. The internal carotid artery and (lateral to it) the abducens nerve *course through the cavernous sinus.*

The cavernous sinus arises in the embryonic period from a venous plexus which surrounds the internal carotid artery and the abducens nerve. The veins of the plexus fuse into a uniform, cavernous (sinuous) spatial system so that the above-mentioned conduction pathways are incorporated into the inferior of the sinus.

The *cavernous sinus*, which communicates with the basilar plexus, *receives* basal cerebral veins and the sphenoparietal sinus. The drainage of blood takes place via the narrow-lumined superior petrosal sinus into the initial part of the sigmoid sinus and via the inferior petrosal sinus into the internal jugular vein. The superior and inferior ophthalmic veins normally also transport their blood into the cavernous sinus, but form at the same time a vascular connection with the drainage area of the facial vein or maxillary vein.

The *sphenoparietal sinus* runs along the posterior margin of the lesser wing of the sphenoid and empties into the cavernous sinus.

The venous plexus which connects the cavernous sinus and the petrosal sinuses of both sides with the anterior venous plexus of the vertebral canal is referred to as the *basilar plexus.*

The *superior petrosal sinus* passes along the upper edge of the temporal pyramid from the cavernous sinus to the initial segment of the sigmoid sinus.

The *inferior petrosal sinus* receives the labyrinthine veins (from the internal acoustic meatus), passes farthest medially through the jugular foramen and, immediately after leaving the skull, opens into the internal jugular vein or, more rarely, into the bulb of the superior jugular vein.

The *drainage of blood from the dural sinus* takes place mainly via the sigmoid sinus into the internal jugular vein. With suitable pressure relationships, drainage is also possible from the cavernous sinus into the angular vein (and thus into the facial vein) via the superior ophthalmic vein, as well as via the inferior ophthalmic vein into the pterygoid plexus (and thus into the maxillary vein). Connections of venous pathways with the external veins of the head occur more or less regularly via the emissary veins, which also communicate with the diploic veins.

The **emissary veins** pass through openings in the skull bones. They probably serve as a means of adjusting pressure.

The following occur with some regularity:
- the *parietal emissary vein* (Fig. **237**), which flows through the parietal foramen, near the sagittal suture and in front of the lambdoidal suture, and connects the superior sagittal sinus with a branch from the superficial temporal vein;
- the *mastoid emissary vein*, which courses through the mastoid foramen behind the mastoid process and permits blood to flow from the sigmoid sinus into the occipital vein; further,
- the relatively frequent *occipital emissary vein* beside the external occipital protuberance, which passes from the confluence of the sinuses to the occipital vein: and
- the inconstant *condylar emissary vein* (Fig. **274**), which passes through the condylar canal and connects the sigmoid sinus with the external vertebral venous plexus.

Comparable to the emissary veins are the **venous plexuses** (Fig. **241**) which pass through the basicranium in the company of large arteries or nerves.

Of noteworthy significance among them are the following:
- the *venous plexus of the foramen ovale* in the foramen ovale between the cavernous sinus and the pterygoid plexus,
- the *venous plexus of the internal carotid*, a venous plexus in the carotid canal which also connects the cavernous sinus and the pterygoid plexus, as well as
- the *venous plexus of the hypoglossal canal* between the venous plexus around the foramen magnum and the internal jugular vein.

The connections between the venous dural sinuses and the extracranial veins (ophthalmic veins, emissary veins, venous plexuses along the arteries and nerves, diploic veins) have clinical significance because infections can be spread along these paths from the soft parts of the head to the meninges (e.g. risk of spreading pathogens via the superior ophthalmic vein to the cavernous sinus in the case of upper lip and nasal furuncles).

Because of the close interrelationships, disease processes in the region of the cavernous sinus can spread easily to the nerves coursing in the sinus and in the wall of the sinus (e.g. abducens paralysis as a result of a thrombosis of a sinus).

Nerves of the dura. The dura mater is richly supplied with sensory nerve fibers. In contrast to brain substance – at least in the region of the basal dura and the venous dural sinuses, as well as their tributaries – it is sensitive to pain. The *meningeal rami* arise from the three branches of the trigeminal nerve (for the dura in the anterior and middle cranial fossae and at the roof of the skull) and from the vagus nerve (for the dura of the posterior cranial fossa).

The *tentorial ramus* leaves the ophthalmic nerve still inside of the cranial cavity, gives off branches to the dura above the cribriform plate, accompanies the trochlear nerve retrograde and ramifies at the tentorium cerebelli and at the posterior portion of the falx cerebri.

The *meningeal ramus* (*middle*) branches off from the maxillary nerve before the latter passes through the base of the skull in the foramen rotundum. It spreads out to each part of the dura which is supplied by the anterior branch of the middle meningeal artery.

The *meningeal ramus* (*mandibular nerve*) first separates from the mandibular nerve extracranially, returns to the middle cranial fossa through the foramen spinosum with the middle meningeal artery (Fig. **241**) and ramifies at the dura with the arterial branches.

The *meningeal ramus* to the dura of the posterior cranial fossa leaves the superior ganglion of the vagus and returns to the cranial cavity through the jugular foramen.

Positional relations of the conduction pathways to the dura mater (Fig. **240**). In contrast to the meningeal arteries which remain extradural, the conduction pathways to or from the brain must also pass through the dura. The dural passage can lie closely adjacent to the openings in the bone (optic canal, jugular foramen, hypoglossal canal), or the site of entry into the dura and bones can be more or less far removed from one another (secondary entrance points: cribriform plate, superior orbital fissure, foramen rotundum). In the latter case, the nerves and vessels course for a time between the dura and bone (extradural, but intracranial). Thus, for example, the trigeminal nerve passes through the dura near the apex of the temporal pyramid and only then forms – between the meningeal and periosteal layer – the trigeminal ganglion and the three main branches. The cavum trigeminale, which protrudes from the trigeminal impression at the apex of the temporal pyramid to the posterior margin of the greater wing of the sphenoid, is thus largely separated from the true dural sac.

Operative procedures (injections, coagulations) at the trigeminal ganglion can be undertaken – from the external base of the skull – without opening the dura.

Arachnoid

The **arachnoid** (Fig. **237**), which lies close to the inside of the dura, covers the entire uneven surface of the brain. It remains separated from the pia by an external, cerebrospinal fluid-containing cavity, the *subarachnoid space*, which is wide in places. The subarachnoid space is permeated by numerous delicate connective tissue trabeculae. It is continuous with the subarachnoid space of the vertebral canal at the foramen magnum.

The subarachnoid space permits a circulation of cerebrospinal fluid over a wide area (→ flow of cerebrospinal fluid, p. 158). Therefore, infectious processes can spread here rapidly (leptomeningitis).

Where an evagination of the arachnoid pushes into the cavum trigeminale, the trigeminal ganglion is bathed in cerebrospinal fluid.

Arachnoid (Pacchionian) granulations are button-shaped, often closely crowded, vascular connective tissue tufts in the vicinity of the large dural sinuses. These Pacchionian bodies penetrate the meningeal layer of the dura and the external layers of the sinus wall and protrude into the lumen of the sinus without breaking through the endothelium. Blood and cerebrospinal fluid are separated from each other only by a thin connective tissue layer. Granulations occur especially in the region of the lateral lacunae of the superior sagittal sinus; they can even be attached to the inner layer of the cranial bones and indent the diploic veins. The granular pits at the inside of the calvaria correspond to the arachnoid granulations.

Subarachnoid cisternae, dilated portions of the subarachnoid space, are formed where the cephalic arachnoid lying adjacent to the dura stretches over recesses at the surface of the brain.

The *cerebellomedullary cistern*, the largest of such cerebrospinal fluid spaces, lies below the cerebellum on the dorsal side of the medulla oblongata. The remaining cisterns are almost all localized at the base of the brain; they are slightly developed at the convex side of the cerebrum.

The cerebellomedullary cistern can be punctured between the atlas and the posterior margin of the foramen magnum (suboccipital puncture).

The *chiasmatic cistern* (in the region of the decussation of the optic nerves) and the *interpeduncular cistern* (between the cerebral peduncles) are basal dilatations of the subarachnoid space which are grouped clinically under the expression "basal cisterns". The *cistern of the lateral fossa of the cerebrum* lies in the lateral sulcus of the cerebrum between the frontal, temporal and parietal lobes.

The **cephalic pia mater** (Fig. **237**) conveys blood vessels to the brain and, at the same time, forms the connective tissue layer of the choroid plexus (*tela choroidea*). It penetrates deeply between the quadrigeminal plate and the posterior end of the corpus callosum and forms the continuous tela choroidea for the choroid plexus of the 3rd ventricle and the lateral ventricles. At the 4th ventricle, it pushes forward toward the epithelial lamina between the cerebellum and the medulla oblongata and forms the tela choroidea of the 4th ventricle.

Vessels and nerves of the arachnoid. The *arteries* and *veins* of the arachnoid are the *cerebral vessels*; they course in the pia mater to their places of entry at the surface of the brain (→ p. 157). The nerves of the arachnoid are restricted largely to the pia mater. In it – in contrast to the arachnoid – numerous fine nerve branches appear. They are given off to the pia partly by cranial nerves leaving the brain stem, partly as twigs of vasomotor nerves. Although end organs of different structural types could be demonstrated, there are only conjectures regarding their function (recording of pressure and volume changes in the subarachnoid space?). Vasomotor nerves course in the wall and in the vicinity of the arteries and veins of the pia mater.

e) Intracranial Course of Blood Vessels of the Brain

The **arteries of the brain** (→ Vol. 2) arise from two different sources and are (almost) completely separated from the arteries of the dura mater. The *internal carotid artery* supplies the frontal and parietal lobes, superior and middle temporal gyri, basal ganglia and midbrain, as well as the contents of the orbit. Both *vertebral arteries* and the *basilar artery* formed by their union give off branches to the brain stem, to the cerebellum, to the occipital lobes and to the basal portion of both temporal lobes.

The *circulus arteriosus* (circle of Willis, Fig. **239**), an arterial ring situated at the base of the brain, connects the two arterial systems of the same and the opposite sides with one another. These anastomoses represent an important safeguard for the blood supply of the brain. Since the connecting branches (communicating arteries) are small in diameter, they cannot guarantee, of course, the blood supply of the adult brain in the case of a *sudden* closure of an internal carotid artery. The significance of the circulus arteriosus lies chiefly in the supply of the basal parts of the brain (midbrain).

The *internal carotid artery*, surrounded by its venous plexus, passes through the carotid canal and arrives in the middle cranial fossa at the apex of the temporal pyramid. In the carotid canal, it gives off fine *caroticotympanic arteries* to the arterial network at the base of the tympanic cavity. Above the foramen lacerum, which is closed by cartilage, the artery passes below the dura into the carotid groove at the

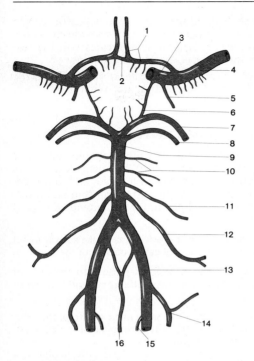

1 Anterior cerebral artery
2 Anterior communicating artery
3 Internal carotid artery
4 Middle cerebral artery
5 Anterior choroid artery
6 Posterior communicating artery
7 Posterior cerebral artery
8 Superior cerebellar artery
9 Basilar artery
10 Pontine arteries
11 Labyrinthine artery
12 Anterior inferior cerebellar artery
13 Vertebral artery
14 Posterior inferior cerebellar artery
15 Posterior spinal artery
16 Anterior spinal artery

Fig. 239 **Arterial circle of cerebrum**, cerebral arteries, basilar artery and intracranial branching of vertebral arteries

lateral surface of the body of the sphenoid and is enclosed by the cavernous sinus. In this section of its course, in which the carotid artery takes an S-shaped bend (carotid siphon), it dispatches small branches to the wall of the cavernous sinus, to the trigeminal ganglion and to the hypophysis. Medial to the anterior clinoid process, the artery passes through the dura, gives off the *ophthalmic artery* in the subarachnoid space and then divides into the *cerebral arteries.*

The *vertebral artery* penetrates into the subarachnoid space through the posterior atlanto-occipital membrane behind the lateral mass of the atlas and enters the cranial cavity through the foramen magnum. Intracranially, it gives off the *anterior spinal artery* (and, more rarely, the *posterior spinal artery*) to the spinal cord, *meningeal branches* to the dura of the posterior cranial fossa and the *posterior inferior cerebellar artery* to the posterior portion of the lower surface of the cerebellum. The two vertebral arteries merge on the clivus at the level of the posterior margin of the pons to form the unpaired *basilar artery*, which provides branches to the cerebellum, pons and inner ear before it bifurcates into the two *posterior cerebral arteries* on the anterior margin of the pons.

The **veins of the brain** ($\rightarrow$ Vol. 2) empty into the *dural sinuses* (Fig. **278**), which carry the blood (chiefly) to the internal jugular vein.

f) Intracranial Course of the Cranial Nerves

The **cranial nerves** pass from the brain into the subarachnoid space as a (more or less) uniform trunk or with a number of "rootlets" (e.g. nerves IX–XII). The sites of passage through the arachnoid and dura are identical, the length of the intradural and the extradural (but still intracranial) section of their course is quite different for the individual cranial nerves (Figs. **238, 240** and **241**).

Of all the cranial nerves, the trochlear has the longest course in the subarachnoid space and the abducens the longest in the cranial cavity outside of the dura.

The *olfactory nerves* pass through the cribriform plate into the cranial cavity and, after a short distance there, enter the olfactory bulb located in the subarachnoid space.

The *anterior ethmoidal nerve* and the artery of the same name exit from the orbit through the anterior ethmoidal foramen to the cribriform plate of the ethmoid, remain extradural and pass into the nasal cavity through one of the anterior openings of the ethmoidal plate. This course shows that the cribriform plate is a secondary floor of the skull.

In the case of the *optic nerve*, which passes through the optic canal into the cranial cavity, the bony and dural passage sites coincide. Above the prechiasmatic groove, usually on the diaphragma sellae, the fibers cross in the optic chiasma from the nasal half of the retina and pass into the optic tract with the uncrossed fibers of the opposite side.

The *dural* exits of all the following cranial nerves lie in the region of the posterior cranial fossa, whereas the *bony* exits for the three ocular muscle nerves (III, IV and VI) and for the three branches of the trigeminal are located in the middle cranial fossa. Since the floor of this fossa is a secondary floor of the skull, these nerves have a longer extradural course. Passage through the dura and exit from the bones lie a considerable distance apart.

The *oculomotor nerve* passes in front of the pons from the medial surface of the cerebral peduncle, penetrates the dura lateral to the posterior clinoid process and courses in the upper lateral wall of the cavernous sinus to the superior orbital fissure where it leaves the cranial cavity and enters the orbit.

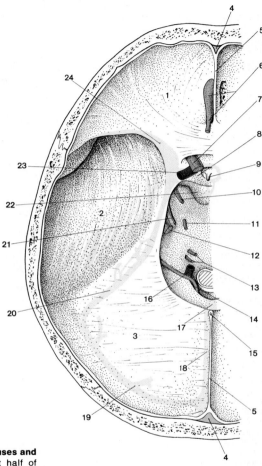

Fig. 240. **Dura, venous sinuses and cranial nerves**, on the left half of skull base, superior view

1 Anterior cranial fossa
2 Middle cranial fossa
3 Tentorium cerebelli
4 Superior sagittal sinus
5 Falx cerebri, cut margin
6 Olfactory bulb and tract
7 Optic nerve
8 Cavernous sinus
9 Hypophysial stalk
10 Oculomotor nerve
11 Abducens nerve
12 Trigeminal nerve
13 Hypoglossal nerve

14 Accessory nerve
15 Inferior sagittal sinus
16 Vertebral artery
17 Great cerebral vein
18 Straight sinus
19 Transverse sinus with junctions of
   inferior cerebral veins
20 Superior petrosal sinus
21 Trochlear nerve
22 Basilar plexus
23 Internal carotid artery
24 Sphenoparietal sinus

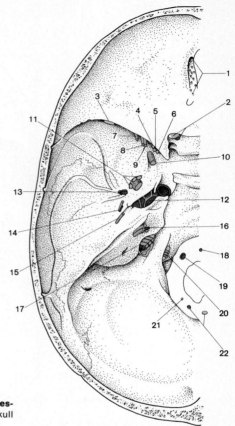

Fig. 241. **Exit sites of intracranial vessels and cranial nerves**, left half of skull base, superior view

1 Olfactory nerves
2 Optic nerve and ophthalmic artery
3 Superior ophthalmic vein
4 Abducens nerve
5 Oculomotor nerve
6 Nasociliary nerve
7 Lacrimal nerve
8 Frontal nerve
9 Trochlear nerve
10 Maxillary nerve
11 Mandibular nerve and venous plexus of foramen ovale
12 Internal carotid artery and internal carotid plexus
13 Middle meningeal artery and meningeal branch of mandibular nerve
14 Superior tympanic artery and lesser petrosal nerve
15 Greater petrosal nerve
16 Facial nerve, labyrinthine artery and vein and vestibulocochlear nerve
17 Inferior petrosal sinus, glossopharyngeal nerve, vagus nerve, accessory nerve and internal jugular vein
18 Anterior spinal artery
19 Vertebral artery
20 Hypoglossal nerve and venous plexus of hypoglossal canal
21 Spinal roots of accessory nerve
22 Posterior spinal artery and spinal vein

The *trochlear nerve* is the only cranial nerve to originate on the dorsal side of the brain behind the quadrigeminal plate; it winds around the brain stem in the subarachnoid space to the basal side and, somewhat posterior to the oculomotor nerve, passes through the dura into the lateral wall of the cavernous sinus, in which it passes to the superior orbital fissure.

The *abducens* leaves the brain at the posterior margin of the pons and passes through the dura behind the dorsum sellae, on the clivus. It accompanies the internal carotid artery, adhering closely to the artery laterally, into the cavernous sinus before it passes from the skull into the orbit through the superior orbital fissure.

The *trigeminal nerve* arises from the brain in the border region of the pons and middle cerebellar peduncle and is organized into a *sensory root* (large, flat, more basally and caudally situated) and a *motor root* (thinner, round, in front of and somewhat toward the parietal side of the sensory root). The nerve passes into the middle cranial fossa near the apex of the temporal pyramid, enclosed by a pouch-like dural process. In this dural outpocketing the *trigeminal ganglion* resides, at whose convex side the three branches of the trigeminal nerve emerge.

The motor root crosses below the sensory root and the ganglion. It is attached to the 3rd trigeminal branch, the mandibular nerve. The trigeminal ganglion lies outside of the subarachnoid space, but, like the "root pieces" of the three trigeminal branches, it is enclosed by a process of the arachnoid, as well as by the periosteal layer (from the basal side) and by the meningeal layer of the dura.

The *ophthalmic nerve* (V$_1$ nerve) courses rostrally from the cavum trigeminale in the inferior lateral wall of the cavernous sinus and – dividing into its branches – passes through the superior orbital fissure into the orbit. The *maxillary nerve* (V$_2$ nerve) arrives in the pterygopalatine fossa through the foramen rotundum at the floor of the cavum trigeminale. The *mandibular nerve* (V$_3$ nerve) leaves the skull through the foramen ovale and gives off branches in the infratemporal fossa.

At the anterior surface of the temporal pyramid directed toward the middle cranial fossa, the greater and lesser petrosal nerves leave the petrous temporal and pass anteromedially in the direction of the foramen lacerum. These nerves remain extradural for their entire course.

The *facial nerve*, the part of the facial attached to it (*nervus intermedius*), and the *vestibulocochlear nerve* pass side by side from the brain stem at the posterior margin of the pons. An outpocketing of the arachnoid and a process of the dura cover the nerves up to the floor of the internal acoustic meatus so that they are still surrounded by cerebrospinal fluid also in the meatus.

The dural and osseous exits of cranial nerves IX–XII correspond to one another.

The *glossopharyngeal nerve* arises with its rootlets from the medulla oblongata dorsal to the olive, and the *vagus nerve* attaches caudally. Both nerves leave the cranial cavity through the jugular foramen together with the *accessory nerve*, whose origin reaches down into the cervical cord.

The *hypoglossal nerve* – as is typical for the anterior root of an occipital spinal nerve – exits from the anterior lateral sulcus of the medulla oblongata and courses through the hypoglossal canal above the margin of the foramen magnum.

5. Viscerocranium

The bony frame of the orbit and nasal cavities, of the infratemporal and pterygopalatine fossae is formed by several skeletal elements. The spaces mentioned lie between the neurocranium and the viscerocranium and are thus bordered both by cranial and by facial bones. The orbit and nasal cavities are definitive structural parts of the "bony face". Important pathways to the face pass through the infratemporal and pterygopalatine fossae. Moreover, in the infratemporal fossa there are parts of the masticatory apparatus. These spaces are therefore grouped together in the "viscerocranium" section.

a) Bony Orbit

The bony walls of the **orbit** (Figs. **227, 229** and **242**) resemble a quadrangular hollow pyramid, the base of which is directed anteriorly and the apex posteriorly and medially. The longitudinal axes of the orbit coursing through the optic canal pass between the dorsum sellae and the internal occipital protuberance.

The size of the orbit varies individually. The distance from the middle of the pyramidal base to the optic canal amounts to 40–50 mm in the adult.

The *base* of the pyramid is simultaneously the entrance (*aditus*) of the orbit. The upper margin (*supra-orbital margin*) is formed by the frontal bone, the lower margin (*infra-orbital margin*) by the maxilla and zygomatic bone. The aditus is marked off medially chiefly by the frontal process of the maxilla and laterally by the zygomatic bone.

On the medial aspect of the supra-orbital margin, there are the frontal notch and, somewhat lateral to it, the supra-orbital notch, each of which can be closed into a foramen. The medial and lateral rami of the supra-orbital nerve (from V_1 nerve) pass through these notches (or openings).

The *roof* of the orbit (*superior part*) is formed by the orbital part of the frontal bone and by the lesser wing of the sphenoid. Quite posteromedially, the optic canal (for nerve II) opens into the orbit. Laterally, just behind the supra-orbital margin, the roof of the orbit is recessed to form the fossa for the lacrimal gland.

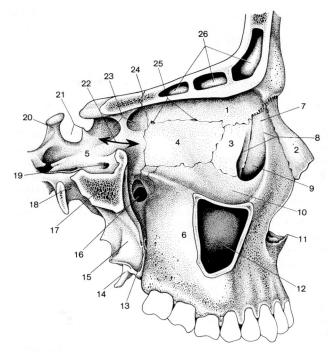

Fig. 242. **Medial wall of orbit and pterygopalatine fossa** (lateral wall of orbit removed, maxillary sinus opened)

1 Orbital part of frontal bone
2 Nasal bone
3 Lacrimal bone
4 Orbital plate of ethmoid
5 Sphenoid
6 Maxilla
7 Frontal process of maxilla
8 Anterior lacrimal crest (maxilla) and posterior lacrimal crest (lacrimal bone)
9 Fossa for lacrimal sac
10 Orbital surface of maxilla
11 Anterior nasal spine
12 Maxillary sinus
13 Pterygomaxillary fissure
14 Pterygoid hamulus

15 Lateral plate of pterygoid process
16 Sphenopalatine foramen
17 Root of greater wing of sphenoid (cut surface)
18 Foramen ovale
19 Foramen rotundum
20 Dorsum sellae
21 Sella turcica with hypophysial fossa and tuberculum sellae
22 Arrow in superior orbital fissure
23 Optic canal
24 Spheno-ethmoidal suture
25 Anterior and posterior ethmoidal foramina
26 Frontal sinus

The composition of the almost sagittally-directed *medial wall* (*medial part*) involves (from front to back): the frontal process of the maxilla, the lacrimal bone, the orbital plate of the ethmoid, the body of the sphenoid, and the root of the lesser wing of the sphenoid.

At the superior margin of the orbital plate of the ethmoid are the *ethmoidal foramina* for the anterior and posterior ethmoidal nerves and the accompanying vessels. The anterior lacrimal crest of the maxilla and the posterior lacrimal crest of the lacrimal bone border the *fossa for the lacrimal sac*, which continues downward into the nasolacrimal canal (for the nasolacrimal duct).

The *floor* of the orbit (*inferior part*) is formed by the orbital surfaces of the maxilla and zygomatic bone and, posteromedially, by the small orbital process of the palatine bone.

At the boundary of the floor and lateral wall of the orbit is the opening of the *inferior orbital fissure* (entry of infra-orbital nerve and artery, connection of inferior ophthalmic vein with the pterygoid plexus), which is bordered posteriorly by the greater wing of the sphenoid, laterally by the zygomatic bone, anteriorly by the maxilla and by the orbital process of the palatine bone. The infra-orbital vessels and nerve course anteriorly in the infra-orbital groove, which closes to form the infra-orbital canal.

The *lateral wall* of the orbit (*lateral part*) is formed anteriorly by the zygomatic bone, superiorly by the zygomatic process of the frontal, and posteriorly by the greater wing of the sphenoid.

The *superior orbital fissure* between the greater and lesser wings of the sphenoid lies at the boundary of the lateral wall and roof of the orbit (passage of nerves III, IV, V_1 and the superior ophthalmic vein).

The zygomatico-orbital foramen at the inner side of the zygomatic bone marks the beginning of a canal which divides within the bone and ends with the zygomaticofacial and zygomaticotemporal foramina (branches of the zygomatic nerve from V_2).

The walls of the orbit are so thin in the vicinity of the paranasal sinuses that disease processes can spread into the orbit from these sites.

b) Bony Nasal Cavity

Right and left **nasal cavities** (Figs. **243–245**) are separated by the *nasal septum*. The common anterior opening of the bony nasal cavities (*piriform aperture*, Fig. **253**) is bordered by both maxillae and both nasal bones. The paired posterior openings (*choanae*) lead into the nasopharynx.

The pneumatic *paranasal sinuses* communicate with the main space of the nasal cavities. They develop between the main supporting columns of the skeleton in spaces not required mechanically and lead to harmonization between the functional shape of the skull and its external form.

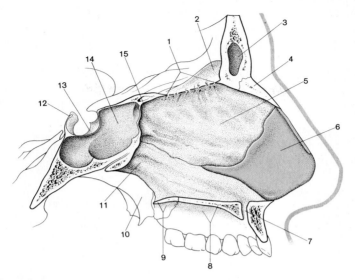

Fig. 243. **Medial wall of nasal cavity**.
Nasal septum

1 Lamina cribrosa
2 Crista galli
3 Frontal sinus
4 Nasal bone
5 Perpendicular plate of ethmoid
6 Cartilaginous nasal septum
7 Incisive canal
8 Palatine process of maxilla

9 Horizontal plate of palatine bone
10 Median plate of pterygoid process
11 Vomer
12 Dorsum sellae
13 Hypophysial fossa
14 Sphenoidal sinus
15 Spheno-ethmoidal recess

The *roof* of the osseous nasal cavity is narrow and is formed by the cribriform plate of the ethmoid. The nasal part of the frontal bone and the nasal bone are attached anteriorly and slightly sloping.

Posteriorly, the roof merges into the short *posterior wall*, the rather steeply-positioned anterior surface of the body of the sphenoid.

By means of the cribriform plate, the olfactory nerves pass into the cranial cavity, and the anterior ethmoidal nerve enters the nasal cavity with its accompanying vessels.

At the *medial* wall (*nasal septum*), the *osseous nasal septum* (perpendicular plate of the ethmoid, vomer) and the *cartilaginous nasal septum* are distinguished.

The osseous part of the wall is completed above by the narrow surface of the sphenoidal crest and the rostrum sphenoidale, below by the lateral surface of the nasal crest of the maxilla and of the palatine bone.

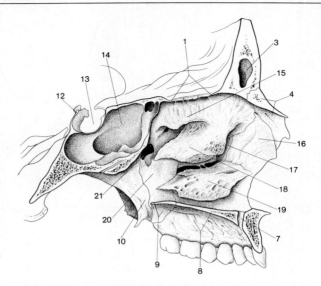

Fig. 244. **Lateral wall of left nasal cavity** after removal of nasal septum

1–14 → Fig. 243
15 Superior nasal concha
16 Frontal process of maxilla
17 Lacrimal bone

18 Middle nasal concha
19 Inferior nasal concha
20 Perpendicular plate of palatine bone
21 Sphenopalatine foramen

The *floor* of the nasal cavity is also the roof of the mouth (palate). It is formed anteriorly by the palatal process of the maxilla and posteriorly by the horizontal plate of the palatine bone. In front, near the septum, the nasal floor is penetrated by the incisive canal.

The following elements are involved in the construction of the *lateral* wall of the bony nasal cavity (from front to back): nasal bone, frontal process and body of the maxilla, lacrimal bone, lacrimal process and ethmoidal process of the inferior concha, uncinate process, ethmoidal bulla and orbital plate of the ethmoid, as well as the perpendicular plate of the palatine bone.

Three *nasal conchae* are rooted in the lateral wall and project downward and medially into the nasal cavity as flat protrusions. They divide the lateral part of the cavity into three *nasal meatuses* (→ p. 686).

Above the superior nasal concha and in front of the body of the sphenoid, the upper portion of the main cavity forms the *spheno-ethmoidal recess*, into which the sphenoidal sinus opens. Behind the middle concha and below the body of the

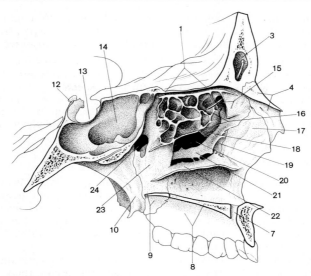

Fig. 245. **Lateral wall of left nasal cavity** after removal of nasal conchae

1–14 → Fig. 243
15 Middle nasal concha (resected),
   probe in opening of frontal sinus
16 Ethmoidal cells
17 Frontal process of maxilla
18 Ethmoidal bulla

19 Lacrimal bone
20 Hiatus semilunaris
21 Uncinate process of ethmoid
22 Inferior nasal concha (resected)
23 Perpendicular plate of palatine bone
24 Sphenopalatine foramen

sphenoid, the *sphenopalatine foramen* is located, through which the sphenopalatine artery and the posterior superior nasal branches (from the maxillary nerve)
arrive at the posterior part of the nasal cavity.

c) Infratemporal Fossa

The **infratemporal fossa** (Fig. **268**) lies at the external basicranium as the
continuation of the temporal fossa and extends out especially in a frontal
direction. It is only accessible when the zygomatic arch and the muscular
process of the mandible are removed and the masseter and temporalis
muscles are folded back.

The roof of the infratemporal fossa is formed primarily by the horizontal
part of the lower surface of the greater wing of the sphenoid. Medially,
the fossa reaches to the lateral plate of the pterygoid process; anteriorly, it
is bordered by the infratemporal surface of the maxilla; the lateral closure
is effected by the ramus of the mandible.

The infratemporal fossa contains the pterygoid muscles, the continuation of the buccal fat pad, a large part of the course of the maxillary artery, the pterygoid plexus, and the branching off of the mandibular nerve.

The infratemporal fossa possesses the following bony passages for communication with other areas of the head: the foramen spinosum (for the middle meningeal artery) and the foramen ovale (for V_3) upward into the cranial cavity; the pterygomaxillary fissure (for the terminal part of the maxillary artery) medially into the pterygopalatine fossa; and the inferior orbital fissure (for the veins between the pterygoid plexus and the inferior ophthalmic vein) anteriorly into the orbit.

d) Pterygopalatine Fossa

The **pterygopalatine fossa** (Fig. **246**) is a narrow space which is indented between the tuber of the maxilla and the anterior margin of the pterygoid process. Medially, the perpendicular plate of the palatine covers this space. Superiorly, the pterygopalatine fossa is bordered by the body of the sphenoid and by the root part of the greater wing. Laterally, it openly communicates with the infratemporal fossa via the pterygomaxillary fissure. Since the vertical plate of the palatine bone (in the region of the sphenopalatine notch) does not extend to the basicranium (body of the sphenoid), a communication between the pterygopalatine fossa and the nasal cavity remains above the free upper margin of the perpendicular plate of the palatine bone (sphenopalatine foramen, Fig. **245**). Through this opening, vessels and nerves pass into the nasal cavity. Downwards, the pterygopalatine fossa narrows into the greater palatine canal (for the

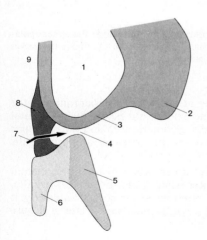

Fig. 246. **Schematic horizontal section in region of pterygopalatine fossa**
1 Maxillary sinus
2 Maxilla
3 Tuber of maxilla
4 Pterygomaxillary fissure
5 Lateral plate of pterygoid process
6 Medial plate of pterygoid process
7 Arrow leads from nasal cavity through sphenopalatine foramen into pterygopalatine fossa
8 Palatine bone
9 Nasal cavity

descending palatine artery and the palatine nerves), which opens at the palate with the greater palatine foramen.

Posterosuperiorly, the foramen rotundum (for V_2) and the pterygoid canal (for the nerve of the pterygoid canal) lead into the pterygopalatine fossa. Anteriorly, connections exist to the orbit via the infratemporal fossa and the inferior orbital fissure (for the infra-orbital vessels and the infra-orbital nerve).

In the pterygopalatine fossa are the parasympathetic pterygopalatine ganglion and the pterygopalatine nerves that arise from the maxillary nerve shortly after its emergence from the foramen rotundum.

6. Masticatory Apparatus

a) Articulation of the Jaw

The **jaw joint** (*temporomandibular articulation*, Figs. **247** and **248**) is the movable union of the head of the mandible with the mandibular fossa of the squamous part of the temporal bone, both articular surfaces being separated by an *articular disc*.

The articulation of the jaw of nonmammals is formed by two parts of the mandibular arch, the quadrate and the articular: quadrato-articular joint =

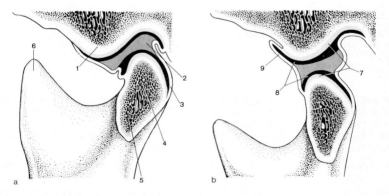

Fig. 247. Schematic sagittal section through temporomandibular joint, medial view
a With mouth closed
b With mouth open

1 Articular tubercle
2 Articular disc
3 Posterior wall of capsule
4 Head of mandible
5 Neck of mandible

6 Coronoid process
7 Articular cartilage
8 Joint cavity
9 Anterior wall of capsule

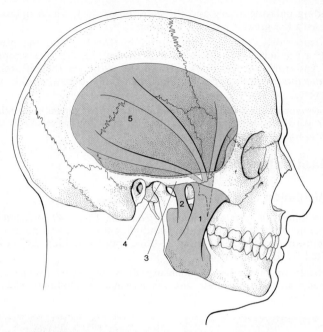

Fig. 248. **Temporalis and masseter muscles**, lateral view

1 Superficial part ⎫
2 Deep part ⎬ of masseter
3 Zygomatic arch ⎭

4 Temporomandibular joint
5 Temporalis

primary jaw articulation (Fig. **214**). In contrast to this, the jaw articulation of mammals, including man, is phylogenetically a new formation between two membrane bones: the squamosal (later squamous part of the temporal bone) and the dentary (future mandible). They come in joint contact (appositional joint) and form the squamoso-dentary joint = secondary jaw articulation.

The *head of the mandible* (Fig. **233**) is cylindrical and extends relatively far medially. The greatest axes of the articular heads of both sides intersect at about the anterior margin of the foramen magnum. The angle formed is quite variable (110–178°).

The *mandibular fossa* (Fig. **235**) is considerably more extensive than the head of the mandible. In this way, an adequate mobility of the cylinder is possible, also around a vertical axis. Only the anterior portion of the mandibular fossa forms the articular surface. The posterior part is covered by compact connective tissue and lies outside of the capsule.

Anteriorly, the articular surface of the socket is covered by fibrocartilage and continues onto the articular tubercle.

The *articular tubercle* lies within the articular capsule. It is concave in the transverse direction and curved convexly in the sagittal direction.

The relatively flaccid *articular capsule* extends posteriorly to the petro-tympanic fissure. It is fused with the circumference of the disc. At the mandible, the capsule passes downward over the head to the neck of the mandible. The capsule is particularly flaccid in front (risk of luxation anteriorly).

The *articular ligaments* are not very distinct. The strong external collateral ligament (*Lateral [temporomandibular] ligament*) courses from the zygomatic process (anterosuperior) downward and posterior to the neck of the mandible and inhibits displacement of the head in the direction of the external acoustic meatus. Extreme lateral deviations are prevented by this ligament.

At the inner side of the joint, there are two weaker ligamentous tracts which, in contrast to the external collateral ligament, are not intertwined with the capsule. The *sphenomandibular ligament* (Figs. **261** and **282**) courses from the sphenoidal spine to the lingula of the mandible and lies in the connective tissue between the medial and lateral pterygoid muscles. The *stylomandibular ligament* connects the styloid process with the angle of the mandible.

The *pterygomandibular raphe*, a tendinous band between the pterygoid hamulus and the mandible (attachment in the region behind the 3rd molar), also passes over the temporomandibular joint at the medial side. The buccinator muscle originates at the anterior side of the raphe, and a part of the superior pharyngeal constrictor (buccopharyngeal part) arises behind it.

The *articular disc*, as a biconcave, fibrocartilaginous intra-articular disc, separates the two articular surfaces of the temporomandibular joint. It can be very poor in cartilage cells, that is, almost purely fibrous. By means of the disc, the joint space is divided into an upper and a lower chamber. The disc covers the articular head and forms the true socket in the functional sense. In gliding movements forward, it is displaced together with the articular head.

The **movement possibilities in the temporomandibular joint** are abundant, but can be reduced to three basic movements. Displacements always occur simultaneously in both joints since the articular heads are coupled to one another as parts of an unpaired mandible.

When the *jaw is opened*, both articular heads advance forward and downward on the articular tubercle. It involves the combination of a hinge movement with a sliding movement (rotary gliding), whereby the compromise axis goes through the mandibular foramen, i.e. the site of entrance of nerves and vessels into the mandible is the least moved point of the entire skeletal piece. Nerves and vessels are not affected by the movement.

The *forward sliding movement* is accompanied by an insignificant depression of the mandible. This movement is always conducted twofold, by the articular tubercle and by the teeth. Corresponding to the variable shape of the tubercle and the plane of occlusion, the extent and course of this movement differ very much individually.

In *grinding movements*, the mandible undergoes alternate movements obliquely to the right and to the left. These movements, however, do not involve a true lateral displacement. The mandibular heads are never raised equally at the same time during grinding movements. Taken as a whole, the mandible thus comes into an oblique position.

The head of the mandible on the side toward which the jaw is displaced stops in the articular fossa and is rotated around its vertical axis. At the same time, the head of the opposite side is displaced forward and downward and finally arrives at the tubercle. In mastication, the corresponding movement then follows immediately on the opposite side.

The side of the apparently "resting" head is the *working side* since on this side the masticatory pressure is exerted among the molar teeth. The side of the wandering head is designated as the *balancing side*. A continuous alternation between working and balancing sides characterizes the grinding movement and brings about the breaking down of food particles.

In *mastication* itself, the partial movements described are combined. Its course depends on the condition of the food and on individual factors. In toothless infants and senile jaws, the course of movement exhibits peculiarities (preference of forward-backward displacement, important in sucking), and the partial loss of teeth also leads to modifications. The movements of the head of the mandible can be easily palpated in front of the ear.

A true hinge movement does not occur in the human temporomandibular joint as a rule, but can be learned by practice. In the cadaver, such a true rotary movement can be passively executed – without a simultaneous sliding movement. The continuous combination of rotary and gliding movements when opening the jaw in the living is thus not predetermined by the shape of the bones or the joints, but is produced by the interplay of the muscles and by nervous coordination.

b) Organization and Innervation of the Masticatory Musculature

Four muscles on each side are designated as *masticatory muscles* (in the narrow sense); they originate at the base and lateral wall of the skull and insert at the mandible: temporalis, masseter, medial and lateral pterygoids. They are innervated by the 3rd branch (mandibular nerve) of the trigeminal nerve. In addition to these, other muscles are active in the masticatory process (musculature of the cheek, floor of the mouth and tongue).

The masticatory muscles represent the musculature of the first pharyngeal arch, as do the anterior belly of the digastric and the mylohyoid, tensor tympani and tensor veli palatini.

Fasciae. The masticatory muscles are enclosed in a fascial sac which separates them from the neighboring organs. By means of this connective tissue compartmentation, the muscles retain the space allotted to them, and the neighboring organs are protected against excessive distortion and crushing during muscular contraction. Especially well-developed are the *temporalis fascia* and the *masseteric fascia* (→ p. 665).

The **temporalis muscle** (Figs. **248** and **262**) originates fan-shaped in the temporal fossa and from the temporalis fascia. The fibers converge and attach with a stout tendon at the coronoid process of the mandible.

The tendon of attachment extends upwards far into the muscle flesh. The temporalis muscle courses below the zygomatic arch to its attachment. Because of the extensive length of its fibers, at has considerable contractive potential and is the true "biting muscle".

Innervation: deep temporal nerves from the mandibular nerve.

The nerves pass from the depth of the infratemporal fossa above the lateral pterygoid muscle along the inferior surface of the temporalis muscle.

At the **masseter muscle** (Figs. **248** and **262**), the *superficial part* arises at the anterior two-thirds of the zygomatic arch, courses obliquely backward and downward to the insertion at the angle of the mandible, and is covered by a superficial aponeurosis. The fibers of the shorter *deep part* pass almost perpendicularly downward from the posterior portion of the zygomatic arch to the outer surface of the ramus of the mandible.

Innervation: masseteric nerve from the mandibular nerve.

The nerve arises from the branching of the mandibular nerve in the infratemporal fossa and passes over the lateral pterygoid muscle and through the mandibular notch along the inferior surface of the masseter.

The **medial pterygoid muscle** (Figs. **249** and **250**) originates in the pterygoid fossa of the sphenoid bone and inserts at the inner surface of the angle of the mandible. The muscle thus courses at the inner side of the mandible in a direction similar to the superficial portion of the masseter coursing on the outside. Both muscles have the same working direction and are synergistic.

Innervation: medial pterygoid nerve from the mandibular nerve.

The short nerve approaches the muscle from the inside (Fig. **264**) and sends out small branches to the tensor veli palatini and tensor tympani muscles beforehand.

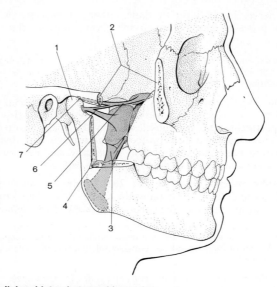

Fig. 249. **Medial and lateral pterygoid muscles,**
lateral view (temporalis and masseter muscles removed)

1 Head of mandible
2 Zygomatic arch (cut surface)
3 Medial pterygoid
4 Ramus of mandible (cut surface)
5 Lateral pterygoid, upper portion
6 Lateral pterygoid, lower portion
7 Insertion of lateral pterygoid at articular
  disc and joint capsule.

The **lateral pterygoid muscle** (Figs. **249** and **250**) is two-headed. The upper head comes from the inferior surface of the greater wing of the sphenoid. The lower head arises at the lateral plate of the pterygoid process of the sphenoid. It passes through the infratemporal fossa and inserts at the condylar process of the mandible (in the pterygoid fovea); the upper head also attaches at the articular disc and the joint capsule.

Innervation: lateral pterygoid nerve from the mandibular nerve.

The nerve frequently arises in common with the buccal nerve and passes medially into the lower head of the muscle, from which the fibers ascend to the upper head.

c) Mastication

In **mastication,** different groups of muscles act together in a well-synchronized manner in order to shape, agitate and break down food particles. *Tongue, lip* and *cheek muscles* have the task of moving and retaining food between the rows of teeth so that the pressure produced by

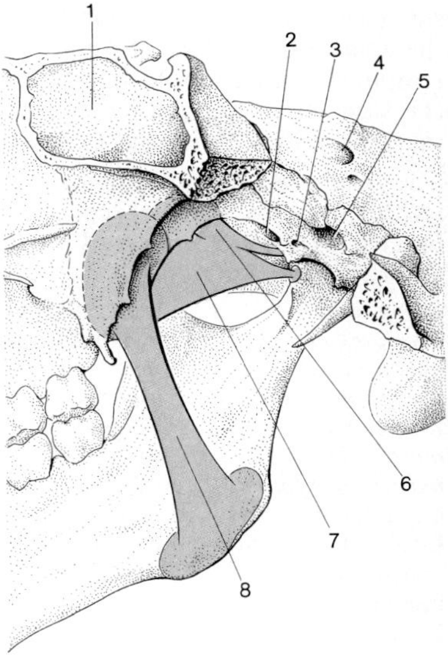

Fig. 250. **Medial and lateral pterygoid muscles**, medial view
1 Sphenoidal sinus
2 Foramen ovale
3 Foramen spinosum
4 Opening of internal acoustic meatus
5 External opening of carotid canal
6 Lateral pterygoid, upper portion
7 Lateral pterygoid, lower portion
8 Medial pterygoid

the *masticatory muscles* (*sphincter muscles of the jaw*) can be effective and can crush the food. The *muscles of the floor of the mouth*, together with the force of gravity, cooperate decisively in the *opening of the jaw*. Their state of tonicity determines at the same time the "initial condition" of the tongue movements.

By contractions on both sides, the mandible can be:
– *dropped* (opening of the jaw) – in cooperation with the lower head of the lateral pterygoid muscle – by the muscles of the floor of the mouth and the force of gravity, whereby the sphincter muscles (temporalis, masseter and medial pterygoid) decrease their tonus and, in the case of extreme opening, the nuchal muscles dorsiflex the head and strengthen the cervical lordosis;
– *lifted* (closing of the jaw) by the masseter, medial pterygoid and temporalis, whereby the upper head of the lateral pterygoid is also contracted;
– *pushed forward* by the traction exerted by the lower head of the lateral pterygoid muscle; and
– *pulled backward* by the fibers of the lower third of the temporalis muscle, which course approximately horizontally.

During *grinding movements*, the mandible is alternately carried obliquely forward by the lower head of the lateral pterygoid muscle of the balancing side (with slight cooperation from the masseter and medial pterygoid on the same side), while on the opposite side the lower fiber tracts of the temporalis muscle hold back the articular head of the working side. At the same time, the sphincter muscles of the working side generate the masticatory pressure that is essential here between the rows of teeth.

The *temporalis*, as an individual muscle, is the strongest jaw constrictor; its torque, however, is exceeded by the momentum of the muscle sling formed by the *masseter* and *medial pterygoid muscles.*

The *force of mastication* generated by the constrictor muscles of the jaw is defined as the total force with which both rows of teeth can be pressed against each other. The *pressure* produced by these muscles is represented as the portion of the masticatory force per 1 cm² of occlusal surface. (Both concepts are frequently used synonymously.) From the physiological cross sections of the temporalis, masseter and medial pterygoids of both sides, a *theoretically possible* vertical *masticatory force* of over 150 kp (= about 1500 N) can be computed. The *masticatory force* that is *physiologically* possible is distinctly lower, since, among other factors, the sensory innervation of the periodontium reflexly prevents a further increase above a fixed limit. The *physiologically essential masticatory force* depends on a series of different factors (among others, the manner and degree of mixing the food with saliva). As a rule, it amounts to only 2–3, 5 kp (= about 20–35 N).

The inferior head of the *lateral pterygoid* pulls the head of the mandible forward. With a paralysis of the muscles of the floor of the mouth, it can open the jaw by itself by contracting on both sides. The upper head contracts simultaneously with the sphincters of the jaw.

7. The Skull as a Whole

Functional structure of the skull (Fig. **251**). The skull is an architectonic unit of different parts that are also functionally definable from one another. The brain capsule with the attached otic capsules, the two orbits, the paired nasal cavities, and the teeth-bearing plates are connected with one another as the basic structural parts. Since considerable pressure and traction forces can appear, however, in the region of the masticatory apparatus, strong supports and pillar-like, by-pass constructions develop around the eye and nose. The *frontal-nasal pillar* from the region of the canine teeth between the nasal opening and the orbit and the *zygomatic arch pillar* from the region of the molars across the lateral margin of the orbit act as frontal reinforcements. In the zygomatic bone, the *zygomatic arch* branches off toward the temporal bone as a horizontal pillar. The pterygoid-*palate pillar* can be followed upward to the base of the cranium from the region of the 3rd molar across the palatine bone and the massive anterior part of the pterygoid process.

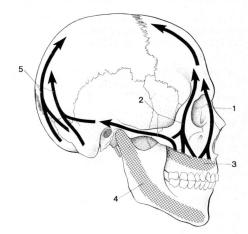

Fig. 251. **Functional structure of skull**
Pillar-like struts as mechanically efficient reinforcements
1 Frontal-nasal pillar
2 Zygomatic arch pillar with vertical and horizontal branches
3 Basal arch in upper jaw
4 Basal arch in lower jaw
5 Occipital pillars

The construction of the *basal arch* in the mandible was already mentioned. A corresponding strengthening of the base can also be shown in the dental plate above the maxillary teeth.

Frontal-nasal pillar and the vertical shank of the zygomatic arch pillar are continued into the curvature of the roof of the cranium and are absorbed into its arched construction. A posterior pillar-like strengthening of the skull is provided by the mastoid process and the posterior margin of the foramen magnum. The curvature of the skull is braced and protected by the duplication of the dura, especially by the falx cerebri.

The bony substance in the skull is distributed unequally. Beside the massive strengthening pillars, there are regions which are less stressed mechanically and in which the bone is very thin or osseous tissue is absent. In tubular bones, the inner space of the tube is not mechanically stressed and is filled with adipose tissue (yellow marrow); in the skull, mechanically neutral spaces can be *pneumatized*. The cavities lined with mucous membrane contain air. Such air-containing (= pneumatic) spaces appear with the formation of the previously mentioned by-pass structures.

Pneumatization can take place only where the formation of air-containing sacs is possible from a mucosal surface, e.g. paranasal sinuses arise in the region of the nasal cavity, tympanic and mastoid air cells are formed as accessory tympanic spaces in the region of the tympanic cavity. Accessory cavities always retain their connection with the main cavity from which they have arisen. The opening of an accessory cavity corresponds to its site of origin during development.

A further function of the accessory cavities is in the equalization of shaping forces acting at the inside and outside of the skull (among other effects: influence on brain shape and size, masticatory apparatus, absolute body size, p. 568).

Weak points of the basicranium. The bony basicranium is variably thick and thus – viewed absolutely – not everywhere equally strong. Between massively shaped bony parts, there are more or less thin-walled bony areas. A well-developed median longitudinal trabecula passes from the dorsum sellae through the clivus, curves around the foramen magnum and continues on the roof of the skull at the internal occipital pro-tuberance, along the groove for the superior sagittal sinus. A stronger, roughly triangular bony frame which courses along the upper edge of the temporal pyramid and both grooves of the transverse sinus communi-cates with the longitudinal trabecula at the internal occipital protuber-ance. An additional transverse trabecula lies at the posterior border of the anterior cranial fossa.

Between these reinforcements of the basicranium, the bone is relatively thin and in addition is perforated for the passage of vessels and nerves. Weak points are the cribriform plate of the ethmoid, the roof of the orbit, the floor of the sella turcica, the osseous tissue of the greater wing of the sphenoid bordering foramina, the region of the mandibular fossa, and the thinner lateral parts of the occipital squama.

Fractures of the basicranium are critically determined by the type, size, place and direction of the trauma. The fracture lines favor the weak points of the basicranium. In the anterior cranial fossa, they frequently course in the cribriform plate or toward the optic canal. In the middle cranial fossa, they can connect the successive nerve exit sites. Transverse fractures in the region of the sella turcica usually lie near the dorsum sellae. Since the temporal pyramid is made up of bone of different strength, fractures, usually of the "transverse" variety, can also occur there. In the occipital region, fracture lines course in the lateral parts of the occipital squama or (in the case of an axial direction of the trauma) circularly around the foramen magnum.

Conduction pathways are endangered when their sites of passage are included in the course of the fracture lines. Extravasation of cerebrospinal fluid or brain tissue are definite signs of a skull fracture. Bleeding in the connective tissue of the eye and in the eyelids (spectacle-like hematoma), from the ear, nose or throat are frequent accompanying symptoms.

Ossification. The ossification of the human skull begins with the appearance of the *membrane bones*. Bony trabeculae are demonstrable in embryos with a length of 15 mm first in the mandible and shortly thereafter in the maxilla. In embryos of 37 mm, all membrane bones are established. The first ossific nucleus in the *chondrocranium* develops in the endochondral part of the occipital squama in embryos of about 30 mm. By the end of the 3rd month of pregnancy, ossific centers have been formed in all cartilage models. Most skull bones arise from two or more ossific centers which fuse with one another. Cartilage and membrane bones merge into a unit, the "skull", in the course of ontogenesis.

The growth of membrane bones takes place at the margins in the cranial sutures by apposition of osseous tissue. The enlargement of cartilage bones occurs by the formation of appositional bone which is not preformed in cartilage. An essential component of skull growth is the change in proportions and surface curvatures. This remodeling requires synchronized, often simultaneous, deposition and resorption processes in different segments of the same bone.

At the end of fetal development, the membrane bones are separated by narrow sutures. Larger skeletal gaps closed by connective tissue (fontanelles, → p. 000) are still found only at these points where more than two bones border on each other. With the exception of the anterior fontanelle, they close in the 1st postnatal year. The suture between the two frontal bones ossifies, as a rule, in the 2nd year; the remaining sutures synostose only in later life (after the age of 40). At the time of birth, a part of the otic capsule is still cartilaginous. The separately-formed ossific loci of a cartilage bone (e.g. the sphenoid) are connected at first by cartilaginous bridges. As remnants of the chondrocranium, cartilaginous joints are preserved between cartilage bones (e.g. spheno-occipital synchondrosis) into the second decade of postnatal life.

The **skull of the newborn** (Fig. **252**) is distinguished from the adult especially in the different proportions of the brain and facial skeleton (Figs. **216** and **217**). The relatively strong development of the brain, eyes and hearing organ causes a proportionately large, highly arched cranium. On the other hand, the viscerocranium which surrounds the still weakly developed portions of the respiratory and digestive tracts is less developed. The volume ratio of brain and facial parts amounts to 8:1 in the newborn child and 2:1 in the adult.

At the roof of the skull, the paired frontal and parietal eminences appear distinctly behind the external occipital protuberance so that the contour of the cranium resembles an oblong pentagon. The bony external acoustic meatus and the mastoid process are completely absent; the occipital protuberances lie close to the anterior margin of the foramen magnum. The transverse axis of the condyles in the newborn child lies nearly at the posterior margin of the external ear opening and divides the longitudinal axis of the skull approximately in the middle. By way of contrast, the center of gravity of the adult head lies distinctly in front of the transverse axis of the condyles. The articular tubercle is not yet formed at the birth, and the articular fossa is not very pronounced. The chin recedes in relation to the maxilla, and the viscerocranium is strikingly low (absence of teeth, poorly developed masticatory apparatus).

The inner base of the skull in the newborn child is still relatively small and narrow. The cribriform plate, however, exhibits almost the same dimensions as in the adult. The middle cranial fossa seems relatively large and, owing to the strong development of the temporal pyramid, also deep. The posterior cranial fossa is

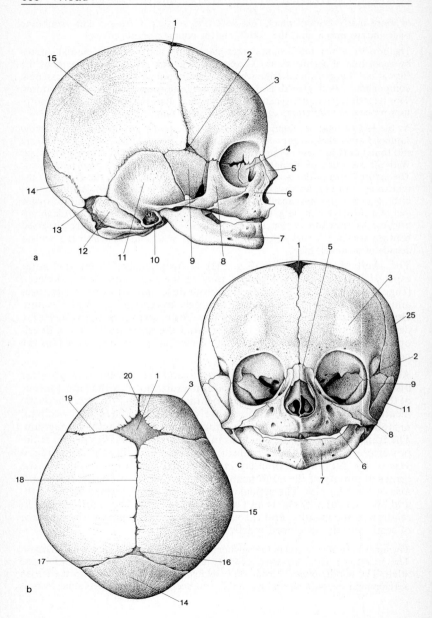

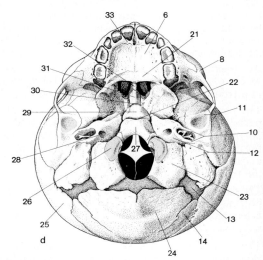

Fig. 252. **Skull of newborn**

a Lateral view
b Superior view
c Anterior view
d Inferior view

1 Anterior fontanelle
2 Sphenoidal (anterolateral) fontanelle
3 Frontal eminence
4 Lacrimal bone
5 Nasal bone
6 Maxilla
7 Mandible
8 Zygomatic bone
9 Greater wing of sphenoid
10 Tympanic ring ⎫
11 Squamous part ⎬ of temporal bone
12 Petrous part ⎭
13 Mastoid (posterolateral) fontanelle
14 Squamous part of occipital bone (upper part)
15 Parietal eminence
16 Posterior fontanelle
17 Lambdoidal suture

18 Sagittal suture
19 Coronal suture
20 Frontal (metopic) suture
21 Palatine bone
22 Spheno-occipital synchondrosis
23 Lateral part of occipital bone
24 Squamous part of occipital bone (lower part)
25 Parietal bone
26 Occipital condyle
27 Basilar part of occipital bone (basi-occipital)
28 External opening of carotid canal
29 Posterior sphenoid, basisphenoid
30 Intersphenoid synchondrosis
31 Anterior sphenoid, presphenoid
32 Vomer
33 Incisive suture

extraordinarily flat in the early months of postnatal life. The foramen magnum is pear-shaped and narrows posteriorly, whereas in the child of 6 or 7 years it has attained the definitive rounded oval shape.

B. Surface Anatomy of the Head

A detailed regional segmentation of the head is necessary for practical medical reasons – especially for specialists. No other part of the human body, for example, is the subject of so many special medical disciplines or diagnostic measures as the head. In the region of the roof of the skull, the *frontal, parietal, temporal* and *occipital regions* are distinguished; in the area of the face, there are the *regions of the nose, mouth, chin, eye, cheek, zygoma* (zygomatic arch) and *parotid gland*.

An *orientative examination* of the head can start with a division into an *anterior head* and a *posterior head*, the border between the two parts lying in a frontal plane behind the external ear.

The *posterior head* shelters the brain stem with the cerebellum and – as parts of the cerebrum – the paired occipital lobes and the posterior portions of the parietal and temporal lobes. The *anterior head* comprises the *face*, in addition to the frontal lobes on each side behind the forehead and temple and the anterior parts of the parietal and temporal lobes of the telencephalon.

The *posterior head* and that *part of the anterior head* enclosing the anterior portion of the telencephalon can be defined as the *cerebral part of the head*; the *face* and the *nasal and oral cavities* concealed behind it represent the *facial part of the head*.

The *cerebral part of the head* consists, therefore, of a largely closed bony capsule the brain surrounded by it and by meninges, and of a uniform soft tissue covering, the scalp.

The *facial part*, on the other hand, is polymorphic and provided with openings for the large sense organs, as well as for the respiratory and digestive passages.

1. Surface Relief of the Head and Palpable Bony Parts

The **surface relief** (Fig. **253**) is determined largely by the roof of the skull between the forehead and external occipital protuberance with the temporal region padded by the temporalis muscle, which is distinctly visible during masticatory movements.

The **face** (Fig. **253**) extends from the eyebrows over the zygomatic arch and ears to the lower margin of the mandible; it receives its typical shape from the facial skeleton, which is covered in the anterior region of the face by a soft tissue mantle of varying thickness. The buccal fat pad contributes to modelling the *cheek*; the shape of the lateral facial and temporal regions is influenced by the masticatory musculature.

The facial profile is determined by the *nose* with its root, bridge and apex. Below the alae of the nose, the nasal openings (*nares*) are separated by the end of the nasal septum. Between the eyelids (*palpebrae*) is the opening of the *palpebral fissure*, between the lips (*labia oris*), the *oral fissure*.

The mouth, nose and lower eyelids are bordered in part by *furrows*. The chin-lip furrow (*mentolabial furrow*) marks the border between the lower lip and the chin (*mentum*); the nose-lip furrow (*nasolabial furrow*) passes between the upper lip and the nose; and the lower lid furrow (*infrapalpebral furrow*) extends between the lower lid and the cheek. The upper lid is marked off from the eyebrow (*supercilium*) by a skin fold.

The *obliteration* of the nasolabial fold or the mentolabial fold can be an indication of inflammatory processes in the region of the upper or lower jaw or can signal a facial paralysis.

The groove which runs from the nose to the middle of the upper lip is referred to as the *philtrum*. In the prolongation of the philtrum, the upper lip has a berry-shaped swelling which fits in a furrow of the lower lip.

The *external ear* (pinna), which surrounds the opening of the external acoustic meatus as a sound funnel, adheres more or less to the temporal squama and the mastoid process with its external arched margin. The *ear lobe* extends laterally down to the level of the posterior circumference of the parotid gland.

The ear lobe is raised by a swelling of the parotid gland.

The *natural* symmetry of any face must be distinguished from an abnormal asymmetry resulting, for example, from paralyses, growth disturbances, inflammation or tumors.

With the exception of the forehead, the cerebral part of the head exhibits a *terminal hairiness*. *Facial hairiness* is sex-specific.

The hint of facial hairiness (beard) and the beginning of baldness in the frontal region (frontal alopecia) are symptoms of an overproduction of the male sex hormone in females (e.g. in tumors of the adrenal cortex).

In light-skinned individuals, the typical pale red *facial coloration* is produced predominantly by arterial blood.

A bluish *discoloration* of the face indicates in an especially striking manner an oxygen deficiency of the arterial blood, e.g. in the case of cardiac insufficiency. Strong facial pallor appears in circulatory collapse or in strong sympathetic tone (e.g. reaction to fright).

In the case of wasting of the tissues of the body (*cachexia*), e.g. in the terminal stage of a carcinomatosis, "the temples cave in" (disappearance of storage fat between the two layers of the temporalis fascia) and "the eyes recede" (disappearance of structural fat in the orbit).

Palpable bony points (Fig. **253**). The bony roof of the skull – except the temporal region – and the facial skeleton can be palpated relatively well through the soft tissue mantle, which is only moderately thick. Bony prominences and edges, like the external occipital protuberance and the mastoid process, the zygomatic arch and the circumference of the orbit, the mental protuberance and the angle of the mandible, facilitate the orientation. The hard palate is palpable from the oral cavity. A finger inserted into the external acoustic meatus can register the positional changes of the head of the mandible during different jaw movements.

In the newborn and infant, the fontanelles are visible and palpable.

Projection of the surface of the brain on the surface of the head (Fig. **254**). An approximate orientation of the position of definite points of the

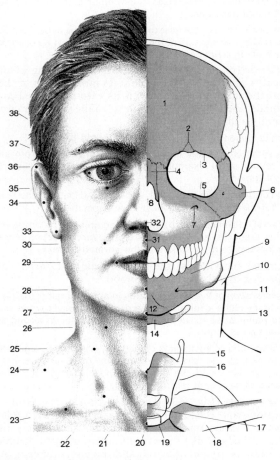

Fig. 253. **Surface relief of head and neck** (right side) **and palpable bony points** (left side)

cerebral surface or the course of the middle meningeal artery and its branches can be obtained with the help of a system of coordinates projected on the external surface of the head.

A straight line, for example, through the lower margin of the orbit and the upper margin of the external acoustic meatus designated as the *Frankfurt horizontal* plane indicates the approximate border between the occipital lobe of the cerebrum and the cerebellum, as well as the course of the transverse sinus; in the temporal region, it marks the lower contour line of the temporal lobes. At the intersection of a line placed parallel to it through the upper margin of the orbit (*upper horizontal plane*) and a perpendicular line through the middle of the zygomatic arch, the approximate lower end of the lateral cerebral sulcus is projected and thus the upper boundary of the temporal lobe at the temporal pole of the cerebrum. The posterior branch of the middle meningeal artery is also found in the vicinity of this intersection.

2. Cutaneous Vessels and Nerves of the Head

a) Cutaneous Arteries

The *arteries* which pass to the skin of the head (Figs. **255, 261** and **277**) simultaneously supply the soft tissue mantle ($\rightarrow$ p. 671). They arise primarily from branches of the *external carotid artery*, since the *internal carotid artery* provides branches only to the frontal region and the bridge of the nose. Anastomoses are formed between the arteries of one side and between the two opposite sides.

1 Squama of frontal bone
2 Frontal notch (medial) and supra-orbital notch (lateral): pressure point for V_1 nerve
3 Supra-orbital margin
4 Nasal bone
5 Infra-orbital margin
6 Zygomatic arch
7 Infra-orbital foramen: pressure point for V_2 nerve
8 Piriform aperture
9 Alveolar part of mandible
10 Angle of mandible
11 Mental foramen: pressure point for V_3 nerve
12 Mental protuberance
13 Greater horn, hyoid bone
14 Body of hyoid bone
15 Upper margin of thyroid cartilage lamina
16 Superior thyroid notch
17 Arch of cricoid cartilage
18 Sternal end of clavicle

19 Jugular notch of sternum
20 Jugular fossa
21 Laryngeal prominence
22 Lesser supraclavicular fossa
23 Omoclavicular triangle
24 Bulge of trapezius muscle
25 Bulge of sternocleidomastoid muscle
26 Carotid triangle
27 Chin (mentum)
28 Mentolabial furrow
29 Angle of mouth (angulus oris)
30 Nasolabial furrow
31 Philtrum
32 Apex of nose
33 Lobule of ear
34 Anthelix
35 Infrapalpebral furrow
36 Helix
37 Eyeball in palpebral fissure
38 Eyebrow

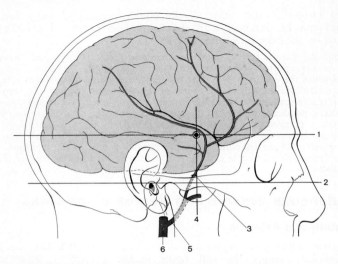

Fig. 254. Projection of middle meningeal artery and cerebral surface onto surface of head

1 Upper horizontal plane
2 Frankfort horizontal plane
3 Foramen spinosum, entrance of middle meningeal artery into cranial cavity
4 Perpendicular line through middle of zygomatic arch
5 Maxillary artery
6 External carotid artery

The *scalp* is supplied

in the *frontal region* by the:

– *supratrochlear* (medial) and *supra-orbital* (lateral) *arteries*, both of which are branches of the ophthalmic artery (from the internal carotid artery);

in the *temporal region* by the:

– *superficial temporal artery*, the smaller, cranial terminal branch of the external carotid artery which passes in the temporalis fascia to the temple between the head of the mandible and the external acoustic meatus;

behind and *above the ear* by the:

– *posterior auricular artery*, a direct branch of the external carotid artery, which ramifies in front of the mastoid process; and

in the *occipital region* by the:

– *occipital artery*, which also originates from the external carotid artery.

The *soft tissue mantle* of the facial part is supplied

in the *anterior region of the face* by the:
- *dorsal nasal artery*, the descending terminal branch of the ophthalmic artery (from the internal carotid artery) which passes downward to the bridge of the nose, and the
- *facial artery* (from the external carotid artery), which gives off the *inferior labial artery* to the lower lip and the *superior labial artery* to the upper lip and which anastomoses as the *angular artery* with branches of the ophthalmic artery in the medial angle of the eye;

in the *lateral region of the face* by the:
- *transverse facial artery* parallel to the lower margin of the zygomatic arch, and the
- *zygomatico-orbital artery* parallel to the upper margin, both arteries being branches of the superficial temporal artery (from the external carotid artery).

b) Cutaneous Veins

The **cutaneous veins** of the head (Figs. **255** and **278**) are also veins of the soft tissue mantle ($\rightarrow$ p. 671 f.). The veins of one side anastomose both with each other and with the veins of the opposite side.

Venous drainage takes place both extracranially and intracranially (through the orbit). The *facial* and *retromandibular veins* carry blood to the *internal jugular vein* from the frontal and temporal regions and from the face; the *occipital vein* conducts it from the region of the occiput to the *external jugular vein* (and also to the *deep cervical vein* via anastomoses). A large part of the blood from the frontal part flows to the *superior ophthalmic vein* and into the *cavernous sinus* (via the *nasofrontal vein*, which connects the *angular* and *superior ophthalmic veins*).

From the wide-meshed venous network of the soft tissue mantle, blood is drained

from the *frontal region* to the facial vein via:

- the *supratrochlear veins* (medial) and the *supra-orbital vein* (lateral), which merge at the medial angle of the eye as the *angular vein*;

from the *face* to the facial vein via:
- the *external nasal veins* (from the bridge of the nose), and
- the *superior labial vein* and *inferior labial veins* (from the upper and lower lips);

from the *temporal region* to the retromandibular vein via:
- the *superficial temporal vein*, which communicates with the venous ring at the margin of the orbit via the *middle temporal* and *transverse facial veins*;

from the *retro-auricular region* to the external jugular vein via:
- the *posterior auricular vein*; and

from the *occipital region* into the external jugular vein and the deep cervical vein via:
- the *occipital vein*.

c) Superficial Lymphatic Pathways

The **superficial lymphatic pathways** of the head (Figs. **256** and **272**) carry lymph from both the skin and the soft tissue mantle. They conduct to *regional lymph nodes below the chin* in the *vicinity of the submandibular* and *parotid glands, behind the external ear* and *at the occiput*, after which deep cervical nodes are inserted.

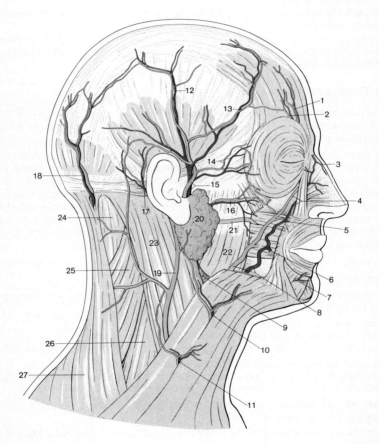

Fig. 255. **Cutaneous arteries and veins in head and neck** (facial musculature partially removed; for designations of facial muscles → Fig. 258)

The *lymphatic vessels* pass

from the *frontal* and *temporal regions* to:
– the *superficial* and *deep parotid lymph nodes* on and in the parotid gland;

from the *face* to:
– the *submandibular lymph nodes* at the submandibular gland, partly via the variably developed *facial lymph nodes* (*buccinator node* on the buccinator muscle, *nasolabial node* below the nasolabial furrow, *malar node* in the cheek region, *mandibular node* at the facial vein on the body of the mandible), and
– the *submental lymph nodes* (especially from the lower lip) below the chin;

from the region *posterior* and *superior to the pinna* to:
– the *mastoid lymph nodes* on the mastoid process; and

from the region of the occiput to:
– the *occipital lymph nodes* behind the attachment of the sternocleidomastoid muscle at the superior nuchal line.

Lymphatic tracts lead directly or indirectly from the lymph nodes mentioned to the *deep, lateral cervical lymph nodes* (along the internal jugular vein). From the deep cervical lymph nodes, the lymph is carried on the right side by the *jugular trunk* to the *right lymphatic duct*, on the left side into the *thoracic duct* or else, on either side, directly into the venous angle.

d) Cutaneous Nerves

In the *face* and at the *part of the scalp situated in the anterior head region*, the skin is innervated by the *three branches of the trigeminal nerve* (Figs. **257** and **259**). A branch of the *great auricular nerve* passes at the angle of the jaw. At the scalp of the posterior head region, the skin is supplied by the *lesser occipital nerve* (from the dorsal ramus of the 2nd cervical nerve). The border between the regions of innervation of the

---

◀ 1 Supratrochlear artery (ascending terminal branch of ophthalmic artery) and supratrochlear vein
2 Supra-orbital artery and vein
3 Dorsal nasal artery (descending terminal branch of ophthalmic artery)
4 Angular artery and vein
5 Superior labial artery
6 Inferior labial artery
7 Mental artery (from inferior alveolar artery) and mental vein
8 Facial artery and vein
9 Retromandibular vein
10 Cutaneous branches of superior thyroid artery and vein
11 Cutaneous branches of superficial cervical artery and vein

12 Parietal branch ⎞ ot superficial temporal
13 Frontal branch ⎠ artery and vein
14 Zygomatico-orbital artery and vein
15 Superficial temporal artery and vein
16 Transverse facial artery and vein
17 Posterior auricular artery and vein
18 Occipital artery and vein
19 External jugular vein
20 Parotid gland
21 Parotid duct
22 Masseter
23 Sternocleidomastoid
24 Semispinalis capitis
25 Splenius capitis and levator scapulae
26 Scalenus medius
27 Trapezius

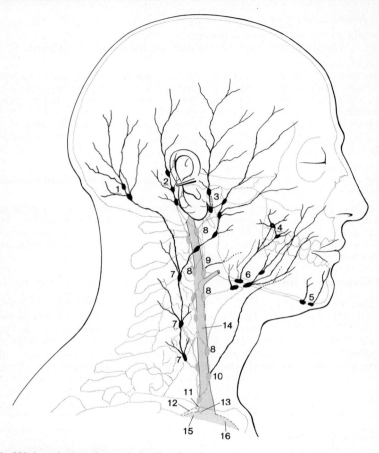

Fig. 256. **Lymphatic pathways in head and neck**
(retropharyngeal lymph nodes not shown)
Superficial lymphatic routes and nodes ———
Deep lymphatic routes and nodes ———

1 Occipital lymph nodes
2 Mastoid lymph nodes
3 Superficial (and deep) parotid lymph nodes
4 Buccinator lymph nodes
5 Submental lymph nodes
6 Mandibular and submandibular lymph nodes
7 Superficial lateral cervical lymph nodes
8–10 *Deep lateral cervical lymph nodes*

9 Jugulodigastric lymph node
10 Jugulo-omohyoid lymph node
11 Jugular trunk
12 Subclavian trunk
13 Right lymphatic duct
14 Internal jugular vein
15 Subclavian vein
16 Brachiocephalic vein

trigeminal nerve and the occipital nerves runs from the crown of the head to the ear.

The *soft tissue mantle* receives sensory innervation

in the *frontal region* from:
– the thin *supratrochlear nerve* (from the frontal nerve) at the lateral side, which passes at the inner angle of the eye toward the forehead, and
– the thick *supra-orbital nerve* (also from the frontal nerve) at the medial side, which divides below the roof of the orbit into the *medial branch* (through the frontal notch) and the *lateral branch* (through the supra-orbital notch);

in the region of the *eyelids* by:
– the *lacrimal nerve* at the lateral angle of the eye and at the upper eyelid,
– the *supra-orbital nerve* at the upper lid,
– the *supratrochlear nerve* at the medial angle of the eye,
– the *infratrochlear nerve* (from the nasociliary nerve) at the medial angle of the eye, and
– branches of the *infra-orbital nerve* at the lower eyelid;

above the *zygomatic arch* by:
– the *zygomaticofacial ramus* (from the zygomatic nerve);

in the region of the *external nose*, at the *maxilla* and at the *upper lip* by:
– the *external nasal branch* of the *anterior ethmoidal nerve* (from the nasociliary) at the bridge of the nose, and

– branches of the *infra-orbital nerve*,
  which pass as *external nasal rami* to the external side of the ala of the nose and as *superior labial rami* to the upper lip;

in the region of the *mandible*, *cheek* and *upper lip* by:
– branches of the *mandibular nerve*, whereby the *mental nerve* ramifies at the chin and upper lip and the *buccal nerve* passes to the cheek, and
– the *anterior ramus* of the *great auricular nerve* (from the cervical plexus) at the angle of the jaw;

in the *anterior temporal region* by:
– the *zygomaticotemporal ramus* (from the zygomatic nerve), which exits from the opening of the same name of the zygomatic arch;

in the *posterior temporal region* by:
– the *auriculotemporal nerve* (from the mandibular nerve), which passes toward the parietal region between the pinna and the superficial temporal artery and which spreads out (in front of and above the ear) with the *anterior auricular nerves* at the anterior surface of the pinna and with the *superficial temporal rami* at the skin of the temple;

behind the ear by:
– the *lesser occipital nerve*, which passes cranialwards along the posterior

margin of the sternocleidomastoid muscle and branches off (into two larger branches) at the lateral occipital region; and

in the *medial region of the occiput* by:

– the *greater occipital nerve*, which penetrates the tendon of the trapezius,

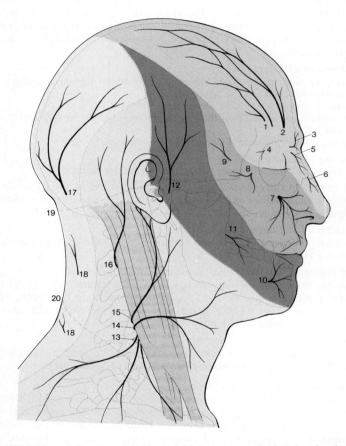

Fig. 257. **Cutaneous nerves and anatomical cutaneous nerve fields in head and neck**

Anatomical cutaneous nerve territories

of ophthalmic nerve	of vagus nerve
of maxillary nerve	of nerves of cervical plexus
of mandibular nerve	of dorsal branches of cervical nerves

enters the subcutaneous tissue medial to the occipital artery, and by this point has ramified into several branches.

3. Soft Tissue Mantle of the Head

The **soft tissue mantle at the cerebral part of the head** is formed by the *scalp*.

At the forehead and in the region of the skin of the head covered by hair, the soft tissues are formed uniformly. A tendinous plate (*galea aponeurotica*; *epicranial aponeurosis*) stretches over the bony roof of the skull and serves for the attachment of muscles radiating from the forehead, temple and occiput (occipitofrontalis, temporoparietalis), which together are referred to as the **epicranius muscle** (Fig. **258**).

The *occipitofrontalis muscle* passes to the central tendon (epicranial aponeurosis) with its *frontal belly* (frontalis muscle) from the region of the eyebrows and glabella and with its *occipital belly* (occipitalis muscle) from the supreme nuchal line. The muscle is able to move the scalp backward and forward. Its anterior belly can raise the eyebrows and "wrinkle" the forehead; the posterior belly "smooths" the forehead.

The *temporoparietalis muscle* passes from the temporal region to the galea. Its posterior portion is referred to specially as the *superior auricular muscle* and is attached to the pinna.

Innervation of epicranius: facial nerve

Perpendicularly ascending connective tissue tracts of the subcutaneous tissue anchor the galea aponeurotica immovably to the skin of the head so that a uniform soft tissue layer arises, the **scalp**.

Adipose tissue is deposited between the bundles of collagenous fibers in the subcutaneous tissue, which gives the scalp a compact, taut quality. The hair follicles reach into the superficial subcutaneous layer.

◀ 1–6 *Branches of ophthalmic nerve*
1 Lateral branch ⎫ of supra-orbital
2 Medial branch ⎭ nerve
3 Supratrochlear nerve
4 Lacrimal nerve
5 Infratrochlear nerve
6 External nasal branch of anterior ethmoidal nerve
7–9 *Branches of maxillary nerve*
7 Infra-orbital nerve
8 Zygomaticofacial branch ⎫ off zygomatic
9 Zygomaticotemporal branch ⎭ nerve
10–12 *Branches of mandibular nerve*
10 Mental nerve

11 Buccal nerve
12 Auriculotemporal nerve
13–16 *Nerves of cervical plexus*
13 Supraclavicular nerves
14 Transverse cervical nerve
15 Great auricular nerve
16 Lesser occipital nerve
17 Greater occipital nerve
18 Dorsal branches of 3rd and 4th cervical nerves
19 Boundary line of 2nd and 3rd cervical segments
20 Boundary line of 3rd and 4th cervical segments

The galea aponeurotica and the pericranium are movably united by loose connective tissue. The subaponeurotic displacement space extends over the entire roof of the skull and ends where the soft parts of the head are fixed at the pericranium: at the upper margin of the orbit, at the zygomatic arch and at the external occipital protuberance.

Cut wounds of the head region gape only mildly if they do not sever the galea completely. Subcutaneous bleeding, therefore, does not spread significantly into the surrounding tissues. The blood vessels fixed in the subcutaneous connective tissue can hardly be retracted when severed (consequently, purse-string closure instead of ligation in the case of injury).

Injuries to the scalp, in which the galea aponeurotica is completely severed, (usually) gape widely. When subjected to traumatic violence, the scalp can be detached in toto over a wide distance. Hemorrhages and effusions below the galea spread extensively into the subaponeurotic space, especially since the tension of the galea exerts pressure on the accumulation of fluid (danger of rapid spread of infection).

Hemorrhages between the pericranium and bone occur as birth injuries (cephalic hematomas) and lead to a detachment of the pericranium from the roof of the skull. As a rule, they do not extend beyond the edges of the bones because the pericranium merges into the connective tissue of the osseous sutures and is anchored firmly to the margins of the bones.

The **hairs of the head** (*capilli*) are characterized especially by their life span (2–4 years) and growth (1 cm per month) in length (→ adult hairs, p. 173).

The **soft tissue mantle of the face** consists mainly of *muscle* and *skin*. The superficial layer of the cervical fascia continues into the face only in its lateral region over the mandibular margin (→ p. 736). The anterior part of the face in front of the masticatory musculature and the buccinator muscle remains free of the superficial fascia of the body. The muscular plate (*facial musculature*) spread out here below the facial skin is knit together with the facial skin at many places by short elastic tendons, but is attached to the facial skeleton only at a few points. Contractions of the facial muscles, the mimicking musculature, therefore, produce movements of the facial skin which serve as a means of communication, *facial expression*. Vessels and nerves of the anterior region of the face spread partly below, partly within the soft tissue mantle.

Unphysiological ultraviolet radiation leads to premature aging of the elastic tissue elements with increasing development of folds of the facial skin.

a) Fasciae in the Head Region

The **parotid fascia** (Fig. **258**) surrounds the parotid gland with a superficial layer, the continuation of the superficial layer of the cervical fascia, as well as with a deep layer, a splitting off of the fascia. The deep layer covers the parotid gland in the deep lateral facial region from behind and below. In front, the parotid fascia merges into the masseteric fascia.

The **masseteric fascia** (Fig. **258**), a firm connective tissue layer on the outer surface of the masseter muscle, is attached above to the zygomatic arch. At the lower margin of the mandible, it goes over into the superficial layer of the cervical fascia, which splits and also covers the lower surface of the medial pterygoid muscle so that a fascial pocket is formed which opens backwards and upwards – toward the deep lateral region of the face.

The osteofibrous space for the temporalis muscle communicates with the facial pocket of the masseteric fascia below the zygomatic arch. Pus formation (suppuration) in the compartment of the temporalis muscle can thus spread downward and arrive at the surface in the cheek region below the anterior margin of the masseter.

The **temporalis fascia** (Figs. **258** and **259**) covers the temporalis muscle. It is firm and penetrated by aponeurotic connective tissue tracts, from which the superficial bundles of fibers of the temporalis muscle originate. The fascia is attached to the superior temporal line above the origin of the temporalis muscle and divides downward into two layers. The superficial layer attaches at the outer surface, the deep layer at the inner side of the zygomatic arch. The tent formed by the two layers encloses a fat body (storage fat).

The **buccopharyngeal fascia** covers the buccinator muscle as a thin layer of connective tissue, merges posteriorly into the pterygomandibular raphe and, finally, into the connective tissue layer which covers the outside of the constrictor muscles of the pharynx.

b) Organization and Innervation of the Muscles of Facial Expression

The muscles of facial expression – like the platysma – are derived from the 2nd pharyngeal arch and are, therefore, innervated by the *facial nerve*. Around the *palpebral* and *oral fissures*, they form flat, extended, ring-shaped constrictor muscles. These are deformable and can be moved together with the attached skin by muscle tracts which are fastened to them. At the *nasal apertures* and *pinna*, the muscles of facial expression are only rudimentarily developed.

Muscles around the Palpebral Fissure (Fig. 258)

The **orbicularis oculi** surrounds the palpebral fissure approximately in the shape of a circle. Three parts can be distinguished. The *palpebral part* lies within the upper and lower eyelids and originates from the medial palpebral ligament and the adjacent bones; it regulates the finer movements of the lids. The *lacrimal part* passes along the lacrimal sac and influences the drainage of tears (sucking and squeezing). The extensive *orbital part* arises from the nasal part of the frontal bone, at the frontal process of the maxilla and at the medial palpebral ligament; it effects a squeezing together of the palpebral fissure.

The **corrugator supercilii muscle** comes from the nasal part of the frontal bone, penetrates the fiber bundles of the frontal belly of the occipitofrontalis muscle in the medial marginal region and attaches to the skin of the eyebrow laterally. It draws the skin in the direction of the root of the nose and produces perpendicular folds on the forehead.

The **depressor supercilii muscle**, situated superficially on the frontal belly of the occipitofrontalis, passes from the bridge of the nose perpendicularly upward to the forehead. It produces deep transverse folds over the root of the nose.

Muscles around the Oral Fissure (Fig. 258)

The **orbicularis oris muscle** forms the muscular foundation of the lips. Its fiber bundles surround the oral fissure and simulate a sphincter muscle. The upper and lower parts of the lips, however, are each paired so that the muscle consists of four quadrants.

Its fibers arise partly from a connective tissue band, which is anchored almost perpendicularly to the mucous membrane lateral to the angle of the mouth, partly via fine intermediate tendons from fiber bundles of adjacent facial muscles (especially the buccinator), which converge toward the angle of the mouth and form a "muscle knot" (gelosis) there. In the middle part of the upper and lower lips, the muscle fibers are intertwined, extending partly beyond the median plane, and form a longitudinally-directed fibrous mat. Superficial bundles enter the skin.

The *marginal part* borders on the oral fissure with narrow, densely-lodged bundles and turns back externally toward the skin below the red portion of the lip. The peripherally situated main part of the sphincter, the *labial part*, is only indefinitely marked off and consists of thick tracts of fibers.

Only microscopically-demonstrable fibers penetrate the marginal part of the orbicularis oris as the *rectus labii muscle* and pass from the skin to the mucous membrane.

The **buccinator** represents the muscular foundation of the cheek and attaches at the orbicularis oris in the region of the angle of the mouth. The buccinator arises in a bow-shaped line from the alveolar process of the maxilla in the region of the molar teeth and posteriorly from the alveolar process of the mandible. The distance between upper and lower jaw is bridged over by the tendinous *pterygomandibular raphe* (Fig. **268**), which is also the origin of the muscle. A part of the superior pharyngeal constrictor originates at the back of this raphe.

Near the angle of the mouth, the fiber tracts cross so that the portions situated superiorly in the cheek arrive largely at the lower lip and vice versa. The buccinator, which is penetrated by the parotid duct at the level of the 2nd upper molar tooth, is the only facial muscle to have a superficial fascia (*buccopharyngeal fascia*) that separates it from the buccal fat pad.

The *buccinator muscle* pushes food particles which have arrived between the rows of teeth and buccal mucosa once more between the rows of teeth and thus has an important function in mastication and in the shaping of food particles. The muscle constricts the vestibule of the oral cavity and forces air or fluid through the oral fissure (blow bubbles, whistle, expectorate: "trumpeter muscle"). Contraction of the muscles of both sides leads to a lateral withdrawal of the angle of the mouth.

In a *paralysis* of the buccinator muscle, the air current when whistling is deflected toward the side.

The **depressor labii inferioris muscle** radiates from the platysma obliquely into the lower lip from inferolateral to superomedial. The muscle, which is covered by the depressor anguli oris, draws the upper lip downward and sidewards (expression of displeasure).

The **depressor anguli oris muscle** courses from the lower margin of the mandible converging to the angle of the mouth. The superficially-situated muscle draws the angle of the mouth downward and stretches the upper part of the nasolabial furrow (expression of dissatisfaction or of sorrow).

The **transversus menti muscle** represents a fibrous tract coursing transversely below the chin between the left and the right depressor anguli oris muscles.

The **risorius muscle,** a very weak and variable muscle bundle, passes from the parotid fascia and the buccal skin in an almost horizontal direction to the angle of the mouth. It produces the "laughing dimple" of the cheek and broadens the oral fissure.

The **mentalis muscle** lies below the depressor anguli oris and arises at the mandible in the region of the lateral incisor. It courses obliquely medially and downward to the skin of the chin, produces the chin dimple, and participates in the protrusion of the lower lip together with the orbicularis oris (pouting of children).

The **levator anguli oris muscle** passes to the angle of the mouth from the canine fossa above the canine tooth and below the infra-orbital foramen.

The **levator labii superioris muscle** courses medially downwards to the upper lip from the lower margin of the orbit above the infra-orbital foramen.

The **levator labii superioris alaeque nasi muscle** arises from the frontal process of the maxilla and inserts in common with the previously-mentioned muscle.

The **zygomaticus major muscle** passes from the zygomatic arch medially downwards to the upper lip and to the angle of the mouth. It lifts the angle of the mouth and draws it outward (true "laughing muscle").

The **zygomaticus minor muscle** originates medial to the zygomaticus major and inserts at the upper lip. It is closely allied with the orbicularis oculi. In common with the two levators, the muscle deepens the nasolabial furrow ("crying").

The **platysma** also continues above the margin of the mandible into the facial region for a varying distance (→ p. 726).

Muscles around the Nasal Aperture (Fig. 258)

The **nasalis muscle** is only weakly developed. It arises at the alveolar wall of the upper canine tooth and passes to the wing of the nose (*alar part*, dilatation of the nostrils) and to the cartilaginous part of the bridge of the nose (*transverse part*, narrowing of the nostrils). The muscles of both sides are connected transversely across the bridge of the nose by a tendinous plate.

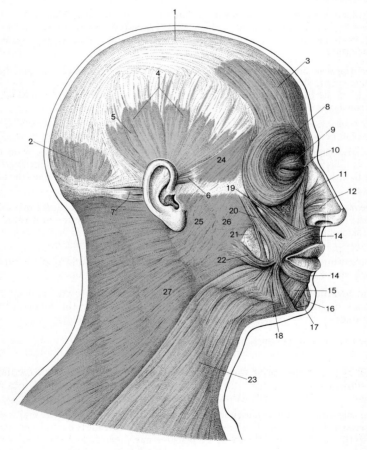

Fig. 258. **Facial musculature and platysma**

The **depressor septi muscle** is represented as a sparse fibrous tract which arises from the alveolar process above the middle incisor, attaches at the end of the cartilaginous nasal septum, and draws the apex of the nose downward.

The **procerus muscle** courses as a short bundle of fibers from the root of the nose to the skin above the nose. The muscle draws the frontal skin toward the root of the nose.

Muscles of the External Ear (Fig. 258)

The *muscles of the external ear* are rudimentary in humans and functionally insignificant. Three muscles are distinguished which attach in front, above and behind the root of the pinna.

The **auricularis anterior muscle** arises at the temporal fascia. The **auricularis superior muscle** comes from the galea aponeurotica. The **auricularis posterior muscle** originates from the mastoid process.

Innervation of the muscles of facial expression: facial nerve

The facial nerve divides in the parotid gland into two large branches which are connected by finer branches in the form of a plexus (*intraparotid plexus*). The branches for the muscles of facial expression proceed from the two branches and take a divergent course – ascending, passing horizontally forward or descending.

c) Conduction Pathways in the Soft Tissue Mantle of the Face

In the soft tissue mantle of the face, arteries, veins and nerves course for the most part separately. The fine branchings of the facial nerve are joined in many ways to the terminal ramifications of the sensory branches of the trigeminal nerve.

The **facial artery** (Figs. **259** and **277**) arises at the level of the hyoid bone from the anterior wall of the external carotid artery, in 18% of the cases

---

◀ 1 Galea aponeurotica
2–5 *Epicranius*
2–3 Occipitofrontalis
2 Occipital belly (occipitalis)
3 Frontal belly (frontalis)
4 Temporoparietalis
5 Auricularis superior (occipital part of temporoparietalis)
6 Auricularis anterior
7 Auricularis posterior
8, 9 Orbicularis oculi
8 Orbital part
9 Palpebral part
10 Procerus and medial palpebral ligament
11 Levator labii superioris alaeque nasi
12 Nasalis

13 Levator labii superioris
14 Orbicularis oris
15 Depressor labii inferioris
16 Mentalis
17 Transversus menti
18 Depressor anguli oris
19 Zygomaticus major
20 Zygomaticus minor
21 Buccal fat pad
22 Risorius
23 Platysma
24 Temporalis fascia
25 Parotid fascia (on parotid gland)
26 Masseteric fascia (on masseter and parotid duct)
27 Superficial layer of cervical fascia

in common with the lingual artery as the *linguofacial trunk*. It passes below (or through) the submandibular gland to the margin of the mandible and arrives at the facial region in front of the attachment of the masseter. Covered by the platysma and the superficial facial muscles, it follows a meandering course (reserve length for the expansion of the buccal cavity) past the angle of the mouth and nasal ala to the medial angle of the eye. Near its origin, the facial artery gives off the *ascending palatine artery*, which ascends in the wall of the pharynx between the stylopharyngeus and styloglossus muscles and which also supplies the palatal arches.

The facial artery sends out the *tonsillar branch* to the palatine tonsil, the *submental artery* – with branches to the submandibular gland – at the lower surface of the mylohyoid muscle, and – in the face – the *superior* and *inferior labial arteries* to the upper and lower lips, respectively. Its terminal branch, the *angular artery*, anastomoses with the dorsal nasal artery, a terminal branch of the ophthalmic artery (from the internal carotid artery).

The arterial pulse can be palpated at the lower margin of the mandible.

The **facial vein** (Figs. **255** and **278**) carries blood away from the scalp and from the face. It begins at the medial angle of the eye as the *angular vein* and communicates with veins of the orbit. The facial vein passes obliquely across the face below the levator labii superioris and zygomaticus major muscles, *dorsal* to the facial artery, crosses the lower margin of the mandible, and runs (usually) superficial to the submandibular gland. It receives tributaries from veins of the face, the pharyngeal wall and from

▶

1 Supratrochlear artery and vein and medial branch of supra-orbital nerve
2 Supra-orbital artery and lateral branch of supra-orbital nerve
3 Supratrochlear nerve
4 Dorsal nasal artery and infratrochlear nerve
5 Angular artery and vein (connection with facial vein interrupted)
6 Infra-orbital artery and nerve
7 Superior labial artery
8 Inferior labial artery
9 Mental artery and nerve
10 Facial artery and vein
11 Submental artery and anterior belly of digastric
12 Submandibular gland
13 Zygomatico-orbital artery and temporal branches of facial nerve
14 Transverse facial artery and zygomatic branches of facial nerve
15 Buccal branches of facial nerve and parotid duct at entrance of buccinator muscle
16 Masseter
17 Mandibular marginal branch of facial nerve
18 Retromandibular vein and cervical branches of facial nerve
19 Temporalis fascia
20 Branches of posterior auricular artery
21 Superficial temporal artery and vein and auriculotemporal nerve
22 Parotid gland, removed as far as level of intraparotid plexus
23 Lesser occipital nerve
24 Great auricular nerve
25 External jugular vein and transverse cervical nerve
26 Supraclavicular nerves
27 Occipital artery and vein and greater occipital nerve
28 Dorsal rami of cervical nerves
29 Accessory nerve with fiber contributions from cervical plexus

the external side of the floor of the mouth. Below the angle of the mandible, it joins the retromandibular vein, generally receives the *superior thyroid vein*, and opens into the internal jugular vein at the level of the greater horn of the hyoid bone.

Thrombosing inflammations of veins caused by small skin infections of the upper lip or the nose can penetrate the cavernous sinus via the angular and superior ophthalmic veins and can produce a thrombosis of the sinus, which can be fatal.

The **retromandibular vein** (Fig. **259**) originates in front of the ear. Veins from the temporal and lateral facial regions drain into it, as well as the *maxillary veins*, which communicate with the pterygoid plexus. The

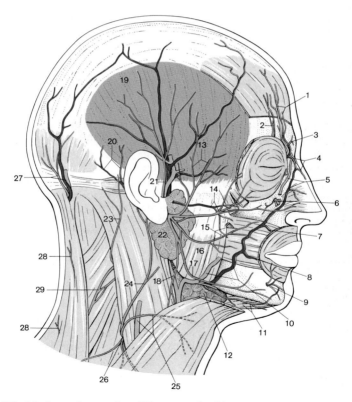

Fig. 259. **Arteries and nerves in soft tissue mantle of face**

retromandibular vein passes downward in the parotid gland and usually opens into the facial vein, more rarely into the internal jugular vein or (additionally) across the sternocleidomastoid into the external jugular vein.

The terminal branches of the **facial nerve** (Fig. **259**), which emerge from the *intraparotid plexus*, enter the soft tissue mantle of the face at the superior and anterior margins of the parotid gland. The following branches are distinguished:

– *temporal branches*, which pass upward to the temple over the zygomatic arch and innervate the frontal belly of the epicranius, the upper portion of the orbicularis oculi, and the anterior and posterior muscles of the external ear;

– *zygomatic branches*, which course anteriorly at the level of the zygomatic arch and supply the lower portion of the orbicularis oculi, as well as the facial muscles below the root of the zygomatic arch;

– *buccal branches*, which pass anteriorly downward into the buccinator and the facial muscles around the opening of the mouth;

– the *marginal mandibular ramus*, which passes at the lower edge of the chin to the facial muscles below the mouth opening; and

– the *cervical (colli) branch*, which courses behind the angle of the mandible to the undersurface of the platysma where it provides motor fibers for this muscle and communicates with the sensory transverse cervical nerve from the cervical plexus.

Considering the divergent radiation of the facial branches, surgeons prefer a radial type of incision for operations of the face.

When the trunk of the facial nerve of one side is lost, all facial branches are affected resulting in *peripheral facial paralysis*.

With *central facial paralysis*, on the other hand, in which the tract (corticonuclear tract) passing from the cerebral cortex to the region of the facial nucleus is interrupted on one side (e.g. in the internal capsule), the branches passing to the temple and forehead are usually still functional. Their cell bodies in the nuclear region of the facial nerve receive excitations from the cerebral cortex of both hemispheres.

With its three branches, the **trigeminal nerve** (Fig. **257**) supplies the facial skin, except for a small area over the angle of the mandible which is innervated by the cervical plexus (anterior ramus of the great auricular nerve).

The area of distribution of the three branches of the trigeminal nerve in the skin of the face is traced back to the development of the face from the frontal eminence, as well as from the maxillary and mandibular processes of the 1st pharyngeal arch.

The *exit sites* from the skull *of the largest cutaneous nerves from each of the three main branches of the trigeminal nerve* lie *paramedian in a vertical line* (Figs. **253** and **259**).

The ophthalmic nerve (V_1) supplies the skin of the forehead via the medial and lateral branches of the *supra-orbital nerve* (main branch of the frontal nerve) which pass through the frontal (medial) and supra-orbital (lateral) notches, respectively, at the upper margin of the orbit. The maxillary nerve (V_2) supplies the skin of the face in the maxillary region via the *infra-orbital nerve*, which traverses the infra-orbital foramen. The mandibular nerve (V_3) innervates the skin of the chin and lower lip via the *mental nerve* (the terminal branch of the inferior alveolar nerve), which passes through the mental foramen.

The places of exit of these cutaneous nerves are "pressure points" at which the disease-altered pain sensitivity of the cutaneous nerves is examined (trigeminal pressure points).

The *sensory nerves of the face* travel predominantly in a *vertical direction*. They cross the course of the *motor nerves of the face* which pass in more of a *transverse direction*.

4. Lateral Region of the Face

The **lateral region of the face** extends upward to the zygomatic arch and caudally to the angle of the mandible. The mandibular ramus divides the lateral facial region into a superficial and a deep area. The *deep lateral region of the face* corresponds to a space, the *infratemporal fossa*.

The **infratemporal fossa** (Fig. 261) contains a fat body superficially (continuation of the buccal fat pad) and is filled largely by the medial and lateral pterygoid muscles. These muscles, together with the tuber of the maxilla and the buccinator muscle, border a pyramid-shaped connective tissue space, a *neurovascular pathway*. It extends from the inner surface of the mandibular ramus to the pterygopalatine fossa and guides the *maxillary artery* deeply into this fossa. The venous networks designated as the *pterygoid plexus* surround the lateral pterygoid muscle at the outer and inner surfaces and convey the blood primarily via the *maxillary veins* (companion veins of the maxillary artery) into the retromandibular vein. The *mandibular nerve* divides within the infratemporal fossa into its large branches, which are normally crossed over by the maxillary artery.

Only part of the vessels and nerves pass from the infratemporal fossa into the superficial lateral facial region. However, for the benefit of a comprehensive presentation, the pathways of the lateral facial region are discussed together (→ p. 677 f.).

a) Superficial Lateral Facial Region

In the **superficial lateral facial region** (Fig. 258), the masseter muscle originates at the lower margin of the zygomatic arch and is covered by the *masseteric fascia*. The *buccal fat pad* (structural fat) lies in front of the masseter on the buccinator muscle; the *parotid gland*, covered by the *parotid fascia*, is attached behind it. This gland lies in the triangle between the temporomandibular joint, the angle of the mandible and the mastoid process, in front of and below the external acoustic meatus.

The **parotid gland** is the largest of the major salivary glands, which also include the *sublingual* and *submandibular glands*. Saliva is also produced by numerous small salivary glands within the oral mucosa, altogether up to 1.5 l daily.

The *parotid gland* (usually referred to only as *parotid* in clinics, Fig. **259**) has grown together firmly with the superficial and the deep layer of the parotid fascia. The largest part of the gland protrudes behind the mandibular ramus into the depth of the parapharyngeal connective tissue space. The styloid process separates the gland from the neurovascular bundle of the neck and from the accessory and hypoglossal nerves. When the jaw is opened, the lower part of the gland is "massaged", and in this way the secretion is emptied in phases.

The parotid is a *pure serous gland*. It produces a "diluting saliva" containing the enzyme *ptyalin*, which breaks down starches.

After a short ascent, the *excretory duct* (*parotid duct*, Fig. **255**) courses horizontally forward across the masseter and the buccal fat pad – about a finger's breadth below the zygomatic arch – to the buccinator, which it penetrates obliquely before opening into the vestibule of the oral cavity opposite the 2nd upper molar tooth. A small accessory salivary gland frequently lies close to the parotid duct.

The parotid duct is endangered in its course on the masseter in the case of facial injuries.

Innervation: parasympathetic from the glossopharyngeal nerve, sympathetic from the superior cervical ganglion.

The *preganglionic, parasympathetic fibers* leave the glossopharyngeal nerve with the *tympanic nerve* at the inferior ganglion and pass in the *tympanic plexus* over the medial wall of the tympanic cavity. From there, they reach the *otic ganglion* as the *lesser petrosal nerve* (through the anterior wall of the petrous temporal and the sphenopetrosal fissure or the foramen ovale). The otic ganglion lies below the foramen ovale at the medial side of the mandibular nerve and gives off *postganglionic* fibers to the parotid gland via the auriculotemporal nerve (from V_3) which reaches the gland directly or by means of an anastomosis with the facial nerve.

The *sympathetic fibers* (from the superior cervical ganglion) come from the *postganglionic* plexus which surrounds the middle meningeal artery, an offshoot of the *external carotid plexus*.

External Ear

The **external ear** comprises the *pinna* and the *external acoustic meatus*. The meatus is separated from the middle ear by the *tympanic membrane* (eardrum).

The **pinna** (*auricle*, Fig. **260**) is a skin fold which contains a plate of elastic cartilage (*auricular cartilage*). It forms a sound funnel. The inner concave surface of the pinna contains numerous prominences and recesses.

The margin of the concavity consists of a ridge (*helix*). The *antihelix*, which begins above the opening of the meatus with two *crura*, courses parallel to it on the inside. A small protuberance, the *tragus*, projects in front of the meatal opening. Continuing downward are the *intertragic notch* and the *antitragus*, which runs out into the *ear lobule*, a cartilage-free skin fold. Between the helix and antihelix is a depression, the *scaphoid fossa*. The *triangular fossa* is embraced by the crura of the antihelix. The deepest depression of the pinna is designated as the *concha*. The *crus of the helix* marks off an upper segment, the *cymba conchae*.

The **external acoustic meatus** (Fig. **260**) consists of an outer *cartilaginous* and an inner *bony* portion. It extends from the pinna obliquely forward and medial and is bent forward. The cartilage of the canal forms a groove in the anterior and inferior walls and communicates continuously with the cartilage of the pinna. The external acoustic meatus is lined by external skin which is firmly united with the perichondrium and periosteum. The skin possesses hairs with sebaceous glands and large apocrine *ceruminous glands*. The tympanic (in front, below and behind) and squamous (above) parts of the temporal bone are involved in the formation of the bony meatus.

When examining the tympanic membrane with an otoscope, the external acoustic meatus is straightened by pulling the auricle backward and upward.

The **tympanic membrane** (Fig. **260**), a thin membrane, is stretched out at the base of the external acoustic meatus and separates it from the cavity of the middle ear. Its margin is folded into the tympanic groove of the tympanic part of the petrous temporal by a *fibrocartilaginous ring*. The larger part of the membrane is rigidly stretched as the tense part (*pars tensa*); only the upper part connected with the squamous temporal is flaccid (*pars flaccida*; Shrapnell's membrane). The border between the tense and flaccid parts is visible as fine limiting bands, the *anterior* and *posterior mallear folds* (→ Vol. 2, Fig. **164**).

The tympanic membrane is not spread out in a flat plane, but is funnel-shaped. Since it is united with two processes of the malleus (hammer), the *manubrium* (handle) and the *lateral process*, the shape of the surface is considerably influenced by these connections. The fusion with the manubrium causes the *mallear stripe*, whereas the lateral process produces a small bulge, the *mallear prominence*, at the border between the tense and flaccid parts. The apex of the manubrium, on the other hand, draws the tympanic membrane inward in a funnel-shape forming the *umbo*, which lies eccentrically near the antero-inferior margin. On the whole, the membrane is placed obliquely, being inclined forward and downward, and is an approximate continuation of the posterior wall of the external acoustic meatus. A plane drawn through the upper and lower margins of

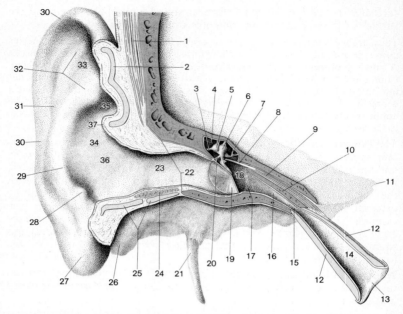

Fig. 260. Schematic "frontal" section through external acoustic meatus, tympanic cavity and auditory tube, anterior view
(Mucosal covering of auditory ossicles not shown)
Cut surface of bone ▢

1 Temporalis muscle
2 Auricular cartilage
3 Posterior ligament of incus
4 Epitympanic recess
5 Body of incus with superior ligament
6 Head of malleus with superior ligament of malleus
7 Stapes
8 Tendon of tensor tympani, attachment at manubrium of malleus
9 Tensor tympani in semicanal for tensor tympani
10 Septum of musculotubal canal
11 Apex of petrous part of temporal bone
12–17 *Auditory tube* in semicanal for auditory tube
12 Cartilage
13 Pharyngeal opening
14 Cartilaginous part
15 Isthmus
16 Bony part
17 Tympanic opening
18 Tympanic cavity

19 Tympanic membrane (cut surface on right side)
20 Lateral ligament of malleus
21 Styloid process of temporal bone
22 Opening of external acoustic meatus
23 External acoustic meatus
24 Ceruminous glands
25 Cartilaginous portion of external auditory meatus
26 Mastoid process
27–37 *Auricle* (pinna)
27 Lobule
28 Antitragus
29 Anthelix
30 Helix
31 Scaphoid fossa
32 Crura of anthelix
33 Triangular fossa
34 Concha
35 Cymba conchae
36 Cavity of concha
37 Crus of helix

the membrane forms an angle of about 45° with the horizontal plane, which opens externally and an angle of about 50° with the median plane, which opens posteriorly. In the newborn, the eardrum lies almost horizontal.

Histology. The main constituent of the tympanic membrane is a compact fibrous connective tissue membrane, the *lamina propria*, containing predominantly radially oriented fibers, except in the flaccid part. The lamina propria is formed by skin continuous with that of the meatus (*cutaneous layer*); the tympanic side of the membrane is covered by a thin mucous membrane (*mucosal layer*).

The **innervation** of the skin at the external ear (Fig. 257) is provided by the following:

– the *auriculotemporal nerve* with *anterior auricular nerves* at the anterior surface of the auricle, with the *nerve of the external acoustic meatus* at the anterior and upper wall of the meatus, with the *branches of the tympanic membrane* on the external surface of the membrane;

– the *vagus nerve* with the *auricular branch* in the region of the auricular concha, as well as at the posterior and inferior wall of the meatus; and

– the *great auricular nerve* (from the cervical plexus) with the *posterior ramus* at the posterior surface and with the *anterior ramus* at the anterior surface of the pinna.

b) Conduction Pathways in the Lateral Facial Region

Vessels and Nerves in the Superficial Lateral Facial Region

In the superficial lateral region of the face, the *parotid gland* resides in a close spatial relationship to vessels and nerves (Fig. 259).

The **external carotid artery** passes *through the gland in a vertical direction*. From the carotid triangle, the artery passes medial to the posterior belly of the digastric between the stylohyoid and styloglossus muscles and enters the gland from below. Within the gland, the external carotid courses upward to the level of the temporomandibular joint and bifurcates into its two terminal branches, the *maxillary* (→ p. 678) and *superficial temporal arteries*. In the lower part of the parotid, the external carotid is accompanied by the **retromandibular vein,** which lies more superficial than the artery.

The **superficial temporal artery** with its companion veins and – towards the occiput – the **auriculotemporal nerve** (→ p. 681) pass directly in front of the auricle at the upper margin of the parotid gland and cross the root of the zygomatic arch below the skin of the temporal region.

The *superficial temporal artery* ramifies in the superficial lateral facial region and in the temporal region. It gives off a *parotid branch* to the parotid gland; the *transverse facial artery* passes toward the cheek below the zygomatic arch and over the masseter muscle; *anterior auricular branches* course to the auricle and to the external acoustic meatus. Above the zygomatic arch, the *zygomatico-orbital artery* courses toward the lateral angle of the eye, whereas the *middle temporal artery* penetrates the temporalis fascia and temporalis muscle and reaches the groove for the middle temporal artery on the temporal squama. On the temporalis fascia, the superficial temporal artery divides into its two terminal branches, the *frontal branch* ascending obliquely across the anterior temporal region and the *parietal branch* passing more perpendicularly toward the temporal region. Both branches anastomose in the region of the scalp with branches from the opposite side and with branches of adjacent arteries.

Lymph nodes. *Superficial* and *deep parotid lymph nodes* (Fig. **256**) lie on and in the parotid gland. They receive lymph from the gland and its surroundings, as well as from the cheek and the scalp.

The **facial nerve** (Fig. **259**) *penetrates the parotid gland in a horizontal direction* superficial to the external carotid artery. Coming from the stylomastoid foramen, it divides within the gland first of all into two main branches, whose fine ramified connections form the *intraparotid plexus*. The fan formed by the terminal branches diverging forward and upward, forward, and forward and downward incompletely divides the anterior portion of the gland into a deep and a superficial section. The facial branches pass from the parotid gland under the masseteric fascia, which they leave only at the anterior margin of the muscle. The branches of the facial nerve diverge from one another like a hand placed on the ear with the five fingers spread out and directed anteriorly.

Only the *posterior auricular nerve* courses dorsally from the stylomastoid foramen between the mastoid process and the external acoustic meatus to the posterior auricular muscle and the occipital belly of the occipitofrontalis muscle. The *digastric branch* passes a short distance downward and enters the posterior belly of the digastric; the *stylohyoid branch* enters the muscle of the same name.

Pathways in and out of the Deep Lateral Facial Region

The **maxillary artery** (Figs. **261**, **268** and **277**), the largest terminal branch of the external carotid artery, proceeds almost at right angles from the bifurcation of this artery. It passes first medial to the neck of the mandible, then continues between the temporalis and lateral pterygoid muscles and over (or through) the lateral pterygoid to enter the pterygopalatine fossa, where it follows a very tortuous course and where it divides into its terminal branches. The maxillary artery supplies the muscles of mastication, the mucous membranes of the oral and nasal cavities, the teeth and the palate, as well as the largest portion of the cranial dura and the bones of the skull.

During the course of the maxillary artery through the lateral deep facial regions, branches arise in *three sections* accompanied by branches of the mandibular nerve in the infratemporal fossa and branches of the maxillary nerve in the vicinity of the pterygopalatine fossa. The *first section* lies medial to the temporomandibular joint, the *second section* courses in the masticatory muscles, and the *third section* forms the terminal division in the pterygopalatine fossa.

Medial to the mandible, the maxillary artery gives off weak branches to the temporomandibular joint, external acoustic meatus and tympanic cavity, as well as the *inferior alveolar artery*, which passes together with the inferior alveolar nerve between the medial pterygoid and the mandibular ramus to the mandibular canal. This artery supplies the roots of the teeth, bones and gingiva and terminates as the *mental artery*, which traverses the mental foramen to supply the chin and lower lip. The *middle meningeal artery*, as a large branch medial to the lateral pterygoid muscle, courses through the foramen spinosum between the dura and bone of the middle cranial fossa and finally divides into *frontal* and *parietal branches*. Both branches course in bony grooves outside of the dura and supply the largest part of the dura, as well as the adjacent skull bones.

Between the masticatory muscles, the maxillary artery sends out muscular branches for the pterygoids, masseter, temporalis and buccinator.

In the pterygopalatine fossa, the maxillary artery divides into several branches. The *posterior superior alveolar artery* passes to the lateral teeth of the maxilla and their gingiva (as well as to the mucosa of the maxillary sinus). The *infra-orbital artery* courses through the infra-orbital groove and canal to the soft parts of the face in the vicinity of the infra-orbital foramen. It dispatches branches to the orbit (inferior rectus and inferior oblique muscles, inferior palpebra), to the mucosa of the maxillary sinus, as well as to the front teeth and their gingiva (*anterior superior alveolar arteries*).

The thin *artery of the pterygoid canal*, which can also arise from the descending palatine artery, passes dorsally through the pterygoid canal to the auditory tube and to the mucous membrane of the upper portion of the pharynx (*pharyngeal branch*).

The *descending palatine artery* arrives at the roof of the oral cavity in the greater palatine canal. It supplies the mucosa of the hard palate and the palatal gingiva of the maxilla as the *greater palatine artery*, the soft palate with the *lesser palatine arteries*, and the tonsillar region with the *pharyngeal branch*. The *sphenopalatine artery* traverses the sphenopalatine foramen and ramifies with the *lateral posterior nasal arteries* and *posterior septal branches* at the (posterior) lateral and the septal mucosa of the nasal cavity.

The **veins** (Fig. **278**) form an extensive network in the infratemporal fossa between the temporalis, medial and lateral pterygoids. Termed the *pterygoid plexus*, it drains into the retromandibular vein via the *maxillary veins*.

The pterygoid plexus receives tributaries from the cranial dura through openings in the basicranium, from the masticatory muscles, from the tympanic cavity and from the external ear. It communicates below the zygomatic arch with the facial vein via the *deep facial vein*.

Lymphatic tracts and lymph nodes (Fig. 272). The lymph from the deep lateral facial region arrives at the *deep lateral cervical lymph nodes* along the internal jugular vein, as well as at the *retropharyngeal lymph nodes* behind the nasopharynx.

The **nerves** (Figs. **261** and **268**) which pass through the infratemporal fossa are branches of the *mandibular nerve*. The *maxillary nerve* passes through the pterygopalatine fossa.

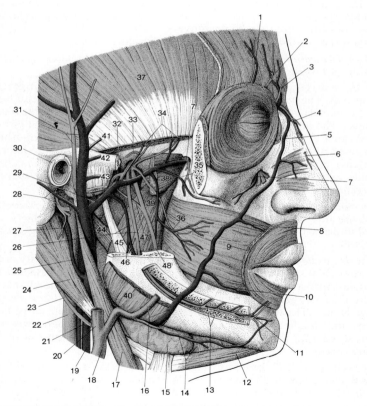

Fig. 261. **Arteries and nerves into and out of deep lateral facial region**
(Zygomatic arch and portion of mandibular ramus removed, mandibular canal opened)

The **mandibular nerve** traverses the foramen ovale from the middle cranial fossa. The trunk, to which the *otic ganglion* is attached medially directly below the base of the skull, divides immediately after entering the infratemporal fossa between the medial and lateral pterygoid muscles. The nerve supplies motor input to the masticatory musculature and the muscles at the floor of the mouth and sensory innervation to the floor of the mouth and the mucosa of the tongue, as well as to the skin over the mandible. The motor branches to the masticatory muscles course with the branches of the middle portion of the maxillary artery.

To the muscles of mastication, the mandibular nerve sends the *masseteric nerve* (through the mandibular notch to the masseter muscle), the *deep temporal nerves* (to the temporalis muscle), the *nerve to the lateral pterygoid* and the *nerve to the medial pterygoid* (to the pterygoid muscles). Motor branches also enter the tensor tympani and tensor veli palatini muscles.

The skin of the cheek is supplied by the *buccal nerve*, which arrives at the external surface of the buccinator through the lateral pterygoid.

The skin of the temple and ear region receive sensory innervation from the *auriculotemporal nerve*. It embraces the middle meningeal artery with

◀ 1 Supra-orbital artery and lateral branch of supra-orbital nerve
2 Supratrochlear artery and medial branch of supra-orbital nerve
3 Supratrochlear nerve
4 Dorsal nasal artery and infratrochlear nerve
5 Angular artery
6 External nasal branch of anterior ethmoidal nerve
7 Infra-orbital artery and nerve
8 Superior labial artery
9 Buccinator
10 Inferior labial artery
11 Mental artery and nerve
12 Anterior belly of digastric
13 Dental branches of inferior alveolar artery and inferior dental branches of inferior alveolar nerve
14 Submental artery and mylohyoid
15 Submandibular gland
16 Facial artery and vein
17 Stylohyoid muscle
18 External jugular vein
19 External carotid artery
20 Retromandibular vein
21 Superior root of ansa cervicalis
22 Internal jugular vein
23 Hypoglossal nerve
24 Posterior belly of digastric

25 Occipital artery
26 Inferior alveolar artery and nerve
27 Digastric branch of facial nerve
28 Posterior auricular artery and facial nerve
29 Maxillary artery and exit of deep auricular and anterior tympanic arteries
30 Cartilaginous external acoustic meatus
31 Superficial temporal artery and auriculo-temporal nerve
32 Middle meningeal artery
33 Masseteric nerve
34 Deep temporal arteries and deep temporal nerves
35 Posterior superior alveolar artery and posterior superior alveolar branches of maxillary nerve
36 Buccal artery and nerve
37 Temporalis (severed)
38 Lateral pterygoid (severed)
39 Medial pterygoid
40 Masseter (severed)
41 Middle temporal artery
42 Zygomatico-orbital artery
43 Transverse facial artery
44 Styloglossus
45 Sphenomandibular ligament
46 Mylohyoid branch of inferior alveolar artery and mylohyoid nerve
47 Chorda tympani
48 Lingual nerve

two roots before passing laterally behind the neck of the mandible toward the temple region. At the replication site, it carries parasympathetic fibers to the parotid from the otic ganglion (*parotid branches*) both directly and via the facial nerve (*communicating rami [of mandibular nerve with facial nerve]*). To a large extent, sensory fibers of the auriculotemporal nerve also course via this anastomosis to the skin of the lateral facial region where they join the facial branches for a short distance.

In the region of the external ear, the auriculotemporal nerve dispatches the *nerve to the external acoustic meatus, branches to the tympanic membrane* and *anterior auricular nerves* (→ p. 677). In the temple region, it branches out into *superficial temporal rami*.

After giving off the motor *nerve to the mylohyoid* (for the mylohyoid muscle and the anterior belly of the digastric), the *inferior alveolar nerve* enters the mandibular canal and supplies the teeth of the mandible. Its terminal branch, the *mental nerve*, passes through the mental foramen to the skin of the chin and the lower lip.

The mucosa of the tongue is innervated by the *lingual nerve* which passes downward medial to the inferior alveolar nerve and receives the *chorda tympani* from behind. The chorda tympani brings preganglionic parasympathetic fibers which will be given off from the lingual nerve to the *submandibular ganglion*. The lingual nerve terminates in the tongue between the mylohyoid and the submandibular duct; it provides taste (chorda tympani) and sensory fibers for the tongue.

The **maxillary nerve** leaves the middle cranial fossa through the foramen rotundum and arrives at the pterygopalatine fossa where it is attached to the *pterygopalatine ganglion* and divides into its three main branches. The maxillary nerve sends sensory branches to the skin of the middle facial region, to the teeth of the maxilla, and to parts of the palatal and nasal mucosa; it carries parasympathetic fibers for the lacrimal gland.

The *infra-orbital nerve*, accompanied by the infra-orbital artery, passes to the facial region via the inferior orbital fissure and the infra-orbital canal. In its passage, it provides *superior alveolar nerves* for the maxillary teeth and the buccal gingiva.

The *zygomatic nerve*, which enters the orbit through the inferior orbital fissure, supplies sensory branches to the skin over the zygomatic bone (*zygomaticofacial ramus*) and in a small region of the temple (*zygomaticotemporal ramus*).

The zygomatic nerve and the zygomaticotemporal ramus also carry postganglionic parasympathetic fibers from the pterygopalatine ganglion which are conducted over the pterygopalatine and maxillary nerves and reach the lacrimal gland via an anastomosis with the lacrimal nerve.

Near its origin, the pterygopalatine ganglion is connected to the maxillary nerve by *pterygopalatine nerves* (usually two) which are now referred to as *ganglionic rami* although their sensory fibers pass by the ganglion or go through it without synapsing. They take up postganglionic parasympathetic and sympathetic nerve fibers, however, which reach the glands of the corresponding mucosal areas via ramifications of the pterygopalatine nerves.

Orbital rami pass through the inferior orbital fissure into the orbit and from there into bony canaliculi to the mucous membrane of the sphenoidal sinus and the posterior ethmoidal air cells. The *pharyngeal ramus* passes dorsally upward to the mucosa of the nasopharynx.

Posterior superior nasal rami reach the mucosa in the posterior region of the nasal cavity through the sphenopalatine foramen and ramify as lateral branches at the lateral wall, as medial branches at the nasal septum. A long branch of the septal branches passes as the *nasopalatine nerve* through the incisive canal to the mucosa of the palate behind the incisor teeth and their palatal gingiva.

The *greater palatine nerve* courses in its canal toward the palate and dispatches *posterior inferior nasal branches* to the mucosa of the middle nasal concha and the two adjoining nasal meatuses before it ramifies in the mucosa of the hard palate and in the palatal gingiva of the lateral teeth. *Lesser palatine nerves* leave the greater palatine canal and reach the mucosa of the soft palate and the tonsillar fossa via the lesser palatine canals.

C. Respiratory Pathway and Digestive Tract in the Head Region

With the development of the face, the primitive (primary) nasal cavity arises from paired olfactory (nasal) sacs. It is converted into a definitive nasal cavity by the inclusion of the much more extensive upper "level" of the primary oral cavity, which was segmented off from the final definitive oral cavity by the formation of a horizontal partition, the secondary palate. The initial sections of the respiratory pathway and the digestive tract thus lie on top of each other in the head region and both lead into the undivided pharynx, where they cross each other.

1. Nasal Cavity

The **main cavities of the nose,** the *nasal cavities*, are the first section of the respiratory system. They serve to prepare the respiratory air, which then passes to the lungs via the pharynx, larynx, trachea and bronchi. The nasal cavities and pharynx comprise the *upper respiratory tract*, in contrast to the *lower respiratory tract* commencing with the larynx. The

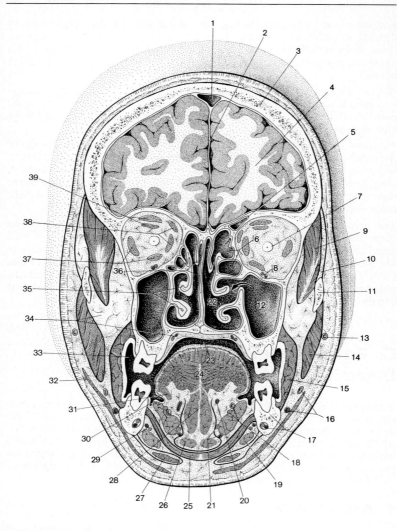

Fig. 262. **Schematic frontal section through head** at level of optic nerve
Anterior view of section surface

1 Superior sagittal sinus
2 Falx cerebri
3 Squamous portion of frontal bone
4 Frontal lobe of cerebrum
5 Frontal sinus
6 Middle and posterior ethmoidal cells
7 Optic nerve and central retinal artery
8 Infra-orbital artery and nerve

paranasal sinuses, which also contain air, communicate with the main cavities of the nose.

a) Main Cavity of the Nose

The paired **nasal cavity** (Figs. **262–265**) begins at the *naris* (*nostril*) which leads to the vestibule of the nose. This is followed by the true nasal cavity which continues into the pharynx at the *posterior nasal aperture* (*choana*). The *nasal septum* separates the right and left nasal cavities from each other.

The **nasal vestibule** is enclosed laterally by the *wing* (*ala*) *of the nose*, medially by the cartilaginous and connective tissue end of the nasal septum. A curved mucosal ridge (*limen nasi*) marks the border to the nasal cavity in the narrow sense. There is a sieve-like corona of coarse hairs (*vibrissae*) growing outward in the vestibule which prevent large pollutants and foreign substances from entering the nasal cavity.

The *nasal cartilages* provide rigid support for the nasal alae and septum. They are mutually displaceable within a layer of connective tissue.

The nasal vestibule is lined by only slightly modified *facial skin*. The stratified squamous epithelium of the epidermis is continuous with the pseudostratified, ciliated columnar (respiratory) epithelium at the limen nasi.

The two **nasal cavities in the narrow sense** lie below the anterior cranial fossa. The *floor* of each cavity rests on the hard palate. The *lateral wall* begins at the floor 10–15 mm lateral to the nasal septum. The nasal cavity is narrowed above like a gable.

---

 9 Temporalis
10 Adipose tissue between two layers of temporalis fascia
11 Zygomatic arch
12 Maxillary sinus, arrow in opening to middle meatus of nose
13 Parotid duct
14 Masseter
15 Buccinator
16 Facial artery and vein
17 Body of mandible, mandibular canal with inferior alveolar artery and nerve
18 Sublingual gland, submandibular duct and lingual nerve (on right side of face before, on left side after crossing submandibular duct)
19 Submandibular gland
20 Arteria profunda linguae
21 Sublingual artery and hypoglossal nerve
22 Nasal cavity: common nasal meatus

23 Oral cavity proper
24 Body of tongue
25 Mylohyoid
26 Geniohyoid
27 Anterior belly of digastric
28 Septum of tongue and genioglossus
29 Submental artery and mylohyoid nerve
30 Sublingual fold
31 Hyoglossus
32 Platysma
33 Vestibule of oral cavity
34 Buccal fat pad, greater palatine artery and nerve
35 Middle and inferior nasal conchae
36 Nasal septum and superior nasal concha
37 Lateral rectus and inferior rectus
38 Medial rectus and superior oblique
39 Superior rectus and levator palpebrae superioris

The groove-shaped *roof* dips forward below the bridge of the nose (*dorsum nasi*) to the nostril. Toward the back, the roof goes over into the obliquely-positioned posterior wall of the nasal cavity, which is surmounted by the body of the sphenoid. Below this site, the choana opens into the nasopharyngeal cavity. The narrow space above the superior concha and in front of the body of the sphenoid is the *spheno-ethmoidal recess*.

The nasal septum represents the medial wall of the nasal cavity (Fig. **243**). Its posterior portion contains bony plates which are attached anteriorly to the *septal cartilage* and the medial crus of the *alar cartilage*. A *ridge* (septal crest) – ascending along the upper angle of the vomer – is formed at the inferior portion of this cartilage-bone junction. At this site, the nasal septum frequently exhibits a sharp bend toward the side (*septal deviation*). The mucosa of the septum contains a cavernous body at the level of the middle nasal meatus.

Nasal breathing is impaired by a strong deviation of the septum or by the enlargement of the cavernous body. Objects which are inserted into the nose – occasionally by children – can slide backwards along the septal ridge (danger of perforating the ethmoid bone).

The *lateral wall* of the nasal cavity is enlarged by the medial projection of three roof-shaped *nasal conchae* which are composed of thin bony plates covered by a mucosa.

Each concha roofs over a *meatus*. The three meatuses communicate medially with one another at the *common nasal meatus* beside the nasal septum.

The *sphenoidal sinus* opens into the spheno-ethmoidal recess.

The *superior nasal meatus* is bordered by the superior and middle nasal conchae and receives 1–2 openings of the *posterior cells* of the *ethmoidal cavity*, which is divided into several chambers.

The *middle nasal meatus* lies between the middle and inferior conchae. The mucosa of the middle meatus continues into the *ethmoidal infundibulum* through the slit-like *hiatus semilunaris* (→ p. 597) bordered by the ethmoidal bulla and the uncinate process. The infundibulum, which bulges toward the maxillary sinus as a shallow mucosal recess, receives the openings of the *frontal sinus* anterosuperiorly, the *anterior ethmoidal air cells* in front of the ethmoidal bulla, and the *maxillary sinus* from below. Occasionally, an additional opening of the maxillary sinus is present behind the main opening. The *middle ethmoidal air cells* (including the ethmoidal bulla) open directly into the middle meatus.

The *inferior nasal meatus*, which is roofed over by the inferior nasal concha, receives the opening of the *nasolacrimal duct* near the anterior end of the concha. It transports lacrimal fluid into the nasal cavity from the conjunctival sac.

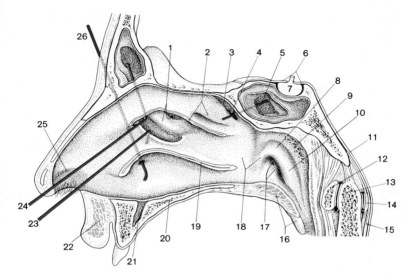

Fig. 263. **Lateral wall of nasal cavity
and nasopharynx** (after Rauber-Kopsch)
Probing of accessory nasal cavities
(middle and inferior conchae resected)

 1 Ethmoidal bulla and entrance into middle
   ethmoidal air cells (arrow)
 2 Superior nasal concha and cut edge of
   middle nasal concha
 3 Spheno-ethmoidal recess
 4 Opening of sphenoidal sinus
 5 Probe in left sphenoidal sinus, large part of
   septum removed
 6 Diaphragma sellae
 7 Hypophysis with hypophysial stalk
 8 Torus tubarius
 9 Pharyngeal tonsil
10 Salpingopharyngeal fold
11 Cephalic dura mater
12 Anterior arch of atlas
13 Dens of axis

14 Transverse ligament of atlas
15 Membrana tectoria
16 Soft palate and ůvula
17 Pharyngeal opening of auditory tube
   (arrow) and torus levatorius
18 Nasopharyngeal meatus (in front) and
   salpingopalatine fold
19 Cut edge of inferior nasal concha
20 Hard palate
21 Nasopalatine nerve in incisive canal
22 Orbicularis oris
23 Probe in hiatus semilunaris, entrance into
   maxillary sinus
24 Probe in frontal sinus
25 Limen nasi
26 Probe in nasolacrimal duct

b) Paranasal Sinuses

All **paranasal sinuses** (Figs. **242**, **245** and **262**) communicate with the main
space of the nasal cavity. Their openings always correspond to the site of
their developmental origin. The development of the paranasal sinuses
occurs relatively late, although the anlagen of the sinuses are already
demonstrable at early embryonic stages. The formation of the accessory
spaces is closely related to the constructive shaping of the facial skeleton.

Since the structuring of the facial skeleton is itself closely related to the development of the deciduous and permanent teeth, it is understandable that the definitive development of the paranasal sinuses takes place only after the conclusion of the second dentition. Quite distinct variations exist individually.

The paranasal sinuses play an important role as the site of infectious processes.

The **maxillary sinus** is the most extensive paranasal sinus. The upper wall borders on the floor of the orbit, the posterior wall corresponds to the tuber maxillae. The anterior wall is formed by the facial surface of the maxilla; the floor has relations to the maxillary teeth. Occasionally, the maxillary sinus can extend into the zygomatic arch and into the bony palate.

The deepest part of the maxillary sinus lies, as a rule, above the roots of the 2nd premolar and the 1st molar teeth. The canine tooth usually has no close topographical relation to the maxillary sinus. The infra-orbital canal courses with the infra-orbital nerve (from V_2) and the infra-orbital vessels in the superior wall of the maxillary sinus. The opening of the maxillary sinus lies near the top, close to the roof.

Since the maxillary sinus opens below the frontal sinus, pus formation in the frontal sinus easily spreads to it. The discharge of an inflammatory exudate from the maxillary sinus is made difficult by the high location of its opening.

The **frontal sinus** is especially variable and often asymmetrically formed. It extends into the medial part of the frontal bone. The extension laterally into the superciliary arch and into the roof of the orbit varies greatly. Both frontal sinuses are separated by the septum, which is usually not straight.

The total of all ethmoidal air cells is referred to as the **ethmoidal sinus**. These irregularly shaped air spaces lie in the labyrinth of the ethmoid bone and are also bordered partly by neighboring bones. The number and size of the cells can vary considerably.

The **sphenoidal sinus** is distinguished in its genesis from the remaining paranasal sinuses since it is segmented off from the posterior portion of the main cavity. Topographically, however, it is closely related to the posterior ethmoidal air cells. The paired sphenoidal sinus opens into the spheno-ethmoidal recess. The opening is surrounded laterally and below by the sphenoidal concha. The septum which separates both cavities is generally formed asymmetrically. Occasionally, the sphenoidal sinus extends into the basal part of the occipital bone. The roof of the sinus has close connections with the optic canal and the chiasmatic groove (upward), as well as to the hypophysis toward the back (operative approach to the hypophysis through the nasal cavity and sphenoidal sinus).

c) Mucous Membrane of the Nasal Cavity

The **mucosa**, which begins at the border of the nasal vestibule, is not structured uniformly; the mucosa of the *respiratory region* can be distinguished from the mucosa of the *olfactory region*. The latter covers the superior concha, the corresponding parts of the roof of the nasal cavity and the nasal septum. The mucous membrane of the middle and inferior conchae, as well as all the remaining portions of the wall belongs to the respiratory region, together with the mucosa of the paranasal sinuses.

Because of the *surface enlargement* of the lateral portions of the wall of the nasal cavity, *respiratory air* comes into extensive contact with the nasal mucosa and is somewhat *warmed* by the venous plexus incorporated in it.

The secretion of the mixed glands *moistens* the air and simultaneously effects a *preliminary purification*. Suspended matter which adheres to the nasal secretion is transported with it to the pharynx by the ciliary action of the respiratory epithelium. The *olfactory organ* and the *sensory nerves* of the nasal mucosa control the respiratory air for harmful chemical impurities, which can elicit a nasal reflex. Beyond this, the nasal cavity functions as a *resonator* for speech.

The flow of inspired air passes predominantly through the middle and the inferior nasal meatuses. In "sniffing", whirls (vortices) of air are formed which rise to the olfactory region and prolong the stay of the air in the nasal cavity.

Each deformation of the walls of the nasal cavity affects the proportions of the flow of air. Just like an inflammatory swelling of the nasal mucosa, it leads to an alteration of speech.

The *mucosa of the respiratory region* bears pseudostratified, ciliated, columnar epithelium with goblet cells. The cilia beat toward the pharynx. Numerous small seromucous glands (*nasal glands*) produce a thin liquid secretion containing mucus. The mucosa of the middle and the inferior conchae is extensively infiltrated with *venous plexuses*, cavernous bodies, the filling of which can swell the mucosa up to a thickness of 5 mm.

The **olfactory organ** is formed in the olfactory region by the *olfactory mucosa*. It is distinguished from the mucosa of the respiratory region by its slightly brownish coloration and its greater thickness.

The olfactory mucosa contains *olfactory cells*, which are its primary and specific sensory cells. Their basal processes form the axons of the *olfactory nerves*. The lamina propria of the olfactory mucosa contains serous glands (*olfactory glands*).

d) Vessels and Nerves of the Nasal Cavity

The **arteries** for the walls of the nasal cavity arise from the *maxillary* and *ophthalmic arteries*.

The **maxillary artery** dispatches the *sphenopalatine artery*, which comes from the pterygopalatine fossa through the sphenopalatine foramen, arrives beneath the mucosa of the nasal cavity, and supplies the postero-lateral and medial walls of the nasal cavity with its terminal branches (→ p. 678).

The **ophthalmic artery** gives off the *anterior ethmoidal artery*, which passes first through the anterior ethmoidal foramen of the ethmoid bone into the anterior cranial fossa, then through the cribriform plate into the nasal cavity before ramifying in the anterior part of the nasal cavity at the lateral and medial walls.

The **veins** from the mucosa of the nasal cavity open into veins of the orbit, into the pterygoid plexus and into the facial veins. They communicate via these outlets with venous sinuses of the cranial dura in the cranial cavity.

Lymphatic pathways in the nasal mucosa pass to regional lymph nodes at two widely separated locations: in the region of the angle of the jaw and behind the upper level of the pharynx.

From the anterior part of the nasal mucosa, the lymph – together with lymph from the soft tissue mantle of the face – arrives at the *submandibular lymph nodes*. From the posterior part of the nasal cavity and from the paranasal sinuses, the lymph is conducted to the *retropharyngeal lymph nodes*, which lie behind the pharyngeal wall at the level of the 1st cervical vertebra, and to the upper *deep lateral cervical lymph nodes*.

The *sensory* **nerves** of the nasal cavity (Fig. **264**) arise from the *ophthalmic and maxillary nerves*. In their terminal ramifications, they also conduct autonomic nerve fibers to the mucosal glands.

The **ophthalmic nerve** gives off the *anterior ethmoidal nerve* via the *nasociliary nerve*. The anterior ethmoidal nerve accompanies the anterior ethmoidal artery into the anterior cranial fossa and from there arrives at the nasal cavity through the cribriform plate. It then gives off *lateral internal nasal branches* which supply the mucosa in the anterior region of the middle and inferior conchae, as well as in that part of the lateral wall located in front of the nasal conchae. Its *medial internal nasal branches* innervate the mucosa in the anterior portion of the nasal septum.

The **maxillary nerve** dispatches sensory fibers through the sphenopalatine foramen posterosuperiorly to the medial and lateral walls of the nasal cavity (→ p. 682).

The *parasympathetic* nerve fibers for the glands of the nasal mucosa arise (like those for the lacrimal gland) from the *greater petrosal nerve*. The postganglionic fibers from the *pterygopalatine ganglion* join the sensory fibers in the pterygopalatine fossa.

The *sympathetic* postganglionic nerve fibers from the carotid plexus, which course with the maxillary artery, also pass to the sensory fibers in the pterygopalatine fossa.

The **olfactory nerves** (Fig. **264**) pass from the olfactory region through the cribriform plate of the ethmoid bone to the *olfactory bulb* in the cranial cavity.

2. Oral Cavity

In the oral cavity, food is broken down into small pieces by the teeth, moistened by the saliva and, with the help of the tongue and cheek, packed and lubricated into morsels capable of being swallowed.

The *saliva* contains the enzyme, ptyalin, which breaks down starches. At the outlet of the oral cavity into the pharynx, the *swallowing reflex* is triggered. The character of the food is controlled by the well-developed *tactile sense* of the lips and the oral mucosa, as well as by the *sense of taste* in conjunction with the *sense of smell*. In the mouth, tones produced in the larynx are transformed into *speech*.

The **oral cavity** (Figs. **262** and **265**) begins at the *oral fissure* with the lips and extends to the oropharyngeal isthmus. The antero-lateral wall of the oral cavity is formed by the lips and cheeks, the roof by the hard and soft palates, the floor by muscles and other organ parts resting on them.

The two rows of teeth and the alveolar processes of the maxilla and mandible covered by the gingiva divide the oral cavity into the *vestibule* between the lips or cheeks and the rows of teeth and into the *oral cavity proper* inside of the rows of teeth. The vestibule and oral cavity proper communicate, apart from the interdental spaces, only between the last molar and the ramus of the mandible.

a) Vestibule of the Oral Cavity

The lips and cheeks – actively deformable with the help of their muscles – form the external wall of the vestibule. This wall can be expanded by food, fluid, and air; the contents of the "cheek pouch" thus formed can be moved by contraction of its musculature.

The **lips** (*labia oris*, Figs. **258** and **265**) are formed by the orbicularis oris muscle and are covered on the outside by facial skin, on the inside by oral mucosa. The transition zone bears the epithelium of the red of the lips. Laterally, at the transition to the cheek, the lips are united at the *angle of the mouth*. The facial skin of the lips possesses adult hair.

The *red of the lips* begins with a sharp boundary. It is covered by weakly cornified, stratified squamous epithelium, into which the lamina propria of the mucosa projects deeply with capillary loops in high papillae; the red color of the blood shines through the epithelium. Glands are absent, the epithelium being moistened when speaking and ingesting food. The red of the lip merges into the labial mucosa without a sharp border.

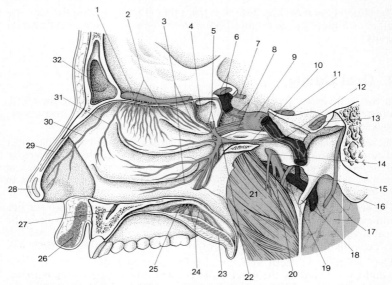

Fig. 264. **Pterygopalatine ganglion and nerves of lateral wall of nasal cavity** (after *Rauber-Kopsch*)

 1 Olfactory bulb
 2 Olfactory nerves
 3 Lateral and inferior posterior superior nasal branches
 4 Sphenoidal sinus
 5 Medial posterior superior nasal branches (severed)
 6 Optic nerve and internal carotid artery
 7 Oculomotor nerve
 8 Ophthalmic (upper) and maxillary (lower) nerves
 9 Trigeminal ganglion
10 Nerve of pterygoid canal, formed by union of greater petrosal and deep petrosal nerves
11 Trigeminal nerve
12 Internal carotid artery and internal carotid plexus
13 Facial and vestibulocochlear nerves at entrance into internal acoustic meatus

14 Mandibular nerve
15 Middle meningeal artery
16 Mastoid process
17 Facial nerve and parotid gland
18 Maxillary artery and styloid process
19 Chorda tympani and inferior alveolar nerve
20 Lingual nerve and nerve to medial pterygoid
21 Medial pterygoid muscle
22 Pterygopalatine ganglion
23 Soft palate
24 Lesser palatine nerves
25 Branches of greater palatine nerve
26 Orbicularis oris
27 Nasopalatine nerve in incisive canal
28 Greater alar cartilage
29 Lateral cartilage of nose
30, 31 Lateral internal nasal branches from anterior ethmoidal nerve
32 Frontal sinus

In an unconscious person, the danger that the lips become parched can be counteracted by an attendant's moistening them.

The *labial mucosa* is loosely connected with the orbicularis oris. Within the loose mucosal connective tissue, there are small salivary glands, (*labial glands*). At the time of puberty, sebaceous glands about the size of the head of a pin frequently develop, which can form a row extending into the buccal mucosa. Upper and lower lips are each connected with the gingiva by a median mucosal fold, the *inferior* and *superior labial frenulum*.

The **cheek** (Fig. 262) contains the buccinator muscle as a muscular foundation. Externally, the *buccal fat pad* adjoins this muscle in front of the anterior border of the masseter muscle.

The *buccal mucosa* is constituted like the labial mucosa; it possesses small salivary glands (*buccal glands*). The opening of the parotid duct projects into the vestibule opposite the 2nd upper molar tooth as a small mucosal papilla (*parotid papilla*).

Labial and buccal mucosae merge into the gingiva at the superior and inferior borders of the lip-cheek pocket.

The **gingiva** (Fig. 267), the mucous membrane over the alveolar processes, is firmly knit with the bone and extends into the interdental spaces in the form of interdental papillae. The gingival epithelium, which surrounds the neck of the tooth, is called *border epithelium*.

The rigid attachment of the gingiva at the alveolar process does not permit the spread of (e.g. inflammatory) fluid accumulations. In the looser mucosal connective tissue of the lips and cheeks, on the other hand, accumulations of fluid or blood can spread easily and lead to extensive swelling.

Malformations in the lip-jaw region. As a relatively frequent malformation (about 15% of all malformations), a cleft (*cleft lip, harelip*) appears in the lateral portion of the upper lip (border of medial nasal prominence and maxillary process). In severe degrees of cleft formation, a *cleft jaw* arises. A cleft formation of the palate behind the incisive fossa is designated as a *cleft palate*; it can be combined with a cleft lip. Depending on the extension of the palatal cleft, sucking is made difficult or impossible, and phonation is disturbed.

b) Dentition

The **teeth** separate the oral vestibule from the oral cavity proper (Fig. 262). The teeth in the upper and lower rows fit close together with their crowns and have no spaces (diastemae) in between except for small interdental spaces at the base of the crowns (Fig. 266).

In humans, *deciduous* (*milk*) *teeth* are formed first and subsequently superseded by *permanent teeth*; human teeth are *diphyodont*.

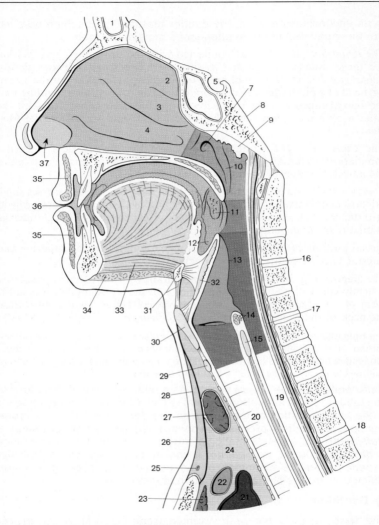

Fig. 265. **Organization of respiratory and digestive tracts in head and neck region**
Sagittal section near median plane, medial view

Vestibule of nasal cavity	☐	Oral cavity proper ☐
Nasal cavity	☐	Faucial isthmus ☐
Vestibule of larynx	☐	Nasopharynx ☐
Ventricle of larynx	☐	Oropharynx ☐
Infraglottic cavity	☐	Laryngopharynx ☐
Vestibule of oral cavity	☐	Connective tissue space of neck ☐

The **teeth** in humans are *variously formed* and fulfill varying functions. Of the front teeth, the chisel-shaped *incisors* serve to cut, whereas the adjoining pointed *canines* serve to hold fast. The lateral teeth (*molars*) are provided with blunt, broad, crowned surfaces for grinding the food. The human teeth are *heterodont*.

The two rows of teeth form the *upper* and the *lower dental arches*. The dental arch of the maxilla resembles a half ellipse, the lower arch a parabola. As a rule, the upper dental arch is somewhat broader than the lower so that the crowns of the maxillary teeth project over those of the mandibular teeth anteriorly and laterally.

Occlusion represents the position which both rows of teeth occupy with respect to each other when the jaw is closed; the crowns contact one another in the *occlusal plane*.

In lateral view, the occlusal plane forms (very often) an arch convex below (*curve of Spee*). It corresponds to the segment of a circular line which courses through the head of the mandible. The central point of the circle lies in the orbit.

In the case of *eugnathia*, the normal case, the two rows of teeth contact each other in the *normal bite*. In so doing, the crowns of the maxillary teeth are directed slightly obliquely outward toward the vestibule, the crowns of the mandibular teeth slightly inward toward the tongue. The cutting edges of the upper and lower incisors cut past each other like the blades of scissors. When the jaw is closed (closed occlusion), the cutting edges of the upper incisors lie in front of those of the lower. In the case of

---

◀ 1 Frontal sinus
2 Superior nasal concha
3 Middle nasal concha
4 Inferior nasal concha
5 Hypophysial fossa
6 Sphenoidal sinus
7 Pharyngeal opening of auditory tube, surrounded by salpingopalatine folds (in front), torus tubarius (above and behind) and torus levatorius (below)
8 Clivus
9 Pharyngeal tonsil
10 Salpingopharyngeal fold
11 Palatine tonsil between palatoglossal (in front) and palatopharyngeal (behind) arches
12 Epiglottic vallecula
13 Aryepiglottic folds
14 Arytenoid (oblique and transverse)
15 Lamina of cricoid cartilage
16 Prevertebral layer of cervical fascia
17 "Retrovisceral space" ("retropharynx")
18 Endothoracic fascia (as continuation of prevertebral layer of cervical fascia)

19 Esophagus
20 Trachea
21 Aortic arch, exit of left common carotid artery
22 Left brachiocephalic vein
23 Thymus
24 Previsceral space
25 Venous jugular arch in "suprasternal space"
26 Pretracheal layer of cervical fascia
27 Isthmus of thyroid gland
28 Superficial layer of cervical fascia
29 Arch of cricoid cartilage
30 Lamina of thyroid cartilage
31 Body of hyoid bone and median thyrohyoid ligament
32 Epiglottis
33 Geniohyoid
34 Mylohyoid
35 Orbicularis oris in lips of mouth
36 Aperture of mouth
37 Naris (nostril)

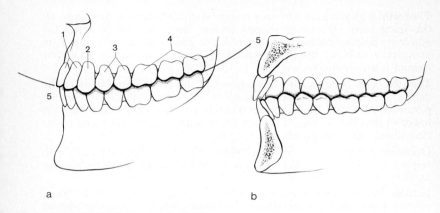

Fig. 266. **Adult dentition in occlusion**
a Left half of dentition, lateral view
b Right half of dentition, medial view
1 Incisors
2 Canines
3 Premolars

4 Molars
5 Plane of occlusion (Spee's curve)

the molars, the external masticatory margin of the upper teeth covers the lower, whereas the inner masticatory margin of the lower teeth projects toward the tongue.

An *end-to-end* (*forceps*) *bite* represents an arrangement in which the cutting edges of the upper incisors strike those of the lower. This type of bite rarely occurs as a *normal biting pattern* (racial characteristic). It occurs mostly as a *defective position*.

Dysgnathia (faulty position of teeth in the case of an anomaly of the jaw) is the result of an abnormal development in the masticatory system which usually affects all parts of the system – teeth, holding apparatus of the teeth, maxilla and mandible, temporomandibular joint, muscles of mastication and of facial expression, tongue.

Prognathism (protrusion of the mandible), which is usually inherited, is characterized by an abnormal prominence of the chin and a reciprocal supraocclusion (overbite) of the front teeth.

In the case of a **complete overbite** (back position of mandible, deep overbite), also usually inherited, the upper front teeth completely cover the lower. A strong sagittal development of the middle of the face (large nasal profile) and the maxilla, with a less-developed mandible, is associated with this condition.

Occlusion abnormalities cause disturbances in swallowing, nasal respiration and the forming of speech.

Antagonists. The cooperation of the teeth in biting is called *articulation*. Since the maxillary teeth are displaced distally against the mandibular teeth by not quite the width of half a tooth, three teeth always cooperate during mastication. The same teeth of both jaws form the *main antagonists*; the third partner of the triad is the *accessory antagonist*. Only the lower 1st incisor and the 3rd upper molar have only one antagonist. If a tooth loses its antagonists, it grows out over the occlusion plane of the remaining teeth.

The movements of both dental arches carried out against one another in **articulation** are designated as *protrusive occlusion, lateral excursion, closure occlusion* (resting position). During articulation, a physiological *grinding* of the teeth occurs which contributes to the maintenance of a broad contact of both rows of teeth in closure occlusion.

Orientation of the teeth in the jaw. The masticatory surface of the tooth is the *occlusal surface*. The external surface turned toward the oral vestibule is designated as the *vestibular surface* (*labial* or *buccal*); the internal surface directed toward the oral cavity proper is referred to as the *lingual surface*. The crowns of adjacent teeth touch with the *contact surface* (approximal surface). The approximal surface turned toward the median plane is *mesial* (proximal), whereas the approximal surface turned away from the median plane is *distal*.

Teeth and Tooth Holding Apparatus

Structure of the tooth (Fig. 267). Three parts can be differentiated in each tooth. The *crown* (*corona*) projects into the oral cavity and bears the cutting edge or the masticatory surface. The *root* is implanted in the dental alveolus. The marginal zone between the crown and root, which is embraced by the gingiva, is the *neck* (*cervix*).

The hard substances of the tooth surround the *pulp cavity*. This cavity contains the *pulp* and continues toward the root into the *root canal* which opens at the *apex of the root* as the *apical foramen*.

Each tooth consists of three *hard substances*: dentin, enamel, cementum. The *dentin* forms the main mass, the nucleus of the tooth, and borders the pulp cavity. In the region of the crown, the dentin is overlaid by *enamel*; at the root, it is covered by *cementum*. In the cementum, the bundles of collagenous fibers are anchored to the periodontal membrane.

The zone of contact between enamel and cementum at the neck can be formed differently on the four sides of the same tooth. Usually, the enamel overlaps the cementum (45%). The enamel and cementum can meet (30%) or not make contact (15%, dentin lies exposed). Rarely, the enamel is covered by the cementum (10%).

Dentin contains the same chemical constituents as osseous tissue, but in different ratios. In contrast to enamel, it can be formed throughout life as *substitute dentin* deposited by odontoblasts and consisting of a calcified

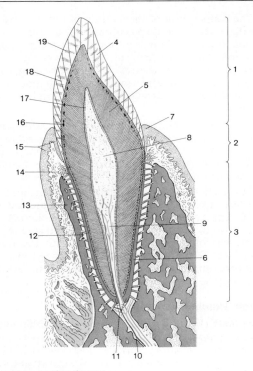

Fig. 267. Tooth and supporting tissues
Schematic sagittal section through lower incisor, mesial view of cut surface

1 Crown (clinical crown)
2 Neck
3 Root
4 Enamel
5 Dentin
6 Cementum
7 Gingiva
8 Pulp cavity with pulp
9 Root canal
10 Vessels and nerves to pulp and periodontium

11 Apex of root and apical foramen
12 Periodontal ligament
13 Alveolar arch (alveolar part of mandible, vestibular side)
14 Circular ligament of tooth
15 External and internal border epithelium
16 Interglobular dentin
17 Layer of odontoblasts
18 Incremental lines of Retzius
19 Hunter-Schreger lines

ground substance (cement substance), in which bundles of collagenous fibers are deposited. These course predominantly in the longitudinal direction of the tooth. The *odontoblasts* lie as an epithelial sheet at the predentin-pulp border (predentin = uncalcified precursor of dentin).

Odontoblasts dispatch long cytoplasmic processes (*Tomes' fibers*) into the dentinal tubules. These fibers course radially – ascending slightly in the region of the crown – to the irregularly shaped, humpbacked enamel-dentin border; in part, they also enter the enamel for a short distance.

The portion of the inorganic substance (predominantly hydroxyapatite) is just about 70% lower than in the enamel, the hardness correspondingly less (but somewhat greater than in bone). After eruption – dependent on the extent of abrasion of the crown – substitute dentin develops so that the pulp cavity is not opened.

Enamel is avascular and aneural and consists of enamel prisms, which course from the enamel-dentin border to the enamel surface and which are united by a calcified organic cement substance. On non-abrased teeth, a resistant cuticle (*cuticula dentis*) about 1 μm thick covers the enamel surface.

The enamel, the hardest substance of the human body, consists of 96–97% inorganic substance (about 90% in the form of hydroxyapatite). Longitudinal ground sections show alternating dark and light stripes (*Hunter-Schreger bands*) near the dentin based on interference. Transverse ground sections exhibit the incremental *lines of Retzius* running parallel to the surface and caused by the rhythmic depositions of calcium.

In its construction and content of about 65% inorganic substances, *cementum* corresponds closely to network bone. It covers the dentin of the entire root. In the cementum, the bundles of collagenous fibers are anchored to the periodontal membrane.

The *dental pulp* fills up the pulp cavity with a gelatinous connective tissue.

The precapillary artery entering the root canal through the *apical foramen* ramifies just above the foramen into several branches which form an extensive capillary network below the layer of odontoblasts. From a network of poorly myelinated nerve fibers also situated below this layer, fine fibrils pass between the odontoblasts into the predentin and for a distance into the dentin within the dentinal tubules. These nerves perceive the pressure exerted by the masticatory muscles when the tooth is under stress and influences reflexly the tonicity of these muscles.

By means of the **periodontium**, a system of collagenous fibers, the tooth is anchored like a spring in the alveolus (gomphosis). The fibers course in different directions between the alveolar wall and the cementum. The periodontal membrane is covered and protected by the gingiva.

From the alveolar margin, tracts of fibers descending obliquely towards the apex of the root offer resistance against the masticatory pressure. Fibers which ascend toward the crown to the neck of the tooth counteract a traction at the tooth. The fiber bundles radiate, for the most part, tangentially into the cementum so that the tooth cannot be turned (enough to mention) in the alveolus around its longitudinal axis. Above the alveolar margin, horizontal fibers which course from the cementum to the cementum connect neighboring teeth. In the connective tissue layer of the gingiva, there are strong fibrous tracts which radiate into the margin of the gingiva from the cementum to the enamel-cementum border, but which also embrace the neck in a circular and figure-of-eight fashion (*ligamentum circulare dentis*).

The periodontal membrane possesses a rich *vascular network* in the spatial gaps between the fiber bundles. The network is fed by lateral twigs of the artery entering the apical foramen and vessels in the marrow spaces of the alveolar processes. The periodontal membrane is also supplied by *sensory nerves* (pressure sensitive).

The **holding apparatus of the teeth** (*periodontium*) is formed by all structures participating in the attachment of the tooth: *cementum, alveolar wall, periodontal membrane* and *gingiva*. They experience their typical molding jointly with the development of the root and the eruption of the tooth.

Movements of the tooth in the alveolus occur during mastication. The tooth is moved insignificantly in the longitudinal direction and is tilted toward the vestibule or oral cavity around a transverse axis which lies roughly in the middle of the root. The tooth thus acts as a two-armed lever; pressure and traction zones arise between the tooth and the alveolar wall. Insignificant tilting movements in the mesial or distal direction are absorbed by adjacent teeth via contact points of the approximal surfaces.

The loss of a neighboring tooth leads to increased mobility of a tooth and to damage of the tissue at the alveolar entrance which can be so considerable that the tooth is inclined into the adjacent space (diastema). Early replacement of a lost tooth is indicated.

Dental Formula and Eruption

Dental formula. The *permanent human dentition* consists of $4 \times 8 = 32$ *permanent teeth*. In each half of the jaw there follows from mesial to distal (Fig. **266**):

2 *Incisors* (I) ⎱
1 *Canine* (C) ⎰ Frontal Teeth

2 *Premolars* (P) ⎱
3 *Molars* (M)   ⎰ Lateral Teeth

The *number and sequence of individual teeth* of the dentition can be expressed in brief form by the *dental formula*, which is noted for only one half of the jaw when there is a symmetrical formation of the dentition in the upper and lower jaw. For the *permanent teeth* it reads:
I2, C, P2, M3.

For the *designation of a tooth*, it was customary earlier to *count* the teeth of each half of the jaw (each fourth of the dentition = quadrant) *from mesial to distal* and to identify each tooth with a perpendicular line in relation to the *median line* and with a horizontal line in relation to the *occlusal plane*.

Example:

⌐ 3 is the left lower canine.

Now there is an international agreement for the *identification of the individual tooth* as a two-digit number which can be typewritten and stored in a computer. Each half of the jaw is coded by a number to which the number of the individual tooth is added. In permanent dentition, the right half of the maxilla is coded with the number 1, the left half of the maxilla with the number 2. The left half of the mandible is identified with the digit 3, the right half of the mandible with the digit 4. With this international system, the left lower canine tooth is thus clearly identified by the number 33.

The quadrants of the deciduous dentition are designated by the digits 5 (= right maxillary half and following clockwise), 6, 7 and 8.

The *deciduous dentition* contains 4 × 5 = 20 *deciduous teeth*; from mesial to distal they are: 2 *incisors*, 1 *canine*, 2 "deciduous molars".

Tooth development and eruption. The deciduous and permanent teeth are already programmed during fetal development. The teeth break through in two phases: the deciduous teeth in the *1st dentition*, the permanent teeth in the *2nd dentition*. The *deciduous teeth* erupt, as a rule, between the 6th and the 24th postnatal month, the permanent teeth between the 6th (7th) and 14th (30th) year. The mandibular teeth usually erupt somewhat earlier than the corresponding maxillary teeth. The *time of eruption*, however, can vary considerably.

The following data present the average pattern:

		Tooth Eruption		Sequence
1.	Dentition:	I	6–8th month	1	
		II	8–12th month	2	
		III	15–20th month	4	
		IV	12–16th month	3	"1st deciduous molar"
		V	20–40th month	5	"2nd deciduous molar"
2.	Dentition:	1	6–9th year	2	
		2	7–10th year	3	
		3	9–14th year	5	
		4	9–13th year	4	
		5	11–14th year	6	
		6	6–8th year	1	"six-year molar"
		7	10–14th year	7	"twelve-year molar"
		8	16–30th year	8	"wisdom tooth"

During the second dentition, the *incisors* and *canine teeth*, as well as the "*deciduous molars*" are replaced by teeth of a 2nd dental generation, by *substitute teeth*. The deciduous teeth serve as proxies for the substitute teeth. The three *molars* of the

2nd dentition, however, are actually teeth of the 1st generation which erupt "belatedly" and are therefore designated as *incremental teeth*. Incremental teeth can erupt depending on the growth of the jaw. If the jaw is retarded in growth, the 3rd molar does not erupt.

Shape of Teeth (Figs. 266 and 274)

The individual teeth are distinguished with regard to their form and task. The shape of the individual teeth, their arrangement in the jaw and the construction of the temporomandibular joint and masticatory musculature conform to the versatile, *omnivorous* feeding habits of man.

The **incisors** serve to bite off bits of food; they have a chisel-shaped crown with a sharp horizontal cutting edge.

Through use and as a result of occlusion, this edge is ground off behind in the upper teeth and in front in the lower. The oral surface bears a projection, the *dental tubercle*. The lateral surfaces of the crown are approximately triangular. Incisors have a long, conical root, somewhat flattened laterally. The upper incisors are broader than the lower.

The **canines** serve to tear and grasp the food. As the longest tooth, they are protected against tilting stress by a long root, especially the canines of the maxilla in the frontal-nasal pillar of the facial skeleton.

The crown has two cutting edges which run toward the *masticatory apex*. The root is simple, strong, long and flattened laterally.

The **premolar teeth** carry out grinding movements; they possess a *masticatory surface* (occlusion surface) and a two-cusped crown.

The root is longitudinally grooved on the approximal side; in the *upper* premolars, it is frequently split into a vestibular and an oral root. Even if the division is absent, two root canals are (usually) formed. The root of the *lower* premolar tooth is not divided; a double root canal is rare.

The **molar teeth** perform the greatest part of the masticatory work. They lie in, or approximately in, the course direction of the masticatory muscles so that a strong masticatory pressure can be produced between the masticatory surfaces which is absorbed by the division of the root and the enlargement of the periodontium. The *masticatory surface* of the molars bears (usually) four cusps which are so positioned that in the closure of the dentition, the cusps of the upper molars fit into the furrows between the cusps of the lower molars and vice versa.

The 1st molar has the largest grinding surface. The *upper* molars have two vestibular roots and an oral root: the *lower* molars have a mesial (anterior) and a distal (posterior) root. The 3rd molars (wisdom teeth) vary considerably in the formation of their crowns and roots.

To distinguish between symmetrical right and left teeth, the following characteristics are used:
– *curvature*: corresponding to the form of the dental arch, the distal portion of the

vestibular surface of the crown of the tooth is more weakly curved than the proximal portion;

- *root*: the roots are directed somewhat obliquely distally;
- *angle*: masticatory edges and contact surfaces form a sharp angle mesially; distally the transition is rounded.

All three characteristics can be demonstrated at the upper incisors; they are lacking in the lower middle incisors. The lower lateral incisors usually exhibit the angle characteristic, whereas the canines show the curvature and root characteristics. The premolars can be distinguished generally on the basis of their root characteristic; in the molars, the curvature characteristic can be used.

With the exception of the "deciduous molars", the **deciduous teeth** resemble the permanent teeth in their form. In distinction to the latter, the deciduous teeth appear bluish-white and exhibit porcelain-like transparency. They are less strongly calcified than the permanent teeth. The bulky arrangement of the roots of the "deciduous molars" is of practical importance: the primordium of the substitute tooth always lies between these roots.

c) Vessels and Nerves of the Teeth and the Periodontium

The **arteries** to the teeth, the alveolar processes and the gingiva (Fig. **277**) are branches of the *maxillary artery*. The *posterior superior alveolar artery* supplies the upper lateral teeth; branches of the *infra-orbital artery* pass to the upper frontal teeth; the *inferior alveolar artery* courses in the mandibular canal to the teeth of the mandible.

The **veins** (Fig. **278**), which course in company with the arteries, carry the blood to the *pterygoid plexus*.

The **lymphatic tracts** (Fig. **272**) from the alveoli and from the buccal gingiva of the maxilla pass across the check to the *submandibular lymph nodes*; those from the oral gingiva drain into the *deep lateral cervical lymph nodes*. From the mandibular alveoli and from the mandibular gingiva, the lymph flows anteriorly to the *submental lymph nodes*, laterally to the *submandibular lymph nodes*.

The **nerves** to the maxilla (Figs. **268** and **273**) arise from the *maxillary nerve*, those to the mandible (Figs. **261** and **269**) from the *mandibular nerve*.

Superior alveolar nerves from the *infra-orbital nerve* pass to the *maxilla*. They form the *superior dental plexus*, which sends out the *superior gingival branches* to the buccal gingiva and the *superior dental branches* to the roots of the teeth. Branches of the *greater palatine nerve* pass to the palatal gingiva; only in the region of the incisor teeth is the palatal gingiva innervated by the *nasopalatine nerve*.

To anesthetize the teeth and gingiva of the maxilla, the anesthetic must be injected in several places.

In the *mandible*, the *inferior alveolar nerve* forms the *inferior dental plexus* in the mandibular canal. It innervates the mandibular teeth with the *inferior dental branches* and the vestibular gingiva with the *inferior gingival branches*, except for the region of the 2nd premolar and 1st molar, where the buccal gingiva of the mandible, like the buccal mucosa, is supplied by the *buccal nerve*.

To anesthetize the mandibular region, nerve blocks must be placed both for the inferior alveolar nerve (at the mandibular foramen) and for the buccal and lingual nerves.

d) Oral Cavity Proper

The **oral cavity proper** (Figs. **262** and **265**) is the space between the rows of teeth and the oropharyngeal isthmus. It is bordered above by the *roof of the oral cavity*, the hard and the soft palate, below by the *floor of the oral cavity* and is filled up mainly by the *tongue*. At the floor of the mouth, the sublingual gland with its excretory duct bulges the mucosa on both sides of the tongue. The *palatine tonsils* are inserted between each of the two palatal arches on the right and left sides of the oropharyngeal isthmus.

The **oral mucosa** is composed of noncornified stratified squamous epithelium (except for the "cornified" apices of the filiform papillae) and mucosal connective tissue, which in places sends tall connective tissue papillae into the epithelium. A muscularis mucosae is absent. The *submucosa* consists of loose connective tissue in which adipose tissue, salivary glands and conducting paths are embedded. The submucosa is absent at the hard palate and the gingiva; at the back of the tongue, it is replaced by a compact connective tissue plate, the *lingual aponeurosis*.

Floor of the Oral Cavity

The **muscular floor of the oral cavity** consists of the mylohyoid, geniohyoid and digastric muscles. They communicate directly or indirectly with the hyoid bone and, as the *higher suprahyoid muscles*, are opposed to the lower infrahyoid musculature of the neck. The stylohyoid also belongs to the suprahyoid muscles. It influences the position and the state of tension of the floor of the mouth and, therefore, will be discussed with the remaining suprahyoid muscles.

The primordia for the suprahyoid muscles arise from different sources, from the mandibular arch, the hyoid arch and from the somatic musculature. Accordingly, the muscles are innervated differently.

The **mylohyoid muscle** (Figs. **262**, **268** and **275**) arises bilaterally at the inner side of the mandible in the region of the mylohyoid line. Both muscle parts converge behind and unite at a medial raphe to form a muscular plate which attaches at the body of the hyoid and connects both mandibular halves. The two mylohyoid muscles form the *diaphragma oris*.

Innervation: mylohyoid nerve from the mandibular nerve.

The **geniohyoid muscle** (Figs. **262**, **268** and **271**) lies above the mylohyoid (toward the oral cavity). It passes from the mental spine at the inner surface of the chin to the body of the hyoid bone.

Innervation: ramus to the geniohyoid muscle (fibers from the ventral rami of the 1st and 2nd cervical nerves, which are attached to the hypoglossal nerve for a long distance).

The **digastric muscle** (Figs. **262**, **275** and **280**) arises with its posterior belly at the mastoid notch of the temporal bone and passes obliquely forward and downward. Near the hyoid bone it goes over into an intermediate tendon which is embraced by the clefted stylohyoid muscle and which is fixed to the hyoid bone by a tendinous band. The anterior belly – located toward the skin from the mylohyoid – originates from the intermediate tendon and inserts in the digastric fossa at the inner surface of the mandible near the lower margin.

Innervation of the anterior belly from the mylohyoid nerve and of the posterior belly from the facial nerve.

The **stylohyoid muscle** (Figs. **275** and **280**) arises from the styloid process of the temporal bone. Its belly divides and embraces the intermediate tendon of the digastric. It inserts at the body and greater horn of the hyoid bone.

Innervation: facial nerve.

Action of the suprahyoid muscles. The upper hyoid muscles, acting in unison with the infrahyoid muscles, suspend the hyoid bone in a certain position, thus determining the position and state of tension of the floor of the mouth at the same time.

The *muscles of the floor of the mouth* draw the hyoid forward and upward during the *act of swallowing*. The contracted mylohyoid muscles form the support for the tongue, for example, when it presses food against the hard palate.

The *geniohyoid muscle* (in cooperation with the mylohyoid muscle) draws the hyoid bone forward, whereas the *stylohyoid muscle* draws it backward and upward.

The hyoid bone is raised by the *digastric muscle*. During positional changes of the hyoid bone, the tongue is moved into a favorable initial position parallel with the bone.

The *muscles at the floor of the mouth* that are attached at the mandible can lower the mandible (*open the jaw*) by contracting bilaterally. This opening movement occurs in synchronization with the sphincter muscles of the jaw (masticatory muscles) and is supported by the inferior head of the lateral pterygoid and, when the body is held erect, by the force of gravity.

Conduction paths at the floor of the mouth (Figs. **268** and **270**). The loose and fat-rich connective tissue in which the sublingual gland is embedded

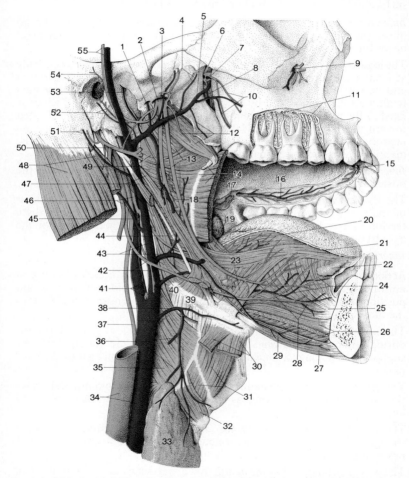

Fig. 268. **Arteries and nerves at floor of mouth and pharyngeal wall** (skeletal and muscular presentation partly after *Pernkopf*)

carries conduction tracts. The *submandibular duct* passes across the posterior margin of the mylohyoid on the floor of the mouth.

The **lingual nerve** crosses the submandibular duct at the level of the 3rd lower molar, lateral to the hyoglossus, from lateral posterosuperior to medial antero-inferior and then passes upward into the lingual mucosa. The *submandibular ganglion* lies close to the lingual nerve near the posterior border of the mylohyoid.

The **hypoglossal nerve** passes beneath the submandibular duct and laterally past the hyoglossus muscle into the musculature of the tongue.

◀ 1–5 *Vessels and nerves in infratemporal fossa*
1 Middle meningeal artery
2 Mandibular nerve
3 Masseteric artery and nerve
4 Deep temporal arteries and nerves
5 Maxillary artery
6 Maxillary nerve
7 Pterygopalatine ganglion
8 Descending palatine artery (right) and greater palatine artery (right)
9 Infra-orbital artery and nerve
10 Branches of posterior superior alveolar artery and posterior superior alveolar branches of infra-orbital nerve
11 Superior dental and superior gingival branches of superior dental plexus
12 Tensor veli palatini, buccal artery and nerve
13 Levator veli palatini and lingual nerve
14 Pterygoid hamulus, pterygomandibular raphe, buccinator (severed)
15 Nasopalatine nerve
16 Greater palatine artery (left) and greater palatine nerve (left)
17 Lesser palatine arteries (left) and nerves (left)
18 Inferior alveolar artery and nerve with exit of arterial branch and mylohyoid nerve
19 Palatine tonsil and palatoglossus
20 Dorsales linguae branches of lingual artery and branches of glossopharyngeal nerve
21 Lingual aponeurosis
22 Anterior lingual glands
23 Hyoglossus and submandibular ganglion
24 Branches of arteria profunda linguae and lingual branches of lingual nerve
25 Genioglossus
26 Geniohyoid and mylohyoid (severed)
27 Anterior belly of digastric
28 Lingual branches of hypoglossal nerve
29 Submental artery and mylohyoid nerve
30 Hyoid bone, sternohyoid and omohyoid muscles (severed)
31 Thyrohyoid and sternothyroid (sectioned)
32 Cricothyroid
33 Thyroid gland with anterior and posterior glandular branches of superior thyroid artery
34 Common carotid artery and internal jugular vein (sectioned)
35 Inferior pharyngeal constrictor
36 Sternocleidomastoid and posterior glandular branch of superior thyroid artery
37 Vagus nerve
38 Superior thyroid artery
39 Infrahyoid branch of superior thyroid artery, superior laryngeal artery and internal branch of superior laryngeal nerve
40 Lingual artery
41 Internal carotid artery with carotid sinus, branch to carotid sinus and carotid body
42 Hypoglossal nerve and superior root of ansa cervicalis
43 Middle pharyngeal constrictor, external carotid artery and facial artery with exit of ascending palatine artery
44 Stylohyoid ligament
45 Occipital artery
46 Glossopharyngeal and accessory nerves (severed)
47 Styloglossus, stylohyoid (severed) and stylopharyngeus
48 Sternocleidomastoid and posterior belly of digastric (severed)
49 Superior pharyngeal constrictor and pharyngobasilar fascia
50 Facial nerve (severed) with exit of digastric and stylohyoid branches as well as entrance of communicating branches with facial nerve
51 Posterior auricular artery and nerve
52 Deep auricular artery and nerve of external acoustic meatus
53 Anterior tympanic artery and chorda tympani
54 Anterior auricular nerves of auriculotemporal nerve
55 Superficial temporal artery and auriculotemporal nerve

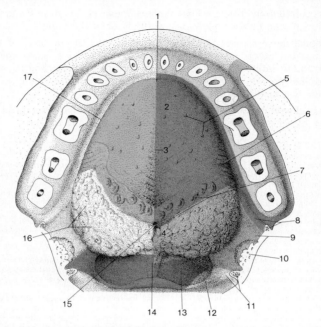

Fig. 269. **Surface of tongue**, schematic horizontal section at level of mouth orifice and necks of teeth

Innervation of mucous membrane of lower lip, cheeks and tongue, as well as gingiva and teeth of mandible (innervation regions partly after *Scharlau*; overlappings of maximal regions not considered)

Sensory innervation regions of:

Trigeminal nerve   ☐ ☐ ☐ ◼
   Mental   ☐
   Buccal   ☐
   Inferior alveolar   ☐
   Lingual   ◼
Glossopharyngeal nerve   ☐
Vagus nerve   ◼

Sensory innervation regions
(taste fibers) of:
Nervus intermedius portion of facial
nerve (chorda tympani)   ☐
Glossopharyngeal nerve   ☐
Vagus nerve   ◼

The hypoglossal nerve is accompanied by the **companion vein of the hypoglossal nerve**. The **lingual artery** courses to the tongue, on the other hand, medial to the hyoglossus muscle.

Tongue

During mastication, the tongue moves the food particles between the rows of teeth and crushes them against the hard palate. It presses the food into the pharyngeal isthmus during *swallowing*, creates a subatmospheric pressure during *sucking* (carrying back of the tongue like an ejector piston) and, as an *organ of speech*, assists in the formation of consonants. The rich innervation of the mucosa transforms the tongue into a highly sensitive *tactile instrument*, and the development of taste buds makes it the main *gustatory organ*.

The **tongue** (Figs. **262** and **269–271**) lies on the floor of the mouth. It consists of a muscular body which is covered by a mucous membrane. The *extrinsic muscles* radiating from the mandible, hyoid and styloid process equip the tongue on the whole with great *mobility*; the *interior muscles* – partly processes of the extrinsic muscles – give it a great *deformability*.

The tongue comprises a posterior part, the *root*, and an anterior portion, the *body*, which runs out into the rounded *apex*. A superficially-visible boundary between the root and body exists at the *back* (*dorsum*) *of the tongue* in the V-shaped *sulcus terminalis*, whose apex is directed posteriorly.

The **root of the tongue** borders on the pharynx and larynx. Its dorsal surface, which lies posterior to the sulcus terminalis and is designated as the *pharyngeal* (postsulcal) *part*, is not visible even in the outstretched tongue. In the resting position of the tongue, with the body held erect, it is directed vertically dorsad and is referred to as the *base of the tongue*. The surface configuration of this area is determined by the *lingual tonsil*.

The *lingual tonsil* consists of subepithelial accumulations of lymphatic nodules (*lingual follicles*) which are organized around *crypts* and give the base of the tongue a bosselated appearance. The individual elevations with a diameter of 1–5 mm are called *lingual nodules*. *Posterior lingual glands* can open into the crypts of the lingual nodules.

---

1 Apex of tongue
2 Dorsum of tongue, oral (presulcal) part
3 Median lingual groove
4 Dorsum of tongue, pharyngeal (postsulcal) part
5 Fungiform papillae
6 Foliate papillae
7 Vallate papillae and sulcus terminalis
8 Palatoglossal arch and palatoglossus muscle

9 Triangular fold
10 Palatine tonsil
11 Palatopharyngeal arch and palatopharyngeus muscle
12 Lateral glosso-epiglottic fold
13 Vallecula
14 Median glosso-epiglottic fold
15 Foramen caecum
16 Lingual tonsils
17 Margin of tongue

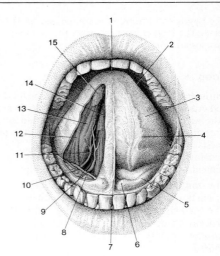

Fig. 270. **Inferior surface of tongue and floor of mouth** (mucous membrane removed on right side, anterior lingual and sublingual glands visible)

 1 Apex of tongue
 2 Margin of tongue
 3 Inferior surface of tongue
 4 Plica fimbriata
 5 Sublingual fold
 6 Sublingual papilla
 7 Frenulum
 8 Sublingual gland
 9 Arteria and vena profunda linguae
10 Submandibular duct
11 Lingual nerve
12 Hyoglossus
13 Inferior longitudinal muscle of tongue
14 Genioglossus
15 Anterior lingual gland

At the **body of the tongue**, the part of the dorsum situated in front of the sulcus terminalis is designated as the *oral (presulcal) part*. At rest, it lies horizontally and faces the palate. The shallow *median lingual groove* divides this part of the dorsum of the tongue into right and left halves. At the apex of the sulcus terminalis, there is a small depression, the *foramen caecum*. It marks the site of origin of the thyroid gland (point of exit of the thyroglossal duct).

The *margin of the tongue (lingual margin)* marks off the dorsum from the *inferior surface of the body*. On the inferior surface, the *frenulum of the tongue* passes from the floor of the mouth as a median mucosal fold. Laterally, there is a raised mucosal fold with a jagged margin, the *fimbriated fold (plica fimbriata)*, which is not always distinctly visible and which is a remnant of the inferior tongue of prosimians. Medial to it, the large *vena profunda linguae* shines bluish through the mucosa. The *anterior lingual glands* lie at the apex of the tongue on both sides of the frenulum.

The **tongue muscles** insert primarily at the *lingual aponeurosis*, a strong connective tissue plate below the mucosa of the dorsum of the tongue. Muscle fibers also radiate into the *lingual septum*, a vertically oriented connective tissue layer which incompletely divides the tongue in the median plane. Extrinsic and intrinsic muscles are aligned in the muscular body of the tongue in three main spatial directions.

Innervation of the extrinsic and intrinsic muscles of the tongue: hypoglossal nerve.

The **extrinsic muscles** (Figs. **262**, **268** and **271**), the *genioglossus, hyoglossus* and *styloglossus*, collectively move the tongue.

From its origin at the mental spine of the mandible, the **genioglossus** spreads fan-like into the muscular body of the tongue and attaches at the aponeurosis.

The muscle lies on the geniohyoid and is separated medially from the same-named muscle of the opposite side by the lingual septum; it is covered laterally by the hyoglossus muscle.

The **hyoglossus muscle** spreads out as a rectangular muscular plate between the greater horn of the hyoid bone, as well as a small portion of the body of the hyoid, and the lateral margin of the lingual aponeurosis.

The hyoglossus is separated from the genioglossus by the inferior longitudinal muscle of the tongue (an intrinsic muscle) and – when present – by the chondroglossus muscle; laterally, it is covered by the mylohyoid, digastric and stylohyoid muscles.

The **chondroglossus** is a variably-formed, delicate muscle which passes from the lesser horn of the hyoid to the lingual aponeurosis. It lies on the genioglossus and is covered by the hyoglossus.

The **styloglossus muscle** radiates from the styloid process (and the stylomandibular ligament) into the tongue at the level of the palatopharyngeal arch.

The main portion of the fibers courses at the margin of the tongue to the apex of the tongue (longitudinal tract of muscle); individual bundles of fibers bend around medially and attach to the fibers of the transverse muscle of the tongue (an intrinsic muscle).

Action of the muscles on the tongue. The *tongue* is:
- *brought forward* by the bilateral contraction of the longitudinal fiber tracts of the genioglossus anchored at the base of the tongue, so that it can be projected out of the oral cavity with the help of the intrinsic muscles; at the same time, the geniohyoids draw the hyoid bone forward and bring the tongue into a favorable initial position;
- *drawn backward* by the styloglossus of both sides which act like a bridle, while the simultaneous contraction of the hyoglossus presses the tongue toward the floor of the mouth; the hyoid bone is drawn backward by the stylohyoid muscle; and
- *led to one side* by the contraction of the styloglossus of the same side and the genioglossus of the opposite side.

The *apex of the tongue* is:
- *raised* by the contraction of the styloglossi muscles, together with the fibers of the genioglossi muscles attaching at the base of the tongue; and
- *depressed* by the most anterior fiber bundles of the genioglossus.

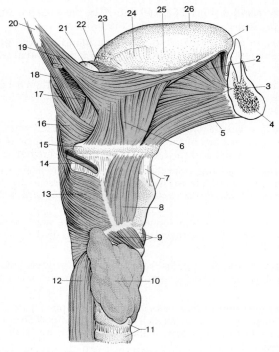

Fig. 271. **Lingual and pharyngeal musculature** (after *Rauber-Kopsch*)

1 Apex of tongue
2 Inferior longitudinal muscle
3 Genioglossus
4 Mandible
5 Geniohyoid
6 Hyoglossus
7 Laryngeal prominence and median thyrohyoid ligament
8 Thyrohyoid
9 Cricothyroid muscle and cricothyroid ligament
10 Thyroid gland
11 Trachea
12 Esophagus, longitudinal muscle layer
13 Inferior pharyngeal constrictor

14 Superior laryngeal artery and internal branch of superior laryngeal nerve
15 Hyoid bone, greater horn
16 Middle pharyngeal constrictor
17 Superior pharyngeal constrictor
18 Stylopharyngeus
19 Styloglossus and stylohyoid muscle (severed)
20 Styloid process
21 Palatine tonsil
22 Palatoglossus
23 Vallate papillae
24 Foliate papillae
25 Margin of tongue
26 Dorsum of tongue, oral part

The *margin of the tongue* of the same side is:
– *depressed* by the unilateral contraction of the hyoglossus muscle.

The **intrinsic muscles** deform the tongue. They consist of:
– *vertical* fiber tracts, **vertical muscle of the tongue**, which, in the non-contracted state, course slightly arched to the lingual aponeurosis;

- *longitudinal* bundles of muscle which, as the **superior longitudinal muscle of the tongue**, pass into a uniform muscular layer below the lingual aponeurosis and which, as the paired **inferior longitudinal muscle of the tongue**, course from the root of the tongue to its apex between the genioglossus and hyoglossus muscles; and
- *transverse* muscle fibers, the **transverse muscle of the tongue**, which attach mostly at the lingual septum, a smaller number passing through the septum without interruption.

In the *deformation of the tongue*, usually two of the intrinsic muscles act as antagonists of the third; in their contraction, they force its elongation. By the contraction of the *transverse* and *vertical* fiber tracts, the longitudinal muscles are extended, and the tongue becomes narrow and long. By the contraction of the *longitudinal* and *transverse* muscles, the vertical muscles are stretched, and the tongue becomes short and high. When the *longitudinal* and *vertical* muscles are contracted, it stretches the transverse muscles, and the tongue becomes short, low and broad.

Paralysis of the hypoglossal nerve on one side causes the outstretched apex of tongue to point to the side of the paralysis, to which it is directed by the contracted genioglossus of the healthy side.

The **mucous membrane of the tongue** is loosely connected with the *inferior side* of the body of the tongue and, in the middle, forms the frenulum, which passes to the gingiva of the mandible. On the *dorsum of the tongue*, the mucosa is attached immovably at the compact *lingual aponeurosis* (Figs. **262** and **269**); the mucosal epithelium is firmly invaginated by *high papillae* from the mucosal connective tissue. The epithelium of the mucosa is stratified squamous, nonkeratinized.

Lingual glands are formed as:
- mucous glands at the base of the tongue (*posterior lingual gland*) and at the posterolateral margin of the tongue;
- serous gustatory glands of the vallate and foliate papillae; and
- *anterior lingual gland* (Blandin-Nuhn's gland), a paired, mixed salivary gland which is located in the tongue musculature at the inferior side of the apex of the tongue and opens on both sides of the frenulum.

The **lingual papillae** (Fig. **269**) are macroscopically visible; they lie in the oral part of the dorsum of the tongue and at the lateral margin. They comprise *gustatory papillae*, vallate, foliate and fungiform, as well as *tactile filiform papillae*. Each papilla consists of a *connective tissue core* and an *epithelial covering*. Numerous sensory nerve endings are present in the core of the filiform papillae; taste buds are found in the epithelium of the gustatory papillae.

The *vallate (circumvalate) papillae* are 7–12 wart-like gustatory papillae with a diameter of 1–3 mm projecting only a little over the surface of the tongue. They lie at the back of the oral part of the dorsum of the tongue and form a V-shaped row in front of the sulcus terminalis. Each papilla is surrounded by a moat. The lingual epithelium lining the moats contains *taste buds* along the entire height of both sides of the moat. *Serous irrigating glands* (Ebner's glands) open into the moat; their secretions wash away the taste-provoking substances.

The *foliate papillae* are transverse foldings of the mucosa at the posterior, lateral margin of the tongue. The mucosal epithelium which lines the folds contain *taste buds*; *irrigating glands* open at the depth of the folds.

The *fungiform papillae* are dispersed on the margin and the apex of the tongue. They are raised 0.5–1.5 mm above the surface of the tongue. In newborn and small children, numerous *taste buds* reside in their epithelium, which partly regress later.

The *filiform papillae* are scattered over the entire dorsum of the tongue. Their epithelium forms small pharyngeally-directed pointed tips, which are only weakly cornified in man. Acting as small levers, these *tips* transmit mechanical stimuli to the endings of the numerous sensory nerve fibers terminating in their connective tissue core. Beyond that, the papillae must also act as fine rasps.

With strong desquamation and swelling of the cornified substances, the filiform papillae give a whitish appearance to the surface of the tongue.

Nerves of the Tongue

The entire *musculature of the tongue* is supplied by the *hypoglossal nerve* (Fig. **269**). From the *lingual mucosa, sensory* fibers course from the oral part via the *lingual nerve*, from the pharyngeal part via the *glossopharyngeal nerve* and from the region between the base of the tongue and the larynx via the *vagus nerve* (Figs. **268** and **269**). The *taste fibers* come from the gustatory organs and are connected to the three nerves mentioned below.

The **gustatory organ** is formed by the *taste buds*. In newborn children and infants, they are found on the palate and in the region of the laryngeal entrance, as well as on the gustatory papillae. Yet, in later life, they regress (variably) at these places.

The *taste buds* infiltrate the entire height of the stratified epithelium as small oval organs. Among the cells arranged longitudinally in the taste buds are *sensory cells* and *supporting cells*. The sensory cells (receptor cells) are secondary sensory cells.

The qualities of taste (sweet, sour, bitter, salty) are preferentially perceived at different parts of the tongue: sweet at the margin in front, salty in the middle, sour at the back and bitter in the region of the vallate papillae. Presumably different kinds of receptors correspond to the four qualities of taste. However, up to now only one type of receptor cell is known.

Peripheral pathway of taste (Fig. **269**). The 1st neuron of the afferent pathway attaching to the sensory cells passes to the gustatory nucleus at the floor of the 4th ventricle:

– from the *fungiform papillae* (and partly from the *foliate papillae*) via the *chorda tympani* with the *facial nerve* (cell bodies in the geniculate ganglion);

– from the *foliate* and *vallate papillae* with the *glossopharyngeal nerve*; and
– from the *region of the laryngeal entrance* with the *vagus nerve*.

Blood Vessels and Lymphatic Vessels of the Tongue

The **arteries** for the tongue (Fig. 277) are branches of the *lingual artery*, which enters the body of the tongue medial to the hyoglossus muscle and at the anterior margin of the muscle gives off the *sublingual artery* to the sublingual gland and to the mucosa of the floor of the mouth. *Dorsal lingual branches* pass to the base and dorsum of the tongue; the *arteria profunda linguae* courses below the apex of the tongue as the terminal branch between the genioglossus and the inferior longitudinal muscle.

Only capillary connections exist through the lingual septum between the right and left sides of the tongue so that when the lingual artery is ligated after the exit of the sublingual artery, one half of the tongue can remain largely bloodless for a longer period. However, the sublingual arteries of both sides communicate with each other and with branches of the ascending palatine and ascending pharyngeal arteries so that necrosis does not occur if the lingual artery becomes occluded before the exit of the sublingual artery.

The **veins** from the tongue (Fig. 278) empty into the facial vein via the *lingual vein*.

Lymphatic drainage (Fig. 272). The lymphatic pathways from the *apex of the tongue* pass to the *submental lymph nodes* below the chin. The *lymph* from the *remaining parts of the tongue*, from the sublingual gland and from the floor of the mouth arrives bilaterally at the upper *deep lateral cervical lymph nodes* along the internal jugular vein, and especially at the *jugulo-omohyoid node* at the crossing of the vein and omohyoid muscle. Some lymphatic vessels from the margin of the tongue can enter into the *submandibular lymph nodes*. Lymph from the *root of the tongue* flows preferentially to the *jugulodigastric node*, which lies below the digastric muscle behind the angle of the mandible.

The lymphatic vascular network of both sides possesses extensive anastomoses beyond the midline so that, for example, the metastatic spread of a tongue carcinoma can occur via the lymphatic pathways of the opposite side.

Roof of the Oral Cavity

The **roof of the oral cavity** (Figs. 273 and 274) is formed by the *hard palate* in the anterior two-thirds and by the *soft palate* in the posterior third.

The **hard palate** serves as a support for the tongue. The mucosa is immovably fixed to the periosteum, a submucosa layer being absent. *Transverse palatine folds* act as an "abrasive ledge", but become indistinct, however, in older individuals. A median longitudinal ridge or *raphe* indicates the suture at which the palatal processes are fused during

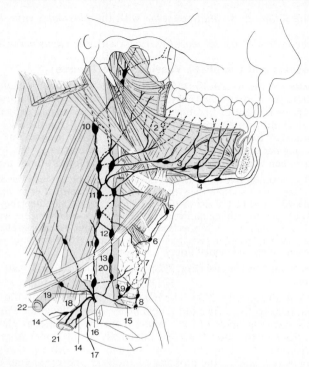

Fig. 272. Lymphatic drainage of tongue and neck, scheme (for designations of muscles →
Fig. 268)

1 Retropharyngeal lymph nodes
2 Lingual lymph nodes (inconstant)
3 Submandibular lymph nodes
4 Submental lymph nodes
5–9 Deep anterior cervical lymph nodes
5 Infrahyoid lymph node
6 Prelaryngeal lymph node
7 Thyroid lymph nodes
8 Pretracheal lymph nodes
9 Paratracheal lymph nodes
10–14 Deep lateral cervical lymph nodes
10 Jugulodigastric lymph node

11 Lateral jugular lymph nodes
12 Jugulo-omohyoid lymph node
13 Anterior jugular lymph nodes
14 Supraclavicular lymph nodes
15 Parasternal trunk
16 Right lymphatic duct
17 Anterior mediastinal trunk
18 Subclavian trunk
19 Jugular trunk
20 Internal jugular vein
21 Subclavian vein
22 Subclavian artery

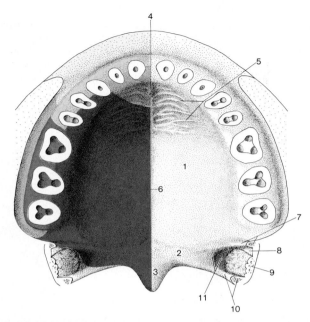

Fig. 273. **Mucous membrane of palate,** schematic horizontal section at level of mouth orifice and necks of teeth

Innervation of mucosa of palate, upper lip and cheek, as well as gingiva and teeth of upper jaw (innervation areas after *Scharlau*; overlapping of maximal regions not considered)

Right half of jaw: **sensory** innervation areas of:

Superior labial branches of infra-orbital nerve

Buccal nerve

Anterior superior alveolar branches and middle superior alveolar branch (superior dental plexus)

Posterior superior alveolar branches

Nasopalatine nerve

Greater and lesser palatine nerves

1 Hard palate
2 Soft palate
3 Palatine uvula
4 Incisive papilla
5 Transverse palatine folds
6 Median raphe

7 Palatoglossal arch and palatoglossus muscle
8 Triangular fold
9 Palatine tonsil
10 Palatopharyngeal arch and palatopharyngeus muscle
11 Semilunar fold and intratonsillar cleft

development. Behind the middle incisor teeth, the *incisive papilla* is elevated above the incisive fossa, which contains the incisive canal. Traversing this canal from the nasal cavity to the oral cavity are a branch of the sphenopalatine artery and the terminal branch of the nasopalatine nerve. In the posterior portion of the hard palate and in the soft palate, numerous mucous glands (*palatine glands*) are embedded in the mucosa.

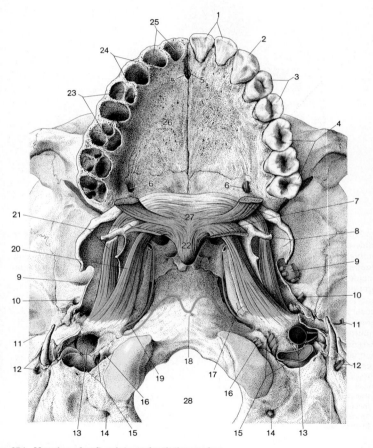

Fig. 274. **Muscles of soft palate and palatine arches**
Alveoli of teeth (right half of upper jaw) and exit sites of blood vessels and nerves at the external base of skull (left side of skull)
Line of junction of pharyngeal wall at base of skull ——

The **soft palate** (*velum palatinum*) is a movable fibromuscular fold which extends posteriorly into the unpaired, median *uvula*. The soft palate hangs down "at rest" from the posterior margin of the hard palate so that the uvula rests on the base of the tongue when the mouth is closed. During swallowing, the uvula presses against the arched posterior wall of the pharynx and closes off the food pathway from the respiratory tract. The base of the soft palate forms a tendinous plate (*palatine aponeurosis*), which is formed by the continuation of the periosteum of the bony palate and the tendons radiating into it.

The *mucosa of the soft palate* is part of the oral and nasal mucosa. The stratified squamous epithelium which lines the oral cavity is continued on the upper surface of the soft palate turned toward the nasopharynx (epipharynx) and goes over with a sharp boundary into the typical pseudostratified ciliated epithelium of the respiratory tract only in the vicinity of the choanae. On the oral side, extensive accumulations of mucous glands (*palatine glands*) lie in the submucosa and are separated from the lamina propria by an elastic bounding layer. On the nasal surface of the soft palate, the elastic fibrous layer lies below the glands, a submucosal layer not being delimited.

The *innervation of the palatine mucosa* and the palatine glands takes place at the hard palate largely via branches of the *greater palatine nerve*, behind the incisor teeth via the *nasopalatine nerve* and at the soft palate via the *lesser palatine nerves.*

1 Incisor teeth
2 Canine tooth
3 Premolar teeth
4 Molar teeth
5 Incisive foramen in incisive fossa: nasopalatine nerve
6 Greater palatine foramen: greater palatine artery and nerve
7 Palatoglossus (oral) and palatopharyngeus (both muscles severed)
8 Pterygoid hamulus (medial, fulcrum for tendon of tensor veli palatini) and lateral plate of pterygoid process
9 Foramen ovale: venous plexus of foramen ovale and mandibular nerve
10 Foramen spinosum: middle meningeal artery and meningeal branch of mandibular nerve
11 Petrotympanic fissure: anterior tympanic artery and chorda tympani
12 Styloid process and stylomastoid foramen: stylomastoid artery and facial nerve
13 Carotid canal: internal carotid artery and internal carotid plexus
14 Condylar canal: condylar emissary vein
15 Jugular foramen: inferior petrosal sinus, glossopharyngeal, vagus and accessory nerves, posterior meningeal artery and internal jugular vein
16 Hypoglossal canal: venous plexus of hypoglossal canal and hypoglossal nerve
17 Cartilaginous and membranous parts of auditory tube
18 Pharyngeal tubercle
19 Pharyngeal recess
20 Levator veli palatini
21 Tensor veli palatini
22 Musculus uvulae
23 Interradicular septa
24 Interalveolar septa of alveolar process
25 Dental alveoli
26 Hard palate
27 Soft palate
28 Foramen magnum

The **muscles of the soft palate**, the *tensor veli palatini* and the *levator veli palatini* (Figs. **268** and **274**), function as tensor and levator of the soft palate, respectively.

The **tensor veli palatini** arises from the scaphoid fossa, from a narrow band at the lower surface of the greater wing of the sphenoid and from the membranous outer wall of the auditory tube. At the level of the pterygoid fossa, the muscle already goes over into its tendon, which turns around the pterygoid hamulus and radiates horizontally into the palatine aponeurosis.

Innervation: tensor veli palatini muscle nerve from the mandibular nerve of the trigeminal.

The **levator veli palatini**, which lies behind the tensor veli palatini, comes from the lower surface of the petrous part of temporal bone in front of the carotid canal and from the cartilage of the auditory tube. It passes obliquely along the auditory tube forward and downward into the soft palate. The tendinous fibers of the muscle of both sides are intertwined and form a muscular loop whose height is adjustable.

Innervation: from the pharyngeal plexus (vagus and glossopharyngeal nerves), possibly also participation of fibers from the facial nerve.

Action of muscles on the soft palate and auditory tube. The *tensor veli palatini* stretches the soft palate and lifts it to the level of its hypomochlion (fulcrum), the pterygoid hamulus. The *levator veli palatini* also stretches the soft palate. It can raise it, however, beyond the line connecting the two pterygoid hamuli and press it effectively against the posterior pharyngeal wall. Both muscles enlarge the lumen of the tube: the tensor veli palatini by traction at the membranous wall, the levator by pushing against the cartilage of the torus tubarius with its muscle belly that has been thickened by contraction.

The **musculus uvulae** (Fig. **274**) arises paired from the aponeurosis of the soft palate, occasionally also from the posterior margin of the horizontal plate of the palatine bone, on both sides of the nasal spine. The paired origins form a uniform muscular cone which, when contracted, shortens the uvula.

Innervation: from the pharyngeal plexus, sometimes also from the facial nerve.

e) Oral Salivary Glands

The salivary glands of the oral cavity produce *saliva*. It is secreted reflexly – daily up to 1.5 l – by stimulation of the olfactory and taste senses, by masticatory movements and by psychological reflexes.

The **oral salivary glands** are *eccrine* (merocrine) *glands*. They possess partly *serous acini*, partly *mucous tubules* as their terminal secretory units. The serous portions secrete the salt-rich and protein-rich diluted saliva which contains ptyalin (α-amylase), a starch-splitting enzyme. The mucous portions produce mucus, an important lubricating agent in saliva.

Large and *small* salivary glands are distinguished. The saliva is given off mostly by the *three large salivary glands*, the *parotid* ($\rightarrow$ p. 674), the *sublingual* and the *submandibular glands*.

The parotid and the submandibular glands lie outside of the oral cavity. They transport their secretion into the vestibule or into the oral cavity proper by means of a long excretory duct.

The **small salivary glands**, numerous pinhead-sized glands, lie throughout the oral mucosa. They possess short excretory ducts and are named according to the part of the mucosa that they occupy (Table 5).

The **sublingual gland** (Figs. **262** and **270**) is 3–4 cm long and bulges the mucosa of the oral cavity between the mandible and tongue to form the *sublingual fold*. The gland can extend backward almost as far as the hook-like glandular (deep) process of the submandibular gland, which goes around the posterior margin of the mylohyoid to the superior side of it. At the medial aspect of the sublingual fold near the lower edge of the frenulum, there is a small elevation, the *sublingual papilla*, on which the *submandibular duct* and the *major sublingual duct* open, usually in common.

The sublingual gland consists of numerous *individual glands* (*minor sublingual glands*) and a large *main gland* (*major sublingual gland*). Through movements of the tongue, the individual glands can be pushed against one another. Part of the small glands opens directly into the oral cavity along the sublingual fold, part into the *duct of the major sublingual gland*. The sublingual gland is a mixed, predominantly mucous gland.

Innervation: parasympathetic from the *facial nerve* (nervus intermedius), sympathetic from the *superior cervical ganglion*.

Table 5. Oral Salivary Glands

	Composition	Place of Discharge
Large Salivary Glands		
Parotid	Pure serous	Oral vestibule
Submandibular	Mixed, mostly serous	Ora cavity proper
Sublingual	Mixed, mostly mucous	Oral cavity proper
Small Salivary Glands		
Labial		
Buccal	Mixed	Oral vestibule
Molar (buccal glands opposite molars)		
Lingual	Mixed (apex)	
	Pure serous (gustatory)	Oral cavity proper
	Pure mucous (base)	
Palatine	Pure mucous	

The *preganglionic, parasympathetic* fibers arrive at the *lingual nerve* via the *chorda tympani*. They leave the lingual nerve near the posterior margin of the mylohyoid and pass to the 2nd neuron in the *submandibular ganglion* (Fig. **268**). From there, postganglionic fibers pass to the sublingual gland.

Sympathetic fibers come from the *postganglionic* plexus of fibers (an offshoot of the *external carotid plexus*) that surrounds the maxillary artery.

The **submandibular gland** (Figs. **261** and **262**) lies below the floor of the mouth in the *submandibular triangle*, which is bordered by the anterior and posterior bellies of the digastric, as well as by the mandible. The gland, together with the submandibular node, is embedded in a fascial compartment of the superficial layer of the cervical fascia. Its excretory duct passes dorsally from the posterior margin of the mylohyoid to the upper side of the floor of the mouth. The *submandibular duct* (Fig. **270**) is frequently accompanied by a hook-shaped glandular process. The submandibular gland is a mixed, predominantly serous gland.

Innervation: like the sublingual gland.

f) Faucial Isthmus

The **faucial** (*oropharyngeal*) **isthmus** (Fig. **265**) connects the oral cavity with the oropharynx. The narrowing of the food pathway is effected by the *anterior* and the *posterior palatal arches* (*palatoglossal* and *palatopharyngeal arches*). The palatal arches are pushed forward into the lumen like a stage backdrop – more or less far depending on the state of contraction of the muscles.

The anterior and posterior palatal arches of each side form a triangular recess between themselves which is filled up almost completely by the palatine tonsil. A small fossa above the tonsil, the *supratonsillar fossa* (intratonsillar cleft, Fig. **273**), is a remnant of the embryonic tonsillar sinus formed from the 2nd pharyngeal pouch. Its upper border forms the *semilunar fold*, an arched mucosal fold coursing from the anterior to the posterior palatal arch and containing a connective tissue framework rich in lymphocytes.

The palatoglossal arch broadens toward the tongue into a triangular field, whose free posterior margin can somewhat cover the front of the palatine tonsil as a *triangular fold* (Fig. **273**). Lymphatic nodules can also infiltrate the triangular fold.

Muscles of the palatal arches. The two palatal arches are produced by the *palatopharyngeus* and *palatoglossus muscles*.

The **palatoglossus** (Figs. **268** and **274**) continues the fiber bundles of the transversus linguae muscle into the anterior palatal arch to the palatal aponeurosis.

The **palatopharyngeus** (Fig. **274**) passes in the posterior palatal arch from the soft palate to the wall of the pharynx (→ p. 761).

Innervation of both muscles: glossopharyngeal nerve.

Action of the muscles of the palatal arches. Together with the transversus linguae, the *palatoglossi* of both sides form a muscular ring whose contraction narrows the faucial isthmus. If a bolus of food of appropriate size passes through the faucial isthmus, the palatoglossi muscles, supported by the *palatopharyngei* muscles, block off the bolus.

When the tongue is fixed, the *palatoglossi muscles* can act as antagonists of the tensor and levator veli palatini and draw the soft palate downward. The *palatopharyngeus* is, beyond that, an elevator of the pharynx, with a circular fibrous tract also a "pharyngeal constrictor" ($\rightarrow$ p. 761).

The **palatine tonsil** (Figs. **268** and **269**) lies on both sides in the triangular recess between the anterior and the posterior palatal arches; its medial surface borders the faucial isthmus. Around the lateral surface of the palatine tonsil, the fascia of the superior pharyngeal constrictor forms a connective tissue capsule in which the tonsil can be removed in toto. The large vessels and nerves in the parapharyngeal connective tissue space are separated from the tonsil by the superior pharyngeal constrictor.

In the case of surgical removal of the palatine tonsil (*tonsillectomy*), the internal carotid artery is relatively protected by the superior pharyngeal constrictor.

The palatine tonsil consists of a covering of nonkeratinized stratified squamous epithelium and a substrate of lymphatic tissue 1–2 cm thick. The surface of the tonsil turned toward the faucial isthmus is enlarged by pit-like invaginations (*tonsillar fossulae*) that branch out into the substance of the tonsil to form the *tonsillar crypts*.

The epithelium of the wall of the crypt is frequently disaggregated and invaded by lymphocytes and granulocytes. Wandering white blood cells, desquamated epithelial cells and bacteria accumulate in the lumen of the fossulae and form the whitish tonsillar thrombi.

The paired *palatine tonsils*, the *pharyngeal tonsils* (adenoids) and the *lingual tonsil* are grouped together under the designation **lymphatic tonsillar ring**. It represents an important outpost in the sense of an "early warning system" of the defense system at the beginning of the respiratory and digestive tracts.

Vessels of the palatine tonsil. Arteries (Fig. **277**). The palatine tonsil is supplied by a large *tonsillar branch* that is given off by the *ascending palatine artery* or directly by the *facial artery* and that passes through the superior pharyngeal constrictor. Smaller branches to the palatine tonsil arise from the *lingual* and the *ascending pharyngeal arteries*.

The **veins** from the palatine tonsil drain into the *pharyngeal plexus* at the wall of the pharynx.

Lymph from the palatine tonsil is carried to the superior *deep lateral cervical lymph nodes*, e.g. to the *jugulodigastric lymph node* (Fig. **272**).

12. Neck

The **neck** is the movable connecting stalk between the head and trunk. The supporting element is the lordotically-curved cervical vertebral column (in transverse sections situated approximately in the center) that carries the head (Fig. **276**). Dorsally, it is adjoined by the well-developed nuchal musculature (cranial tracts of the erector spinae), as well as the trapezius and levator scapulae muscles passing to the shoulder girdle (in the caudal region also the rhomboideus). The anterior surface of the cervical vertebral body borders on a narrow, muscle-free longitudinal band at the *visceral space*, which is situated ventral to the cervical vertebral column and which is enclosed by the (true) *cervical musculature* and the pretracheal or prevertebral layer of the *cervical fascia*.

The unpaired *visceral tube* (pharynx and cervical part of the esophagus, as well as the larynx and the cervical part of the trachea) and the *endocrine organs* (thyroid and parathyroid glands) lie within the *visceral space*.

In the newborn and in the small child, the thymus (derived from the epithelium of the 3rd pharyngeal pouch) still extends into the neck region from the superior mediastinum.

The large *conduction pathways* that connect the head and the trunk (common carotid artery, internal jugular vein, lymphatic trunks of the neck, vagus nerve, sympathetic trunk) course in the dorsolateral boundary region of the visceral space and are separated from the viscera and the muscular layers by connective tissue tracts (fascial layers).

The conduction pathways of the upper limb use the neck as the region of passage (subclavian vessels, lymphatic trunks of the arm) or arise in the cervical region (brachial plexus); finally, the musculature of the uper limb can be traced back phylogenetically to primordial material from the lower cervical myotomes.

The cranial *border of the neck* is defined by a line that courses along the lower margin of the body of the mandible, passes over the apex of the mastoid process and continues along the superior nuchal line to the external occipital protuberance. The caudal boundary is indicated by the upper margin of the manubrium sterni, by the clavicle, acromion, scapular spine and the spinous process of the 7th cervical vertebra.

The cross-sectional surface of the neck near the head–neck border resembles an oval placed sagittal to the longitudinal axis, whereas at the level of the larynx it is circular. Near the trunk, on the other hand, the cross-sectional surface is once again oval, but assumes a frontal orientation to the greatest axis.

The *neck* (in the narrow sense) and the *nuchal region* are delimited from each other at the body surface by a line coursing on each side from the mastoid process to the acromion.

The composition of the nuchal region was already discussed on p. 000, the anchorage of the upper limb at the thoracic wall and neck on p. 000. The following discussion is concerned primarily with the "neck in the narrow sense". The musculature of the floor of the mouth situated in the submandibular triangle, the submandibular gland and the conduction pathways coursing through this region to the tongue and to the face were described in the corresponding sections of the preceding chapter on the head.

A. Wall of the Neck

1. Locomotor Apparatus of the Neck

Of the locomotor apparatus of the neck, the cervical vertebral column and the nuchal musculature have already been discussed. Still to be considered are the hyoid bone and its tendinous connections as the passive portion and the (true) cervical muscles as the active portion.

a) Hyoid Bone and Tendinous Connections

The **hyoid bone** (Fig. 283) is shaped like a horseshoe. The slender *greater horn (cornu)* – directed backward and somewhat outward – is attached on both sides to the *transverse body* and ends with a button-shaped thickening. The *lesser horn* projects obliquely backward and upward at the border of the body and greater horn on each side (usually) as a short, conical process.

The body and greater horns are palpable through the skin. When the eyes are directed straight ahead, the hyoid lies at the level of the flexion site at which the vertical contour of the neck goes over into the approximately horizontal contour of the floor of the mouth (apex of the "floor of the mouth-cervical angle", which amounts to about 90° in this position, Fig. **265**). Since the hyoid bone is inserted as a bony inscription into the muscular sling formed by the musculature of the floor of the mouth and the infrahyoid muscles, it possesses a certain range of movement which is of use in swallowing, as well as in the movements of the cervical vertebral column or the tongue. The connective tissue attachments at the base of the skull (by the stylohyoid ligament), however, does not permit the hyoid to advance caudally beyond the fourth cervical vertebra.

A *fracture* of the hyoid bone (or styloid process of the temporal bone, as well as a tear of the stylohyoid ligament) causes the hyoid bone to sink down onto the larynx. Consequently, in swallowing, the hyoid (and larynx) can no longer be drawn upward and forward (below the tongue) in the usual way by the musculature of the floor of the mouth. If the lower respiratory tract is not sufficiently closed, the victim can swallow the wrong way (danger of aspiration pneumonia).

Ossification of the *hyoid bone* begins in the body and greater horn before birth.

The lesser horn can remain cartilaginous for a long time (or permanently). The primordial material for the hyoid bone is derived from the cartilages of the 2nd and 3rd pharyngeal arches.

The **stylohyoid ligament** (Fig. **268**) connects the base of the skull with the hyoid. It passes from the apex of the styloid process, which arises at the lower surface of the petrous temporal, to the lesser cornu. The ligament can ossify partially (rarely completely).

The **thyrohyoid membrane** (Fig. **283**) stretches between the cranial margin of the thyroid cartilage and the hyoid bone, where it passes to the upper margin of the body and greater horn – along the inner surface. The tense membrane determines how far the larynx and hyoid bone can be withdrawn from one another, the thyrohyoid muscle regulating the actual interval.

The middle part of the membrane not covered by muscle (between the superior thyroid notch and the body of the hyoid bone) is strengthened by elastic longitudinal tracts into the *median thyrohyoid ligament* and can be palpated through the skin as a springy resistance. In the posterior margin of the membrane (between the superior horn of the thyroid cartilage and the posterior end of the greater horn of the hyoid), elastic strengthening tracts are likewise embedded. This portion of the membrane is referred to separately as the *lateral thyrohyoid ligament* and generally contains a grain-sized nodule of elastic cartilage (*cartilago triticea*) that frequently ossifies during middle age.

The *retrohyoid bursa* lies as a mucous bursa between the thyrohyoid membrane and the inner surface of the body of the hyoid. In males, it is pushed forward usually below the pretracheal layer of the cervical fascia, which is fixed at the lower border of the hyoid bone, and facilitates sliding movements of the membrane against the body of the hyoid and the infrahyoid musculature.

b) Organization and Innervation of the Cervical Musculature

The **cervical musculature** can be organized into a

superficial layer, consisting of the

- *platysma* and the *sternocleidomastoid*, as well as the
- *infrahyoid muscles* (= rectus, or straight, group of the neck), and a *deep layer*, consisting of the
- *scalene muscles* (step-like muscles) and the
- *prevertebral cervical muscles* (longus group)

Superficial Layer of Cervical Muscles

The **platysma** (Fig. **258**) represents that part of the superficial facial musculature remaining in the cervical region that is derived from the muscular primordia of the 2nd pharyngeal arch (hyoid arch).

All of the remaining superficial facial musculature has shifted completely into the head region and forms the muscles of facial expression.

The platysma is a very thin, muscular plate located directly beneath the skin. It extends from the border of the mandible up to the level of the 2nd (3rd) rib and as far as the acromion.

The platysma lies on the superficial layer of the cervical fasica and passes over the external jugular vein that courses there (Fig. 276). Cranially, the muscle fibers are attached at the mandible and at the facial skin; numerous bundles are intertwined with fiber tracts of the muscles of facial expression. Caudally, the platysma ends with scattered bundles of varying length in the subcutaneous tissue, partly also in the cutaneous connective tissue. The medial fibers of the muscles of both sides cross over each other, generally under the chin, and diverge caudally so that a triangular median surface of the anterior cervical region remains uncovered by the platysma.

Innervation: cervical ramus of the facial nerve from the parotid plexus via the transverse cervical nerve ($\rightarrow$ p. 672).

The **sternocleidomastoid** (Fig. **275**), a branchiomeric muscle from the 6th pharyngeal arch, arises with two heads (sternal and clavicular) which embrace the supraclavicular fossa. The sternal head originates at the upper border of the manubrium sterni, the clavicular head from the sternal end of the clavicle. The muscle belly is ensheathed in the superficial layer of the cervical fascia (Fig. **276**) and courses obliquely upward in a slight helical turn across the lateral surface of the neck before inserting with a well-developed tendon at the mastoid process and at the superior nuchal line. The surface of the muscle, which is directed ventrally at its origin, faces laterally at its insertion.

Innervation: accessory nerve, as well as from ventral branches of cervical nerves 2–4 (especially via the lesser occipital nerve) for the muscle fibers derived from the cervical myotomes.

The accessory nerve enters the musle from the lower side at the border between the cranial and middle third (either comletely or only with the fibers for the sternoclei-domastoid).

The **infrahyoid muscles** (Figs. **275** and **276**) represent the cranial continuation of the rectus system of the trunk (rectus abdominis) and spread between the sternum and hyoid.

The more or less distinctly developed tendinous intersections do not mark off true metameres, but indicate muscle segments which also contain material from adjacent somites (pseudometamerism).

The geniohyoid muscle is the only muscle of the rectus system to course cranially from the hyoid; thus, it belongs in the group of suprahyoid muscles.

Innervation: with the exception of the thyrohyoid, the infrahyoid muscles are innervated by branches of the ansa cervicalis.

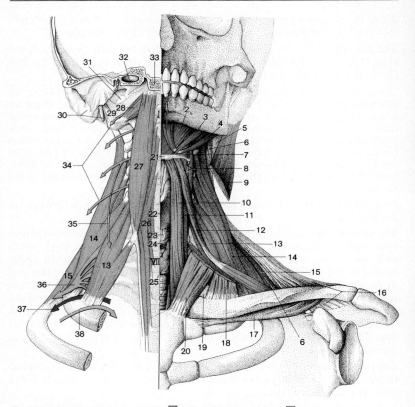

Fig. 275. **Muscles of floor of mouth** ▨ **and neck musculature** ▨, ventral view
Muscles of floor of mouth, sternocleidomastoid and infrahyoid muscles (left side), as
well as scalenes and prevertebral neck muscles (right side). Left sternocleidomastoid
severed above the infrahyoid muscles; right half of skull removed by frontal section in
front of osseous external acoustic canal; right half of hyoid bone, of laryngeal skeleton
and of sternum removed; right clavicle also removed.

I Anterior arch of atlas   VII Body of 7th cervical vertebra

 1 Digastric, anterior belly
 2 Mylohoid
 3 Stylohoid
 4 Digastric, posterior belly
 5 Longissimus capitis
 6 Levator scapulae
 7 Hyoglossus
 8 Thyrohyoid muscle and lateral thyrohyoid ligament
 9 Sternocleidomastoid
10 Sternohyoid
11 Sternothyroid

12 Omohyoid
13 Scalenus anterior
14 Scalenus medius
15 Scalenus posterior
16 Trapezius
17 Subclavius
18 Sternocleidomastoid, clavicular head
19 Lesser supraclavicular fossa
20 Sternocleidomastoid, sternal head
21 Hyoid bone
22 Thyroid cartilage

This nerve loop presents a superior root (fibers of the ventral rami of the 1st and 2nd cervical nerves which temporarily lie on the hypoglossal nerve) and an inferior root (fibers of the ventral rami of cervical nerves 2, 3 [4]).

The thyrohyoid ramus (from Cl, 2) leaves the hypoglossal nerve only after the exit of the superior root of the ansa cervicalis.

The following four muscles are grouped as infrahyoid muscles:

The **sternohyoid** arises from the dorsal surface of the manubrium sterni and from the sternoclavicular joint. It approaches the midline cranially and inserts at the upper margin of the body of the hyoid.

The **sternothyroid** also has its origin on the posterior surface of the manubrium sterni, lying dorsal and somewhat medial to the preceding muscle. It courses steeply upward and attaches at and behind the oblique line of the thyroid cartilage (Fig. **268**).

A tendinous intersection can also be more or less distinctly formed here – as in the sternohyoid – at the level of the upper border of the sternum.

The **thyrohyoid** (Fig. **271**) forms the cranial continuation of the sternothyroid to the hyoid (insertion at the body and ventral half of the greater horn).

The separation of both muscles is incomplete, since the lateral bundles of fibers of the sternothyroid go over into the thyrohyoid and course up to the hyoid.

The variable *levator glandulae thyroideae* can split off from the thyrohyoid muscle. Its bundles of fibers pass from the caudal part of the muscle, from the thyroid cartilage or from the hyoid bone to the isthmus of the thyroid gland or to a pyramidal lobe.

The **omohyoid** originates at the upper margin of the scapula, medial to the scapular notch, as well as at the superior transverse scapular ligament and passes to the body of the hyoid. It is organized into a *caudal* and a *cranial belly* by an intermediate tendon.

The muscle corresponds to the lateral marginal band of a broad muscular plate in reptiles, which has extended its origin up to the scapula and whose medial portion is preserved as the sternohyoid muscle. This explains the lateral origin of the omohyoid at the upper border of the scapula – a deviation from the remaining muscles of the rectus group. The tendinous intersection lies above the clavicle,

23 Cricothyroid muscle and cricothyroid ligament
24 Cricoid cartilage
25 Thyroid gland
26 Longus colli
27 Longus capitis
28 Rectus capitis anterior
29 Rectus capitis lateralis
30 Mastoid process and styloid process of temporal bone
31 Jugular foramen
32 Carotid canal
33 Basi-occipital, sawed surface
34 Roots of cervical plexus: ventral rami of cervical nerves I–IV
35 Phrenic nerve
36 Roots of brachial plexus: ventral rami of cervical nerves V–VIII and thoracic nerve I
37 Subclavian artery in the scalenus gap
38 Subclavian vein in front of scalenus anterior

behind the sternocleidomastoid, and crosses the great vessels of the neck. The superior belly forms a blunt angle with the inferior belly – open dorsocranially – and inserts at the body of the hyoid lateral to the sternohyoid. The two muscle bellies are enclosed by the pretracheal layer of the cervical fascia, which is firmly fused with the intermediate tendon and thus unites the muscle with the clavicle.

Deep Layer of Neck Muscles

The **scalene muscles** (Figs. **275** and **276**) form a tent-like roof over the pleural cupola and close the dorsolateral portion of the superior thoracic aperture cranially. In the cervical region, the muscles take the place of the intercostal muscles and their derivatives; they are closely related to the dorsal group of the shoulder girdle muscles.

Innervation: from the ventral rami of spinal nerves C4–8 (T1), partly via the dorsal scapular nerve.

The **scalenus anterior** arises at the anterior tubercles of the transverse processes of C3–6 and passes to the scalene tubercle on the surface of the 1st rib.

The **scalenus medius**, the best-developed of the scalariform muscles, has its origin (in the groove located between the anterior and posterior tubercles) at the transverse processes of C3–7 and often exhibits accessory slips of origin from the atlas and axis. The muscle inserts at the 1st rib dorsolateral to the groove for the subclavian artery, occasionally also with some bundles of fibers at the external surface of the 2nd rib.

The subclavian artery and the brachial plexus pass through the **scalenus gap**, which is bordered by the scalenus anterior and scalenus medius (Figs. **275** and **277**). The subclavian vein passes over the 1st rib in front of the attachment of the scalenus anterior. The scalenus gap can be divided by the inconstant **scalenus minimus**, which arises from the anterior tubercle of the transverse process of C(6)7. Its fibers are attached – directly dorsal to the scalenus anterior – at the 1st rib (inner margin) and radiate into the suprapleural membrane. The subclavian artery courses ventral to the scalenus minimus, the caudal "roots" of the brachial plexus (C(6)7, T1) passing through the scalenus gap dorsal to it.

The **scalenus posterior** originates from the posterior tubercles of the transverse processes of C5 and C6, turns around the dorsal margin of the scalenus medius ventrally with its muscle belly and attaches at the external surface of the 2nd, sometimes also the 3rd rib.

Prevertebral cervical muscles (Fig. **275**). The three muscles of the "longus group" fill the groove that is formed by the anterolateral surfaces of the bodies of the cervical, as well as by the three cranial thoracic vertebrae and their transverse processes.

The **rectus capitis anterior** lies farthest cranially between the atlas and the occiput (→ p. 493). It is generally a unisegmental muscle that is supplied only by the ventral ramus of the 1st cervical nerve.

The *longus capitis* and *longus colli* are often not distinctly delimited from one another. They possess a complicated pennate structure with longitudinal and oblique tracts of fibers. Their muscle mass is usually incompletely penetrated by tendinous intersections.

The **longus capitis** passes from the transverse processes of C3–6 to the basilar part of the occipital bone.

Innervation: ventral rami of cervical nerves 1–5(6).

The **longus colli** arises at the vertebral bodies of the three lower cervical and three upper thoracic vertebrae, as well as at the transverse processes of C2–5. Its fibers insert at the transverse processes of C5–7, at the cervical vertebral bodies 2–4 and at the anterior tubercle of the atlas.

Innervation: ventral rami of cervical nerves 2–6.

c) Action of the Neck Musculature

Corresponding to the different types of "working points" of the cervical musculature, their action is quite different and versatile. Facial and cervical skin are moved directly by the platysma. The shape of the neck, however, is changed also by lowering the mandible (with the cooperation of the infrahyoid muscles) or by forward flexion of the head and neck (by the prevertebral muscles).

The cervical and nuchal muscles act together in head movements and bring each of the large sense organs in the head into a favorable position. Depending on the type of body movement, the head carries out collateral movements and countermovements (for the maintenance of balance) which involve the cervical muscles (sternocleidomastoid, scalenes, prevertebral muscles). Neck movements and the head movements connected with them are frequently characteristic movements of expression.

The scalene muscles are essential for the elevation of the ribs during relaxed respiration. The infrahyoid muscles play an important role in the masticatory process and in swallowing. At the same time, they determine the position of the larynx between the hyoid and the superior thoracic aperture.

The **platysma** is able to influence facial expressions by its attachment to the skin of the cheek and the lower lip. Through a very powerful and sudden contraction, involuntary in most individuals (e.g. when terrified), the cranial and caudal ends of the fibers approach each other, the skin of the neck is compressed and pressed forward (the neck appears thickened) and the jaw is drawn downward.

The contraction of the platysma leads to an enlargement of the superficial veins. In the region of the carotid triangle, this also involves the deep veins situated below the superficial fascial layer and thus promotes the return of blood from the head into the thorax.

When contracted unilaterally, the **sternocleidomastoid** turns the face toward the opposite side and flexes the head toward the same side. Together with the nuchal muscles, the two sternocleidomastoids regulate the position of the head. When there is a sudden strong exertion of the muscles, the head is "thrown against the neck".

Together with the suprahyoid muscles, the **infrahyoid muscles** determine the position of the hyoid by means of their tonus.

The *sternothyroid* and *thyrohyoid* regulate the distance of the larynx from the hyoid. The infrahyoid muscles can draw the hyoid downward. Together with the suprahyoid muscles and the inferior head of the lateral pterygoid, they are able to open the jaw also when there is resistance. They can lower the head and flex the vertebral column, as long as the nuchal muscles reduce their tension. By contraction of the *omohyoid muscles*, the angle formed by the two muscle bellies is increased and the pretracheal layer of the cervical fascia is stretched.

Deep muscles of the neck. The *scalene muscles* raise the (cranial) ribs and thus contribute to inspiration (→ p. 528). With unilateral contraction, they are able to pull the cervical vertebral column laterally and to turn it slightly toward the same side. The scalenus anterior muscles assist in the flexion of the cervical vertebral column.

The *longus colli* can flex the cervical vertebral column and, through unilateral contraction, can turn it somewhat toward the same side. The *longus capitis*, together with the *rectus capitis anterior*, bends the head forward.

Paralyses: An isolated paralysis of the *sternocleidomastoid* is very rare. The flexion of the head toward the damaged side and the rotation of the face toward the healthy side are then possible even in a diminished form since the failure of the sternocleidomastoid is partly compensated for by the action of the nuchal muscles passing to the head and atlas.

The *infrahyoid muscles* become paralyzed only through the complete destruction of the entire ansa cervicalis, in which case the thyroid cartilage deviates toward the healthy side.

When the *scalenes* are paralyzed, thoracic respiration is not affected permanently, at least not to an extent worth mentioning. The external intercostal muscles can largely compensate for it through their action as rib elevators.

The *sternocleidomastoid* is shortened in the (so-called) congenital muscular *wryneck* (*torticollis*) and degenerates as scarred tissue. The head is bent toward the affected side and turned toward the healthy side. In addition to serious deformities of the cervical vertebral column, asymmetries of the face and head can arise.

2. Cervical Fascia

Cervical fascia (Figs. **258**, **265** and **276**). The connective tissue system that encloses muscles, visceral tubes and conduction pathways in the cervical region, separates them from one another and at the same time connects them with each other is compressed within the different regions into three very strong connective tissue layers. They border important movable clefts and are designated in their totality as *cervical fascia*.

Since the nomenclature of the three layers of the continuous connective tissue system is somewhat troublesome, the clinician speaks only of superficial, middle and deep cervical fascia.

The *superficial* layer of fascia (*superficial cervical fascia*) lies below the platysma. It curves around the ventrolateral surface of the neck and continues in the nuchal region into the nuchal fascia and the superficial dorsal fascia lying on the trapezius. The superficial layer is attached at the anterior surface of the manubrium sterni and clavicle, at the hyoid and at the lower margin of the mandible. Caudally, it communicates with the pectoralis fascia. Above the hyoid, the superficial layer of the cervical fascia encloses the submandibular gland; at the angle of the mandible, it goes over into the masseteric fascia and the parotid fascia. The sternocleidomastoid is ensheathed by the superficial layer. The external investment is very well-developed over the third of the muscle near the attachment site. In the cranial portion of the lateral cervical triangle, the superficial and deep fascial layers are fused with each other.

The *middle* (*pretracheal*) *layer of the cervical fascia* is relatively firm and lies in front of the cervical viscera as a triangular fascial apron. Caudally, the pretracheal layer is attached at the dorsal surface of the two clavicles and the sternum: cranially, it extends to the hyoid. The fascial layer surrounds the infrahyoid muscles. It can be stretched by the omohyoid, whose intermediate tendon has fused firmly with it. In the process, the lumen of the internal jugular vein is enlarged, since the pretracheal layer participates in the formation of the vascular sheath and is connected with the wall of the vein.

Quite commonly, tracts of the middle fascial layer "lift" the traversing superficial cervical veins and the deep veins (from the neck and shoulder regions) covered by the connective tissue layer.

Above the sternum, between the superficial and pretracheal layers of the cervical fascia is a space filled with adipose tissue and veins.

Frequently designated as the *suprasternal space*, it extends laterally to the sternocleidomastoid and cranially approximately to the isthmus of the thyroid gland.

The *deep (prevertebral) layer of the cervical fascia* is attached at the muscle-free middle band of the vertebral column, at the anterior longitudinal ligament, and covers the prevertebral cervical muscles, as well as the scalenes. Cranially, the deep fascial layer is fixed at the base of the

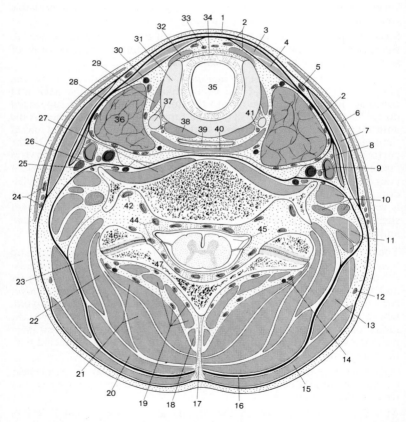

Fig. 276. **Cross section of neck** through body of seventh cervical vertebra and cricothyroid joint, cranial view of cut surface

skull; caudally, it goes over into the endothoracic fascia (connective tissue route to the mediastinum).

From the scalenus medius, the prevertebral layer reaches the clavicle; with the scalenus medius and scalenus posterior, it arrives at the external surface of the thorax and covers the brachial plexus and the subclavian artery – conduction paths to the upper limb.

From the connective tissue system of the neck, especially from the prevertebral layer, connective tissue tracts, which are occasionally strengthened by a tendinous tract from the scalenus anterior, radiate to the suprapleural membrane and contribute to the fixation of the pleura cupola.

The prevertebral layer lies dorsal to the neurovascular bundle from the neck to the head. Lateral to this, it communicates with the fascia of the levator scapulae, with the nuchal fascia and with the superficial layer of the cervical fascia.

◀ 1 Superficial layer of cervical fascia
 2 Pretracheal layer of cervical fascia
 3 Sternohyoid
 4 Sternothyroid
 5 Anterior jugular vein
 6 Platysma
 7 Sternocleidomastoid
 8 Omohyoid
 9 Neurovascular bundle from head to neck: ansa cervicalis, common carotid artery, vagus nerve, internal jugular vein
10 Scalenus anterior and "roots" of brachial plexus
11 Scalenus medius and scalenus posterior
12 Accessory nerve
13 Levator scapulae
14 Deep cervical artery and vein
15 Trapezius
16 Nuchal fascia
17 Ligamentum nuchae
18 Spinalis muscle
19 Multifidus and posterior part of external vertebral venous plexus
20 Splenius (cervicis and capitis)
21 Semispinalis (cervicis and capitis)
22 Longissimus (cervicis and capitis)
23 Illiocostalis cervicis
24 External jugular vein and supraclavicular nerves

25 Lateral jugular lymph node
26 Phrenic nerve and sympathetic trunk
27 Prevertebral layer of cervical fascia, longus colli muscle, vertebral artery
28 Capsule of thyroid gland
29 Lateral crico-arytenoid
30 Anterior branch of superior thyroid artery
31 Cricoid cartilage
32 Cricothyroid
33 Branches of superior thyroid vein
34 Cricothyroid ligament
35 Infraglottic cavity
36 Left lobe of thyroid gland
37 Inferior horn of thyroid cartilage and cricothyroid joint
38 Posterior crico-arytenoid
39 Laryngopharynx
40 Inferior pharyngeal constrictor
41 Inferior laryngeal nerve
42 Vertebral vein
43 Body of seventh cervical vertebra
44 Internal vertebral venous plexus in epidural space
45 Subarachnoid space and denticulate ligament
46 Superior articular process of first thoracic vertebra
47 Arch of 7th cervical vertebra

B. Surface Anatomy of the Neck

1. Superficial Relief of the Neck and Palpable Skeletal Parts

The **surface relief** of the neck (Fig. **253**) is determined in the healthy individual essentially by the amount and distribution of the subcutaneous adipose tissue and by the appearance of the musculature. In males, the *laryngeal prominence* (*"Adam's apple"*) of the thyroid cartilage projects distinctly, whereas the female larynx – approximately one-third smaller – protrudes only slightly into the median contour line of the neck. At the level of the hyoid bone, the border of the floor of the mouth is marked externally by a transverse skin crease (*hyoid crease*) that is distinctly pronounced in infants and small children. At the muscular neck, the sternocleidomastoid bulges forward on each side. At its anterior margin – at about the middle of a line connecting the angle of the jaw and the jugular fossa – the pulse of the common carotid artery can be palpated. The skin is depressed in the region of the jugular fossa and above the clavicle.

When not enlarged, the thyroid gland produces no conspicuous thickening of the neck. It can be marked off more or less distinctly during the act of swallowing, when it moves craniad, together with the larynx, and again descends.

In the case of *goiter*, the skin of the neck bulges out depending on the degree of enlargement of the thyroid gland.

The neck appears long and slender when the superior thoracic aperture is placed distinctly oblique. The contour of the trapezius is decidedly concave and there is only moderate development of the subcutaneous fat. If the upper margin of the sternum lies relatively high, the marginal line of the trapezius courses laterally in a flat arch and subcutaneous fat is strongly developed; the neck appears short and thick.

Palpable skeletal parts (Fig. **253**). At the neck, the osseous "borders" (upper margin of the sternum, clavicle, acromion; lower margin of the mandible, mastoid process) can be readily palpated. The body and greater horn of the hyoid bone, the upper margin and lamina of the thyroid cartilage and the arch of the cricoid cartilage are likewise accessible to the palpating finger. If the transverse portion of the thyroid gland is only weakly developed, the trachea can be followed into the depth of the jugular fossa.

The sternocleidomastoid forms an important landmark for subdividing the neck into **discrete regions**. The area situated over the muscle is designated as the *sternocleidomastoid area*; the deepened triangular field enclosed by its two heads and the clavicle is referred to as the *lesser supraclavicular fossa* (Fig. **275**).

The *middle triangle of the neck*, the unpaired *anterior cervical region*, is bordered by the two sternocleidomastoid muscles and the lower margin of the mandible. The cervical viscera and the neurovascular route connecting the head and trunk lie in this region.

The *lateral triangle of the neck*, the paired *lateral cervical region*, extends between the sternocleidomastoid and trapezius, as well as the clavicle. In its basal portion, the branches of the brachial plexus and the subclavian vessels are bound together into the neurovascular bundle of the arm.

Within the large triangle of the lateral cervical region, a small field located medially and caudally is marked off by the inferior belly of the omohyoid and designated as the *omoclavicular triangle* (*greater supraclavicular fossa*). The subdivisions of the anterior cervical triangle are the *submandibular triangle* (bordered by the anterior and posterior bellies of the digastric, as well as by the mandible) and the *carotid triangle* (framed by the sternocleidomastoid, posterior belly of the digastric and the superior belly of the omohyoid). In the depth of the carotid triangle, the common carotid artery bifurcates into the internal and external carotids.

2. Cutaneous Vessels and Nerves of the Neck

a) Cutaneous Veins

The **cutaneous veins of the neck** (Figs. **276** and **278**) lie on the superficial layer of the fascia and are covered by the platysma. They empty into two larger veins, the *external jugular* and the *anterior jugular*, that pass deeply in the lower part of the neck at the posterior or anterior margin of the sternocleidomastoid and are braced in their course and held open by fascial tracts (especially the pretracheal layer). During inspiratory enlargement of the thorax, therefore, blood can be sucked in and carried back to the heart. Like the internal jugular veins (and the subclavian vein), the danger of an air embolism also exists for these veins in the case of perforating injuries. Venous valves are very sparse in cutaneous veins; occasionally they are completely absent.

The **external jugular vein** proceeds from the *posterior auricular vein*, which can unite with the *occipital vein*, and a large lateral branch of the retromandibular vein. It courses caudally below the platysma and over the sternocleidomastoid, enters the omoclavicular triangle through the superficial and the middle layer of the cervical fascia and opens into the subclavian vein or into the venous angle, more rarely into the internal jugular vein.

A venous valve usually lies at the site of the opening.

The **anterior jugular vein** is formed at about the level of the hyoid bone by the union of several cutaneous veins from the region of the floor of the mouth. The vein can pass downward along the anterior border of the sternocleidomastoid and then communicate with the vein of the opposite side above the jugular notch of the sternum via the *jugular venous arch* (Fig. **265**). The anterior jugular vein crosses below the sternocleidomastoid and opens into the external jugular vein or into the subclavian vein. However, it can also course near the midline or in the midline and form a paired or unpaired *median cervical vein.*

b) Cutaneous Nerves

The **innervation of the skin** of the neck (Fig. **257**) takes place via the four cutaneous branches of the *cervical plexus* which pass to the surface through the superficial layer of the cervical fascia at the posterior margin of the sternocleidomastoid (approximately in the middle of the muscle) and radiate backward and upward (as far as the occiput), cranially, ventrally and laterally.

The skin receives sensory innervation

behind the ear and *at the occiput* via
– the *lesser occipital nerve*;

in the region of the *pinna* via
– the *great auricular nerve* (*posterior ramus* to the posterior surface and to the adjacent area; *anterior ramus* to the ear lobule, to the anterior surface of the pinna – together with the *anterior auricular nerves* from the *auriculotemporal nerve* – and to the neighborhood of the angle of the jaw);

in the area of the *anterior cervical region* via
– branches of the *transverse cervical nerve*, which divides into *superior rami* to the skin of the floor of the mouth and *inferior rami* for the half of the anterior cervical region located below the hyoid;

in the area of the *lateral cervical region* (as well as in the clavicular and the anterior shoulder regions) via the
– *medial, intermediate* and *lateral supraclavicular nerves.*

Segmental relations of the skin. The cutaneous branches of the cervical plexus carry sensory fibers from the ventral rami of cervical nerves 2–4 (C1 dispatches no sensory fibers to the skin). Accordingly, three segmental zones follow in the region of the neck from cranial to caudal, whereas segments C2–8 are developed in the nuchal region (→ Fig. **57 a**). Since the ventral portions of segments C5–T1 have shifted to the upper limb, a segmental discontinuity (*hiatus*) exists between C4 and T2. The overlapping of cutaneous segments is not as distinctly pronounced in the cervical region as in the trunk.

The ventral segment C2 borders on the sensory area of the trigeminal nerve and is limited largely to the cutaneous field between the pinna and the crown of the head. C3 protrudes cranially somewhat over the margin of the mandible, extends over the entire anterior cervical region and spreads out laterally beyond the sternoclei-domastoid region into the lateral cervical region. C4 supplies the basal portion of the lateral cervical region and a cutaneous band of the thoracic wall (to about the level of the 1st intercostal space) where it borders on the ventral segment of T2.

C. Connective Tissue Space of the Neck: Incorporation of Conduction Pathways and Organs

The *muscular mantle* of the neck encloses the paired *conduction pathways* for the head and the upper limb, as well as the unpaired, centrally-situated *visceral space*. Pathways of conduction and visceral space are embedded in the *connective tissue system of the neck*, which is compressed into three layers of the cervical fascia. They separate the *connective tissue spaces* and at the same time connect them with one other.

Previsceral and retrovisceral movable spaces. The pretracheal layer and the middle part of the prevertebral layer border the *visceral space* (Fig. 276). The loose connective tissue that unites the cervical viscera with the two fascial layers facilitates extensive displacements of the digestive tract and the lower respiratory tract in relation to the vertebral column, as well as the organ systems against each other. The movable space situated between the pretracheal layer and the cervical viscera is also called the *previsceral space*; the space between the posterior wall of the pharynx and the prevertebral layer is designated as the **retropharyngeal (retrovisceral) space** (Fig. 265). This sliding space is directly continuous caudally with the posterior part of the superior mediastinum.

The *parapharyngeal* (*lateropharyngeal*) *space* represents the triangular (in cross section) movable space situated lateral to the pharynx in the transitional region of the head and neck. It is limited laterally by the connective tissue capsule of the parotid gland and the pterygoid muscles, dorsally by the prevertebral layer of the cervical fascia. Connective tissue tracts divide it medially from the *retropharyngeal space* and pass from the deep cervical fascia to the external fascial covering of the pharynx, while at the same time forming the medial wall of the connective tissue sheath of the neurovascular bundle to the head. Cranially, the parapharyngeal space extends to the base of the skull; caudally, it is continuous with the connective tissue layer of the carotid triangle without any boundary mark. Retropharyngeal and parapharyngeal spaces are grouped together under the generic term *peripharyngeal space*.

The *styloid process* projects from the base of the skull into the parapharyngeal space. The fascial covering of the muscles arising at this process broadens out into a frontally placed connective tissue plate (*stylopharyngeal fascia*) that reaches to the wall of the pharynx and divides the parapharyngeal space into an anterior and a posterior portion. The *anterior part* contains fat traversed only by smaller vessels (e.g. the ascending palatine artery), whereas the *posterior portion* is penetrated by large conduction pathways, the neurovascular bundle of the neck to the head, as well as by cranial nerves (glossopharyngeal, accessory and hypoglossal).

In the deep layer of the cervical fascia, the cervical part of the sympathetic trunk (Fig. **276**) lies in front of the longus colli muscle.

Below the deep layer of the cervical fascia, the phrenic nerve courses on the scalenus anterior to the mediastinum. Posterolateral to the neurovascular trunk from the neck to the head and lateral to the sympathetic trunk, the cervical plexus exits between the upper slips of origin of the scalenus anterior and scalenus medius into the sternocleidomastoid region. The brachial plexus and the subclavian artery follow caudally and, together with the subclavian vein (situated in front of the deep fascial layer), form the neurovascular bundle from the neck to the arm.

Within the movable spaces and in the connective tissue routes along the conduction pathways, inflammation and bleeding can spread relatively unhindered into the cervical region. Suppurations (pus formations) and phlegmons in the retropharyngeal space (e.g. proceeding from the retropharyngeal lymph nodes) or in the parapharyngeal space (as a consequence of a suppurative angina) can rapidly penetrate into the mediastinum and lead to threatening symptoms.

Additional paths for spreading inflammations run along the brachial plexus and the subclavian vessels through the lateral triangle of the neck into the axilla. Gravitation abscesses that proceed from the cervical vertebral column and penetrate into the prevertebral muscles, on the other hand, are retained for a long time by the deep layer of the cervical fascia.

1. Neurovascular Bundle from the Neck to the Upper Limb

The **neurovascular bundle** *from the neck to the upper limb* consists of the *subclavian artery* and *vein*, the *subclavian trunk* and the *brachial plexus*; it passes through the lateral triangle of the neck to the axilla.

The *brachial plexus* and the *subclavian artery* (Fig. **275**) course in the *connective tissue route* that leads from the scalene gap between the anterior and middle scalene muscles through the lateral cervical triangle into the axilla. The connective tissue route proceeds from the deep layer of the cervical fascia.

On the other hand, the connective tissue that accompanies the *subclavian vein* in front of the scalenus anterior communicates directly both with the middle and with the deep fascial layers. The typical connective tissue sheath of the neurovascular bundle to the arm arises in the axilla just below the clavicle.

The **subclavian artery** (Figs. **25** and **277**) carries blood to a part of the neck, to the anterior thoracic wall, to the shoulder girdle and to the arm, as well as to a part of the brain and to the cervical part of the medulla. It arises from the brachiocephalic trunk on the right side, from the aortic arch on the left, and crosses over the first rib in the scalene gap. Beyond the 1st rib, it continues as the axillary artery, which is surrounded by the cords of the brachial plexus and is covered by processes from the deep layer of the cervical fascia.

The branches of the subclavian artery exhibit a number of variants with regard to their origin and distribution. As a rule, the *vertebral artery*, the *internal thoracic artery* and the *thyrocervical trunk* branch off medial to the scalenus anterior, whereas the *costocervical trunk* branches off behind it. At their origin and in their course near the origin, they are covered by the deep layer of the cervical fascia.

The *vertebral artery* (Fig. **277**), which – together with the internal carotid artery – feeds the arteries to the brain, arise at the posterior wall of the subclavian artery as a large vessel medial to the scalenus anterior; after a short course, it enters the foramen transversarium of the 6th cervical vertebra. Extracranial branches → p. 496, intracranial branches → Vol. 2.

The *internal thoracic artery* (Fig. **193**) arises from the underside of the subclavian artery and passes toward the diaphragm (about 1 cm) lateral to the sternal border at the inner surface of the anterior thoracic wall (→ p. 520).

The *thyrocervical trunk* (Fig. **277**) leaves the subclavian artery at the anterior (medial) margin of the scalenus anterior and divides (usually) into three branches, which can also arise, however, from the subclavian artery separately and independently.

The *suprascapular artery* crosses in front of the scalenus anterior laterally and behind the clavicle, sends the *acromial branch* through the attachment of the trapezius to the level of the shoulder, enters the supraspinatus *over* the superior transverse scapular ligament and, together with the circumflex scapular artery (from the subscapular artery), forms the scapular anastomosis. The *transverse cervical artery* courses – often between the cords of the brachial plexus – through the scalene gap toward the nuchal region. It divides into the *superficial branch*, which arrives at the undersurface of the trapezius together with the accessory nerve, and into the *deep branch*, which passes with the dorsal scapular nerve to the rhomboids and the latissimus dorsi.

The *transverse cervical artery* is very variable. The superficial branch can be replaced by the *superficial cervical artery* coursing ventral to the scalenus anterior, the deep branch by the *dorsal scapular artery*.

The *inferior thyroid artery*, the main branch of the thyrocervical trunk, first continues the latter's route and ascends at the anterior margin of the scalenus anterior. It then arches medially, penetrates the deep layer of the cervical fascia and ramifies at the lower pole and at the posterior surface of the thyroid gland (*glandular branches*), at the wall of the laryngo-pharynx (*pharyngeal branches*), as well as at the cervical part of the esophagus (*esophageal branches*) and trachea (*tracheal branches*). It dispatches the *inferior laryngeal artery* to the mucosa of the posterior wall of the larynx and to the posterior crico-arytenoid muscle.

The *ascending cervical artery* originates from the initial section of the inferior

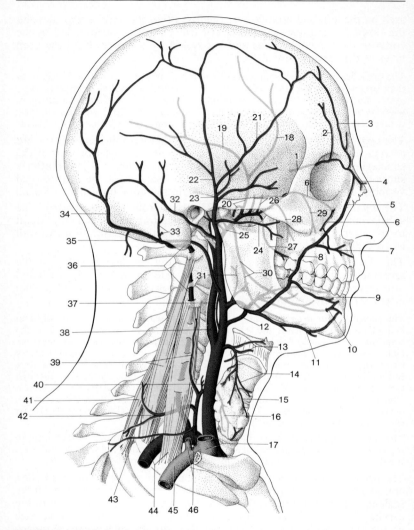

Fig. 277. **Arteries to head and neck**
Branches of external carotid artery, anastomoses between external and internal
carotid arteries, branches of subclavian to neck and central nervous system

1 Ophthalmic artery
2 Supra-orbital artery
3 Supratrochlear artery

4 Dorsal nasal artery
5 Angular artery
6 Infra-orbital artery

thyroid artery, more rarely directly from the trunk, and passes cranially medial to the phrenic nerve. It gives off branches to the scalene muscle (and to the musculature of the back) and sends *spinal branches* into the vertebral canal for the spinal cord via the intervertebral foramina.

The *costocervical trunk* ($\rightarrow$ Vol. 2, Fig. **6**) leaves the scalene gap at the posterior wall of the subclavian artery – as the common stem of the *deep cervical* and *highest intercostal arteries* – and sends branches to the nuchal muscles and to the upper two intercostal spaces.

The *deep cervical artery*, frequently a large artery, penetrates dorsally into the semispinal capitis muscle between the transverse processes of the 7th cervical and 1st thoracic vertebra, runs upward on its dorsal side and supplies the nuchal muscles.

The *highest* (*supreme, superior*) *intercostal artery* passes in front of the 1st and 2nd ribs and bifurcates into the *posterior intercostal arteries I* and *II*, which course ventrally in their corresponding intercostal spaces. Each gives off a *dorsal branch* to the muscles and skin of the back and a *spinal branch* to the spinal cord through the intervertebral foramina.

The **subclavian vein** (Fig. **278**) is a continuation of the axillary vein (toward the heart) in the lateral triangle of the neck and extends from the 1st rib to the union with the internal jugular vein (behind the sternoclavicular joint) to form the brachiocephalic vein. Covered by the middle layer

---

7 Superior labial artery
8 Facial artery
9 Inferior labial artery
10 Mental artery
11 Submental artery
12 Lingual artery with dorsales linguae branches, divides into sublingual artery and arteria profunda linguae (not labelled)
13–15 *Superior thyroid artery*
13 Infrahyoid branch and superior laryngeal artery
14 Sternocleidomastoid branch, posterior glandular branch and cricothyroid branch
15 Anterior glandular branch
16 Inferior thyroid artery
17 Common carotid artery and internal jugular vein
18 Frontal branch } of middle
19 Parietal branch } meningeal artery
20 Middle meningeal and masseteric arteries
21 Frontal branch } of superficial
22 Parietal branch } temporal artery
23 Superficial temporal artery with exit of middle temporal (cranial) and zygomatico-orbital arteries (both not labelled)
24 Transverse facial artery
25 Maxillary artery with exit of deep auricular (to external acoustic meatus) and anterior tympanic arteries (both not labelled)

26 Deep temporal arteries
27 Buccal artery
28 Posterior superior alveolar artery
29 Anterior superior alveolar arteries
30 Inferior alveolar artery with exit of mylohyoid branch (not labelled)
31 Ascending palatine artery
32 Posterior auricular artery
33 Auricular branch of occipital artery with mastoid branch (into mastoid foramen)
34 Occipital artery
35 Descending branch of occipital artery
36 Vertebral artery
37 Ascending pharyngeal artery
38 Internal carotid artery and carotid sinus
39 Ascending cervical artery and scalenus medius
40 Pharyngeal branches of inferior thyroid artery
41 Scalenus posterior
42 Transverse cervical artery (on scalenus medius) with superficial branch and deep branch
43 Suprascapular artery
44 Subclavian artery and scalenus anterior
45 Subclavian vein
46 Thyrocervical trunk and external jugular vein

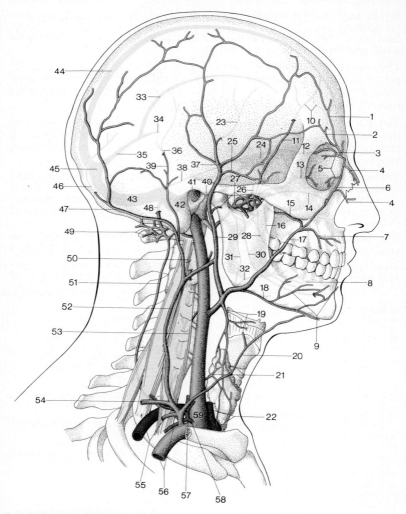

Fig. 278. **Veins of head and neck**
Tributaries of internal jugular vein, venous pathways and cervical branches of
subclavian and brachiocephalic veins

1 Supratrochlear vein
2 Supra-orbital vein
3 Nasofrontal vein
4 External nasal veins
5 Superior and inferior palpebral veins
6 Angular vein
7 Superior labial vein
8 Vena profunda linguae

of the cervical fascia, the subclavian vein courses in front of the scalenus anterior and behind the clavicular insertion of the sternocleidomastoid. Its direct tributaries (*pectoral, dorsal scapular* and *thoraco-acromial veins*) carry blood from the pectorales, rhomboid and deltoid muscles.

The *vertebral vein*, companion vein of the vertebral artery, leaves the canal formed by the foramina of the transverse processes of the cervical vertebrae (usually) through the foramen transversarium of C6 and empties dorsally into the brachiocephalic vein.

The *deep cervical vein* (Fig. **278**) connects the suboccipital venous plexus with the vertebral vein or directly with the brachiocephalic vein and courses behind the transverse processes of the cervical vertebrae, between the semispinalis capitis and cervicis muscles.

The **subclavian trunk** (Fig. **272** and **278**) accompanies the subclavian vein. It carries lymph from the arm and the trunk wall above the umbilicus – via the *axillary lymph nodes* ($\rightarrow$ p. 210 and Fig. **112**) – on the right side into the right lymphatic duct, on the left side into the thoracic duct.

The **brachial plexus** ($\rightarrow$ Fig. **87**), following directly caudad to the cervical plexus, arises from the ventral rami of cervical nerves 5–8, as well as part of the 1st (2nd) thoracic and occasionally the 4th cervical nerve. The fibers from the ventral spinal nerve branches first combine into three primary *trunks* at the exit of the scalene gap. The *upper trunk* carries fibers from C(4) 5 and 6, the *middle* from C7 and the *lower* from C8 and T1(2).

◄ 9 Inferior labial veins
10 Frontal diploic vein and anterior temporal diploic vein
11 Deep temporal vein
12 Superior ophthalmic vein
13 Inferior ophthalmic vein
14 Infra-orbital vein
15 Deep facial vein
16 Descending palatine vein
17 Facial vein
18 Submental vein
19 Superior thyroid and superior laryngeal veins
20 Anterior jugular vein
21 Middle thyroid vein
22 Common carotid artery and brachiocephalic trunk
23 Middle temporal diploic vein
24 Cavernous sinus
25 Middle temporal vein
26 Middle meningeal vein
27 Transverse facial vein (severed), maxillary veins and pterygoid venous plexus
28 Buccal vein
29 Retromandibular vein
30 Inferior alveolar vein
31 External palatine vein
32 Lingual vein

33 Inferior sagittal sinus
34 Great cerebral vein
35 Straight sinus
36 Posterior temporal diploic vein
37 Superficial temporal veins
38 Superior petrosal sinus
39 Posterior auricular vein
40 Inferior petrosal sinus
41 Superior bulb of jugular vein
42 Sigmoid sinus
43 Transverse sinus
44 Superior sagittal sinus
45 Confluence of sinuses
46 Occipital diploic vein
47 Occipital vein
48 Mastoid emissary vein
49 Suboccipital venous plexus
50 Vertebral vein
51 Deep cervical vein
52 External jugular vein
53 Anterior vertebral vein
54 Transverse cervical vein
55 Subclavian artery and suprascapular vein
56 Subclavian vein and subclavian trunk
57 Jugular trunk
58 Right lymphatic duct
59 Inferior bulb of jugular vein

The primary trunks each divide into a ventral and a dorsal branch (*ventral divisions* for the genetic flexors, *dorsal divisions* for the genetic extensors) and are organized at the entrance into the axilla and at the approach to the axillary artery into secondary cords (*fasciculi*).

The dorsal branches of all three trunks join together to form the *posterior cord* (C5–8, T1) on the dorsal side of the artery. The ventral branches of the upper and middle trunks form the *lateral cord* (C5–7) at the lateral side of the axillary artery. The *medial cord* (C8, T1) arises alone from the ventral branch of the inferior trunk and is attached to the dorso*medial* side of the artery.

The part of the brachial plexus situated above the clavicle is designated as the **supraclavicular part**; its branches leave the brachial plexus in the lateral triangle of the neck and pass to the muscles of the shoulder girdle.

The *dorsal scapular nerve* (C4, 5) penetrates the scalenus medius, passes underneath the levator scapulae, courses downward beneath the rhomboids – parallel to the medial margin of the scapula – and supplies these muscles.

The *nerve to the serratus anterior* (C5–7[8]) also passes through the scalenus medius, crosses the 1st rib laterally and descends on the external surface of the serratus anterior, which it innervates, approximately at the (mid-)axillary line.

The *nerve to the subclavius* (C[4] 5, 6) penetrates the subclavius from behind and frequently gives off a branch to the phrenic nerve.

The *suprascapular nerve* courses laterally in the omoclavicular triangle at the lateral margin of the brachial plexus to the scapular notch, through which it passes *below* the superior transverse scapular ligament to the supraspinatus and infraspinatus muscles.

The **infraclavicular part** of the plexus is located distal to the upper margin of the clavicle. *Short* branches are given off by its cords (partly also from its trunks): *medial* and *lateral pectoral*, *subscapular* and *thoracodorsal nerves* to the shoulder muscles (→ p. 215). *Long* branches from the infraclavicular part arise from the cords as nerves of the free upper limb (→ p. 215).

2. Neurovascular Bundle from the Neck to the Head:
Nerves and Vessels in the Neck Region

The **neurovascular bundle of the neck** (Fig. **276**), which continues the large axial neurovascular route from the trunk to the head, consists of the *common carotid artery* (medially), the *internal jugular vein* (laterally) and the *vagus nerve* (dorsally between the artery and vein), as well as the lymphatic plexus – along the internal jugular vein – which empties into the venous angle as the *jugular trunk*. Vessels and nerves are enclosed by the compact, connective tissue *neurovascular sheath* (*carotid sheath*), into which fibrous tracts of the pretracheal layer of the cervical fascia radiate, with only loose communication with the prevertebral layer.

In its entire course, the *neurovascular bundle* lies in the connective tissue space lateral to the cervical viscera, in front of the prevertebral layer of the cervical fascia (the direction of its course corresponds somewhat to the line: sternoclavicular joint-middle ear). The bundle passes upward from the superior thoracic aperture, at first still covered by the middle layer of the cervical fascia, behind the sternocleidomastoid (in the *sterno-cleidomastoid region*) and, with the head directed straight ahead, arrives at the *carotid triangle* approximately in the middle of the anterior margin of the muscle. Above the thyroid cartilage, the *internal carotid artery* maintains the direction of the common carotid artery into the para-pharyngeal space.

The distance between the neurovascular bundles of both sides is deter-mined by the width of the neck. It increases from the thyroid gland cranialwards. When the head is rotated, the neurovascular bundle comes to lie at the anterior margin of the sternocleidomastoid on the side from which the face has been averted, whereas on the opposite side it is covered in its entire extent by muscle.

In the caudal half of the bundle, the *ansa cervicalis* from the *cervical plexus* (usually situated medial to the internal jugular vein and in front of the common carotid artery) is enclosed in the connective tissue sheath together with its muscular branches (Fig. **276**). The *superior root* of the ansa cervicalis passes downward inside of the neurovascular sheath ventral to the internal carotid artery (Figs. **261** and **268**), whereas the *inferior root* (usually) loops around the internal jugular vein from the lateral side.

In the *carotid triangle*, the vessels and nerves are regrouped.

As a rule, the **common carotid artery** (Fig. **277**), which arises from the brachiocephalic trunk on the right side and from the aortic arch on the left, gives off no branches. It bifurcates in the carotid triangle (usually) at the level of the 4th cervical vertebra (level of the laryngeal prominence) into the *external carotid artery* (medially in front) and into the *internal carotid artery* (laterally and behind). Whereas the internal carotid artery enters the carotid canal of the base of the skull without giving off branches and feeds the cerebral arteries, the external carotid artery immediately provides branches for the cervical organs, the face and the scalp.

Nerves and receptors. External and *internal carotid nerves* from the superior cervical ganglion of the sympathetic trunk pass to the carotid bifurcation, as well as to the internal and external carotid arteries. They form plexuses that pass to the target organs with the branches of the arteries.

The dilatation of the internal carotid artery at its origin from the common carotid (and also often the carotid bifurcation) is referred to as the *carotid sinus*. The wall of the carotid sinus contains pressure receptors that respond to changes in the tension of the vascular wall as the result of a change in blood pressure ("blood pressure governor"). The *carotid body* (Fig. **268**), a millimeter-sized, reddish-brown nodule, lies in the carotid bifurcation and, as a chemoreceptor, controls the oxygen content of the blood. Both receptors are connected with the glossopharyngeal nerve by a thin nerve, the *carotid sinus ramus*.

In the carotid triangle, the **external carotid artery** (Fig. **277**) gives off as *anterior* branches the *superior thyroid, lingual* and *facial arteries*. It dispatches *medially* the *ascending pharyngeal artery, dorsally* the *occipital* and *posterior auricular arteries* before it divides into its terminal branches, the *maxillary* and *superficial temporal arteries* below the temporomandibular joint and behind the neck of the mandible.

The *superior thyroid artery* arises caudal to the greater horn of the hyoid and descends medially in a narrow arch to the thyroid gland where it supplies blood to the ventral portion of the gland via the *anterior glandular branch*, to the lateral glandular portion via the *lateral glandular branch* and to the upper pole at the anterior and posterior surfaces via the *posterior glandular branch*.

The superior thyroid artery dispatches the *infrahyoid branch*, which passes along the hyoid bone and anastomoses with the same-named artery of the opposite side. It also gives rise laterally to the muscular, *sternocleidomastoid branch*.

Two branches of the superior thyroid artery pass to the larynx. The *superior laryngeal artery* is attached caudally to the internal ramus of the superior laryngeal nerve, passes through the thyrohyoid membrane (usually) in common with the nerve and supplies the greatest part of the muscles and mucous membrane of the larynx with blood.

The weak *cricothyroid branch* arises near the lower border of the thyroid cartilage, courses on the cricothyroid muscle, to which it sends branches, anastomoses medially with the same-named artery of the opposite side and sends 1–2 twigs through the cricothyroid ligament to the anterior, inferior mucosa of the larynx.

The *lingual artery* – as the 2nd anterior branch – leaves the external carotid artery at the level of the greater horn of the hyoid. In almost one-fifth of the cases, it arises in common with the facial artery via the *linguofacial trunk*. The artery gives off the *suprahyoid branch* before it passes – covered by the hyoglossus muscle – to the tongue and the floor of the mouth.

The *facial artery*, the 3rd anterior branch of the external carotid artery, reaches the submandibular triangle medial to the stylohyoid and digastric muscles, is covered by the submandibular gland and arrives at the face at the anterior margin of the masseter above the margin of the mandible.

The *ascending pharyngeal artery* arises at the medial aspect of the external carotid artery, occasionally also from the occipital artery, and passes craniad along the pharyngeal wall medial to the neurovascular bundle and to the stylopharyngeus muscle as far as the base of the skull.

It gives off *pharyngeal branches* to the wall of the pharynx, dispatches the *inferior tympanic artery* through the tympanic canaliculus to the medial wall of the tympanic cavity and, with its terminal branch, the *posterior meningeal artery*, passes through the jugular foramen to the dura mater of the posterior cranial fossa.

The *occipital artery*, as the 1st posterior branch of the external carotid artery, leaves at about the level of exit of the facial artery. It courses between the stylohyoid and the posterior belly of the digastric to the transverse process of the atlas, passes into the groove for the occipital artery at the medial surface of the mastoid process and ramifies at the bones and scalp of the occiput, as well as in the nuchal musculature ($\rightarrow$ p. 496).

The *posterior auricular artery* also arises posteriorly, covered by the parotid gland, and arrives – across the stylohyoid muscle and styloid process – behind the pinna on the mastoid process where it divides into the *auricular branch* (to the posterior surface of the pinna, with perforating branches also to the anterior surface) and the *occipital branch* (to the occiput, anastomoses with branches of the occipital artery).

Beforehand, it gives off a *parotid branch*, muscular branches and – into the stylomastoid foramen – the *stylomastoid artery*, which accompanies the facial nerve into the facial canal and enters the dura at the hiatus of the canal for the greater petrosal nerve. The *posterior tympanic artery*, a branch of the stylomastoid artery, passes with the chorda tympani through the small canal of the chorda tympani to the mucosa of the middle ear cavity (including the tympanic membrane) and supplies the mucosa of the mastoid air cells with the *mastoid branches* and the stapedius muscle with the *stapedial branch*.

The **internal jugular vein** (Fig. **278**) carries blood away from the venous sinuses of the base of the skull, from the face and from organs of the neck. It is generally larger on the right side than on the left and – as a continuation of the sigmoid sinus – begins in the jugular foramen with a dilatation, the *superior bulb of the jugular vein*. It also receives the *vein of the cochlear aqueduct* and the *venous plexus of the hypoglossal canal*, more rarely the *inferior petrosal sinus* (junction usually distally directly into the internal jugular vein). The internal jugular vein courses first dorsally, then downward, lateral to the internal carotid artery, and, enclosed in the neurovascular sheath, enters the cervical region laterally in front of the common carotid artery. Shortly before it unites with the subclavian vein to form the brachiocephalic vein at the venous angle, the vein is dilated into the *inferior bulb of the jugular vein*, which possesses a single or bipartite venous valve.

The tributaries of the internal jugular vein vary in number, depending on whether the "root" veins gather first into venous trunks or empty separately. It receives *pharyngeal veins* from the venous *pharyngeal plexus* at the dorsal wall of the pharynx and the *lingual vein* and – as variants – its tributaries (*dorsal lingual veins, companion vein of the hypoglossal nerve* as the end portion of the *sublingual vein, vena profunda linguae*) from the region of the tongue, provided they do not flow into the facial or retromandibular veins.

The *superior thyroid vein*, which courses with the artery of the same name, receives the *superior laryngeal* and *sternocleidomastoid veins* (as long as these do not open independently) and can convey blood from the thyroid gland to the internal jugular vein (or the facial vein). The *middle thyroid veins*, which do not accompany an artery, conduct blood from the lower portion of the thyroid lobe into the internal jugular vein, which occasionally receives the *external jugular vein* close to this opening.

The *facial vein* enters the internal jugular vein at the level of the greater horn of the hyoid. It collects blood from the anterior facial region, passes *behind* the facial artery over the border of the mandible and arrives at the carotid triangle superficial to the submandibular gland. As long as the *retromandibular vein* does not open directly into the internal jugular vein, the facial vein also carries off blood from the scalp, as well as from the superficial and the deep lateral regions of the face.

The **jugular trunk** (Figs. **272** and **278**) conducts lymph from the head and neck indirectly – over the terminal sections of the right lymphatic duct on the right side, the thoracic duct on the left side – or also directly into the venous angle. The short lymphatic trunk arises from efferent lymphatic tracts of the deep lateral cervical lymph nodes and accompanies the portion of the internal jugular vein near the opening.

The **groups of lymph nodes in the cervical region** are organized (recently) into *anterior* and *posterior* (lateral) *cervical lymph nodes*. In both groups, *superficial* and *deep* lymph nodes can be distinguished – corresponding to their position. The superficial cervical lymph nodes are regional lymph nodes; they discharge lymph into the deep lymph nodes. The deep cervical lymph nodes form the second filter station for the lymphatic tracts in the head-neck region, but also receive direct lymphatic tributaries from their surroundings. They are thus collecting lymph nodes and regional lymph nodes at the same time.

The *superficial anterior cervical lymph nodes* lie along the anterior jugular vein. They receive lymph from the skin of the anterior region of the neck (below the hyoid bone) and send it on to the deep anterior cervical lymph nodes. The *deep anterior cervical lymph nodes* are arranged along the lower respiratory pathway, the *prelaryngeal lymph nodes* on the cricothyroid ligament, the *thyroid lymph nodes* at the thyroid gland, the *pretracheal* and *paratracheal lymph nodes* in front of and beside the trachea. The lymph which they receive from the superficial lymph nodes and which, at times, is directly conducted to them from the surroundings is carried off to the deep cervical lymph nodes.

The *lateral* cervical lymph nodes lie in the vicinity of the sternocleidomas-toid and extend into the omoclavicular triangle. The *superficial lateral cervical lymph nodes* are arranged along the external jugular vein. As regional lymph nodes, they receive lymph from the region of the ear lobule, the floor of the external acoustic meatus, as well as from the skin over the angle of the jaw and over the lower part of the parotid gland. The *deep lateral cervical lymph nodes* filter (almost) the entire lymph from the head and neck. They can be organized into several groups (Fig. **272**).

The *lateral* and *anterior jugular lymph nodes* lie along the internal jugular vein. The *jugulodigastric node* (at the crossing of the internal jugular vein and the posterior belly of the digastric) receives (as a regional lymph node) lymph from the palatine tonsil and from the base of the tongue. Lymph flows to the *jugulo-omohyoid node* (at the crossing of the internal jugular vein and the superior belly of the omohyoid) from the tongue and – via connected *submandibular* and *submental lymph nodes* – from the middle and the lower parts of the face. The group referred to as the *supraclavicular lymph nodes* (along the subclavian vein in the omoclavicular triangle) receives lymph from the arm.

Closely allied with the internal carotid or the common arteries, the **vagus nerve** (Fig. **268** and **276**) passes caudad – in the neurovascular bundle from the neck to the head – and enters the mediastinum between the subclavian artery and brachiocephalic vein.

At the level of its inferior ganglion, it gives off the *auricular ramus* to the skin in the infundibulum of the pinna and the skin of the external auditory meatus and dispatches *pharyngeal rami* which traverse between the internal and external carotid arteries to the nerve plexus on the external surface of the middle con-strictor of the pharynx. This *pharyngeal plexus* receives contributions from bran-ches of the glossopharyngeal nerve and the cervical sympathetic trunk.

The *superior laryngeal nerve* leaves the vagus at the lower end of the inferior ganglion and passes through the medial cervical region to the larynx (→ p. 779). The only other vagal branches in the cervical region are the *superior* and *inferior cervical cardiac rami*, which pass to the cardiac plexus.

The *right recurrent laryngeal nerve* (Fig. **280**) first branches off from the vagus nerve ventral to the subclavian artery, courses dorsally below the subclavian artery – medial to the origin of the vertebral artery – and finally passes cranially in the right furrow between the trachea and esophagus. It gives off *tracheal* and *esophageal rami* and reaches the larynx as the *inferior laryngeal nerve*. The *left recurrent laryngeal nerve* arises in front of the end of the arch of the aorta, bends around the ligamentum arteriosum, crosses beneath the arch of the aorta (Fig. **280**) and thus reaches the left furrow between the trachea and esophagus.

The **cervical plexus** will be discussed here since the *superior root of the ansa cervicalis* and the *ansa cervicalis* belong to it and course in the neurovascular sheath.

The *cervical plexus* arises near the cervical vertebral column from the ventral rami of cervical nerves 1–4 between the superior origins of the anterior and middle scalenes. The nerves emanating from the plexus (Fig. **279**) supply the skin of the neck, the infrahyoid muscles and the diaphragm.

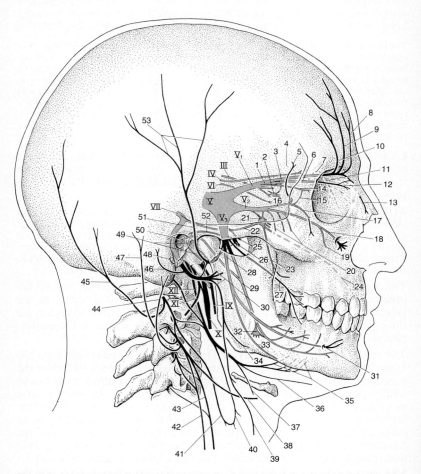

Fig. 279. **Nerves of head and neck**, schematic diagram of selected cranial nerves and cranial nerve branches, as well as the cervical plexus
(for the sake of clarity, nerves and nerve rami only partially depicted)

Fibers from the ventral rami of C1 and 2 are temporarily attached to the hypoglossal nerve. Cervical fibers thus arrive via the 12th cranial nerve – as *geniohyoid muscular rami* – at the geniohyoid and – as *thyrohyoid rami* which branch off at the posterior border of the hyoglossus – at the thyrohyoid muscle.

The *superior root of the ansa cervicalis* already leaves the hypoglossal nerve at the entrance into the carotid triangle where the latter crosses over the external carotid artery (Figs. **261** and **268**) and passes downward in the carotid sheath medial to the internal jugular vein, in front of the internal carotid artery. The *inferior root* (C1–3), which courses caudad outside of the neurovascular sheath lateral to the internal jugular vein, forms a nerve loop with the superior root, the *ansa cervicalis*, at differing levels, usually at the lower angle of the carotid triangle or behind the omohyoid. From the ansa, branches pass to both bellies of the omohyoid and to the sternohyoid and sternothyroid muscles.

The **nerves to the skin of the neck** course through the superficial layer of the cervical fascia in a limited area at the posterior margin of the

---

III	Oculomotor nerve	21	Pterygopalatine ganglion
IV	Trochlear nerve	22	Greater petrosal nerve
V	Trigeminal nerve	23	Greater and lesser palatine nerves
V_1	Ophthalmic nerve	24	Nasopalatine nerve
V_2	Maxillary nerve	25	Masticatory nerves
V_3	Mandibular nerve	26	Otic ganglion
VI	Abducens nerve	27	Buccal nerve
VII	Facial nerve	28	Inferior alveolar nerve
IX	Glossopharyngeal nerve	29	Lingual nerve
X	Vagus nerve	30	Intrapartoid plexus of facial nerve
XI	Accessory nerve	31	Mental nerve
XII	Hypoglossal nerve	32	Submandibular ganglion
1	Frontal nerve	33	Mylohyoid nerve
2	Ciliary ganglion	34	Marginal mandibular branch of facial nerve
3	Supra-orbital nerve	35	Lingual branches of hypoglossal nerve
4	Posterior ethmoidal nerve	36	Geniohyoid branch
5	Zygomaticotemporal branch of zygomatic nerve	37	Thyrohyoid branch
6	Nasociliary nerve	38	Transverse cervical nerve of the neck
7	Anterior ethmoidal nerve	39	Cervical branch of facial nerve
8	Supratrochlear nerve	40	Superior root of ansa cervicalis
9	Medial branch of supra-orbital nerve	41	Inferior root of ansa cervicalis
10	Lateral branch of supra-orbital-nerve	42	Supraclavicular nerves
11	Nasal branches of anterior ethmoidal nerve	43	Phrenic nerve
12	Infratrochlear nerve	44	Great auricular nerve
13	External nasal branch of anterior ethmoidal nerve	45	Greater occipital nerve
14	Lacrimal nerve	46	Posterior auricular nerve
15	Communicating ramus (of lacrimal nerve with zygomatic nerve)	47	Lesser occipital nerve
16	Zygomatic nerve	48	Auricular branch of vagus nerve
17	Zygomaticofacial branch of zygomatic nerve	49	Tympanic nerve, tympanic plexus
18	Infra-orbital nerve	50	Chorda tympani
19	Anterior superior alveolar branches	51	Auriculotemporal nerve
20	Middle and posterior superior alveolar nerves	52	Lesser petrosal nerve
		53	Superficial temporal branches

sternocleidomastoid, at the level of its middle third at the so-called *nervous point*.

The delicate *lesser occipital nerve* (C2, 3) courses along the sternocleidomastoid in the region of the mastoid process and divides into its branches, which pass toward the crown of the head, supply a variable large cutaneous region at the occiput and anastomose with branches of the greater occipital and great auricular nerves.

The *great auricular nerve* (C3) passes perpendicularly upward on the surface of the fascia and divides into the *posterior ramus* for the skin at the posterior surface of the pinna and a variable adjacent area and into the *anterior ramus* for the anterior surface of the pinna and the skin at the angle of the jaw.

The *transverse cervical (colli) nerve* (C3) first cuts across the sternocleidomastoid toward the midline beneath the platysma and divides into *superior rami* for the skin above the hyoid bone and *inferior rami* for the skin of the lower part of the neck. The cervical ramus of the facial nerve provides several anastomoses to the motor fibers of the superior rami (altogether also designated as the *ansa cervicalis superficialis*) for the innervation of the platysma.

The *supraclavicular nerves* (C3, 4) appear in several tracts underneath the sterno-cleidomastoid, radiate fan-shaped and penetrate at varying heights through the fascia and platysma above the clavicle. The *medial supraclavicular nerves* supply the skin over the medial third of the clavicle and the adjacent thoracic skin. The *intermediate supraclavicular nerves* pass to the skin over the middle third of the clavicle and the thoracic wall up to the 4th rib. The *lateral (posterior) supraclavicular nerves* innervate the skin over the acromion and the deltoid muscle.

As the "accessory phrenic nerve", the **phrenic nerve** (C[3], 4) usually receives fibers from the ventral ramus of the 5th cervical nerve which have been temporarily attached to the nerve to the subclavius. After a long spiral on the "anterior surface" of the scalenus anterior, the phrenic nerve crosses from the "lateral" to the "medial" margin, advances through the superior thoracic aperture into the thoracic cavity behind the subclavian vein and in front of the artery. Here it supplies motor innervation to the diaphragm, sensory innervation to the pericardium via its *pericardiac ramus* and to the peritoneum of the upper part of the abdomen (epigastrium) via its *phrenico-abdominal rami*.

To a varying extent, motor fibers (C2–4) from the cervical plexus pass to the accessory nerve and are deposited in front of the entrance into the sternocleido-mastoid and at the lower surface of the trapezius. They innervate the parts of the muscle arising from the upper cervical myotomes and are branched off from the lesser occipital nerve for the sternocleidomastoid, from a supraclavicular nerve or as direct branches from C3 and C4 for the trapezius.

The short nerves to the prevertebral cervical muscles and the contributions to the innervation of the scaleni anterior and medius, as well as the levator scapulae, arise directly from ventral rami of the corresponding spinal nerves and are, strictly speaking, not branches of the cervical plexus.

The **glossopharyngeal nerve** is closely adjacent to the vagus after exiting from the jugular foramen (Fig. **268**). However, it is not enclosed in the neurovascular bundle, but reaches the dorsolateral surface of the stylopharyngeus between the internal carotid artery and the internal jugular vein, before passing to the root of the tongue between this muscle and the styloglossus.

The inferior ganglion of the glossopharyngeal gives rise to the *tympanic nerve* and *communicating rami* to the auricular ramus of the vagus. The tympanic nerve courses in the tympanic canaliculus to the mucosa of the tympanic cavity, ramifies into the *tympanic plexus* from which it dispatches preganglionic, parasympatheic fibers to the otic ganglion as the *lesser petrosal nerve.*

Distal to the inferior ganglion, the glossopharyngeal nerve gives rise to the *stylopharyngeal muscular ramus, pharyngeal rami* to the pharyngeal plexus (for the innervation of the superior pharyngeal constrictor and the mucosal area associated with it) and the *carotid sinus ramus* to the carotid sinus and carotid body. *Tonsillar rami* innervate the mucosa of the palatine tonsil and the palatal arches; *lingual rami* supply the foliate and vallate papillae, as well as the mucosa of the root of the tongue.

The **accessory nerve** (Fig. **268**) enters the posterosuperior angle of the carotid triangle beneath the sternocleidomastoid in front of the internal jugular vein, innervates the former and passes through the lateral cervical triangle to the trapezius (Fig. **259**).

The **hypoglossal nerve** (Fig. **263**) arrives at the carotid triangle underneath the posterior belly of the digastric between the internal jugular vein and the internal carotid artery and finally crosses the lingual and facial arteries in an arc (hypoglossal arch) superficial to the external carotid artery and to its anterior branches. The nerve passes lateral to the hyoglossus muscle on the floor of the mouth and penetrates the body of the tongue.

The *superior root of the ansa cervicalis* leaves the hypoglossal nerve high up at the beginning of the hypoglossal arch; the *thyrohyoid ramus* to the thyrohyoid muscle exits at about the middle of the arch. The superior thyroid artery usually arises from the external carotid below the hypoglossal arch, whereas the sternocleidomastoid artery crosses over it to reach the muscle.

The *hypoglossal arch* courses farthest caudally of the three nerve arches passing to the tongue. The other two, formed by the *lingual* and the *glossopharyngeal nerves*, lie at different depths in the *submandibular triangle.*

With its three cervical ganglia, the *cervical part* of the *sympathetic trunk* (Fig. **276**) is embedded in the deep layer of the cervical fascia in front of the longus capitis and longus colli muscles. The *superior cervical ganglion*, a flat, spindle-shaped body 2.5–3 cm long, lies behind the internal carotid artery about 2 cm below the base of the skull. The *middle cervical ganglion*, often only weakly developed, is adjacent to the inferior thyroid artery at the level of the 6th cervical vertebra. The *inferior cervical ganglion* usually fuses with the 1st thoracic ganglion to form the *cer-*

vicothoracic ganglion (→ Vol. 2, Figs. **6** and **7**); it lies above the pleural cupola in the fossa between the transverse process of C7 and the 1st rib, dorsal to the subclavian artery, lateral to the origin of the vertebral artery and medial to the scalenus anterior. From the middle cervical ganglion, two interganglionic rami usually pass to the inferior cervical ganglion or the cervicothoracic ganglion. In so doing, the weaker ventral interganglionic ramus curves around the subclavian artery from the front so that a nerve loop, the *ansa subclavia*, is formed.

From the cervical part of the sympathetic trunk, *cervical cardiac nerves* course through the medial cervical region to the cardiac plexus (→ Vol. 2).

The **pharyngeal plexus**, an autonomic nerve plexus in the wall of the pharynx (at the level of the middle pharyngeal constrictor with cranial and caudal processes), is composed of efferent and afferent fibers from the *glossopharyngeal nerve* (for the upper part) and the *vagus nerve* (for the lower part), as well as efferent fibers that leave the *sympathetic trunk* at the level of the superior cervical ganglion. The motor responses of the pharynx, partly also the swallowing and gag reflexes, are controlled via the pharyngeal plexus.

3. Position of Cervical Organs in the Visceral Space

The **cervical organs** lie in the depth of the medial triangle of the neck between the paired neurovascular bundles to the head. They are covered in front by the middle layer of the cervical fascia and the infrahyoid musculature enclosed in it. The visceral space between the two neurovascular bundles forms the connective tissue stroma for the passage of connection routes between the facial skeleton and the body cavities, for the trachea (in front), pharynx and esophagus (behind).

Independent organs limited only to the neck are the larynx, as well as the thyroid and parathyroid glands which are attached in front of the trachea and lateral to the larynx. The pharynx has close neighborly relations to the cranium and facial skeleton. The trachea and esophagus continue into the mediastinum.

The **pharynx** (Fig. **265**), a 13–15 cm long, fibromuscular tube lined by a mucous membrane, is attached cranially to the base of the skull and lies in front of the vertebral column. At its incomplete anterior wall, it communicates above with the nasal cavity, in the middle part with the oral cavity, in the lower segment with the larynx.

In *anterior rhinoscopy*, the nasal cavities are examined through the nostrils (nares) by means of a nasal speculum. In *posterior rhinoscopy*, the choanae and the posterior part of the nasal cavities are made visible through the mouth and nasopharynx with the help of a laryngoscope.

The **esophagus** (Fig. **265**) is connected to the pharynx at the level of C6–7. The short initial part of the esophagus, the esophageal opening (Fig. **282**), is distinguished in its wall structure from the remaining portions of the esophagus (→ Vol. 2).

The short *cervical part of the esophagus* following the esophageal opening is frequently displaced toward the left and enters the mediastinum behind the trachea.

The **larynx** (Fig. **271**), the initial part of the respiratory pathway, is multistructured of cartilage, ligaments and muscles. The thyroid cartilage at the front supports the other parts of the larynx, which are (almost) completely concealed behind it. Only the arch of the cricoid cartilage lies free in front at the lower border of the thyroid cartilage and – like the latter – is palpable through the skin.

With the larynx in the middle position and the head held erect, the upper margin of the larynx (Adam's apple, *laryngeal prominence*) in males lies at the level of the C5, the transition from the larynx to the trachea at the level of C6–7. The larynx in females lies about half a vertebra and that of the newborn around three vertebrae higher.

The **trachea** (Fig. **265**) continues the respiratory pathway into the mediastinum of the thoracic cavity. Because it follows the lordosis of the cervical vertebral column, the trachea withdraws increasingly from the anterior wall of the neck – at the level of the jugular fossa up to 7 cm. The *anterolateral wall* of the trachea, which is constructed of horseshoe-shaped cartilaginous bars and ligaments (Fig. **283**), can be palpated through the anterior wall of the neck in the jugular fossa below the thyroid gland. The *posterior wall* of the trachea, which consists of muscle and connective tissue, closely adjoins the esophagus.

The **thyroid gland** covers the trachea in front with its narrow, transversely-oriented isthmus at about the level of the 2nd–4th tracheal cartilage (Fig. **265**). The gland widens out on each side of the trachea and larynx into an oval lobe which can extend as far as the upper margin of the thyroid cartilage (Fig. **268**). It follows the positional changes of the larynx.

A goiter can compress the trachea so strongly ("flattened or scabbard trachea") that respiration is hindered. The trachea, esophagus and neurovascular bundle to the head can also be displaced by this.

The **parathyroid glands**, two (or more) pea-sized organs on each side of the thyroid gland, occupy a variable location within the gland, but are usually embedded posteriorly in the capsule – frequently near the upper and the lower poles of each lobe.

D. Organs of the Neck

The displaceable cervical organs in the visceral spaces of the neck (larynx, trachea, pharynx, esophagus and thyroid gland with the parathyroids) are attached to one another at the level of the larynx by connective tissue and muscular tracts as an "organ packet". Therefore, during movements (e.g. swallowing), they are always moved together.

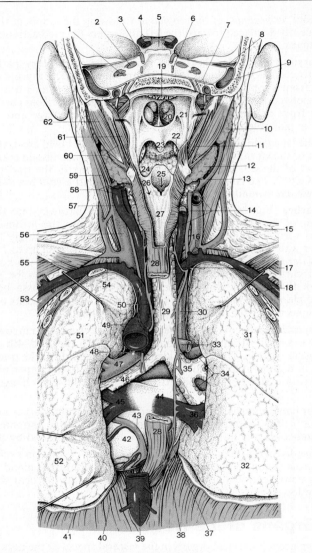

Fig. 280. **Pharynx, superior and inferior mediastinum**, dorsal view (posterior base of skull and vertebral column removed, pharynx opened)

1. Pharynx

The **pharynx** forms the connecting piece on the one hand for the digestive pathway between the oral cavity and the esophagus and on the other for the respiratory pathway between the nasal cavities and the larynx. The two pathways cross in the pharynx.

a) Form and Position of the Pharynx

The **pharyngeal cavity** can be organized into three segments (Fig. **265**). The upper segment, the *nasopharynx* (*epipharynx*), communicates with the nasal cavities at the choanae via the *nasopharyngeal meatus* (Fig. **263**). The middle segment, the *oropharynx* (*mesopharynx*), lies directly behind the oral cavity and is separated from it by the faucial isthmus. The lower segment, the *laryngopharynx* (*hypopharynx*), bears the inlet to the larynx anteriorly.

1 Facial nerve with nervus intermedius portion and vestibulocochlear nerve
2 Trigeminal nerve
3 Oculomotor nerve
4 Ophthalmic artery and optic nerve
5 Sella turcica
6 Abducens nerve
7 Inferior petrosal sinus (medial) and superior bulb of jugular vein
8 Superior petrosal sinus
9 Sigmoid sinus
10 Parotid gland
11 Stylohyoid ligament
12 Submandibular gland
13 Retromandibular vein
14 Right internal jugular vein, right vagus nerve and right common carotid artery
15 External jugular vein
16 Exit of vertebral artery (medial) and thyrocervical trunk
17 Right recurrent laryngeal nerve (passes beneath subclavian artery)
18 Right subclavian artery and vein
19 Pharyngeal tonsil
20 Choana
21 Torus tubarius
22 Palatine tonsil
23 Uvula
24 Lingual tonsil
25 Inlet (aditus) of larynx
26 Piriform recess
27 Laryngopharynx
28 Esophagus (partially resected)
29 Trachea
30 Superior vena cava
31 Superior lobe of right lung
32 Inferior lobe of right lung
33 Azygos vein
34 Branches of right pulmonary artery
35 Right primary bronchus
36 Right pulmonary veins
37 Inferior vena cava
38 Right vagus
39 Thoracic aorta
40 Diaphragm
41 Diaphragmatic pleura
42 Right ventricle of heart
43 Great cardiac vein
44 Left atrium of heart
45 Left pulmonary veins
46 Left primary bronchus
47 Left pulmonary artery
48 Ligamentum arteriosum
49 Arch of aorta
50 Left recurrent laryngeal nerve (loops around ligamentum arteriosum and arch of aorta)
51 Superior lobe of left lung
52 Inferior lobe of left lung
53 Left subclavian artery and vein
54 Insertion of scalenus anterior at first rib
55 Subclavius
56 Left internal jugular vein
57 Left external carotid artery
58 Left internal carotid artery and left vagus nerve
59 Sternocleidomastoid
60 Stylohyoid
61 Stylopharyngeus
62 Digastric, posterior belly

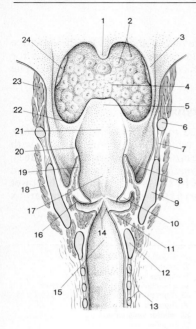

Fig. 281. Frontal section through middle and lower portions of pharyngeal cavity and larynx, dorsal view

1 Palatine uvula
2 Vallate papillae
3 Palatopharyngeal arch
4 Dorsum of tongue, pharyngeal part
5 Epiglottis
6 Hyoid bone
7 Thyrohyoid membrane
8 Fold of laryngeal nerve in piriform recess
9 Thyroid cartilage
10 Vestibular fold with vestibular ligament
11 Vocal fold with vocal ligament and vocalis muscle
12 Cricoid cartilage
13 Tracheal cartilages
14 Rima glottidis
15 Infraglottic cavity
16 Ventricle of larynx
17 Vestibule of larynx
18 Inferior pharyngeal constrictor
19 Quadrangular membrane
20 Aryepiglottic fold
21 Inlet of larynx
22 Pharyngo-epiglottic fold
23 Middle and superior pharyngeal constrictors
24 Palatine tonsil

The **nasopharynx** is closed off cranially by its *fornix*, or roof. The mucosa is attached at the base of the occipital bone, at the apex of the petrous part of the temporal bone and at the sphenoid bone and is laid in longitudinal folds. In the adult, it contains a thin layer of lymphatic tissue, which is abundantly developed, however, in childhood and which bulges into the posterior and lateral walls of the nasopharynx as the pharyngeal tonsil.

The **pharyngeal tonsil** forms the upper part of the lymphatic tonsillar ring.

An inconstant, especially deep indentation between two mucosal folds is designated as the *pharyngeal bursa*.

At the time of its strongest development in early school age, the pharyngeal tonsil can displace the choanae so that respiration and sleep are impaired resulting in over-fatigue and diminished attentiveness in school. A faulty development of the facial skeleton can also result.

The **auditory** (*pharyngotympanic, Eustachian*) **tube**, which unites the pharyngeal and tympanic cavities, opens into the lateral wall of the nasopharynx at about the level of the inferior nasal meatus. The tube opening (*pharyngeal opening of the auditory tube*, Fig. **263**) is surrounded at its

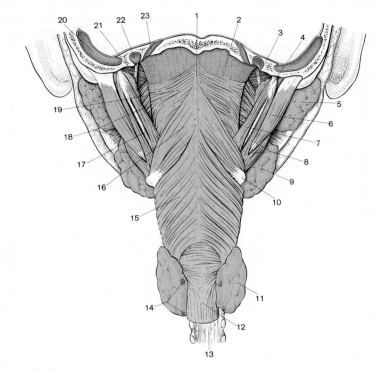

Fig. 282. **Pharyngeal musculature**, dorsal view (after *Rauber-Kopsch*)

1 Pharyngeal raphe
2 Pharyngobasilar fascia
3 Sphenomandibular ligament
4 Styloid process of temporal bone
5 Parotid gland
6 Digastric, posterior belly
7 Stylopharyngeus
8 Stylohyoid
9 Submandibular gland
10 Hyoid, greater horn
11 Thyroid gland
12 Esophagus, muscle layer
13 Trachea
14 Parathyroid glands
15 Inferior pharyngeal constrictor
16 Middle pharyngeal constrictor
17 Stylohyoid ligament
18 Medial pterygoid
19 Superior pharyngeal constrictor
20 Sigmoid sinus
21 Lateral pterygoid
22 Superior bulb of jugular vein
23 Inferior petrosal sinus

posterior and superior circumference by the arch-like tubal elevation (*torus tubarius*) which is formed by the free end of the tubal cartilage. It forms the posterior and the anterior lips of the tube. The *posterior lip* is continued downward into a mucosal fold (*salpingopharyngeal fold*), which contains the salpingopharyngeus muscle and extends into the lateral wall of the pharynx. From the *anterior lip of the tube*, a weaker mucosal fold (*salpingopalatine fold*) passes to the soft palate. The lower circumference of the tubal opening is bordered by the levator eminence (*torus levatorius*) produced by the levator veli palatini muscle.

Behind the torus tubarius, the lateral wall of the nasopharynx evaginates into the *pharyngeal recess* (Rosenmuller's fossa, Fig. **274**), which extends craniad up to the pharyngeal roof.

The **tubal tonsil** is an accumulation of lymphatic tissue around the opening of the auditory tube. This tissue can continue downward strand-like into the lateral wall of the pharynx and form the lymphatic "lateral cord".

The **oropharynx**, which is accessible through the faucial isthmus for direct inspection and study, is separated from the nasopharynx during swallowing by the apposition of the soft palate against the posterior pharyngeal wall. A horizontal plane placed through the upper end of the epiglottis is arbitrarily regarded as the lower boundary of the oropharynx.

In the **larnygopharynx**, the entrance of the larynx is invaginated from the front so that it exhibits a lumen shaped like a half-moon in cross section. A recess, the *piriform recess* (Fig. **281**), bordered against the base of the tongue by the pharyngo-epiglottic folds, is evident on each side of the larynx. By means of this mucosal channel through the pharynx, food from the base of the tongue is said to arrive at the esophageal inlet. The *pharyngo-epiglottic fold* is produced by the stylopharyngeus muscle. In the anterior wall of the piriform recess is a mucosal fold passing almost parallel and somewhat further caudad, the *fold of the laryngeal nerve*. In it, the internal ramus of the superior laryngeal nerve arrives at the larynx.

b) Histology and Function of the Pharynx

The **wall of the pharynx** consists of a *mucosa, submucosa, muscularis* and an external adventitial connective tissue layer. A muscularis mucosae is absent in the entire pharyngeal mucosa.

The **mucous membrane** of the nasopharynx is covered, for the most part, by pseudostratified, ciliated, columnar epithelium. The appositional region of the soft palate at the posterior pharyngeal wall, island-like areas on the folds of the nasopharyngeal tonsils and the entire oral and laryngeal pharynx are covered by a nonkeratinized stratified squamous epithelium. Mixed glands lie in the *lamina propria of the mucosa* lining the pharyngeal roof and around the laryngeal aditus, whereas numerous *mucosal (pharyngeal) glands* reside in the rest of the pharyngeal mucosa. The anterior and posterior walls of the laryngopharynx contain an extensive venous network in their mucosa.

The **submucosa** consists of a compact layer of connective tissue. It is especially well-developed at the upper end of the pharynx, where a muscular layer is absent. Termed the *pharyngobasilar fascia* (Fig. **282**), it attaches the pharyngeal wall to the base of the skull.

The *muscular layer* of the pharynx is surrounded by a thin fascia which goes over into the loose *retropharyngeal connective tissue* on the posterior surface of the pharynx and borders the parapharyngeal space laterally.

Pharyngeal Musculature

The muscles of the pharyx, which arise from the muscle material of pharyngeal arches 3–5, consist of skeletal muscle. The pharyngeal musculature is composed of three large, superficial *constrictors* and three weakly-developed *levators*.

The **pharyngeal constrictors** (*superior, middle* and *inferior*, Figs. **268, 271** and **282**) arise ventral to the skeletal elements of the skull, hyoid and larynx. They enclose the pharyngeal space at the sides and dorsally. Their bundles of fibers attach mostly at the *pharyngeal raphe*, a median tendinous tract especially evident in the cranial portion that attaches at the pharyngeal tubercle of the basicranium.

The **superior pharyngeal constrictor** has a fiber course ascending only slightly toward the middle and can be further subdivided according to the different areas of origin of its parts.

The *pterygopharyngeal part* arises from the posterior margin of the medial lamina of the pterygoid process and from the pterygoid hamulus, the *buccopharyngeal part* from the pterygomandibular raphe. The *mylopharyngeal part* comes from the mylohyoid line of the mandible and the *glossopharyngeal part* from the tongue musculature and the mucosa of the oral cavity. Occasionally, some bundles of fibers arise from the lower surface of the petrous temporal near the apex, the *petropharyngeal part*. The *pharyngobasilar fascia* is attached to the superior pharyngeal constrictor cranially.

Innervation: glossopharyngeal nerve.

The **middle pharyngeal constrictor** covers the lower portion of the superior pharyngeal constrictor.

Its *chondropharyngeal part* arises at the lesser horn of the hyoid, the *ceratopharyngeal part* at the greater horn.

Innervation: glossopharyngeal and vagus nerves.

The **inferior pharyngeal constrictor** has the steepest course of fibers. It covers the middle pharyngeal constrictor dorsally.

Its *thyropharyngeal part* arises from the external surface of the thyroid cartilage, the *cricopharyngeal part* from the lateral surface of the cricoid cartilage (Fig. **284**). Inconstant fibrous bundles come from the 2nd tracheal cartilage.

Innervation: vagus nerve.

The **pharyngeal levator muscles** are represented by the *palatopharyngeus, salpingopharyngeus* and *stylopharyngeus*. They pass from the cranial skeleton and from the auditory tube as thin bundles of muscle fibers and enter the wall of the pharynx from above.

Innervation: glossopharyngeal nerve.

The **palatopharyngeus muscle** (Fig. **274**) is the strongest elevator of the pharynx. It radiates from the palatal aponeurosis and from the pterygoid hamulus and, for the most part, courses downward in the palatopharyngeal arch on the inner surface of the pharyngeal constrictor. Its fibers partly terminate at the posterior margin of the thyroid cartilage and partly form a sling with the muscle of the opposite side in the caudal pharyngeal segment above the pharyngeal raphe, which is only indistinctly evident here. A shortening of the sling lifts the dorsal wall of the pharynx like a pouch. An additional bundle of fibers of the palatopharyngeus muscle coursing on the luminal side of the superior pharyngeal constrictor passes into the posterior wall of the pharynx in an approximately circular direction.

The **salpingopharyngeus muscle** originates from the free end of the tubal cartilage as a weak muscular tract and passes in the salpingopharyngeal fold to the lateral wall of the pharynx.

The **stylopharyngeus muscle** (Fig. **271**) arises near the base of the skull at the styloid process, inserts itself between the upper and the middle pharyngeal constrictor on the inner surface of the muscular tube and reaches the thyroid cartilage together with the fiber bundles from the palatopharyngeus muscle. Some of the fibers end in the submucosa of the pharyngeal wall.

Action of the pharyngeal musculature. The *pharyngeal constrictors* can constrict the pharyngeal space, diminishing the lumen. Since the fiber bundles of the middle and inferior pharyngeal constrictors course mostly obliquely upward to the site of insertion at the pharyngeal raphe (fixed point), their contraction also leads to a shortening of the digestive tube, whereby the hyoid bone and the larynx are lifted.

The more weakly-developed *pharyngeal levators* elevate the pharynx and shorten it. The horizontal bundle of fibers of the *palatopharyngeus* situated on the luminal side of the superior pharyngeal constrictor constricts the pharyngeal wall and presses it against the stretched and raised soft palate during closure of the nasopharynx.

Swallowing

Since the *food* and *air passages cross* in the pharyngeal space, there is the danger during swallowing that food particles can get into the respiratory tract – nose or larynx. This danger is prevented by a *reflex protection of the air passage* which occurs simultaneously with the – likewise reflexive – transport of food. *Swallowing is initiated voluntarily*, the *act of swallowing* being a *uniform process*. For didactic purposes, it can be divided into the (voluntarily initiated) preparation phase, the rapidly occurring true swallowing process and the transport phase of the food through the esophagus.

In the *preparatory phase*, the floor of the mouth is contracted, and the tongue presses the food against the soft palate. The subsequent phases are then elicited by means of the excitation of the receptors in the palatal mucosa.

The *reflex protection of the respiratory tract* takes place by the *closure of the nasopharynx* and the *inlet of the larynx*.

The *nasopharynx* is closed off from the oropharynx by the *elevation* and *stretching of the soft palate* (tensor and levator veli palatini muscles), which is pressed against the posterior *wall of the pharynx*. This wall *bulges forward* (Passavant's cushion) at this level owing to the circumscribed contraction of the superior pharyngeal constrictor and – passing in front of this – a fiber tract of the palatopharyngeus.

The *inlet of the larynx* is closed by two mechanisms. With the contraction of the floor of the mouth (mylohyoid muscles), the hyoid and *larynx are elevated* with the assistance of the digastric and the thyrohyoid muscles, thus bringing the inlet closer to the epiglottis. At the same time, during the carrying back of the base of the tongue, a fat body which lies in the connective tissue in front of and beside the epiglottis presses on the latter. In the process, the *epiglottis is brought closer to the inlet of the larynx*, which is thus (incompletely) closed. Generally, reflex cessation of breathing also occurs for the duration of the act of swallowing.

The *transport of food* through the pharynx and esophagus is likewise guaranteed by several mechanisms.

Pulled by the styloglossus and hyoglossus muscles, the *tongue* presses the food against the faucial isthmus and into the pharynx like a stamper. The *pharynx*, the lumen of which otherwise forms a transversely-directed cleft, is unfolded anteriorly and superiorly by the elevation of the larynx. Most of the food glides through the piriform recess (mainly the masticatory side), but some also passes above the epiglottis.

By the *shortening of the inferior pharyngeal constrictor*, a dorsal protrusion of the posterior wall of the pharynx occurs which – lifted by the contraction of the palatopharyngeus muscle – forms a "sack" to take up the food. The contraction of the pharyngeal constrictors above the food transports it into the esophagus.

The *transport through the esophagus* (e.g. in the case of fluids) can be effected by a jerky, strong contraction of the floor of the mouth and of the superior pharyngeal constrictor as "jet swallow" when the body is held erect or (in the case of solid food) can be produced by continual waves of contraction (*peristalsis*) of the esophagus.

The vital *swallowing* (*deglutition*) *reflex* is also maintained when sleeping and is ensured by several cranial nerves. Afferents and efferents of the swallowing reflex are coordinated in the swallowing center located in the medulla oblongata.

By voluntary disturbance of the mechanisms which ensure the upper and lower respiratory pathways (e.g. by attempting to speak when swallowing), "swallowing the wrong way" can occur.

In the case of *paralysis of the soft palate* (e.g. as a result of diphtheria), food particles can get into the nasal cavity.

c) Vessels and Nerves of the Pharynx

Arteries (Fig. 277). The strongest artery of the pharynx, the *ascending pharyngeal artery*, is a branch of the external carotid. At the pharynx medial to the neurovascular bundle, it passes upward to the base of the skull (→ p. 749). Additional arterial inflow comes from the *ascending palatine artery* (region of the tubal opening) and from the *inferior thyroid artery* (laryngopharynx).

The **venous plexus** (*pharyngeal plexus*) that surrounds the wall of the pharynx has several outlets into the *internal jugular vein*, as well as connections with the *pterygoid plexus* and with the *meningeal veins*.

The **lymphatic pathways** from the pharynx and from the pharyngeal tonsil (Fig. 272) pass to the *retropharyngeal lymph nodes* and the upper *deep lateral cervical lymph nodes*.

Nerves. The pharynx is innervated by the *vagus* and *glossopharyngeal nerves*, as well as by the *sympathetic trunk* (superior cervical ganglion). The nerves form a plexus (*pharyngeal plexus*) at the external side of the pharynx. From this plexus, motor fibers pass to the musculature; sensory and secretomotor fibers pass to the mucous membrane.

Esophagus → Vol. 2.

2. Larynx

The **larynx** is a completly-formed closure apparatus at the beginning of the lower respiratory pathway. Finely coordinated closure possibilities enable it to carry out various functions.

The larnyx is concerned in *swallowing*; the shunt for the passage of food from the oral cavity to the esophagus is placed in the pharyngeal space with the support of the larynx, the entrance into the larynx thereby (largely) closed.

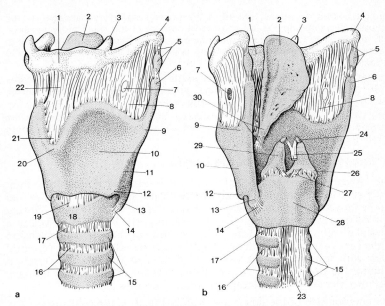

Fig. 283. **Hyoid bone and skeleton of larynx**, connections of skeletal elements
a Left oblique view from in front
b Left oblique view from behind

 1 Body of hyoid bone
 2 Epiglottic cartilage
 3 Lesser horn of hyoid
 4 Greater horn of hyoid
 5 Lateral thyrohyoid ligament and
   cartilago triticea
 6 Superior horn of thyroid cartilage
 7 Opening for superior laryngeal artery and
   internal branch of superior laryngeal nerve
 8 Thyrohyoid membrane
 9 Superior thyroid tubercle
10 Thyroid cartilage, left lamina
11 Oblique line
12 Inferior thyroid tubercle
13 Inferior horn of thyroid cartilage
14 Articular capsule of cricothyroid joint
15 Tracheal cartilages

16 Anular ligaments of trachea
17 Cricotracheal ligament
18 Arch of cricoid cartilage
19 Cricothyroid ligament
20 Laryngeal prominence
21 Superior thyroid notch
22 Median thyrohyoid ligament
23 Membranous part of trachea
24 Corniculate cartilage
25 Cricopharyngeal ligament
26 Muscular process of arytenoid cartilage
27 Articular capsule of crico-arytenoid joint
28 Lamina of cricoid cartilage
29 Arytenoid cartilage, posterior surface
30 Stalk of epiglottis and thyro-epiglottic
   ligament

Foreign bodies or mucus formed in the lower respiratory passage can be removed by *coughing*, i.e. by short-term closure of the respiratory passage with subsequent forceful expiration. Inspiration of harmful substances (e.g. caustic suspended matter) into the lung is prevented by *reflex closure* in the larynx.

Closure of the respiratory tract is a prerequisite for *increasing the internal pressure of the abdominal cavity* (e.g. abdominal pressure during defecation or birth), whereby the glottis in the larynx is usually closed.

With the help of the larynx, finely balanced *tones* can be produced which are formed in the oral cavity by articulation and released at the opening of the mouth as *voiced speech*.

a) Shape and Position of the Larynx

The **larynx** is connected directly with the infrahyoid muscles and indirectly (via the thyrohyoid membrane) with the suprahyoid muscles and can be moved in the connective tissue space of the neck by them. During swallowing, speaking, coughing and straining, the larnyx is moved in a vertical direction about 2–3 cm. With elevation of the head and extension of the cervical vertebral column, the larynx is raised about one vertebral level; with lowering of the head and flexion of the cervical vertebral column, the lower border of the larynx dips into the superior thoracic aperture, the vertical displacement totaling up to 4 cm.

The **anterior side** of the larynx (→ Vol. 2, Fig. 3) is directed toward the middle layer of the cervical fascia and is formed, for the most part, by the *thyroid cartilage*, which projects anteriorly like a ship's bow. In the midline, the "thyroid cartilage bow pushes through" the gap between the infrahyoid muscles of both sides; a notch at the upper edge of the bow, the *superior thyroid notch*, is palpable below the skin (Fig. 253). Below the thyroid cartilage, the *cricoid arch* extends to the anterior side of the larynx. The gap between the lower margin of the thyroid cartilage and the cricoid arch is closed by the elastic cricothyroid ligament.

The **posterior side** of the larynx is lined by mucosa. The laryngeal inlet (*laryngeal aditus*, Figs. 280 and 281) is bordered by two mucosal folds sloping steeply backward (*aryepiglottic folds*) and the *epiglottis*. The mucosal folds course from the upper border of the epiglottis obliquely downward and backward where they meet in an acute angle. Near their posterior end, the aryepiglottic folds are stiffened by two small cartilages which produce small tubercles in the mucosa. The *corniculate tubercle* lies near the midline below, the *cuneiform tubercle* lateral to it and somewhat higher (Fig. 284 b).

From the upper margin of the epiglottis, which projects above the hyoid from behind, a median and two lateral mucosal folds (*median* and *lateral glosso-epiglottic folds*) pass to the base of the tongue (Fig. 269). The three folds border two shallow fossae (*valleculae*).

The *piriform recess* is inserted posteriorly as a mucosal groove between the posterior end of the lamina of the thyroid cartilage (laterally) and the arytenoid cartilage (medially).

The **internal space** of the larynx, the *laryngeal cavity* (Fig. **281**), is divided into three levels (Fig. **265**) by two pairs of horizontal mucosal folds, the *vestibular* (above) and the *vocal* (below), both of which project from the wall into the lumen and lie in a sagittal plane one above the other.

The *vestibular folds* cover the lower free margin of a connective tissue plate, the *quadrangular membrane*. The *vocal folds* ("true vocal cords") project into the lumen further than the vestibular folds. In their shorter posterior region, they contain the muscular process of the arytenoid cartilage; in their anterior part, there is the elastic vocal ligament and the vocalis muscle. At the *rima glottidis* (the interval between the vocal folds and arytenoid cartilages), therefore, the posterior *intercartilaginous part* can be distinguished from the anterior *intermembranous part*.

The *upper portion* of the laryngeal cavity, the *vestibule*, extends from the laryngeal inlet to the vestibular folds. The epiglottis lies in the 4–5 cm high anterior wall of the vestibule; its stalk projects backward to form the *epiglottic tubercle*.

The *middle portion*, about 1 cm high, between the vestibular and vocal folds, is evaginated laterally to form the *ventricles*.

The *lower portion* of the laryngeal cavity, the space below the vocal folds, is widened as the *infraglottic cavity*, which continues into the trachea at the lower border of the cricoid cartilage.

b) Histology and Function of the Larynx

The larynx possesses a cartilaginous *laryngeal skeleton*. The skeletal elements are connected by a *ligamentous apparatus*, articulate with each other at *joints* and are moved by *laryngeal muscles*. The framework of cartilage and the muscles are covered on the dorsal aspect and in the laryngeal cavity by mucosa.

Skeleton of the Larynx

The base of the laryngeal skeleton (Figs. **281** and **284**) is the *cricoid cartilage*. It supports the *thyroid cartilage* on both sides and the two *arytenoid cartilages* behind. The *epiglottis* is attached to the inner side of the thyroid cartilage by connective tissue. The laryngeal skeleton is formed from hyaline cartilage – except for the epiglottis, the vocal process of the arytenoid cartilage, and the small cartilages in the aryepiglottic folds and in the thyrohyoid ligament, which consist of elastic cartilage.

The hyaline laryngeal cartilages can undergo variably strong ossification from the 2nd decade of life.

The **cricoid cartilage** has the form of a signet ring. The *arch* of the ring is in front, the 2–2.5 cm high *lamina* behind. Laterally, the upper margin of the lamina bears an oval articular surface for the arytenoid cartilage on both sides; the lateral margin on each side presents a round articular surface for the lesser horn of the thyroid cartilage.

The **thyroid cartilage** consists of a right and a left plate (lamina), each approximately quadrangular in shape. Both *laminae* are inclined slightly to the outside and are united with each other in front at an approximate right angle (Fig. **286**). The edge of the angle – corresponding to the inclination of the laminae – is directed forward and upward.

At the upper end of the edge, at the *laryngeal prominence*, the deep *superior thyroid notch* cuts between the two thryoid cartilage plates; at the lower end, a flat *inferior thyroid notch* can be delineated.

The external side of each lamina is divided into two facets by an oblique ridge (*oblique line*) directed from posterosuperior to antero-inferior. The thyrohyoid muscle arises from the oblique line; the sternothyroid is attached at the cartilage ridge. At the posterior facet, the field of origin of the thyropharyngeal part of the inferior pharyngeal constrictor is located. The ridge is strengthened above and below by tubercles, the *superior* and *inferior thyroid tubercles*, respectively.

A long upper and a short lower horn, the *superior* and *inferior cornua*, emerge from the posterior aspect of each thryoid lamina. The inferior horn articulates with the lateral edge of the cricoid cartilage; the superior horn is connected with the greater horn of the hyoid by the *lateral thyrohyoid ligament*.

The **arytenoid cartilage** is approximately three-cornered and shaped like a pyramid. It possesses four surfaces and three pronounced processes. *Posterior*, *middle* and *anterolateral surfaces* – each faceted by muscular and ligamentous attachments – are distinguished, as well as a *basal articular surface* which articulates with the lateral part of the upper border of the cricoid lamina.

The superior process, the *apex* of the pyramid, is inclined medially and posteriorly. The *corniculate cartilage* sits on the apex and projects into the *aryepiglottic fold*. The anterior process (*vocal process*) gives origin to the vocal cord. The lateral process (*muscular process*) provides attachment for the posterior and lateral crico-arytenoid muscles.

The **epiglottis** has roughly the shape of a tennis racket. Its stalk (*handle*) is attached at the middle of the inner side of the thyroid cartilage bow by means of connective tissue. The surface of the epiglottis is curved slightly concave backwards.

Joints of the Laryngeal Skeleton

The articular movements influence partly the distance between the vocal processes and the thyroid cartilage, partly the distance between the arytenoid cartilages and their vocal processes.

In the **cricothyroid articulations** (Fig. **283**) of both sides, the joints between the inferior horns of the thyroid cartilage and the cricoid cartilage, mainly tilting movements which alter the distance between the vocal processes and the inner side of the thyroid cartilage bow are executed around a transverse axis (Fig. **285**). Moreover, the articular capsule also permits slight gliding movements in all directions.

The **crico-arytenoid articulation** (Fig. **283**), the joint between the arytenoid and the cricoid, is a modified hinge joint. The articular surface of the arytenoid is concave and groove-shaped, that of the cricoid convex. A restraint by collateral ligaments is absent. The axis is oblique from dorsal-medial-cranial to ventral-lateral-caudal.

Different movements are possible in this joint (Fig. **286**). By displacement of the axis of the hinge, both arytenoids and their vocal processes can be brought closer to each other or withdrawn from each other by about 2 mm. By tilting around the axis of the hinge, the two vocal processes are elevated and withdrawn from one another or depressed and brought nearer to each other. In addition, the loose joint capsule also permits a rotary movement around the longitudinal axis, which likewise influences the distance between the vocal processes.

Laryngeal Ligaments

The ligamentous support of the larynx consists of *intrinsic laryngeal ligaments* that unite parts of the laryngeal skeleton with one another and *extrinsic laryngeal ligaments* by which the larynx is secured to the hyoid and the trachea.

Intrinsic laryngeal ligaments (Fig. **286**). The membrane of dense networks of elastic fibers situated beneath the mucous membrane of the larynx and corresponding to the submucosa is referred to as the *fibro-elastic membrane of the larynx*. It is developed very differently in the three portions of the larynx.

In the region of the *infraglottic cavity*, it is called the *conus elasticus* and is a short tube which begins with a round lumen at the inner surface of the cricoid and ends with a slit-like, sagittally-directed space beneath the mucosa of the left and right vocal folds.

As thickened upper ends of the conus elasticus, the *vocal ligaments* (Fig. **281**) are attached behind at the vocal processes of both arytenoids, in front at the inner side of the thyroid cartilage bow. With the two vocal ligaments, the conus elasticus forms the elastic wall of the tone-producing "lip pipe" in the larynx.

The *cricothyroid ligament* (Fig. **283**) is a firm, anterior, median fibrous tract in the conus elasticus stretched between the cricoid and lower margin of the thyroid cartilage.

Since the cricothyroid ligament lies below the glottis, an incision or puncture through this ligament (*cricothyrotomy, coniotomy*) to circumvent a life-threatening closure of the glottis, e.g. mucosal swelling (*glottic edema*), artificially opens the airway.

The *quadrangular membrane* (Fig. **281**) represents the weakly-developed portion of the fibro-elastic membrane of the larynx which underlies the mucous membrane of the laryngeal ventricle.

The *vestibular membrane* (false vocal cord, Fig. **281**) represents the lower free margin of the quadrangular membrane. The ligamentous marginal zone of the membrane lies in the vestibular fold and is attached on both sides at the anterior side of the arytenoid cartilage and at the inner side of the thyroid cartilage bow, above the insertion of the vocal cord.

The elastic *posterior crico-arytenoid ligament* (Fig. **283**) strengthens the flaccid articular capsule of the crico-arytenoid joint medially.

The *cricopharyngeal ligament* (Fig. **283**) passes from the corniculate cartilages to the posterior side of the cricoid lamina and into the connective tissue of the pharyngeal mucosa located behind it.

The *thyro-epiglottic ligament* (Fig. **283**) fixes the stalk of the epiglottis to the inner side of the bow of the thyroid cartilage.

Extrinsic laryngeal ligaments (Fig. 283). The *thyrohyoid membrane* spreads out between the upper border of the thyroid cartilage and the hyoid bone. Reinforced fiber tracts of the membrane have special names: the *median thyrohyoid ligament* (between the superior thyroid notch and the body of the hyoid bone) and the *lateral thyrohyoid ligament* (between the superior horn of the thyroid cartilage and the posterior end of the greater cornu of the hyoid).

Laryngeal Musculature

The *hyoid muscles* collectively move the larynx; they raise, depress, tilt, and position it at a definite level. The *laryngeal muscles*, on the other hand, move parts of the laryngeal skeleton toward (or against) one another. According to position and origin, the laryngeal musculature can be classified as *external* (cricothyroid, innervated by the *external ramus* of the *superior laryngeal nerve*) and *internal* (all of the remaining laryngeal muscles supplied by the *inferior laryngeal nerve*).

The **cricothyroid muscle** (Fig. **284**) arises anteriorly from the arch of the cricoid and passes with a steep medial and a flatter lateral fiber tract to the lower margin of the thyroid cartilage and to the anterior border of the inferior horn of the thyroid cartilage.

The **posterior crico-arytenoid muscle** (Fig. **284**) courses laterally upward from the posterior surface of the lamina of the cricoid to the muscular process of the arytenoid.

In about 25% of the cases, a lateral separation of the muscle (**ceratocricoid**) unites the inferior horn of the thyroid cartilage with the lamina of the cricoid.

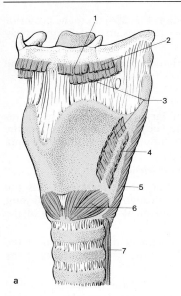

Fig. 284. **Laryngeal musculature**
a Left oblique view from in front
b Left oblique view from behind

1–4 *Insertions or origins of infrahyoid*
muscles
1 Sternohyoid
2 Omohyoid
3 Thyrohyoid
4 Sternothyroid
5 Inferior pharyngeal constrictor
6 Cricothyroid

7 Esophagus, muscle layer
8 Aryepiglottic fold
9 Cuneiform tubercle and cuneiform cartilage
10 Transverse arytenoid
11 Oblique arytenoid
12 Posterior crico-arytenoid
13 Thyro-epiglottic
14 Aryepiglottic

The **lateral crico-arytenoid muscle** (Fig. **276**) arises externally from the lateral portion of the upper margin of the arch of the cricoid and inserts at the muscular process of the arytenoid.

The **vocalis muscle** (Fig. **281**) comes from the posterior surface of the bow of the thyroid cartilage and passes within the vocal fold to the vocal process of the arytenoid.

The **thyro-arytenoid muscle** originates lateral to the vocalis muscle from the posterior surface of the bow of the thyroid cartilage and inserts with thin fibrous tracts at the anterolateral surface of the arytenoid.

The **thyro-epiglottic muscle** (Fig. **284**) forms the upper continuation of the thyro-arytenoid muscle and inserts at the epiglottic cartilage and at the quadrangular membrane.

The **oblique** and **transverse arytenoid muscles** (Fig. **284**) unite the posterior side of both arytenoid cartilages with fiber bundles arranged transversely and crosswise.

The **aryepiglottic muscle** (Fig. **284**) continues the oblique arytenoid muscle beyond the apex of the arytenoid into the aryepiglottic fold.

Action of the Laryngeal Muscles

With respect to function, two types of laryngeal muscles are distinguished: *tensor muscles* which stretch the vocal cord (and thus also the vocal folds) and *positioning muscles* which influence the width of the rima glottidis by way of the arytenoid cartilage.

The **tensor muscles** are the *cricothyroid* and *vocalis*.

With the thyroid cartilage fixed in position, the *cricothyroid* tilts the cricoid around the transverse axis passing through the cricothyroid joint (Fig. **285**) and thus produces a rough adjustment of the tension of the vocal folds.

The *vocalis muscle* influences the fine adjustment of the tension of the vocal folds by isometric contraction and thus the vibrating ability of the vocal folds.

The **positioning muscles** are represented by all of the remaining internal laryngeal muscles attaching to the arytenoid cartilage. Among these muscles, *openers* and *closers* of the rima glottidis are distinguished.

An **opener** of the entire rima glottidis is represented solely by the *posterior crico-arytenoid*. By traction at the muscular process, the arytenoid is rotated externally around the vertical axis between this cartilage and the upper border of the lamina of the cricoid and tilted somewhat laterally. By the action of both sides, the vocal processes and the vocal cords emanating from them are withdrawn from each other and elevated, and the rima glottidis is dilated.

The *lateral crico-arytenoid muscle* functions as an *opener of only the intercartilaginous part* of the rima glottidis by turning the arytenoid inward around the vertical axis, thus moving the apex of the vocal process toward the midline. With both sides contracting, the intercartilaginous part forms a triangular opening.

As a **closer** *of the intermembranous part*, the *lateral crico-arytenoid* simultaneously positions the apices of the vocal processes against one another. The muscle is supported by the *thyro-arytenoid muscle* in rotations of the arytenoid around the vertical axis, i.e. in closing the intermembranous part.

The *oblique* and *transverse arytenoids* also produce a *closure of the intercartilaginous part* of the rima glottidis by drawing both arytenoids toward the midline along the "hinge" axis.

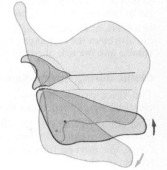

Fig. 285. Rocking movement between cricoid and thyroid cartilages as function of cricothyroid (scheme)
Position of cricoid and arytenoid cartilages with relaxed vocal cords ——
Position of cricoid and arytenoid cartilages with contraction of cricothyroid muscles, vocal cords (and thus also vocal folds) stretched ——

Laryngeal Mucosa

The *mucosal lining of the laryngeal cavity* can exhibit typical structural differences in the different portions of the larynx.

The stratified, nonkeratinized *squamous epithelium* that lines the pharynx and the side of the epiglottis facing the oral cavity is continued into the laryngeal vestibule for a varying distance. A variable broad zone of stratified, columnar epithelium is continuous with the pseudostratified ciliated epithelium (with numerous goblet cells) that lines the respiratory pathways as far as the small bronchioles. The *vocal folds* form the *exception*. They are lined by stratified squamous, partly also keratinized, whitish epithelium which provides the strong mechanical quality needed for phonation.

Mixed tubulo-alveolar *glands* lie on the laryngeal side of the epiglottis, in the vestibular folds and in the mucous membrane at the level of the transverse arytenoid muscle. Their secretions keep the vocal folds moistened. The *vocal folds* are *devoid of glands*; only at their posterior end does a gland occur almost regularly.

In orators, incomplete moistening of the vocal folds can lead to hoarseness.

The *connective tissue of the mucous membrane* is loosely formed at the inlet and in the vestibule of the larynx. At the vocal folds, on the other hand, the mucosa has grown together firmly with the vocal ligaments.

A diseased fluid accumulation in the mucosal connective tissue of the laryngeal inlet and vestibule (*glottic edema*) can lead to suffocation.

Closure of the Laryngeal Inlet during Swallowing

During swallowing, the laryngeal inlet is largely closed. The effective mechanisms for this, the "base of the tongue-epiglottis mechanism" and the "fat pad-epiglottis mechanism", were discussed on p. 764.

Moreover, the contraction of the aryepiglottic and thyro-epiglottic muscles should aid in lowering the epiglottis.

In infants, in whom the epiglottis still projects over the margin of the tongue, fluids can also enter the esophagus, but only by passing through the piriform recess, thus eliminating the risk of swallowing the wrong way.

Glottis during Respiration and Phonation

The voice-producing part of the wall of the larynx bordering the rima glottidis is referred to as the **glottis**.

The *rima glottidis* (Fig. **286**) consists of an anterior two-thirds, the *intermembranous part* bordered by the *vocal folds*, and a posterior one-third, the *intercartilaginous part* limited by the arytenoid cartilage. The shape of the rima varies according to the manner of respiration or phonation.

The rima glottidis in males is 2.0–2.4 cm long; it is 0.5 cm wide during quiet respiration and up to 1.4 cm wide during vigorous respiration. In females and in children, the dimensions are smaller. The angle formed by both laminae of the thyroid cartilage amounts to about 90° in males and usually more than 120° in females. The size of the larynx and the vocal pitch dependent on it are among the secondary sexual characteristics and develop their typical quality at puberty.

During *laryngoscopy*, the intercartilaginous part appears in the laryngoscope at the bottom, the intermembranous part and the epiglottis at the top. The pale vocal folds protrude medially from the red vestibular folds. The cuneiform and corniculate tubercles are evident in the aryepiglottic fold on both sides of the epiglottis.

Respiration (Figs. **286a–c**). In *quiet respiration* and in *whispering*, the intermembranous part is closed, while the intercartilaginous part is opened in the form of a triangle (traction of the lateral crico-arytenoid muscle). During *medium respiration*, the intermembranous and intercartilaginous parts are opened slightly (traction of the posterior crico-arytenoid muscle), and the entire rima glottidis forms an acute-angled triangle. In *extermely violent respiration*, the intermembranous and intercartilaginous parts are opened in the shape of a rhombus (extreme traction of the posterior crico-arytenoid).

For **voice production** (Fig. **286 d**), the rima glottidis is first closed, the *closure of the glottis* representing the phonation position. From this position, the vocal folds – simultaneously stretched – are caused to vibrate by an expiratory blast of air current, thus producing sound waves.

The *volume* is determined by the strength of the air current, the *pitch* by the frequency of the vibrations. As in a stringed instrument, the frequency of the vibration depends on the length, tension and thickness of the vocal folds, which are adjusted coarsely by the cricothyroid muscle and the muscles attaching to the muscular process and then finely tuned by the vocalis muscles. The cavities of the pharynx, mouth and nose – as passages attached to the larynx – serve as *resonators* for the tones arising at the glottis. The air column vibrating in these passages determines the quality (*timbre*) of the tone.

If parts of these attached tubes are closed, e.g. the nasal cavity during a cold, the timbre is altered.

Speech. The position of the larynx makes it possible for humans to control the expiratory, tone-carrying air current at the organs of speech (palate, tongue, teeth and lips) and to articulate the tones into *speech*. The *vowels* are formed by alterations within the attached passages, the *consonants* as sounds with the help of the organs of speech.

Sound not produced by the glottis, e.g., by the vestibular folds after operative removal of the vocal folds, or by swallowed air ("belch language", esophageal speech) after the removal of the larynx, can be formed into speech in the mouth.

When coughing, the closed rima glottidis is opened by a explosive-like expiration.

c) Vessels and Nerves of the Larynx

Arteries (Figs. **268** and **277**). The *superior laryngeal artery* arises from the superior thyroid artery cranial to the upper margin of the lamina of the thyroid cartilage, penetrates the thyrohyoid membrane, generally together with the internal ramus of the superior laryngeal nerve, and supplies the greatest portion of the mucosa and the musculature of the larynx.

Occasionally, a *thyroid foramen* is formed in the lamina of the thyroid cartilage below the superior thyroid tubercle for passage of the superior laryngeal artery and vein.

The thin *cricothyroid branch* (also from the superior thyroid artery) gives off fine branches to the anterior, lower laryngeal mucosa. The weak *inferior laryngeal artery* (from the inferior thyroid artery) passes upward behind the cricothyroid joint to the mucosa of the posterior wall of the larynx and to the posterior crico-arytenoid muscle.

Veins (Fig. **278**). The *superior laryngeal vein* accompanies the artery of the same name; the *inferior laryngeal vein* drains blood from the *thyroideus impar plexus*, which surrounds the lower pole of the thyroid lobes and the initial portion of the trachea.

The **lymphatic drainage** takes place in separate paths. Lymph from the supraglottic region of the mucosa reaches the *anterior jugular lymph nodes* through the thyrohyoid membrane – via *infrahyoid lymph nodes* when present as variants – and thence to the *deep lateral cervical lymph nodes*. From the portion below the glottis, the lymph flows off through the cricothyroid ligament, first to the *prelaryngeal* and *paratracheal lymph*

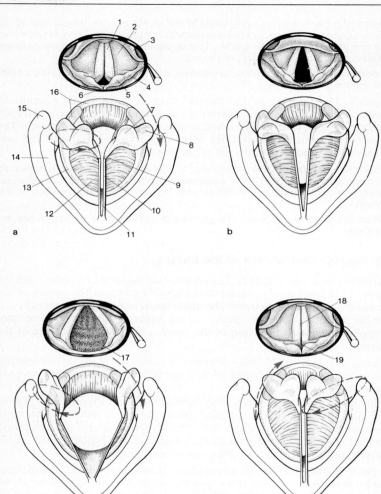

Fig. 286. **Larynx** (after *Pernkopf*)
Shape of rima glottidis in laryngoscope (above)
Position of vocal cords in skeletal preparation (below)
a In quiet respiration and whispering
b In medium respiration
c In forced respiration
d In voice production (phonation position)
Arytenoid articular surface ☐

nodes (nodes of the *deep anterior cervical lymph nodes*) and then to the caudally-situated *deep lateral lymph nodes.*

In the region of the vocal folds, only a sparsely formed, fine lymphatic capillary network is developed which is connected predominantly to the lymphatic tracts of the supraglottic region, but also to the lower region of lymphatic vessels. Connections with the opposite side exist for lymphatic vessels situated near the median plane.

Nerves. The *superior laryngeal nerve* leaves the vagus at the level of the inferior ganglion and immediately gives off the thin *external ramus,* the motor branch of the superior laryngeal nerve, which dispatches short twigs to the inferior pharyngeal constrictor and passes downward along the larynx to the cricothyroid muscle. The main sensory branch (*internal ramus,* Fig. **268**) penetrates the thyrohyoid membrane and supplies the *laryngeal mucosa above the glottis.*

The *inferior laryngeal nerve* (Fig. **276**) ascends to the larynx in the sulcus between the trachea and esophagus as the terminal branch of the recurrent laryngeal nerve. It penetrates the inferior pharyngeal constrictor beside the lesser horn of the thyroid cartilage and innervates all of the *intrinsic laryngeal muscles,* as well as the *mucosa below the glottis.*

Trachea → Vol. 2.

3. Thyroid and Parathyroid Glands

The thyroid and parathyroid glands, both endocrine, are of different derivation, yet they stand in intimate spatial relationship to each other – an important factor in surgery of the thyroid gland. Both organs, therefore, are discussed together.

a) Form and Position of the Thyroid and Parathyroid Glands

The **thyroid gland** (Figs. **271**, **276** and **282**), a soft, reddish-brown organ weighing 18–60 g, consists of two oval, cup-shaped glandular lobes, *right* and *left,* and the transversely-placed *isthmus* that unites the two lobes. The lobes and isthmus together form roughly the letter H. In about 50%

◄ 1 Vocal fold
2 Vestibular fold
3 Margin of epiglottis
4 Cuneiform tubercle
5 Corniculate tubercle
6 Interarytenoid notch
7 Apex ⎫
8 Muscular process ⎬ of arytenoid
9 Vocal process ⎭ cartilage
10 Vocal ligament

11 Cricothyroid ligament
12 Conus elasticus
13 Arch of cricoid cartilage
14 Lamina ⎫ of thyroid
15 Superior horn ⎭ cartilage
16 Lamina of cricoid cartilage and arytenoidal articular surface
17 Posterior wall of trachea
18 Rima glottidis, intermembranous part
19 Rima glottidis, intercartilaginous part.

of the cases, a *pyramidal lobe* is present – a process which, as the remains of the embryonic thyroglossal duct, extends a varying distance craniad from the isthmus in the direction of the hyoid bone.

Scattered islands of thyroid tissue (*accessory thyroid glands*) can appear along the entire earlier course of the embryonic thyroglossal duct – beginning at the foramen caecum at the base of the tongue. Here they can form, in the case of goiter disorders, "small goiters" (up to 1 cm in diameter).

The antero-lateral surface of the thyroid gland is completely concealed behind the middle layer of the cervical fascia. The lobes of the thyroid with their cup-shaped concavity adjoin the cranial tracheal cartilages below, the larynx above, and the lateral wall of the esophagus behind. On both sides, they are thus closely adjacent to the recurrent laryngeal nerve, their posterior surface being closely related to the common carotid artery (Fig. 276).

In operations of the thyroid gland, the recurrent laryngeal nerve must be avoided as much as possible.

Capsule. The thyroid gland is surrounded by a doubled connective tissue capsule, the inner layer of which has grown firmly together with the organ. Connective tissue tracts from this layer subdivide the gland into lobules. The external layer is derived from the pretracheal layer of the cervical fascia and is only loosely attached to the inner layer. The thyroid vessels ramify between the two layers, both of which are attached posteriorly at the trachea.

Parathyroid glands (Fig. 282), as a rule, upper and lower lentil-shaped bodies on each side, about 8 mm long and weighing 30–50 mg, are embedded in the posterior aspect of the thyroid gland between the layers of the capsule, more rarely in the thyroid tissue.

In thyroid operations, the surgeon should preserve a posterior portion of the gland in order to spare the parathyroid glands.

The number and location of the parathyroid glands vary considerably. They can also be found in the cervical connective tissue above and below the thyroid gland.

b) Histology and Function of the Thyroid and Parathyroid Glands

The **thyroid gland** produces two kinds of hormones: *thyroxine* and *calcitonin*. Thyroxine and triiodothyronine – even stronger in its effect – stimulate cell metabolism and growth and sensitize organs for the action of the sympathetic nervous system. *Calcitonin* reduces the blood calcium level and promotes bone formation; it acts antagonistically to the parathyroid hormone.

The *thyroxine-producing*, endocrine, epithelial cells of the thyroid gland are *follicular cells* arranged as vesical-shaped follicles. Depending on the functional phase, the follicles are variably filled with colloid, the carrier substance of the hormone, and the epithelial cells are of different heights so that different *follicular phases* can be distinguished. Individual *somatostatin*-forming cells lie close to the follicular cells; they influence the inhibiting of the secretion.

A *hyperfunction* of the thyroid gland (hyperthyroidism, "soft goiter", Graves' disease) leads to an abnormal increase in cell metabolism, connected with emaciation, elevation of temperature and signs of an elevated sympathetic tonus. In the case of *hypofunction* (hypothyroidism), metabolism, growth and mental alertness are retarded concomitant with a swelling of the subcutaneous connective tissue (myxedema). Congenital hypofunction leads to dwarfism and mental retardation (cretinism). When there is a deficiency of iodine in the food, a benign, simple goiter arises.

The *calcitonin-producing* cells (*C-cells*, parafollicular cells) lie singly or in small groups in the connective tissue near the follicular cells or within the follicular epithelium.

In the **parathyroid gland**, *parathormone* is produced which regulates the metabolism of calcium and phosphates by stimulating the osteoclasts to destroy bone.

The parathyroid gland consists of epithelial nests, little fat and connective tissue, and contains abundant capillaries. Glycogen-rich (thus pale staining) and dark *principal cells* are distinguished, in addition to small amounts (3%) of *oxyphil cells* of unknown significance.

Hyperfunction leads to bone destruction, to an increase in blood calcium levels and to calcium deposition in the blood vascular walls, as well as to the formation of renal calculi and the increased secretion of phosphates. *Hypofunction* causes deficient calcification of the skeleton and teeth, as well as an increase in nerve excitability owing to a decrease in blood calcium levels. Loss of the parathyroid glands leads to spasms, tetany.

c) Vessels and Nerves to the Thyroid and Parathyroid Glands

The *thyroid gland* is supplied with blood vessels on both sides from two sources. *Upper vessels* arise from the *neurovascular trunk of the neck to the head*, *lower vessels* from the *neurovascular trunk of the head to the upper limb*. Only branches of the inferior thyroid artery (as a rule) pass to the two *parathyroid glands* on each side. Lymphatic vessels pass to the upper and lower deep lateral lymph nodes of the neck.

Arteries (Fig. **277**). The *superior thyroid artery*, the first branch of the external carotid, passes to the upper pole of the thyroid lobe and ramifies on its anterior surface. The *inferior thyroid artery*, the largest branch of the thyrocervical trunk, ramifies at the lower pole of the thyroid lobe and on its posterior side. The artery courses medially in the arch behind the neurovascular trunk passing to the head and penetrates the deep layer of the cervical fascia behind the thyroid lobe.

Veins (Fig. **278**). The *superior thyroid vein* carries blood from the superior half of the thyroid gland to the internal jugular vein. In addition, *middle thyroid veins,* pass to the internal jugular vein without accompanying arteries.

The *thyroideus impar plexus* ($\rightarrow$ Vol. 2, Fig. **3**), a large venous plexus at the lower pole of both thyroid lobes and at the isthmus, conveys blood into the left brachiocephalic vein via the strong, unpaired *inferior thyroid vein* in front of the trachea.

The **lymphatic drainage** takes place via *thyroid lymph nodes* into the deep lateral cervical lymph nodes.

From the upper half of the thyroid gland, lymphatic tracts – in part through the interpolation of *prelaryngeal lymph nodes* – pass to the *anterior jugular lymph nodes.* The tracts from the lower half of the gland pass to the caudal *lateral jugular lymph nodes* directly ventral or via *pretracheal lymph nodes,* whereas those from the dorsal glandular part and from the parathyroid glands enter these nodes via the *paratracheal lymph nodes.*

The **nerves** to the thyroid and parathyroid glands originate from the *vagus nerve* and the *cervicothoracic ganglion.*

Index to Volumes 1 and 2

Volume numbers are given in roman numerals (I, II). Page numbers in *italics* refer to illustrations; page numbers in **bold type** refer to the systematic chapters in Volume II. Where there are extended discussions of certain topics, the page numbers given here refer only to the first page on which relevant information about the topic appears. There may be further information on a topic in the pages immediately following.

Bursa, bursae
  prepatellar I: 351, *364*, 373
  retrohyoid I: 726
  of semimembranosus I:
    354, *368*, 373
  subacromial I: *194, 195*,
    198
  subscapular I: *194, 195*,
    198
  suprapatellar I: *364*, 372
  subdeltoid I: *194*, 198
  synovial I: 42
    of shoulder joint I: *194*,
      198
    of tendo calcaneus I: *384*,
      387, *388*
    testicular II: 200
    of triceps brachii tendon I:
      230
  trochanteric I: 325, *345*
  of tibial tuberosity I: 358,
    364
Buttock II: 181

C

Cachexia I: 653
Cajal's tangential cells II: 361
Calamus scriptorius II: 274
Calcaneus I: 394, *396, 402,
  404, 405*
  ossification I: *306*, 398
Calcar avis II: *315*, 331
Calcitonin I: 780
Calices, renal II: *154*, 159
Callus I: 21
Calvaria I: 608, *610, 617*
Canal, canals, adductor I:
  332, *340*
  alveolar I: 601
  anal II: *117*, 118, *212*
  carotid I: *582, 585*, 587,
    589, *718*
  carpal I: 238, 255, 266
  central, of bone I: 16, *17*
    of spinal cord I: *110*,
      123, II: *253*, 254, *273,
      284, 329, 331*
  of cervix of uterus II: *214*,
    220
  chordal, anterior I: 590
  condylar I: 572, *752, 718*
  diploic I: 609
  facial I: *585*, 589

Canal, canals
  femoral I: 337
  hypoglossal I: *572, 572,
    573, 615, 718*
  incisive I: *599*, 602,
    635–637, 687
  infra-orbital I: *599*, 600
  inguinal I: 537, *542*
  mandibular I: *605*, 607
  musculotubal I: *587*, 590
  nasolacrimal I: 601
  obturator I: 304, *308*, 342
  optic I: *579, 592, 615, 633*
  palatine, greater I: *509*,
    601
    lesser I: 602
  palatovaginal I: 603
  pelvic I: 310
  perforating I: 17
  pterygoid I: *577*, 580
  pudendal I: *329*, 348, II:
    178
  pyloric II: *94*, 95, *105*
  radial I: 219
  root, of tooth I: 697, *698*
  sacral I: 461, *462, 463*
  of Schlemm II: 383, *384,
    392*
  semicircular II: *418*, 423
  spiral, of cochlea II: 417,
    418, 420
  supinator I: 243
  vertebral I: 455, 477
    contents I: 480
  vomerovaginal I: 598
Canaliculus, canaliculi, bile
  II: 131, 133
  caroticotympanic I: 587,
    589
  of chorda tympani I: 590
  lacrimal II: *402*, 403
  mastoid I: 587, 590
  tympanic I: 587, 590
Canines I: 695, *696, 700, 702,
  718*
Cannon's ring II: 124
Cap, of duodenum II: *86*, 95,
  104
Capillary, capillaries I: 47
  lymphatic I: *48*, 55
  sinusoidal, of liver II: 131
  structure I: *50*, 53
Capilli I: 172, 664
Capitate bone I: 254,
  256–258, 263
  ossification I: *182*, 255

Capitulum, of humerus I:
  178, 192, *227*
  ossification I: *182*, 193
Capsule, articular *see* Joint,
  capsule
  external II: 343, *370*
  extreme II: 343, *370*
  fibrous, perivascular, of li-
    ver II: 131
  glomerular II: *156*, 157
  internal II: 340, *341, 342,
    366*, 369, *369, 370*
  of kidney, fatty II: *86*, 149,
    152, 153
    fibrous II: 153, *154, 156*
  of lens II: 383
  of prostate II: 208
  splenic II: 143, *144*
  of suprarenal gland II: 164,
    165
  testicular II: 200
  of thyroid gland I: *734*, 780
Caput humeri I: 191
Carina, of trachea II: 20
  urethral, of vagina II: *214*,
    227
Carpal tunnel syndrome I:
  267
Carpals, carpal bones I: 254,
  256–258
  ossification I: *182*, 255
Carpus I: 254
  radiography I: 255
Cartilage, cartilages, alar I:
  686
  articular I: *20, 29*, 30, *30*
  arytenoid I: *767*, 770
  of auditory tube I: *676,
    718*, II: 414
  auricular I: 675, *676*
  corniculate I: *767*, 770
  costal I: 503, *508*
  cricoid I: *734, 760, 767*,
    770, *778*, II: *66*
  cuneiform I: *773*
  epiglottic *see* Epiglottis
  hyaline I: 18
  of larynx I: *767*, 769
  nasal I: 598, 686, *692*
  thyroid I: *760, 767*, 770,
    778, II: *66*
  tracheal I: *767*, II: 18, *19,
    66*
Cartilago triticea I: 726, *767*
Caruncle, lacrimal II: *400,
  402*, 403

Furrow, furrows, brachial *see*
    Sulcus, bicipital
    cerebral II: 321
    dorsal I: 498, *499*
    formation, of cerebral cor-
        tex II: 328
    gluteal I: 326, *499*
    infrapalpebral I: 652, *654*
    inguinal I: 335, *549, 554*
    mentolabial I: 652, *654*
    nasolabial I: 652, *654*
    see also Groove, Sulcus

G

Gait, waddling I: 321
Galea aponeurotica I: *617*,
    663, *668*
Galen's vein II: **523**
Gallbladder II: *6*, 75, *76, 86,
    88, 105, 127*, 137
    arteries II: 138
    lymphatic drainage II: 139
    nerves II: 139
    veins II: 139
Ganglion, ganglia I: 110, *111*
    aorticorenal I: *147*, II: 176,
        590, *593*
    autonomic I: 111, *111, 119,
        142*, 145, *145, 151*
        in retroperitoneal space
            II: **590**
        in subperitoneal pelvic
            space II: 237
    of autonomic plexus II:
        175, **586**, *590*
    basal I: *126*, 128, II: 320,
        340, *341*, 342
        arteries II: 373
        veins II: 380
    cardiac I: *147*, II: 55, **592**
    celiac I: *147*, 175, II: *104*,
        565, *590*, **591**, *593*
    cervical, inferior I: 146,
        755, II: **587**, *588*, **590**
        middle I: 146, 755, II:
            587, *588*, 589, *589*
        superior I: 146, *147*, 755,
            II: *563*, **587**, *588*, **589**
    cervicothoracic I: 146, *147*,
        755, II: *10, 12*, 56, **588**,
        588, **589**, *590*
    ciliary I: *142, 147, 752*, II:
        406, *551*, **552**, *554*, **556**

Ganglion
    of cranial nerves I: *142*, **556**
    of dorsal root II: 254
    geniculate I: *142*, II: **556,
        561**, *562*
    of glossopharyngeal nerve
        I: *142*, II: **556**, *563*, **563**
    of head, organization II:
        551
    impar II: 238, **589**, **591**
    intramural I: 145
    jugular, of glossopharyn-
        geal nerve II: **563**
        of vagus nerve II: **564**
    lumbar II: *150*, 175, **589**,
        591
    mesenteric I: *147*, II: 176,
        590, **593**
    nodose II: **564**
    organ I: 111, 145, *145, 151*
    otic I: *142, 147*, 681, *752*,
        II: **556**, *563*, **563**
    paravertebral I: 146
    pelvic I: *147*, II: 230, 238,
        594
    petrosal II: **563**
    phrenic II: 175, **594**
    prevertebral I: 146, 149,
        151
    pterygopalatine I: *142,
        147*, 682, *692, 706, 752*, II:
        554, **556**, *557*, **561**
    renal II: 176, **593**
    sacral II: 238, **589**, **591**
    semilunar *see* Ganglion,
        trigeminal
    sensory I: 110, *111*
        of cranial nerves I: 141
    spinal I: *117–119*, 132,
        481, II: *253*, 254, **569**
    spiral, of cochlea II: *420*,
        562
    splanchnic I: 57
    stellate *see* Ganglion, cer-
        vicothoracic
    submandibular I: *142, 147*,
        682, *706*, 707, *752*, II: **554**,
        556, **559**, *561*
    of sympathetic trunk I:
        117,118,145,146,*147,151*
    thoracic II: *10, 12*, 56,
        588–590, **590**
        splanchnic II: **591**
    trigeminal I: *142*, 631, *692*,
        II: **552**, *552*, **554**, *556*

Ganglion
    of vagus nerve I: *142*, II:
        564, *565*
    vestibular I: *142*, II: 424,
        562
    vertebral II: **590**
Gap, scalenus I: 730
Gartner's duct II: 218
Geniculum, of facial nerve II:
    560
Genitalia *see* Organs, sex
Gennary's stripe II: 365
Genu, of corpus callosum II:
    312, 315, 354, 368
    of facial canal I: 589
    of facial nerve II: *286*, 292,
        560, *561*
    of internal capsule II: 370,
        370
    valgum I: 356, *357*
    varum I: 356, *357*
Gerdy's line I: 547
Gigantism I: 9
Gingiva I: 693, *698*
Ginglymus I: 33
Girdle, limb, I: 176
    pelvic I: 176, 301
        connections I: 305, *308*,
            309, *309*
        ligaments II: 307, *308*,
            309, *309*
        palpable bony points I:
            239, *240*
        skeleton I: 301
    shoulder I: 176
        action of muscles I: 189
        connections I: *178*, 181
        ligaments I: *178*, 183
        movement possibilities I:
            184
        muscles I: 185, *187, 188*,
            II: **426**
        palpable bony points I:
            290, *291*
        skeleton I: 177, *178, 180*
        surface anatomy I: 289
Glabella I: *592*, 593, *593*
Gland, glands I: 91, *91, 92*
    apocrine, sweat I: 171, *171*
    classification I: 91, *91, 92*
    cutaneous I: 171, *171*
    endocrine I: 91, *91*, 94, *96,
        97*
        connective tissue I: 95
        discharge I: 95
        function I: 94

Hypothalamus
  functions I: 128
  nuclear regions II: 333, *333*
  veins II: 334
Hypothenar I: 272
  muscles I: 275, II: **434**
Hypothyroidism I: 781

I

Ileum II: *80*, 85, 106, *108*
Ileus II: 87
Ilium I: 301, *302*, 303
  ossification I: 305, *306*
Immune system *see* Defense
  system, specific
Immunity, cellular and hu-
  moral I: 77
Immunization I: 78
Immunoblasts, T- I: 78
Impression, impressions, cardiac, of lungs II: *60, 61*, 63
  digital I: 591, 594, 610
  of liver II: *127*, 129
  trigeminal I: 584, *615*
Incisive I: 599
Incisors I: 695, *696*, 700, 702,
  718
Incisure, angular II: 95
  pre-occipital II: 323
Incus I: 571, *676*, II: 411, *412*
Indusium griseum II: *316*,
  328, 350, *356*, 368
Infarct I: 52
Infundibulum, ethmoidal I:
  686
  of hypophysis I: *123, 125,
  142*, II: *269*, 270, 313, *335,
  350*
  of uterine tube II: 191, *214*
Inlet, of larynx I: *758, 760*,
  768
  pelvic I: 311, *311*
    sexual differences I: 312
  thoracic I: *508*, 509
Innervation, of anal closure
  II: 125
  of extrinsic eye muscles II:
  291
  of heart II: 291
  of secretion II: 291
  of smooth musculature II:
  291
  of tongue II: 290

Innervation
  motor, voluntary, of visceral skeletal musculature II:
  291
  segmental I: 133
  see also individual names of
  organs or body parts
Inoculation, prophylactic I:
  78
Insufficiency, of cardiac
  muscle II: 33
  mitral II: 35
  tricuspidal II: 33
  valvular II: 33
Insula II: *311*, 321, 323, *323,
  326, 366*
Insulin II: 139
Integument I: 161, *162*
Intermaxillary I: 599
Interneurons I: *101*, 131, 139,
  II: 256
Internode I: *106*, 107
Interoceptors I: 122
Interparietal bone I: 574
Intersections, tendinous I:
  514, 533
Intestine, large II: 87, 114,
  115
    arteries II: *112*, 122
    form and position II:
    115, *115*
    histology and function
    II: *115*, 119
    lymphatic drainage II:
    114, 123, *124*
    nerves II: 124
    veins II: 123
  small I: 87, II: *80, 82*, 84,
  104
    arteries II: 110, *112*
    convolutions II: 106
    form and position II: 104
    histology and function
    II: 107, *108*
    lymphatic drainage II:
    113, *114*
    nerves II: 114
    veins II: 111
Intumescence, tympanic II:
  563
Iris II: *382, 384*, 386, *400*
  blood vessels II: *392*, 394
Ischemia I: 52
Ischium I: 301, *302*, 304
  ossification I: 305, *306*

Islets, of Langerhans *see* Islets, pancreatic
  pancreatic II: 139
Isocortex II: 359
Isthmus, of cingulate gyrus
  II: 328
  faucial I: *694*, 722
  oropharyngeal I: 722
  of prostate II: 208, *209*
  of thyroid gland I: *694*,
  779, II: *14*
  of uterine tube II: *214*, 217
  of uterus II: *212, 214*, 220

J

Jejunum II: *80*, 85, 106, *108*
Joint, joints I: 27, *29*
  accumulation I: 28
  ball-and-socket I: 32, *33*
  capsule I: 29, *29*, 31
  cartilaginous *see* Synchondroses
  cavity I: 29, *29*
  compound I: 32
  ellipsoid I: 33, *33*
  epiphysial, cartilaginous I:
  23
  fibrous *see* Syndesmoses
  ginglymus I: 33
  hinge I: 33, *33*
  inhibition I: 35
  mechanics I: 34
  membranes I: 31
  movements I: 34
  pivot I: *33*, 34
  saddle I: 33, *33*
  segmentation I: 28
  simple I: 32
  spheroidal I: 32
  structure I: 29, *29*
  surfaces I: 29
    coherence I: 32
  synovial I: 27, 29, *29*
  types I: 32, *33*
Joint, joints, named
  acromioclavicular *see*
  Joint, clavicular
  ankle, inferior I: 401, *402*,
  404, *404*
    movement possibili-
    ties I: 407
    superior I: 401, *402*

Muscle, muscles, named, scalene
function I: 528, 732
sartorius I: *318, 324, 340, 350*, 353, II: *182*, **438**
function I: 333, 373
semimembranosus I: *318, 325, 350*, 354, II: **439**
function I: 333, 373
semispinalis I: 485, *487, 488, 734*, II: **445**
function I: 494
semitendinosus I: *318, 325, 345, 350*, 354, II: **438**
function I: 333, 373
serratus anterior I: 188, *188, 200*, II: **426**
function I: 190
posterior inferior I: *482*, 515, *516*, II: **449**
function I: 515
superior I: 515, *516*, II: **449**
function I: 515
soleus I: *386*, 387, *389*, II: **440**
function I: 412
shpincter, anal
external II: *117, 118*, 121 *180−182*, 188, *190*, 194, 212, 246, **465**
internal II: *117*, 121, *194, 212*
of bile duct II: 137
cardiac, functional II: 23, *24*
choledochal II: 137
of hepatopancreatic ampulla II: 137
pupillae II: *384*, 386
pyloric II: *86, 98*, 100, *105*
urethrae II: *178, 180, 181*, 184, *194, 212*, 242, **466**
function II: 186
urethrovaginal II: 184
vaginae II: 184

spinalis I: *482*, 485, *487, 734*, II: **444**
splenius I: *487, 488*, 490, *497*, II: **447**
function I: 493
stapedius II: 411, *412*, 413, **453**

Muscle, muscles, named
sternalis I: 203, II: **428**
sternocleidomastoid I: *658*, 727, *728, 734*, II: **460**
function I: 190, 494, 732
sternohyoid I: *728*, 729, *734*, II: **460**
sternothyroid I: *728*, 729, *734*, II: **460**
function I: 732
styloglossus I: *706*, 711, *712*, II: **458**
function I: 711
stylohyoid I: 705, *728, 761*, II: **458**
function I: 705, 711
stylopharyngeus I: *706, 712, 761*, 764, II: **463**
function I: 764
subclavius I: *187*, 188, *514, 728*, II: **427**
function I: 188
subcostal I: 513, II: **449**
subscapularis I: *195*, 200, *200, 202*, II: **428**
function I: 204
supinator I: *240*, 241, **431**
function I: 253
suprahyoid I: 704
function I: 705
supraspinatus I: *195*, 198, *199*, II: **427**
function I: 204
suspensory, of duodenum II: 106, *150*
tarsal II: *400*, 406
temporalis I: *640*, 643, II: **453**
function I: 645
temporoparietalis I: 663, *668*, II: **454**
tensor fasciae latae I: *318, 324*, 327, *340, 345*, II: *182*, **436**
function I: 333, 373
tympani I: *676*, II: 411, *412*, 413, **452**
veli palatini I: *706*, 718, 720, II: **459**
function I: 720
teres major I: *199*, 201, *202*, II: **428**
function I: 204
minor I: *195*, 199, *199, 202*, II: **427**
function I: 204

Muscle, muscles, named
thyro-arytenoid I: 773, II: **464**
function I: 774
thyro-epiglottic I: 773, *773*, II: **464**
function I: 776
thyrohyoid I: *712, 728*, 729, II: **461**
function I: 732
tibialis anterior I: 382, *383, 389*, II: **439**
function I: 411
posterior I: *386*, 387, *389, 412*, II: **440**
function I: 411
trachealis II: 19, *19*
transverse, of tongue *see* Muscle, transversus linguae
transversospinal I: 485, *487*
function I: 493
transversus abdominis I: *329, 482, 514*, 533, *535*, II: **450**
function I: 535
linguae I: 713, II: **459**
function I: 713
menti I: 667, *668*, II: **455**
perinei, deep II: *178, 180−182*, 184, *188, 190*, 194, 212, 246, **466**
function II: 185
superficial II: *180, 182*, 185, *246*, **466**
thoracis I: 513, *514*, II: **450**
function I: 515
trapezius I: 186, *187, 202, 488, 728, 734*, II: **426**
function I: 190, 205, 494
of Treitz I: 106
triceps brachii I: *195, 199, 202, 218*, 219, II: **429**
function I: 204, 231
surae I: 385, *386, 404, 405*
function I: 411
urethrovaginal II: 184
uvulae I: *718*, 720, II: **460**
vastus I: *324, 340, 350*, 352, II: **438**
function I: 373
vertical, of tongue *see* Muscle, verticalis linguae